Manual of
Neurologic Therapeutics

Seventh Edition

4/21/06

Sam,
Good luck in
your new career

Martin

Manual of Neurologic Therapeutics

Seventh Edition

Edited by

Martin A. Samuels, M.D., M.A.C.P., F.A.A.N.

Neurologist-in-Chief and Chairman
Department of Neurology
Brigham and Women's Hospital
Professor of Neurology
Harvard Medical School
Boston, Massachusetts

LIPPINCOTT WILLIAMS & WILKINS
A **Wolters Kluwer** Company

Philadelphia • Baltimore • New York • London
Buenos Aires • Hong Kong • Sydney • Tokyo

Acquisitions Editor: James D. Ryan
Developmental Editor: Grace R. Caputo
Production Editor: Frank Aversa
Manufacturing Manager: Colin J. Warnock
Cover Designer: Patricia Gast
Compositor: Techbooks
Printer: R.R. Donnelley–Crawfordsville

© **2004 by LIPPINCOTT WILLIAMS & WILKINS**
530 Walnut Street
Philadelphia, PA 19106 USA
LWW.com

Library of Congress Cataloging-in-Publication Data

Manual of neurologic therapeutics / [edited by] Martin A. Samuels.—7th ed.
　　p. ; cm.
　Includes bibliographical references and index.
　ISBN 0-7817-4646-9
　1. Neurology—Handbooks, manuals, etc.　2. Nervous system—Diseases—Handbooks, manuals, etc.　I. Samuels, Martin A.
　[DNLM: 1. Nervous System Diseases—diagnosis—Outlines.　2. Nervous System Diseases—therapy—Outlines. WL 18.2 M294 2004]
　RC355.M36 2004
　616.8—dc22

　　　　　　　　　　　　　　　　　　　　　　　　　　　　　2003065888

10 9 8 7 6 5 4 3 2

This book is dedicated to the original contributors
to the Manual of Neurologic Therapeutics.
They were all members of a single group of residents
in the neurology training program at the Massachusetts General Hospital
when the idea was hatched almost 30 years ago.
They have all gone on to distinguished careers in neurology.

Telmo M. Aquino
Raymond J. Fernandez
Robert D. Helme
Daniel B. Hier
Richard C. Hinton
Stephen M. Sagar
Thomas M. Walshe
Howard D. Weiss

CONTENTS

CONTRIBUTING AUTHORS

Anthony A. Amato, M.D.
Associate Professor of Neurology, Harvard Medical School; Chief, Neuromuscular Division, Vice-Chairman, Department of Neurology, Brigham and Women's Hospital, Boston, Massachusetts

Robert W. Baloh, M.D.
Professor of Neurology, University of California Medical School; Director, Neurootology Laboratory, University of California Medical Center, Los Angeles, California

Donald C. Bienfang, M.D.
Assistant Professor of Ophthalmology, Harvard Medical School; Chief, Division of Neuroophthalmology, Department of Neurology, Brigham and Women's Hospital, Boston, Massachusetts

Edward B. Bromfield, M.D.
Assistant Professor of Neurology, Harvard Medical School; Chief, Division of Epilepsy and Electroencephalography, Brigham and Women's Hospital, Boston, Massachusetts

Kirk R. Daffner, M.D.
Associate Professor of Neurology, Harvard Medical School; Chief, Division of Cognitive and Behavioral Neurology, Brigham and Women's Hospital, Boston, Massachusetts

David M. Dawson, M.D.
Professor of Neurology, Harvard Medical School; Senior Neurologist, Department of Neurology, Brigham and Women's Hospital, Boston, Massachusetts

Steven K. Feske, M.D.
Assistant Professor of Neurology, Harvard Medical School; Director, Stroke Division, Department of Neurology, Brigham and Women's Hospital, Boston, Massachusetts

Robert B. Fogel, M.D.
Instructor in Medicine, Harvard Medical School; Physician, Division of Sleep Medicine, Brigham and Women's Hospital, Boston, Massachusetts

Robert D. Helme, F.R.A.C.P., Ph.D.
Professor of Neurology, University of Melbourne, Carlton, Victoria; Neurologist, Barbara Walker Centre for Pain Management, St. Vincent's Hospital, Fitzroy, Victoria, Australia

Galen V. Henderson, M.D.
Instructor in Neurology, Harvard Medical School; Director, Critical Care and Emergency Neurology, Department of Neurology, Brigham and Women's Hospital, Boston, Massachusetts

Santosh Kesari, M.D., Ph.D.
Instructor in Neurology, Harvard Medical School; Associate Neurologist, Department of Neurology, Brigham and Women's Hospital, Boston, Massachusetts

Ian Yi-Onn Leong. M.B.B.S., M.R.C.P.
Clinical Tutor, Department of Medicine, National University of Singapore, Singapore; Associate Consultant, Department of Geriatric Medicine, Tan Tock Seng Hospital, Singapore

Christina M. Marra, M.D.
Professor, Department of Neurology and Medicine—Infectious Diseases, University of Washington School of Medicine, Seattle, Washington

Michael Ronthal, M.B.B.Ch., F.R.C.P., F.R.C.P.E.
Associate Professor of Neurology, Harvard Medical School; Senior Neurologist, Department of Neurology, Beth Israel—Deaconess Medical Center, Boston, Massachusetts

Martin A. Samuels, M.D., M.A.C.P., F.A.A.N.
Professor of Neurology, Harvard Medical School; Neurologist-in-Chief and Chairman, Department of Neurology, Brigham and Women's Hospital, Boston, Massachusetts

Egilius L.H. Spierings, M.D., Ph.D.
Associate Clinical Professor of Neurology, Harvard Medical School; Consultant, Department of Neurology, Brigham and Women's Hospital, Boston, Massachusetts

Lewis R. Sudarsky, M.D.
Associate Professor of Neurology, Harvard Medical School; Director, Movement Disorders Division, Department of Neurology, Brigham and Women's Hospital, Boston, Massachusetts

Patrick Y. Wen, M.D.
Associate Professor of Neurology, Harvard Medical School; Director, Division of Neurooncology, Department of Neurology, Brigham and Women's Hospital, Boston, Massachusetts

David A. Wolk, M.D.
Instructor in Neurology, Harvard Medical School; Associate Neurologist, Department of Neurology, Brigham and Women's Hospital, Boston, Massachusetts

John W. Winkelman, M.D., Ph.D.
Assistant Professor of Psychiatry, Harvard Medical School; Medical Director, Sleep Health Center, Newton, Massachusetts; Physician, Division of Sleep Medicine, Department of Medicine, Brigham and Women's Hospital, Boston, Massachusetts

FOREWORD

It is to the classic monographs of Erb, Hughings Jackson, Gowers, K. Wilson, and their contemporaries that all scholars of neurology turn for knowledge of many of the common diseases of the human nervous system. These writings summarize the personal observations—clinical and pathological—of the author himself, expressed in the lucid and elegant language of the era. The author's reputation attested to the verity of the observations. But perusal of these landmark documents reveals little in the nature and future prospects of therapy or means of prevention. As a consequence, neurology became known as a large branch of medicine with a multitude of diagnosable diseases bereft of therapy.

All this has changed. Because of prodigious advances in biochemistry, neuropathology, and genetics, new methods of therapy have been devised, or at least conceptualized, for many of the previously recognized diseases as well as new disorders disclosed by the application of these methods. In fact, such an aggregation of new information about therapies of neurologic diseases has emerged that several neurologists have judged that a monograph devoted to the subject was warranted.

This was surely the reasoning of Professor Martin A. Samuels, who undertook this task many years ago. The success of his venture is reflected in the continued demand for the *Manual of Neurologic Therapeutics*, now in its 7th edition. Professor Samuels, like many others who had received their specialty education in our residency program at the Massachusetts General Hospital, brings to his subject a keen knowledge of neurology and a high motivation to advance the understanding of established methods of therapy in neurology.

As a member of the staff of the neurology service of the Massachusetts General Hospital, I have enjoyed and benefited from my association with Professor Samuels both during the period when he was a graduate student and later, as an esteemed faculty colleague. I applaud his latest medical literary contribution.

Raymond D. Adams, M.D.
Boston, Massachusetts

PREFACE TO THE FIRST EDITION

Until very recently the neurologist's primary task was to categorize and organize the structure and pathologic alterations of the nervous system. In fact, neurology has long been known as a discipline with elegantly precise and specific diagnostic capabilities but little or no therapeutic potentiality. Further, many surgeons, pediatricians, and internists have traditionally thought of the neurologist as an impractical intellectual who spends countless hours painstakingly localizing lesions while ignoring pragmatic considerations of treatment. Perhaps this conception is largely attributable to the peculiar complexity of the nervous system and the consequent relative naivete of physicians in their understanding of its functions.

Many of the classic descriptions of disease states in other medical disciplines were completed in the last century; in neurology, these have only been described in the past generation, and only in the last ten years has neurology begun to be characterized by subcellular mechanistic concepts of disease. This maturity has meant that the neurologist is now as much involved in the therapeutic aspects of his specialty of medicine as any of his colleagues. Certain neurologic diseases, such as epilepsy, have been treatable for relatively long periods of time, but understanding of the subcellular mechanisms of other diseases has led to newer, more effective forms of therapy.

An example of this is the enlarged understanding we now have of the biochemical alterations in Parkinson disease, and the resultant therapeutic implications. Now, much as the endocrinologist treats diabetes with insulin and the cardiologist treats congestive heart failure with digitalis, the neurologist treats Parkinson disease with L-dopa. In all these situations, the underlying condition is not cured; rather, an attempt is made to alter the pathophysiologic processes by utilizing a scientific understanding of the function of the diseased system.

This manual embodies a practical, logical approach to the treatment of neurologic problems, based on accurate diagnosis, that should prove useful to both clinician and student. No attempt is made to reiterate the details of the neurologic examination; it is assumed that the reader is competent to examine the patient—although particularly important or difficult differential diagnostic points are mentioned when appropriate. In this regard, it should be emphasized that this manual is only a guide to diagnosis and therapy, and each patient must be treated individually. The manual is organized to best meet the needs of the clinician facing therapeutic problems. Thus, the first seven chapters are concerned with symptoms, such as dizziness and headache, while the last ten consider common diseases, such as stroke and neoplasms.

I thank the many colleagues and friends whose criticism and comments were useful in the preparation of this book, in particular Drs. G. Robert DeLong, C. Miller Fisher, George Kleinman, James B. Lehrich, Steven W. Parker, Henry C. Powell, E. P. Richardson, Jr., Maria Salam, Bagwan T. Shahani, Peter Weller, James G. Wepsic, and Robert R. Young. In addition I am indebted to Sara Nugent and Helen Hyland for their assistance in the preparation of the many manuscripts, and to Diana Odell Potter, formerly of Little, Brown and Company, for her editorial skills. Jane Sandiford, formerly of Little, Brown, and Kathleen O'Brien and Carmen Thomas of Little, Brown provided invaluable assistance in the final preparation of this material. Deep appreciation goes to Lin Richter, Editor-in-Chief of the Medical Division, Little, Brown and Company, for her support throughout this effort. I further thank Jon Paul Davidson, also formerly of Little, Brown, for his valuable encouragement and help early in the course of this project. Much support and encouragement was derived from my new colleagues in the Peter Bent Brigham Hospital Neurology Section, The Longwood Avenue Neurology Program, and the West Roxbury Veterans Administration Hospital. A great deal of inspiration came from the birth of my daughter Marilyn, and my deepest thanks go to my wife, Linda, who provided constant encouragement, editorial skill, and infinite patience.

Martin A. Samuels

PREFACE

Once the last bastion of therapeutic nihilism, neurology has now clearly entered the era of intense therapy for virtually every class of disease that affects the nervous system. Consequently, the modern neurology department is now subdivided into a dozen clinical subspecialties, each with its own group of experts, often with their own postresidency specialized fellowship training programs. General neurology still exists but it is usually practiced in a consultative mode in either the hospital or the ambulatory setting. Now, the movement disorder specialist is as different from the epileptologist as the hematologist is from the endocrinologist. Basic research in the neurosciences is routinely translated into new drugs, devices, and procedures aimed at ameliorating disorders in almost all the major categories of disease. Even neurodegeneration, traditionally the most therapeutically resistant class of disease, is beginning to crack under the influence of molecular genetics and its translation into drugs that may slow or prevent cell death.

In this context, the original contributors to the *Manual of Neurologic Therapeutics* all agreed that the 7th edition would require a major reorganization and that the sections needed to be written by experts who had dedicated their careers to each of the various areas of concentration. Furthermore, to be optimally accessible in both office and bedside venue, the *Manual* needed to be presented in a format conducive to electronic presentation as well as print reproduction. Thus, the information contained here is presented in a more consistent format than previously, with better use of headings and less reliance on a traditional outline.

The 7th edition contains an entire chapter on neurologic intensive care, now a well-defined subspecialty. Epilepsy management currently involves not only an array of new drugs but also innovative strategies such as vagal nerve stimulation and a greater emphasis on earlier surgical treatment. Neurootology encompasses the common complaint of dizziness, emphasizing both pharmacologic and physical therapy approaches to treatment. Back and neck pain, still among the most common complaints in all of medicine, are now evaluated with much improved diagnostic tests, which lead to more precise treatment. An entire chapter is dedicated to sleep disorders, an enormous area of disability in which major new advances in therapy have occurred. Cancer neurology now involves a complex array of chemotherapy, radiation therapy, and new cutting edge treatments using monoclonal antibodies. No area has changed more substantively than multiple sclerosis, in which fresh magnetic resonance imaging-influenced diagnostic criteria and several immunomodulatory drugs have substantively altered the clinical course of the disease. The area of neuromuscular diseases has been influenced enormously by the use of potent treatment for immune-mediated diseases and better diagnostic precision using molecular techniques applied to blood and muscle biopsy specimens. Pain management has become an art and science of its own, deserving of its own chapter in this edition. The triptan drugs, currently numbering seven, have changed the approach to migraine, and many other headache syndromes are now more clearly classified and specifically treated.

The management of acute stroke has dramatically changed even in the four years since the 6th edition, with widespread use of not only intravenous thrombolytic drugs but also sophisticated interventional techniques aimed at extracting cerebral emboli and opening narrowed vessels with angioplasty and stenting. The advances in Parkinson disease and other movement disorders reflect the widespread availability of new dopamine receptor agonists and the use of deep brain stimulation in advanced and drug-resistant disease. Even Alzheimer disease is now treated with some success using a class of anticholinesterase drugs, and other dementias are more clearly classified and managed. Neuroophthalmology has become a major segment of neurologic practice, a fact that is reflected in an entire chapter now dedicated to that group of disorders. The most prevalent of the toxic and metabolic disorders have undergone an alteration in approach based on a better understanding of the nervous system's reaction to perturbations in its milieu. Moreover, the array of infectious agents affecting the nervous system continues to change as new diseases emerge and the approach with antibiotics undergoes reassessment.

The 17 chapters of the 7th edition of the *Manual of Neurologic Therapeutics* are all brand new; all written by noted experts in the particular area. Emphasis has been placed on practical management, with consideration of the essentials of diagnosis and pathophysiology. The impressive progress in neurologic therapeutics is seen in the increased bulk of the book, now twice its original size.

To complete the quarter century cycle since the book was first published, the foreword to the 7th edition is written by Dr. Raymond D. Adams, to whom the 1st edition was dedicated.

Martin A. Samuels
Boston, Massachusetts

1. COMA, HEAD TRAUMA, AND SPINAL CORD INJURY

Galen V. Henderson

COMA

BACKGROUND

1. *Coma* implies total or near-total unresponsiveness. It is a sleep-like state of unconsciousness from which the patient cannot be aroused by external or internal stimuli.
2. *Stupor* refers to a state of severely impaired arousal with some responsiveness to vigorous stimuli.
3. *Obtundation* refers to a lesser state of decreased arousal with some responsiveness to touch or voice.
4. *Lethargy* (somnolence) refers to a state in which arousal, although diminished, is maintained spontaneously or with repeated light stimulation.
5. *Confusion* refers to a state of impaired attention and implies inadequate arousal to perform a coherent thought or action.
6. *Delirium* usually refers to a state of confusion with periods of agitation and sometimes hypervigilance, active irritability, and hallucinations, typically alternating with periods during which the level of arousal is depressed.

PATHOPHYSIOLOGY

1. Excitatory inputs emanating from the midbrain and rostral pons ascend to the thalamus exciting thalamocortical neurons of the thalamic intralaminar and midline nuclei. The neurons project widely throughout the cerebral cortex and this reticular-activating system supports arousal.
2. These ascending reticulothalamic neurons are cholinergic neurons arising from the mesopontine reticular formation.
3. Attention is thought to depend on the diffuse arousal system and cortical systems for directed attention in various spheres:
   a. Posterior parietal lobes (sensory awareness).
   b. The frontal association cortex (motor attention: directed movements of the eyes, limbs, and body).
   c. Cingulated cortex (motivational aspects of attention).
   d. Lesions that affect these areas multifocally spread down conceptual integration causing global inattention or confusional states.
   e. Acute confusional states.
      1) Diffuse disease in the cerebral cortex
      2) Focal lesions in various regions of the cortex
      3) Thalamic cortical connections
      4) Forebrain and subcortical structures

DIAGNOSIS

Clinical Presentation

1. The goal of the examination of the unresponsive patient is the distinction of coma caused by destruction of brain tissue as in a cerebral hemorrhage or from metabolic coma secondary to disease extrinsic to the brain, such as uremic or hypoglycemic encephalopathy.

TABLE 1-1. GLASGOW COMA SCALE

Points	Eye Opening	Verbal	Motor
6	—	—	Obeys
5	—	Oriented	Localizes to pain
4	Spontaneous	Confused	Withdraws to pain
3	To speech	Inappropriate	Flexion (decorticate)
2	To pain	Unintelligible	Extensor (decerebrate)
1	None	None	None

2. Neurophysiologic function is crucial in determining the level of brain involvement and disease progression.
3. The Glasgow coma scale (GCS; Table 1-1) is a standardized instrument designed for rapid assessment and communication about patients who have coma due to head trauma.
   a. This scale attempts to quantitate the severity of trauma on the basis of patient's best response in three areas: eye opening, motor activity, and language.
   b. The GCS scores range from 3 to 15. When the total score is 8 or less, the patient is considered to be in coma.

Components of the Examination

1. Level of consciousness should be described according to
   a. Unresponsive.
   b. Unresponsive to pain.
   c. Responsive to voice.
   d. Lethargic but spontaneously responsive classifications are best supplemented by a description of the stimuli used and the nature of the responses.
2. Examination of the eyes
   a. Ocular motility
      1) Pupil size and reactivity.
      2) Pupils are the most reliable means of distinguishing metabolic from structural disease.
      3) Preserved pupillary reflexes with absent eye movements to vestibular stimulation or even respiratory depression implicate metabolic coma.
      4) Absent pupillary light reflexes indicate structural brainstem damage with important qualifications.
      5) Symmetric or asymmetric impairment of the pupil's reaction to light usually indicates structural brainstem disease. Pontine infarction or hemorrhages sometimes cause small, "pinpoint" pupils, but they can be seen to react to light under magnification.
      6) Drugs affecting pupillary function
         a) Anticholinergic atropine-like drugs, profound anoxia, hypothermia, or severe barbiturate intoxication can paralyze pupillary reactions.
         b) Atropine-like drugs, tricyclic antidepressants, and lithium toxicity cause large poorly reactive pupils. Such pharmacologic mydriasis can be confirmed by failure of the pupils to constrict to 1% pilocarpine eye drops.
         c) Narcotic intoxication also causes very small pupils. Naloxone administration may be used to reverse this intoxication.
         d) Hallucinogens such as lysergic acid diethylamide (LSD) can dilate the pupils by their sympathomimetic effect.
   b. Optic fundi: If the pupils are small, dilation to view the fundi should be deferred until stability of the patient's condition is assured and a probable cause of unresponsiveness is determined. I do not encourage the dilation of pupils with eye drops, but if it is performed, all caregivers should be notified, a notation made on the chart, and a banner placed on the wall at the head of the bed.

1) Papilledema indicates raised intracranial pressure (ICP), but is often absent in the elderly patient and more sensitive in pediatric patients with high cerebrospinal fluid (CSF) pressure.
2) Retinal hemorrhages and optic disc edema may signify hypertensive encephalopathy.
3) Massive trauma may cause cumulus cloud infiltrates from fat embolism.
4) Subhyaloid blood or a black view indicates retinal bleeding into the vitreous (Terson syndrome) after massive abrupt subarachnoid hemorrhage.
5) Retinal infarcts (cotton-wool spots) indicate vasculitis, intravenous (IV) drug use, or septic emboli.

  c. Eyelids and corneal reflexes
1) The eyes are closed in coma, as in sleep, by tonic contraction of the orbicularis oculi and by inhibition of the levator palpebrae.
2) Absence of orbicularis tonus or failure of lid closure indicates seventh nerve involvement, either central or peripheral. Conversely, the presence of good lid closure and tone indicates that the caudal pons is spared.
3) Reflex spasm of the lids, blepharospasm, occurs with metabolic encephalopathy or posterior fossa lesions.
4) Spontaneous blinking implies sparing of the pontine reticular formation. Occasionally in cases of postictal coma, blinking continues while the lids are closed.
5) Blinking in response to a bright light, even through closed lids, does not indicate sparing of the visual cortex since this reflex may be mediated at a brainstem level.
6) Blinking in response to a loud sound indicates integrity of the lower pons.
7) Absence of blinking to sound, threat, or light indicates severe metabolic compromise or structural damage of the pontine tegmentum.
8) Bilateral lid closure and upward deviation of the eyes in response to strong corneal stimulation assures function from the rostral midbrain right down to the medulla oblongata.
9) A combination of failure of lid closure with spared eye deviation on corneal stimulation signifies destruction of the facial nerve or nucleus.
10) Loss of both lid closure and eye deviation on corneal (pain) stimulation is of little diagnostic help other than indicating that brainstem depression is severe.

3. Skeletal motor and reflex signs
  a. Patients who have hemispheric lesions typically lie in comfortable-appearing, relatively normal postures.
  b. Patients who have brainstem lesions often display abnormal postures. The symmetry of spontaneous movement may give a clue about the side of a focal lesion. Postures with some localizing significance are usually fragmentary and may be elicited by noxious stimuli.
  c. The terms *decorticate* and *decerebrate rigidity* refer to experimental studies of animals and do not accurately reflect the clinicopathologic correlations that they imply.
1) Decorticate posturing: lower extremity extensions and internal rotation with flexion of both upper extremities
2) Decerebrate posturing: lower and upper extremity extensions
  d. Upper extremity flexion reflects more superficial, less severe, and more chronic lesions at the level of the diencephalon or above. Upper and lower extremity extension will often accompany brainstem lesions; however, as mentioned, the upper extremity extension depends on the degree and acuteness of the lesion and being reflexively driven, on the stimulus applied at the time of the examination. The responsible lesions may also be reversible, as in severe toxic and metabolic encephalopathies.
  e. Deep tendon reflexes and plantar responses may also suggest a lateralized lesion, but they, too, are often misleading signs. Careful observation for subtle movements suggesting nonconvulsive seizures should be sought in all cases of coma.

4. Responses respiratory pattern
   a. Hyperventilation is common and has poor localizing value. Differential diagnosis includes
      1) Fever
      2) Sepsis
      3) Metabolic acidosis
      4) Drug toxicity
      5) Cardiopulmonary disease
   b. *Cheyne–Stokes respirations* refer to a periodic breathing pattern of alternating hyperpnea and apnea.
   c. Apneustic.
      1) Characterized by a prolonged pause at the end of inspiration and is also called "inspiratory cramp."
      2) It does localize to a lesion in the mid to caudal pons.
   d. Biot breathing
      1) Characterized by chaotic or ataxic breathing pattern with loss of regularity of alternating pace and depth of inspirations and expirations that may occur when the neurons in the respiratory center are damaged.
      2) Such patients are prone to apnea.
      3) A variety of lesions may cause this pattern.

Level of Consciousness

1. Structural coma can result from primary cerebral hemispheric or primary brainstem involvement.
   a. Purely unilateral cerebral lesions do not produce coma.
   b. Loss of consciousness from unilateral cerebral lesions indicates pressure or displacement of the opposite hemisphere or brainstem as the mass effect shifts across the midline.
   c. Persisting loss of consciousness from cerebral hemispheric disease indicates bilateral cerebral hemispheric damage.
2. As the mass effect builds, it causes coning through the tentorial notch and this herniation distorts the brainstem, interrupting activity ascending to the cerebral hemisphere from the reticular activating system of the rostral midbrain–thalamic area.
   a. Secondary destruction occurs in the brainstem tegmentum. In contrast to primary brainstem hemorrhage, which is usually in the base of the pons, this damage occurs in the tegmentum.
   b. The secondary changes lead to permanent coma and brainstem tegmental signs involving eye movements and the pupils. The supratentorial pressure may compress the posterior cerebral arteries against the incisura of the tentorium, causing infarction of the occipital lobes. Patients may survive this compressive effect to be left with visual-field defects or blindness from damage to the striate cortex or geniculate bodies.
   c. The mass itself may be remote from the visual pathways.

Ocular Response

Gaze Deviation
Deviation of the eyes implicates a structural cause of coma.
1. Tonic horizontal deviation
   a. Eyes deviate conjugately toward the side of massive lesions in the cerebral hemisphere.
   b. This ipsiversive deviation does not specify frontal lobe damage, but occurs more often with massive lesions in the posterior hemisphere, especially the nondominant side.
   c. In the acute phase, the eyes may be brought up to the mid position only by vigorous passive head turning and oculocephalic maneuvers.
   d. In the acute phase, it may be impossible to move the eyes to the opposite side for several hours, then the vestibuloocular reflex (VOR) resumes a full range of

motion. The combination of cerebral hemispheric damage and anticonvulsant or sedative drugs can eliminate the VOR.

2. Contraversive deviation
   a. Unilateral damage in the pontine tegmentum causes contraversive deviation. Version of the eyes to the side opposite cerebral hemispheric lesions (that is, toward the side of hemiparesis) signifies an irritative lesion, such as an epileptic focus.
   b. "Wrong-way deviation" is usually a sign of thalamic hemorrhage and is commonly associated with intraventricular hemorrhage and dissection into the brainstem suggesting that the wrong-way deviation might be caused by the brainstem dissection.
   c. Deviation of the eyes opposite to the lesion is also a feature of acute cerebellar damage.
3. Tonic vertical deviation
   a. Upward deviation occurs in patients with hypoxic–ischemic encephalopathy involving the cerebral hemispheres and cerebellum.
   b. Upward deviation may also occur in the apneic phase of Cheyne–Stokes respiration.
   c. Transient upward deviation is a cardinal feature of oculogyric crises as a side effect of neuroleptic and other drugs.
   d. Downward deviation indicates involvement of the midbrain thalamic junction. This is seen with acute hydrocephalus, medial thalamic hemorrhage, and occasionally metabolic coma, particularly hepatic encephalopathy.

Misalignment of the Eyes

1. In coma as in sleep, small horizontal phorias become evident and are not a pathologic sign.
2. Limited duction of an eye to VOR reflex stimulation confirms that strabismus is paralytic—a heterotropia not a phoria.
3. Limited abduction signifies sixth nerve palsy and limited adduction indicates internuclear ophthalmoplegia (INO) or third nerve palsy.
4. Vertical misalignment of the visual axes indicates skew deviation or fourth nerve palsy. Skew is caused by disruption of otolithic vestibular projections into the ocular motor nuclei. Fourth nerve palsy often follows head trauma.
5. Orbital blowout fractures may also cause vertical strabismus.
6. Metabolic encephalopathy or drug intoxication can rarely cause skew deviation or INO, but they typically indicate structural damage in the brainstem tegmentum.

Vestibuloocular Reflex

1. Distinction of brainstem versus cerebral involvement as the cause of ocular deviation is confirmed by testing the VOR by oculocephalic maneuvers.
2. Passive rocking of the head from side to side in flexion and extension elicits the so-called doll head reflex.
   a. This is predominantly a test of the labyrinthine ocular reflex.
   b. It should not be performed in patients with neck injury or an unstable cervical spine.
   c. Although acute massive cerebral hemispheric lesions may transiently abolish the VOR, persisting VOR paralysis to one side or both indicates involvement of the brainstem tegmentum.
   d. Absence of the doll eyes response indicates either destruction of the brainstem tegmentum or severe metabolic depression. With acute unilateral pontine hemorrhage or infarction the eyes are deviated horizontally to the opposite side and can be brought up to the mid position only.
   e. Caloric stimulation of the VOR is an integral part of the neuro-ophthalmic assessment of the comatose patient.
      1) The head is elevated to 30 degrees on a pillow to make the horizontal semicircular canal vertical. Fifty to 100 mL or more of ice water is injected into the auditory canal until nystagmus or tonic deviation of the eyes occurs.

2) In unconscious patients, nystagmus fast phases are absent and the eyes deviate in the direction of cold stimulation.
3) Failure of deviation indicates structural interruption or severe metabolic depression of brainstem VOR pathways.
4) Drug intoxication can paralyze the VOR in the early stages of coma. Discrete involvement of brainstem connections by structural lesions can cause monocular paresis of adduction (INO).
5) Incomplete adduction as in INO may also result from metabolic- or drug-induced encephalopathy. Delayed downward deviation in response to caloric stimulation of the horizontal VOR is another feature of barbiturate coma.
6) With structural brainstem lesions, the eyes do not deviate at all or they move dysconjugately and incompletely in response to vestibular stimulation.
7) Caloric testing should be combined with oculocephalic maneuvers if the caloric response is indefinite or absent. For example, the patient may have peripheral vestibular damage from ototoxic drugs. In that case, the neck proprioceptive reflexes may move the eyes. Normally the cervico-ocular reflex is negligible or absent. In patients with bilateral peripheral damage, the gain of the cervico-ocular reflex (neck proprioceptive reflex) may be increased to move the eyes normally. When testing the oculocephalic maneuvers, rotation should be brisk since the VOR responds best to high-frequency rotation. Moreover, once deviated in response to oculocephalic maneuvers, the eyes drift rapidly back to the mid position in coma since the eye velocity-to-position integrator is leaky so that the VOR signal is not stored to maintain eccentric gaze. Reflex eye movements are useful in evaluating the outcome of coma.

Roving Eye Movements
1. The presence of slow roving eye movements indicates metabolic coma or supratentorial structural lesions.
2. Roving occurs at a rate of four to six per minute.
3. They are slow drifting movements that may be conjugate or dysconjugate and are predominantly horizontal.

Ocular Bobbing
1. Typical ocular bobbing occurs in patients with intrapontine lesions associated with bilateral sixth nerve palsies or horizontal gaze palsies. It consists of fast downward movement from the mid position followed by delayed slow return.
2. Reverse ocular bobbing, consisting of fast upward movement from the mid position followed by delayed slow return is seen with metabolic encephalopathy.
3. Inverse ocular bobbing is also said to be a manifestation of metabolic encephalopathy, particularly anoxic. Inverse bobbing (also called "ocular dipping") consists of slow downward deviation of the eyes followed after a delay by quick return to the mid position.
4. Converse bobbing (reverse dipping) designates slow upward drift and faster return to the mid position. These variations on bobbing have less reliable localizing value.
5. Dorsal midbrain structural damage may give rise to vertical movements with convergent components, called "pretectal pseudobobbing."

Vertical Pendular Nystagmus
1. Rarely, acute brainstem stroke may cause large amplitude pendular oscillations. More often this type of nystagmus is delayed and accompanies palatal tremor in patients who have recovered from coma or have maintained consciousness after brainstem vascular damage.
2. Ping-pong gaze
   a. Slow alternation of horizontal gaze deviation between sides every few seconds is rarely encountered after bilateral infarcts of the cerebral peduncles or cerebral hemispheres.
   b. Periodic alternating gaze deviation is a similar phenomenon having a cycle of direction change every 2 minutes, and is the counterpart of periodic alternating nystagmus without a fast phase.

Other Coma-like States

Locked-in Syndrome
1. Lesion in the pons.
2. Patient remains awake but unable to talk or move the arms or legs. The patient is "de-afferented" but remains conscious.
   a. The only way the patient can express his or her alertness is by communication through intact voluntary eyelid and vertical eye movements.
   b. Midbrain involvement can cause the locked-in syndrome accompanied by bilateral ptosis and third nerve palsies The only clue that the patient is conscious is some remnant of movement such as the orbicularis oculi in response to command.
   c. These patients require meticulous nursing and psychological care.
   d. Survival may be prolonged and recovery is possible in patients depending on the lesion type and extent of damage.

Vegetative State
1. This state has many eponyms—vegetative state, coma vigil, apallic syndrome, and akinetic mutism.
2. Coma seldom lasts more than 2 to 4 weeks.
3. Eyes eventually open and sleep–awake cycles appear.
4. Caloric and rotational nystagmus quick phases are regained if the brainstem is intact.
5. Patients do not obey verbal commands but they open their eyes on alerting.
   a. Seen with damage of the frontal limbic syndrome, deep midline lesions that disconnect the frontal lobe from the thalamus, or extensive cortical anoxic damage.
   b. If the damage is predominantly frontal, the patient's eyes may follow the examiner (i.e., tracking). It is the eyes open, sometimes with preserved ocular-following responses, that gives the appearance of coma vigil.

Psychogenic Unresponsiveness
The eyes are particularly important in distinguishing psychogenic unresponsiveness and catatonia from coma and the vegetative state.
1. If the patient lies with the eyes closed, lifting the eyelids results in a slow closure in genuine coma but rapid closure of the eyes is nonphysiologic.
2. Roving eye movements are a type of smooth eye movement and smooth eye movements cannot be produced voluntarily.
3. The patient with psychogenic unresponsiveness never has roving eye movements.
4. Caloric testing elicits nystagmus in psychogenic coma but not in coma. Fast eye movements are abolished in genuine coma. Occasional patients who feign unresponsiveness can inhibit caloric-induced nystagmus by concentrated visual fixation. However, they do not exhibit deviation of the eyes without nystagmus fast phases, as does the comatose patient. Similarly, in psychogenic coma during oculocephalic maneuvers visual fixation enhances the VOR so that the eyes move in the orbit, stabilizing the gaze in one spot. In comatose patients, the VOR may be hypoactive or lost with deep metabolic coma or with structural lesions in the pontine tegmentum.
5. Patients with psychogenic unresponsiveness often look away from the examiner, toward the mattress.

Death by Brain Criteria (Brain Death)
(See section on Brain Death.)

TREATMENT

Approach

1. As with all acutely ill patients, the approach to the comatose patient should follow a rapid prioritized algorithm that ensures stabilization and maintenance of vital

TABLE 1-2. APPROACH TO THE ASSESSMENT AND MANAGEMENT OF ACUTE COMA

Stabilization
- Airway control
- Oxygenation and ventilation
- Adequate circulation (includes avoidance of hypotention in strokes)
- Cervical stabilization

Immediate therapies given to all patients
- Thiamine 100 mg IV
- Dextrose 50% 50 mL IV (may be held if immediate fingerstick glucose establishes adequate serum glucose)
- Naloxone 0.4–2 mg IV (may be repeated)
- Obtain blood for CBC, PT/PTT, chemistry panel, toxic screen, blood cultures, anticonvulsant levels

Threatening conditions to be considered for possible early therapy
- Elevated ICP → head CT
- Meningitis, encephalitis or both → antibiotics, LP, blood cultures
- Myocardial infarction → ECG
- Hypertensive encephalopathy → early therapy
- Status epilepticus → EEG
- Acute stroke → consider thrombolytic therapy

IV, intravenous; CBC, complete blood count; PT, prothrombin time; PTT, partial thromboplastin time; ICP, intracranial pressure; CT, computed tomography; LP, lumbar puncture; ECG, electrocardiogram; EEG, electroencephalogram.
From Neurologic Clinics, Neurologic Emergencies, May 1998, with permission.

functions and rapid assessment and therapy for potential disorders that threaten life and independent functions (Tables 1-2 and 1-3).
2. The ABCs (*a*irway, *b*reathing, and *c*irculation) of acute resuscitation top the list.
3. Acute cervical stabilization is crucial whenever there is any possibility of cervical trauma or instability caused by medical disease, as in rheumatoid arthritis.
4. Maneuvers that require neck movement should be modified to minimize movements or should be avoided (oculocephalics stimulation) until after adequate radiographs have eliminated any concern of cervical instability.

HEAD INJURY

BACKGROUND

1. In the Western world, traumatic injuries are the leading cause of death in ages 15 to 40 years.
2. Head injuries account for most morbidity and mortality from trauma and are responsible for over half of the trauma-related deaths.
3. Traumatic brain injury (TBI) in previously healthy young adults peaks in the 15- to 24-year-old age group; males are affected more commonly than are females.
4. There are approximately 1.5 million new brain injuries annually in the United States.
5. Rates of TBI-related hospitalization have declined nearly 50% since 1980, a phenomenon that may be attributed, in part, to successes in injury prevention, high-quality prehospital paramedic systems, helicopter transport systems, and comprehensive acute care in an intensive care unit (ICU).

TABLE 1-3. SOME CAUSES OF COMA

1. Focal disease
   a. Trauma (contusion, ICH)
   b. Nontraumatic ICH
   c. Ischemic stroke
   d. Infection (abcess, subdural empyema, focal encephalitis)
   e. Tumor
   f. Demyelination (MS, ADEM)
2. Nonfocal disease
   a. Trauma (elevated ICP, diffuse axonal injury)
   b. Vascular syndromes
      i. SAH
      ii. Aneurysm in posterior fossa with mass effect
      iii. Hypoxic–ischemic encephalopathy
      iv. Stroke (focal strokes with nonfocal presentations, posterior fossa infarct with mass effect, hydrocephalus
      v. Hypertensive encephalopathy
   c. Infection (meningitis, diffuse encephalitis)
   d. Tumor related
      i. Tumor (brainstem invasion, posterior fossa mass, elevated ICP, and hydro-cephalus), paraneoplastic syndromes (brainstem encephalitis, vasculitis)
   e. Toxic and metabolic
      i. Toxic
      ii. Metabolic
      iii. Withdrawal symptoms
      iv. Nutritional deficiencies
      v. Disordered temperature regulation
   f. Seizures (postictal state, nonconvulsive status epilepticus)
   g. Others
      i. Basilar migraines
      ii. Transient global amnesia
      iii. TTP and other syndromes of medical illness
      iv. Sleep deprivation
      v. Situational (i.e., ICU psychosis)
      vi. Psychiatric (conversion, depression, mania, catatonia)

ICH, intracranial hemorrhage; MS, multiple sclerosis; ADEM, acute disseminated encephalomyelitis; ICP, intracranial pressure; ICU, intensive care unit; SAH, subarachnoid hemorrhage; T TP, thrombotic thrombocytopenic purpura.
From Neurologic Clinics, Neurologic Emergencies, May 1998, with permission.

6. Approximately 200,000 patients experience severe TBI (i.e., present in coma); 80,000 to 90,000 survive with varying degrees of disability.
   a. In 1993 the reported mortality from the Traumatic Coma Data Bank (TCDB) was about 33%.
   b. While some suggest that contemporary management of patients with severe TBI should limit the mortality rate to approximately 20%, leaving only 50,000 deaths per year, some continue to report mortality rates as high as 37%, 51%, or 60%.
7. The direct cost estimate is around $4 billion annually.

PATHOPHYSIOLOGY

1. TBI is a heterogeneous pathologic entity.
2. TBI is typically classified as primary or secondary.
   a. Primary injuries are mechanical events such as acceleration, deceleration, rotational, penetrating, and blunt forces that occur at the moment of impact.
   b. Secondary injuries can occur from the time of the initial event to minutes, hours, and even days after primary injury.

   c. Patients with traumatic injuries are particularly susceptible to secondary cerebral insults because of associated pulmonary and circulatory physiologic abnormalities. For example, hypotensive events, with or without hypoxia, double the mortality and significantly increase the morbidity of severe head injury. Hypotension occurring in the initial phase of resuscitation is significantly associated with increased mortality following brain injury, even when episodes are relatively brief. About 6% of patients with severe TBI as the main presenting feature also have a cervical spine injury. About 24% of patients with cervical spine injury as the main presenting feature also have a TBI. The degree of permanent brain damage and disability caused by a TBI depends on the severity of the primary injury (i.e., the mechanical disruption of brain tissue at the time of impact) and the secondary injury (i.e., damage due to physiologic and metabolic abnormalities caused by the primary injury).

Scalp Laceration

1. Tend to bleed profusely because of the ample blood supply and poor vasoconstrictive ability of the scalp vasculature.
2. They should be inspected, palpated, irrigated, débrided, and sutured.

Skull Fractures

1. Linear fractures are usually benign unless they occur in the area of (or involve) the middle meningeal artery or dural sinus, which may result in epidural or subdural hemorrhages, respectively.
2. Depressed fractures may cause dural tears and injury to underlying brain tissue.
3. Comminuted fractures are multiple linear fractures with depression at the site of impact.

Basal Skull Fractures

1. Linear fracture that extends into the anterior, middle, or posterior cranial fossa at the skull base.
2. They are often difficult to visualize on plain skull films or axial computed tomography (CT) scans. The diagnosis is often based on clinical signs and symptoms.
3. There is a risk of meningitis if the dura is penetrated; however, prophylactic antibiotics are not indicated.
4. Anterior fossa fractures generally involve the frontal bone and ethmoid and frontal sinuses.
   a. Characterized by bilateral periorbital ecchymosis ("raccoon eyes").
   b. Anosmia from damage to the olfactory apparatus is common.
   c. Rhinorrhea occurs in 25% of patients, usually lasts 2 to 3 days, and is often self-limiting with conservative measures (e.g., elevating the head of the bed, cautioning the patient against blowing his/her nose, lumbar drain placement).
5. Middle fossa fractures are characterized by ecchymosis over the mastoid process behind the ear that may not appear for up to 24 hours (Battle sign) and otorrhea.
   a. Otorrhea indicates tympanic membrane rupture that allows free flow of CSF through the ear; this problem is often self-limiting with conservative measures (e.g., elevating the head of the bed).
   b. May be associated with cranial nerve (CN) VI, VII, and VIII palsies.
6. Never insert a nasogastric tube (NGT) into a patient with a suspected basal skull fracture.
   a. This warning should probably be applied to all comatose patients with TBI.
   b. Use an orogastric tube instead.

Concussion

1. Patients may or may not have loss of consciousness.
2. Patients should have "normal" CT scan findings.

3. Patients commonly complain of headache, dizziness, irritability, short-term memory loss, and/or short attention span. These "minor" head injuries may have sequelae that may be devastating to activities of daily living.

Contusion

1. A contusion is bruising of brain tissue.
2. Contusions may be caused by coup or contrecoup injuries.
3. They most commonly involve the tips of the frontal and temporal lobes, and often enlarge over the first 24 to 48 hours after injury.
4. It is important to check coagulation studies (e.g., prothrombin and partial thromboplastin times) and platelet counts and support clinically important abnormalities.

Subdural Hematoma

1. Classification
   a. "Acute" is used for those less than 3 days old.
   b. "Subacute" if they are 3 days to 3 weeks old.
   c. "Chronic" if they are more than 3 weeks of age.
2. Acute subdural hematoma (ASDH) is the most common traumatic intracranial hematoma and carries the highest associated mortality (as high as 60% in some series).
3. ASDHs usually arise from venous bleeding caused by tearing of bridging veins in the subdural space between the dura and the arachnoid.
4. There is a fourfold increase in the mortality rate if surgery to evacuate the hematoma was delayed 4 hours or more after injury compared with patients who had surgery within 2 hours.
5. Surgical treatment options include burr holes or formal craniotomy and evacuation of the clot.

Epidural Hematoma

1. Epidural hematoma (EDH) is most commonly caused by arterial bleeding into the epidural space, between the skull and dura.
2. Associated with temporal bone fractures causing a tear in middle meningeal artery. Arterial blood rapidly accumulates, and patients can deteriorate quickly (so-called "talk and die").
3. Acute EDH carries a 5% to 10% mortality, but emergent surgical intervention is necessary.
4. Determinants of outcome include GCS score, age, presence of pupillary abnormalities, associated intracranial lesions, presence of traumatic subarachnoid hemorrhage, time between deterioration and surgery, and ICP.
5. Acute EDH is seen in 2.7% to 4% of patients with TBI.
   a. Nine percent of patients who are comatose after injury have an EDH requiring craniotomy.
   b. The peak incidence of EDH occurs in the second decade of life, and it is rare after age 50.
   c. The mean age for EDH in children is 6 to 10 years, and EDH is less frequent in very young children and neonates.
   d. As with TBI in general, 53% (range, 30%–73%) of EDHs are traffic-related; falls account for 30% (range, 7%–52%) and assaults 8% (range, 1%–19%).
   e. Acute EDH results from injury to the middle meningeal artery (36%) or a venous structure (32%) such as the middle meningeal vein, diploic veins, or one of the venous sinuses, and this explains why the most common locations are temporoparietal or temporal lobes.
6. The clinical presentation of EDH is focal deficits, hemiparesis, and decerebration. From 22% to 56% of patients are comatose on admission.
   a. The classic "talk and die" lucid interval is seen in 47%; this is where the patient is unconscious, wakes up, and then deteriorates.

1) Twelve percent to 42% remain conscious; 18% to 44% with pupillary abnormalities.
2) Three percent to 27% present neurologically intact.
3) Eight percent present with seizures.
7. Treatment
    a. Patients with EDH should undergo urgent evacuation if they have a GCS score less than 9 or if they have anisocoria or more than 30 mL of EDH, regardless of GCS score.
    b. Those who may be considered for nonoperative management include those with an EDH that is
        1) Less than 30 mL in volume, less than 15 mm thick, and less than 5 mm of midline shift, as long as the GCS score is above 8.
        2) These patients should undergo serial CT scanning and close observation.

Intracerebral Hematoma

1. Intraparenchymal hemorrhages (IPHs) are unusual in nonpenetrating head trauma.
2. Enlarging cerebral contusions can coalesce into frank intraparenchymal clots requiring surgical intervention.
3. It is more common to see IPH with penetrating injuries (i.e., gunshot and stab wounds).
4. The lesion size and patient status dictate treatment.

Diffuse Axonal Injury

1. Deceleration and rotation of the brain may result in shearing of nerve axons.
2. Mortality after diffuse axonal injury (DAI) is as high as 50%.
3. DAI is the most common cause of a posttraumatic vegetative state.
4. The findings of the initial CT scan are normal in 50% to 85% of patients.
5. Magnetic resonance imaging (MRI) is more sensitive than CT scanning for detecting the hallmark small punctate hemorrhages that are caused by shearing of small perforating arteries.
6. Many believe that involvement if the corpus callosum is a sine qua non of DAI.

Cerebral Edema

1. Cerebral edema leads to increased brain volume from increased water content.
2. Steroids should not be used to treat posttraumatic edema (see below).

Herniation Syndromes

1. Herniation is the shifting of brain tissue to an abnormal area and is secondary to ICP differentials.
2. The associated signs and symptoms depend on the location of herniation and anatomy of the structures being compressed.
3. The most commonly seen syndromes are cingulate/subfalcine herniation, uncal/tentorial herniation, and tonsillar herniation.
    a. Cingulate (or "subfalcine") herniation
        1) Characteristic of unilateral space-occupying lesions in the frontal lobe that force the cingulate gyrus under the falx cerebri.
        2) Compression of the anterior cerebral artery (ACA) may occur, resulting in ischemia/infarction.
        3) No clinical signs or symptoms are specific to cingulated herniation; involvement of the legs is not uncommon.
    b. Uncal (or "tentorial") herniation
        1) Most commonly seen with expanding mass lesions in the middle cranial fossa causing the uncus of temporal lobe to herniate between the brainstem and the tentorial edge.

2) Signs and symptoms include
  a) Decreased consciousness from compression of the reticular formation in the rostral brainstem
  b) Dilated ipsilateral pupil from compression of CN III
  c) Contralateral hemiplegia from direct compression of the cerebral peduncle
c. Tonsillar herniation ("cerebellar herniation")
  1) Arises from expansion of posterior fossa lesions (or supratentorial lesions invading the posterior fossa) causing the cerebellar tonsils to herniate through the foramen magnum into the upper spinal canal, compressing the medulla.
  2) Signs and symptoms include
    a) Guarding against neck flexion
    b) Systemic hypertension
    c) Cardiorespiratory impairment or arrest

TREATMENT

Prehospital Management

1. The evaluation and treatment of traumatic injuries should be initiated from the time prehospital emergency personnel arrive at the scene and continue during transport and through acute management in the emergency department.
2. The priorities for assessment and treatment of the patient with a head injury can be summarized as the ABCs: airway, breathing, and circulation.
  a. Airway/breathing
    1) Securing and maintaining an airway is top priority to ensure adequate oxygenation and ventilation.
    2) Airway patency is often compromised by the presence of foreign objects; obstruction by the tongue and/or pharyngeal/laryngeal soft tissue; accumulation of blood, secretions, or vomitus; and airway collapse by direct trauma.
    3) Ventilation can be compromised by pulmonary contusions, rib fractures (flail chest), diaphragmatic rupture, presence of hemo- or pneumothorax, brainstem injury affecting the respiratory centers, or cervical cord injury affecting phrenic nerve function.
    4) In the absence of airway obstruction, supplemental oxygen should be given via face mask. Otherwise, an airway should be secured via endotracheal or nasotracheal intubation.
    5) Direct tracheotomy or cricothyroidotomy offer alternatives in the presence of massive facial trauma or upper airway swelling.
    6) If needed, respiration can be supported with bag ventilation either via face mask or tracheal tube.
    7) Do not prophylactically hyperventilate. Present evidence, including a randomized clinical trial that demonstrated an adverse effect on neurologic outcome in patients with head injury undergoing prophylactic hyperventilation, strongly suggests that aggressive prophylactic hyperventilation may actually worsen tissue hypoxia and lead to secondary brain injury.
  b. Circulation
    1) In concert with securing the airway and procuring ventilation, blood flow to the brain and other organs must be rapidly and aggressively supported.
    2) Hemodynamic collapse in the trauma setting is most often associated with blood loss, although cardiac dysfunction and neurogenic causes are also common.
    3) External hemorrhage should be controlled via direct wound pressure—tourniquets are not recommended for limb hemorrhage.
    4) Internal hemorrhage can only be addressed in the hospital setting.
    5) The current dogma is that hypovolemic shock is best treated with aggressive IV volume replacement.

6) The advanced trauma life support (ATLS) guidelines state that estimated blood loss should be replaced at a 3:1 ratio with crystalloid.

7) Blood products such as whole blood and packed red blood cells are ideal for volume resuscitation, although storage and handling requirements make their field use impossible.

   a) Isotonic crystalloid IV solutions are currently the only option available to paramedics in the field.

   b) Large-volume crystalloid fluid resuscitation is used to restore hemodynamic parameters until O negative or cross-matched blood is available.

   c) Blood is generally considered the "gold standard" for resuscitation, it is not typically available in the prehospital setting. Furthermore, there are significant concerns with compatibility, disease transmission, and storage requirements associated with banked blood.

Surgical Management

1. Surgical treatment of TBI is the oldest and one of the most important aspects of neurotrauma care. However, there are multiple unresolved issues. For example, should hemorrhagic contusions be removed? Should dominant lobe intraparenchymal hematomas be evacuated? What is the role of decompressive craniotomy in the treatment, or avoidance, of intracranial hypertension?

2. In 1995, the Brain Trauma Foundation, the American Association of Neurological Surgeons (AANS), and the Joint Section on Neurotrauma and Critical Care of the AANS and Congress of Neurological Surgeons first published an evidence-based tome to improve nonpenetrating TBI care. Table 1-4 is a brief outline of those guidelines, which were updated in 2000. There are similar monographs for penetrating head injury and prehospital care, and one pending regarding surgical management of TBI.

ACUTE SPINAL CORD INJURY

BACKGROUND

1. Spinal cord injury in North America occurs in about 11,000 people per year, and the prevalence in the United States is approximately 200,000 patients.

2. Ten thousand people per year die from the complications associated with spinal cord injury.

3. Most cases occur in males aged 15 to 30 years.

4. Twenty-five percent of spinal cord injuries occur in children.

PATHOPHYSIOLOGY

1. The causes of spinal cord injury are multiple and vary within geographic regions within each country. In industrialized nations, motor vehicle collisions are the most common cause of spinal cord injuries.

2. Of those who experience trauma to the spinal column, approximately 15% will have a neurologic injury.

   a. The cervical spine is at greatest risk, with 50% of cervical spine fractures or ligamentous disruptions resulting in neurologic injury.

      1) In children, the distribution of injury is different, as close to half the trauma to the spine occurs in the cervical spine (42%).

TABLE 1-4. GUIDELINES FOR MANAGING TRAUMATIC BRAIN INJURY

Degrees of Certainty
   Standards—Accepted principles of patient management that reflect a high degree of
      clinical certainty.
   Guidelines—A particular strategy or range of management strategies that reflect
      moderate clinical certainty.
   Options—The remaining strategies for patient management for which there is unclear
      clinical certainty.

Initial Management
   Standard: None.
   Guideline: None.
   Option: Rapid, physiologic resuscitation–sedation and neuromuscular blockade for
      specific indications (e.g., airway compromise, elevated ICP). Mannitol or
      hyperventilation (never to $Paco_2$ < 25 mm Hg) only if there are signs of
      life-threatening herniation.

Resuscitation of Blood Pressure and Oxygenation
   Standard: None.
   Guideline: Avoid SBP < 90 mm Hg arterial oxygen saturation < 90%.
   Option: Maintain SBP to keep CPP (the mean arterial pressure less the intracranial
      pressure) > 70 mm Hg. Endotracheal intubation if GCS score is <8 (coma).

Indications for ICP Monitoring
   Standard: None.
   Guideline: Severe TBI (GCS<8) with an abnormal CT scan, or with a normal CT if
      >40 years old, posturing, or SBP <90 mm Hg; ICP monitoring may be used in
      selected noncomatose patients.

ICP Pressure Treatment Threshold
   Standard: None.
   Guideline: Treat ICP at an upper threshold of 20–25 mm Hg.
   Recommendations for ICP monitoring technology: Ventriculostomy is the "gold
      standard."
   Intraparenchymal monitors (e.g., fiberoptic, strain gauge) may be used when the
      ventricles are not accessible.

CPP
   Standard: None.
   Guideline: None.
   Option: Maintain CPP > 70 mm Hg.

Hyperventilation
   Standard: Avoid prolonged or profound ($Paco_2$ < 25 mm Hg) hyperventilation.
   Guideline: Early hyperventilation compromises CPP when CBF is reduced.
   Option: Use brief hyperventilation ($Paco_2$ 31–35 mm Hg) for acute neurologic
      deterioration.

Use of Mannitol
   Standard: None.
   Guideline: Mannitol (0.25–1 g/kg) is effective for control of raised ICP
   Option: Use with ICP monitoring and signs of tentorial herniation or progressive
      neurologic deterioration.
         Avoid hypovolemia, maintain euvolemia
         Keep serum osmolarity <320 mOsm

Use of Barbiturates in Control of Intracranial Hypertension
   Standard: None

(continued)

TABLE 1-4. (*continued*)

Guideline: High-dose barbiturate therapy may be considered in patients with severe TBI with intracranial hypertension refractory to maximal medical and surgical therapy.

Role of Steroids
Standard: The use of steroids is not recommended in severe TBI.
Guideline: None.
Option: None.

Role of Antiseizure Prophylaxis
Standard: Prophylactic use of anticonvulsants is not recommended to prevent late (> 7 d) posttraumatic seizures.
Guideline: None.
Option: Phenytoin and carbamazepine are effective in preventing early (< 7 d) posttraumatic seizures. Stop prophylaxis 7 d after injury. There is no evidence that antiseizure prophylaxis improves outcome.

Nutrition
Standard: None.
Guideline: Provide 140% of estimated calories to nonparalyzed and 100% of estimated calories to paralyzed patient with severe TBI.
Option: Utilize jejeunal alimentation.

ICP, intracranial pressure; SBP, systolic blood pressure; CPP, cerebral perfusion pressure; GCS, Glasgow coma scale; TBI, traumatic brain injury; CT, computed tomography; CBF, cerebral blood flow. From the Brain Trauma Foundation, the American Association of Neurological Surgeons (AANS), and the Joint Section on Neurotrauma & Critical Care of the AANS and Congress of Neurological Surgeons.

---

    2) Sixty-seven percent of cervical spine injuries in children occur in the upper cervical spine.
  b. The most common mechanisms of spinal cord injury are hyperflexion, hyperextension, axial loading, and penetrating injury.
  c. Spinal cord injuries are classified as complete or incomplete.
    1) Complete injuries imply loss of all motor, sensory, and reflex function below the level of the injury.
    2) Incomplete injury implies some intact neurologic function below the level of the injury.
      a) Central cord injury
        • Most commonly results from hyperextension.
        • Greater motor dysfunction is seen in the upper extremities compared with the lower extremities.
        • Most commonly seen in those with preexisting acquired stenosis such as spondylotic disease.
        • The central part of the cord is the watershed area and is more susceptible to ischemia.
      b) Anterior cord syndrome
        • Anterior cord syndrome has classically been described as resulting from a traumatic disc herniation.
        • The disc damages the anterior and lateral areas of the spinal cord, leaving the posterior columns intact.
      c) Brown–Sequard syndrome
        • Contralateral loss of pain and temperature sensation, as well as ipsilateral loss of motor function and proprioception.
        • Typically results from penetrating wounds or severe unilateral fractures leading to a hemisection of the spinal cord. In this syndrome, for injuries that result in quadriplegia, the 5-year survival rate is 85%.

TREATMENT

Care at the Scene of the Accident

1. Treatment in the field begins with the ABCs, which are followed by a brief neurologic examination.
2. It is important that all trauma victims be treated as a patient with a spinal cord injury.

Management in the Hospital

1. Starts by repeating what was done in the field—the ABCs are reassessed, and further respiratory support is given via supplemental oxygen with a nasal canula or intubation.
   a. Blood pressure management may include the use of fluids and pressors.
   b. Placement of an NGT
   c. Foley catheter
   d. Warming blankets help to lower associated morbidity in spinal cord injury.
   e. Mast trousers are sometimes used to combat refractory hypotension from spinal shock.
   f. A detailed neurologic examination helps identify the extent and probable location of the injury. Medications such as methylprednisolone are commonly started.
2. Radiographs of the spine are obtained, and decisions on closed or open reduction are made. Multiple surgical approaches exist, however, great controversy exists in the timing of surgery.

Pharmacologic Treatment

1. For acute spinal cord injury, pharmacologic therapy is routine in medical centers.
   a. This resulted from the National Acute Spinal Cord Injury Studies (NASCISs) no. 2 and no. 3, which were both double-blind, randomized controlled trials. NASCIS 2 compared methylprednisolone and naloxone. NASCIS 3 compared 24-hour methylprednisolone and tirilazad mesylate and 48-hour methylprednisolone. Modest clinical improvement was seen at 6 weeks and 6 months in the treatment groups when compared with those treated by placebo. However, in patients in whom methylprednisolone was begun after 8 hours, no significant neurologic improvement over placebo was noted.
   b. Methylprednisolone protects the spine from lipid peroxidation and decreases the accumulation of water and sodium. Lazaroids (tirilazad) are synthetic nonglucocorticoids with a strong antioxidant potential. Gangliosides are thought to stabilize the cells' lipid bilayer.
   c. All three drugs have undergone human trials, but methylprednisolone is the only medication that showed statistical clinical benefit. The lazaroids and gangliosides have not been shown to be clinically effective and are not currently part of the standard care of spinal cord injury.
2. Methylprednisolone
   a. Standard dosage 30 mg/kg initial bolus administered IV over a 15-minute period, followed by a 45-minute pause, then begin treatment with 5.4 mg/kg/h infusion for 23 hours, if infusion is started less than 3 hours from the time of the injury.
   b. The infusion should continue for 48 hours if started between 3 and 8 hours from the time of the accident.
   c. Contraindications
      1) Not to be given for open injuries, such as gunshot wounds, due to an increased risk of wound infection and lack of proven neurologic benefit.
      2) Outcomes are worse if methylprednisolone is administered more than 8 hours after injury.

   d. Main drug interactions
      1) Methylprednisolone increases circulating glucose levels.
      2) Decreases effect of phenytoin and phenobarbital.
      3) Rifampin increases clearance of methylprednisolone.
   e. Main side effects
      1) Hypersensitivity
      2) Increased risk of infection

Surgical Treatment

1. The role of surgery in the treatment of acute spinal cord injury remains controversial.
2. The goals of surgery for spinal cord injuries are spinal cord decompression, correction of spinal column deformity, and spinal column stabilization.
3. The goals sound straightforward; however, little evidence supports exactly how or when this should be done.
4. Surgical stabilization and decompression
   a. Anterior operations or posterior operations.
   b. Instrumentation such as plates, wires, and rods plays an important role in ensuring spinal column stabilization.
   c. Instrumentation can be placed either through an anterior procedure or a posterior procedure.
   d. In the absence of definitive data, the selection of the most appropriate procedure and its timing remains the realm of individual surgical judgment.

Prevention of Complications

1. Aspiration precautions: Placement of a nasogastric tube is used to reduce the risk of aspiration and pneumonia.
2. Urinary retention: Placement of a Foley catheter reduces the risk of hydronephrosis and renal impairment.
3. Warming blanket: Hypothermia can promote systemic complications and is commonly seen in trauma victims and patients with spinal cord injury.
4. Cervical immobilization
   a. The short-term goal of immobilization is to prevent further misalignment and additional injury to the spinal cord.
   b. Immobilization can be achieved by bed rest, traction, or spinal orthosis.
   c. Orthosis for immobilization of the spine allows early mobilization of the patient and can help in achieving spinal column alignment.
5. Cervical collar for treatment of cervical spine injuries.
   a. Standard procedure: Initially, all patients are placed in a firm cervical collar (I consider using Philadelphia or Miami J).
   b. Contraindications: associated tracheal injury or soft-tissue injury in the neck.
   c. Complications: skin ulceration caused by pressure from the collar.
   d. Special points:
      1) The Philadelphia collar can be used to treat stable fractures.
      2) A sterno-occipitomandibular immobilization (SOMI) brace or halo device is used for unstable fractures.
6. Braces for treatment of thoracic and lumbar spine injuries.
   a. Standard procedure: A brace such as the thoracic lumbar sacral orthosis (TLSO), or Jewett brace is used to treat fractures of the thoracic spine. In the lumbar spine, a corset brace, Boston overlap hard-shell brace, or body cast is used.
   b. Contraindications: severe thoracic or abdominal trauma.
   c. Complications: skin ulceration from the brace.
   d. Special points:
      1) Once these braces are in place, a flat and upright lateral thoracic spine or lumbar spine radiograph should be obtained.
      2) If movement of the spinal column is noted, the patient is placed back on bed rest and surgical stabilization is considered.

7. Oxygenation: Respiratory complications are the largest cause of morbidity and mortality in the patient with spinal cord injury. Since half the patients with spinal cord injuries arrive with complete injuries, the need for respiratory support is high. The goals are to guard against respiratory failure and to ensure adequate oxygenation to the injured spinal cord.

   a. Standard procedure: A nasal cannula or face mask to provide supplemental oxygen should be used in the acute phase of treatment in those patients who do not require intubation.

   b. Endotracheal intubation is warranted in those patients with respiratory distress. Impending respiratory failure should be suspected in those patients with absent chest wall movement and excessive abdominal wall movement.

   c. If the blood gas has a Po_2 less then 70 mm Hg, or a Pco_2 greater that 45 mm Hg, intubation should be accomplished.

   d. Contraindications: In the case of major facial or skull base trauma, tracheotomy should be preformed instead of nasal or endotracheal intubation.

   e. Complications: Endotracheal intubation may worsen a cervical spine cord injury in cases with unstable cervical spine fractures or ligament injury.

   f. Special points: Most high cervical injuries will require intubation.

      1) Intubation is indicated with lesions at or above C-3 because there is no diaphragmatic or intracostal muscle function.

      2) Lower cervical or upper thoracic injuries may require intubation because of delayed ascending cord swelling.

8. Blood pressure: The treatment objective is to maintain or enhance blood flow to the injured cord, and treat shock if present.

Patient Placement, Catheters, and Vasopressors

1. Neurogenic shock can happen with injuries above T-6.

   a. The sympathetic outflow tracts are found from T-1 to L-2.

   b. Lesions at T-6 (or above) disrupt a significant proportion of these tracts, which results in the loss of sympathetic nervous system control over peripheral vascular tone. This results in pooling of blood and reduces central venous return.

   c. Examination reveals warm extremities, good urine output, and vital signs that show bradycardia and hypotension.

2. Standard procedure: Placement of the patient in Trendelenburg position (head down) helps reduce the pooling of blood in the lower extremities.

   a. A Swan–Ganz catheter or central venous catheter is used to assess and regulate fluid status.

   b. Vasopressors are used to augment blood pressure.

3. Contraindications: relative contraindication in those patients with impaired cardiac function.

4. Complications: development of heart failure from fluid overload.

5. Special points: Hypovolemic shock is commonly seen in patients with spinal cord injury and additional systemic trauma. Treatment for this type of shock is fluid replacement and transfusion of red cells if there are active losses.

   a. It is possible to have both neurogenic and hypovolemic shock in the same patient.

6. Dopamine

   a. Standard dosage: Dopamine is the agent of choice for treatment of neurogenic shock, and is started at 5 μg/kg/min, and titrated to effect.

   b. Contraindications: Use of dopamine in the face of hypovolemia could lead to end-organ damage.

   c. Main drug interactions: Monoamine oxidase inhibitors increase the effects of dopamine.

   d. Main side effects: tachycardia and cardiac ectopy.

   e. Special points: Goal is a systemic blood pressure (SBP) of 110 mm Hg to 140 mm Hg, and a pulmonary capillary wedge pressure (PCWP) of 12 mm Hg to 16 mm Hg.

7. Atropine
   a. Standard dosage: Symptomatic bradycardia is treated with 0.4 mg atropine administered IV.
   b. Contraindications: unstable cardiovascular status; acute angle closure glaucoma.
   c. Main drug interactions: Diphenhydramine is addictive with synergetic effects. Scopolamine also is addictive with synergetic effects.
   d. Main side effects: May precipitate ventricular fibrillation in patients with cardiac history.
   e. Special points: Central nervous system side effects such as confusion and hallucinations can confuse the clinical picture if an associated head injury exists.

Reduction
The goals of reduction are restoration of spinal column alignment and the release of continuing pressure on the spinal cord. Reduction can be achieved by closed or open methods.
1. Closed reduction
   a. Standard procedure: typically done in the emergency department for cervical facet dislocations or significant subluxation.
   b. The halo device has largely replaced tongs to achieve reduction.
      1) The halo ring is attached to weights, which are added in 5- to 10-lb increments.
      2) Sequential cross-table lateral films or fluoroscopy are used throughout the reduction.
      3) Once the reduction is complete, the weight is removed and the halo vest is put into place.
   c. Contraindications: Major skull fractures that would prohibit halo placement.
   d. Complications: During the course of reduction, an acute disc herniation may occur adding further injury to the spinal cord.
2. Open reduction
   a. Special points: Surgical reduction (open reduction) is indicated in those patients with neurologic compromises because of a compressive lesion. It may be also preformed when closed reduction has failed.
   b. There is controversy about the speed with which reduction should be accomplished. Many neurosurgeons believe that cervical dislocation should be reduced within a few hours, although thoracic and lumbar dislocations (which frequently require extensive surgical procedures) are best treated in a semielective fashion.

Imaging
The patient's clinical history and physical examination findings dictate the radiographs physicians should obtain. The most common radiographs used today are plain films, CT, and MRI.
1. Plain films: A cervical spine series should be obtained on all patients with suspected cervical spine injury.
   a. Odontoid, anteroposterior, and lateral films. All seven cervical vertebrae down to the C7-T1 junction should be seen.
   b. Plain films remain the fastest and least expensive way to obtain an initial assessment that allows visualization of the entire spine.
2. CT: Plain films do not provide detail of the bony anatomy and may not reveal fractures.
   a. CT is the most sensitive method for the detection of spinal column fractures.
   b. CT scan is indicated when an abnormality is identified on initial plain films or can be the initial imaging modality.
3. MRI provides details of the soft tissue including the spinal cord parenchyma.
   a. It has become part of the routine analysis in patients with spinal cord injury.
   b. Its role in the acute pretreatment management of spinal cord injury remains controversial.

1) For cases where MRI can be obtained rapidly in urgent situations, it will provide the greatest amount of information about the spinal cord. However, a delay in obtaining MRI may be harmful to the incomplete or deteriorating patient.
2) Some patients have been reported to deteriorate after reduction of cervical dislocation and are found to have a large disc herniation.

BRAIN DEATH

BACKGROUND

1. In the United States, the principle that death can be diagnosed by two means, cardiac asystole or neurologic criteria (designated as brain death), is the basis of the Uniform Determination of Death Act, although the law does not define any of the specifics of the clinical diagnosis.
2. There is a clear difference between severe brain damage and brain death. The physician must understand this difference, because brain death means that life support is useless, and brain death is the principal requisite for the donation of organs for transplantation.
3. There are many ethical, religious, and philosophical considerations regarding the definition of death.

PATHOPHYSIOLOGY

1. In adults, the chief causes of brain death are traumatic brain injury and subarachnoid hemorrhage.
2. In children, abuse is a more common cause than motor vehicle collisions or asphyxia.

DIAGNOSIS

In 1995, the American Academy of Neurology published suggested practice measures, an evidence-based review. This report specifically addressed the tools of clinical examination and the validity of confirmatory tests and provided a practical description of apnea testing.

Neurologic Examination

1. Before the neurologic examination for the determination of brain death can be performed the following prerequisites are met:
   a. Ruling out the presence of complicated medical conditions that may confound the clinical assessment, such as
      1) Severe electrolyte, acid–base, or endocrine disturbances
      2) Absence of severe hypothermia, defined as a core temperature of 32°C or lower
      3) Hypotension, defined as SBP less then 90 mm Hg
      4) Absence of evidence of drug intoxication, poisoning, or neuromuscular blocking agents
   b. Interpretation of the CT scan is essential for determining the cause of brain death. Usually, CT scanning documents a mass with brain herniation, multiple hemispheric lesions with edema, or edema alone. However, such a finding on the CT scan does not obviate the need for a careful search for confounders. Conversely, the CT scan findings can be normal in the early period

after cardiorespiratory arrest or with patients with fulminant meningitis or encephalitis.
   c. If the clinical suspicion is high, examination of the CSF should be diagnostic for infection in the central nervous system.
2. The clinical neurologic examination remains the standard for the determination of brain death and has been adopted by most countries. The clinical examination of patients who are presumed to be brain dead must be performed with consistency and precision. The declaration of brain death requires:
   a. Serial neurologic examinations
   b. Establishment of the cause of coma
   c. Ascertainment of irreversibility
   d. Resolution of any misleading clinical neurologic signs
   e. Recognition of possible confounding factors
   f. Interpretation of the findings on neuroimaging
   g. Performance of any confirmatory laboratory tests that are deemed necessary

Evaluation of the Comatose Patient

Coma or Unresponsiveness
1. Motor responses of the limbs to painful stimuli may be absent after supraorbital pressure and nail-bed pressure.
2. Motor responses ("Lazarus sign") may occur spontaneously during apnea testing, often during hypoxic or hypotensive episodes, and are of spinal origin.
3. Neuromuscular blocking agents can produce prolonged weakness.
   a. If neuromuscular agents have recently been administered, examination with a bedside peripheral nerve stimulator is needed.
   b. A train of four stimulus should result in four thumb twitches.

Absence of Brainstem Reflexes
1. The response to bright light should be absent in both eyes.
2. Round, oval, or irregularly shaped pupils in brain death are in middle position (4–6 mm, but the size of the pupils may vary from 4 to 9 mm.
3. Dilated pupils are compatible with the brain death because intact sympathetic cervical pathways connected with the radially arranged fibers of the dilator muscle may remain intact.
4. Many drugs can influence pupil size, but light responses remain intact.
   a. In conventional doses, atropine given intravenously has no marked influence on papillary response.
   b. Because nicotine receptors are absent in the iris, neuromuscular blocking drugs do not noticeably influence pupil size.
   c. Topical ocular instillation of drugs and trauma to the cornea or bulbus oculi may cause abnormalities in pupil size and can produce nonreactive pupils.
   d. Preexisting anatomic abnormalities of the iris or effects or previous surgery should be excluded.
5. Ocular movements.
   a. Ocular movements are absent after head turning and caloric testing with ice water. (Testing is only done when no fracture or instability or the cervical spine is apparent, and in patients with head injury, the cervical spine must be imaged to exclude potential fractures, instability, or both.)
   b. The oculocephalic reflex, elicited by fast and vigorous turning of the head from middle position to 90 degrees on both sides, normally results in the eye deviation to the opposite side of the head turning. Vertical eye movements should be tested with brisk neck flexion. Eyelid opening and vertical and horizontal eye movements must be absent in brain death.
   c. Caloric testing should be done with the head elevated to 30 degrees during irrigation of the tympanum on each side with 50 mL of ice water. Tympanum irrigation can be accomplished by inserting a small tube into the external auditory canal and connecting it to a 50-mL syringe filled with ice water. Tonic

deviation of the eyes directed to the cold caloric stimulus is absent. The investigator should allow up to 1 minute after injection, and the time between stimulation on each side should be at least 5 minutes.

    d. Drugs that can diminish or completely abolish the caloric responses are sedatives, aminoglycosides, tricyclic antidepressants, anticholinergics, antiepileptic drugs, and chemotherapeutic agents.

    e. After closed head injury or facial trauma, lid edema and chemosis of the conjunctive may restrict movement of the globes. Clotted blood or cerumen may diminish the caloric response and repeated testing is required after direct inspection of the tympanum. Basal fracture of the petrous bone abolishes the caloric response only unilaterally and may be identified by an ecchymotic mastoid process.

6. Facial sensation and facial motor response.

    a. Corneal reflexes should be tested with a throat swab.

    b. Corneal reflex should be absent.

    c. Grimacing to pain can be tested by applying deep pressure with a blunt object on the nail beds, pressure on the supraorbital ridge, or deep pressure on both condyles at the level of the temporomandibular joint.

    d. Severe facial trauma may limit interpretation of all brainstem reflexes.

7. Pharyngeal and tracheal reflexes.

    a. The gag response, tested by stimulation of the posterior pharynx with a tongue blade, should be absent.

    b. Lack of cough response to bronchial suctioning should be demonstrated.

8. Apnea testing.

    a. Disconnect the ventilator.

    b. Deliver 100% O_2 at 6 L/min. Option: Place a cannula at the level of the carina. Look closely for respiratory movements. Respiration is defined as abdominal or chest excursions that produce adequate tidal volumes. If present, respiration can be expected early in the apnea test. When respiratory-like movements occur, they can be expected at the end of the apnea test, when oxygenation may become marginal. When the result is in doubt, a spirometer can be connected to the patient to confirm that tidal volumes are absent.

    c. Measure arterial Po_2, Pco_2, and pH after approximately 8 minutes and reconnect the ventilator.

    d. If respiratory movements are absent and the Pco_2 is equal to or greater than 60 mm Hg (option: 20-mm Hg increase in Pco_2 over a baseline normal Pco_2), the apnea test result is positive (i.e., it supports the clinical diagnosis of brain death), and the test should be repeated.

    e. If during the apnea testing, the systolic blood pressure is below 90 mm Hg, the pulse oximeter indicates marked desaturation, and cardiac arrhythmias occur, immediately draw a sample, connect the ventilator, and analyze arterial blood gas. The apnea test result is positive if the arterial Pco_2 is above 60 mm Hg or the Pco_2 increase is equal to or greater than 20 mm Hg above baseline normal Pco_2.

Requirements for Death by Brain Criteria

1. Coma of a known cause

2. Absence of motor responses

3. Absence of papillary responses to light and pupils and mid position with respect to dilatation (4–6 mm)

4. Absence of corneal reflexes

5. Absence o f caloric response

6. Absence of gag reflex

7. Absence of coughing in response to tracheal suctioning

8. Absence of respiratory drive at a $Paco_2$ that is 60 mm Hg or 20 mm Hg above the normal baseline values

9. Interval between two examinations according to the patient's age

    a. Usually 6 hours for adults but this time period varies depending on state/country

10. Perform confirmatory tests if required

Neurologic States That Can Mimic Brain Death

1. The locked-in syndrome is usually a consequence of the destruction of the base of the pons.
   a. The patient cannot move the limbs, grimace, or swallow, but the upper rostral mesencephalic structures involved in voluntary blinking and vertical eye movements remain intact.
   b. Consciousness persists because the tegmentum, with the reticular formation, is not affected. The condition is most often caused by an acute embolus to the basilar artery.
2. Guillain–Barré syndrome involving all the peripheral and cranial nerves.
   a. The progression occurs over a period of days, and knowledge of the history should prevent the dangerous error of diagnosing brain death.
3. Hypothermia from prolonged environmental exposure may mimic loss of brain function, but alcohol intoxication and head injury are often major confounders.
   a. Hypothermia causes a downward spiral of loss of brainstem reflexes and pupillary dilatation. The response to light is lost at core temperatures of 28°C to 32°C, and brainstem reflexes disappear when the core temperature drops below 28°C.
   b. These deficits are all potentially reversible, even after extreme hypothermia.
4. Many sedative and anesthetic agents can closely mimic brain death, but aspects of brainstem function, particularly the pupillary responses to light, remain intact. When ingested in large quantities, many drugs can cause a partial loss of brainstem reflexes.
5. A reasonable approach to drug/toxin exposure is as follows:
   a. If it is known which drug or poison is present but the substance cannot be quantified, the patient should be observed for a period that is at least four times the elimination half-life of the substance, provided that the elimination of the drug is not interfered with by other drugs or organ dysfunction.
   b. If the particular drug is not known but high suspicion persists, the patient should be observed for 48 hours to determine whether a change in brainstem reflexes occurs; if no change is observed, a confirmatory test should be performed.

Confirmatory Tests

1. Confirmatory tests are optional in adults but recommended in children younger than 1 year. In several European, Central and South American, and Asian countries, confirmatory testing is required by law. Certain countries (e.g., Sweden) require only cerebral angiography. In the United States, the choice of tests is left to the discretion of the physician, but bedside tests seem to be preferred.
2. Cerebral angiography may document nonfilling of the intracranial arteries at the entry to the skull because the systolic pressure is not high enough to force blood through the intracranial vascular tree.
   a. Perivascular glial swelling and the formation of subintimal blebs caused by ischemia may cause the collapse of smaller vessels, leading to increased intravascular resistance.
   b. Cerebral angiography is performed with an injection in the aortic arch to visualize both the anterior and the posterior circulation. Arrest of flow is found at the foramen magnum in the posterior circulation and at the petrosal portion of the carotid artery in the anterior circulation.
   c. Magnetic resonance angiography and CT angiography may produce similar views.
3. Electroencephalography is used in many countries and remains one of the most well-validated confirmatory tests.
   a. Recordings are obtained for at least 30 minutes with a 16- or 18-channel instrument. In a patient who is brain dead, electrical activity is absent at levels higher than 2 μV with the instrument set at a sensitivity of 2 μV/mm.

b. High levels of sensitivity set on the electroencephalography machine increase artifacts.
4. Transcranial Doppler ultrasonography has a sensitivity of 91% to 99% and a specificity of 100%.
   a. A portable, 2-Hz, pulsed-wave Doppler ultrasonographic instrument is used, insonating both middle cerebral arteries and vertebral arteries.
   b. The absence of a signal may be artifactual if a bone window interferes with insonation.
   c. In patients who are brain dead, transcranial Doppler ultrasonography typically reveals the absence of the diastolic or reverberating flow that is caused by the contractile force of the arteries; the pulsatility index is very high, with systolic velocities that are only a fraction of the normal level.
5. Nuclear imaging with technetium may demonstrate an absence of intracerebral uptake of the tracer. The correlation with conventional angiography is good.

Continuation of Mechanical Ventilation and Support

When mechanical ventilation and support are continued because of ethical or legal objections to their discontinuation, what usually follows is an invariant heart rate from a differentiated sinoatrial node, structural myocardial lesions leading to a marked reduction in the ejection fraction, decreased coronary perfusion, the need for increasing use of inotropic drugs to maintain blood pressure, and a fragile state that leads to cardiac arrest within days or weeks.

INCREASED INTRACRANIAL PRESSURE (INTRACRANIAL HYPERTENSION)

BACKGROUND

1. Increased ICP, or intercranial hypertension, is a pathologic condition common to a wide variety of serious neurologic illnesses (Table 1-5).
2. Proper understanding of the pathophysiology of each entity allows prompt recognition and rational therapeutic goals and hopefully allows better neurologic outcomes.

PATHOPHYSIOLOGY

1. The principles of intracranial hypertension are based on the Monro–Kellie doctrine.
   a. The skull, a rigid compartment, is filled to capacity with noncompressible contents—brain matter (80%), intravascular blood (10%), and CSF (10%).
   b. The volume of these three components remains nearly constant in a state of dynamic equilibrium. If any one component increases the volume, other components must decrease for the overall volume to remain constant, otherwise ICP will rise.
   c. As a result, most therapeutic modalities for the treatment of increased ICP (e.g., CSF drainage, hyperventilation, mannitol) are directed toward reducing intracranial volume.
2. Normal range of ICP is 3 to 15 mm Hg or 5 to 20 cm H_2O.
   a. Elevations above these levels can rapidly lead to brain damage or death by
      1) Global hypoxic–ischemic injury resulting from the reduction of cerebral perfusion pressure (CPP) and cerebral blood flow (CBF).
      2) Mechanical compression, distortion, and herniation of brain tissue by compartmentalized ICP gradients.

TABLE 1-5. CONDITIONS ASSOCIATED WITH INCREASED INTRACRANIAL PRESSURE

Intracranial mass lesions
   Cerebral hemorrhage
   Subdural hematoma
   Epidural hematoma
   Intracerebral hemorrhage
   Subarachnoid hemorrhage
   Brain tumor
   Cerebral abscess

Increased cerebrospinal fluid volume
   Hydrocephalus

Increased brain volume (cerebral edema)
   Benign intracranial hypertension (pseudotumor cerebri)
   Cerebral infarction
   Global hypoxic–ischemia
   Reye syndrome
   Acute hyponatremia
   Hepatic encephalopathy
   Head trauma
   Meningitis
   Encephalitis
   Lead encephalopathy
   Eclampsia
   Hypertensive encephalopathy
   Dural sinus thrombosis

3. Relationship between neurologic decline with elevated ICP.
   a. Depending on the clinical situation, global increases in ICP begin as regional cerebral edema, but regional cerebral edema often causes profound tissue shifts and brainstem distortions without causing global ICP elevations.
   b. Neurologic deterioration correlates with horizontal displacement of the anterior septum and the pineal gland rather than global ICP.
   c. ICP elevation is a terminal and most likely an irreversible circumstance that results when mass expansion exceeds intracranial compliance.
   d. The clinical signs of increased ICP are well known but are highly unreliable. The combined clinical signs are
      1) Depressed level of consciousness
      2) Reflex hypertension, with or without bradycardia
      3) Headache
      4) Papilledema
      5) Vomiting
      6) Cranial nerve palsies
   e. Because these clinical signs are unreliable, it is important to remember that the only way to diagnose increased ICP is to directly measure it.
4. Herniation syndromes (see section on Herniation Syndromes).
5. Prognosis depends on the etiology.

DIAGNOSIS

Recognition of symptoms and treatment is essential because elevated ICP can rapidly lead to irreversible brain damage or death.
1. Only invasive neuromonitoring of ICP can accurately diagnose and monitor efficacy of treatment modalities.

2. Traditional neurologic practice depends on changes in the patient's neurologic examination as the primary monitoring technique. This approach is inadequate in critically ill patients with depressed level of consciousness, in whom early signs of neurologic deterioration cannot be appreciated.
3. The goal of ICP monitoring is to detect abnormal physiologic events before the loss of the neurologic function, therefore allowing clinicians to intervene and avoid additional brain injury.

TREATMENT

Physiologic Principles

1. Intracranial anatomy
   a. The components of volume within the nondistensible cranium of the normal adult brain are brain tissue (1,400 mL), blood (150 mL), and CSF (150 mL).
   b. CSF is produced constantly by the choroids plexus within the ventricles at a rate of 0.34 mL/min.
   c. CSF is transported into the dural sinuses via arachnoid granulations. Normally, this pathway offers little resistance to CSF outflow. As a result, jugular venous pressure is a major determinant in ICP.
2. Intracranial compliance
   a. Because the cranial vault is a rigid and fixed container, any additional intracranial volume can lead to increased ICP. The Monroe–Kellie doctrine states that the volume of the rigid intracranial vault cannot change.
   b. As the volume increases, intracranial contents must be displaced (Table 1-6). As a mass lesion expands in the intracranial vault, there are minimal increases in pressure that occur initially because CSF and blood are displaced.
   c. When these mechanisms become exhausted, intracranial compliance falls sharply, and further small increments in intracranial volume lead to dramatic elevations of ICP (Fig. 1-1).
   d. Intracranial compliance can be described as change in volume divided by the change in pressure.
3. Cerebral perfusion and autoregulation
   a. Brain tissue requires constant perfusion to ensure adequate delivery of substrate, principally oxygen and glucose.
   b. The hemodynamic response of the brain has the capacity to preserve perfusion across a wide range of systemic blood pressures.
   c. CPP, defined as the mean systemic arterial pressure (MAP) minus the ICP, provides the driving force for circulation across the capillary beds of the brain.
   d. Autoregulation refers to the physiologic response whereby CBF remains relatively constant over a wide range of blood pressures as a consequence of alterations of cerebrovascular resistance (Fig. 1-2).

TABLE 1-6. HORIZONTAL DISPLACEMENT OF MIDLINE STRUCTURES ON COMPUTED TOMOGRAPHY SCANS AND LEVEL OF CONSCIOUSNESS

	True Dimensions from Midline (mm)	
Level of Consciousness	Pineal	Septum Pellucidum
Awake	0–3	2–7
Drowsy	3–6	2–10
Stupor	6–9	7–14
Coma	9–15	12–18

From Ropper AH. Lateral displacement of the brain and level of consciousness in patients with an acute hemispheral mass. *N Engl J Med* 1986;314:953–958, with permission.

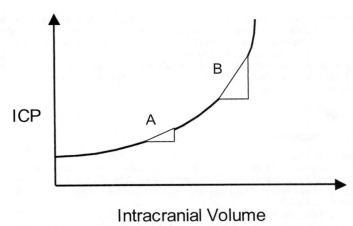

Intracranial Volume

FIG. 1-1. Intracranial compliance curve.

1) If systemic blood pressure drops, cerebral perfusion is preserved through vasodilatation of arterioles in the brain; likewise, arteriolar vasoconstriction occurs at high systemic pressures to prevent hyperperfusion. At the extreme limits of MAP or CPP (high or low), flow becomes directly related to perfusion pressure.
2) CBF is also strongly influenced by pH and P_{CO_2} (Fig. 1-3).
   a) CBF increases with hypercapnia and acidosis and decreases with hypocapnia and alkalosis.
   b) This forms the basis for the use of hyperventilation to lower ICP, and this effect on ICP is mediated through a decrease in intracranial blood volume.
3) Cerebral autoregulation is critical to the normal homeostatic functioning of the brain, and this process may be disordered focally and unpredictably

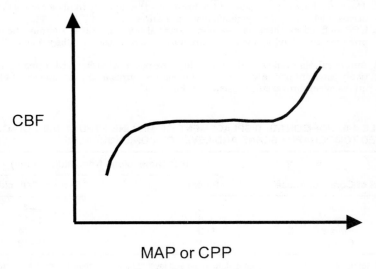

MAP or CPP

FIG. 1-2. Cerebral autoregulation curve.

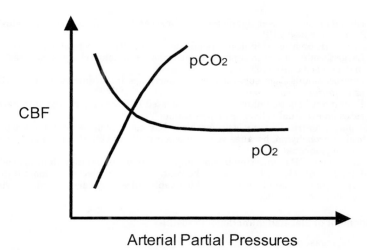

FIG. 1-3. Arterial partial pressures curve.

in disease states such as traumatic brain injury and severe focal cerebral ischemia.

4. ICP waveforms
   a. Normal ICP waveform reflects a transient increase in cerebral blood volume that occurs with each arterial pulse.
   b. Under normal conditions, the amplitude of ICP pulse pressure is relatively small (2–3 mm Hg).
      1) Under pathologic conditions when intracranial compliance is reduced, ICP pulse pressures increase to levels as high as 10 to 15 mm Hg.
      2) Elevation of CSF pulse pressure in patients with mildly increased ICP can be a useful sign of reduced intracranial compliance, indicating that the patient is on a "steep" portion of the ICP–volume curve, and is at risk for sudden elevations of ICP with minor increases in intracranial volume.
      3) In conditions of reduced intracranial compliance and/or inadequate CPP, pathologic CSF pressure waves may occur.
      4) Normally there are three pulse waves seen on ICP tracing:
         a) They are reflections of cardiac systole (P1), diastole (P2), and emptying of the cerebral vessels (P3).
         b) There are normal fluctuations that occur in the ICP with each respiratory cycle.
         c) Two types of pathologic ICP waves have been described. The most important pressure changes are the Lundberg A waves, also called plateau waves, which can occur suddenly, reach levels of 20 to 80 mm Hg, and last from minutes to hours. Lundberg B waves are of lesser amplitude (5–20 mm Hg) and are less dangerous. Clinically, they are a useful marker of inadequate CPP and reduced intracranial compliance, and may be harbingers of plateau waves.

Indications for Intracranial Pressure Monitoring

1. Monitoring of ICP can be an important tool in selected patients. Indications for ICP monitoring, as well as specific types of monitors, vary.
2. In general, patients who should be considered for ICP monitoring are those with primary neurologic disorders, such as stroke or traumatic brain injury, who are not

moribund and who are at significant risk for secondary brain injury due to elevated ICP and decreased CPP:
   a. Severe traumatic brain injury resulting in coma (GCS score of 8 or less).
   b. Large tissue shifts from supratentorial ischemic or hemorrhagic stroke resulting in decreased consciousness.
   c. Hydrocephalus from subarachnoid hemorrhage, intraventricular hemorrhage, or posterior fossa stroke.
   d. Fulminant hepatic failure, in which elevated ICP may be treated with barbiturates or, eventually, liver transplantation.
3. In general, ventriculostomy is preferable to ICP monitoring devices that are placed in brain parenchyma, because ventriculostomy allows CSF drainage as a method of treating elevated ICP.
4. Parenchymal ICP monitoring is most appropriate for patients with diffuse edema and small ventricles (which may make ventriculostomy placement more difficult) or any degree of coagulopathy (in which ventriculostomy carries a higher risk of hemorrhagic complications).

Management of Elevated Intracranial Pressure

1. General measures
   a. Head position elevated 15 to 30 degrees and in a neutral position to avoid jugular compression
   b. Avoid hypotonic fluids
   c. Intubation only to protect airway
   d. Glucose management
   e. Agitation, fever, and seizures should be treated
   f. Blood pressure management to maintain CPP
   g. Neurosurgical consultation
2. Stepwise approach
   a. General measures as noted above.
   b. Insert ICP monitor—ventriculostomy versus parenchymal device.
   c. General goals: maintain ICP below 20 mm Hg and CPP above 70 mm Hg.
      1) For ICP above 20 to 25 mm Hg for longer than 5 minutes.
   d. Drain CSF via ventriculostomy (if in place)
   e. Elevate head of the bed
   f. Osmotherapy: mannitol 25 to 100 g every 4 hours as needed (maintain serum osmolality below 320 mOsm/L).
   g. Glucocorticoids: dexamethasone 4 mg every 6 hours for vasogenic edema from tumor, abscess (avoid glucocorticoids in head trauma, ischemic and hemorrhagic stroke)
   h. Sedation (e.g., morphine, propofol, or midazolam); add neuromuscular paralysis if necessary (patient will require endotracheal intubation and mechanical ventilation at this point, if not before)
   i. Hyperventilation: to $Paco_2$ 30 to 35 mm Hg
   j. Pressor therapy: phenylephrine, dopamine, or norepinephrine to maintain adequate MAP to ensure CPP above 70 mm Hg (maintain euvolemia to minimize deleterious systemic effects of pressors)
   k. Consider second-tier therapies for refractory elevated ICP
      1) High-dose barbiturate therapy ("pentobarb coma")
      2) Aggressive hyperventilation to $Paco_2$ below 30 mm Hg
      3) Hemicraniectomy
3. Throughout ICP treatment, consider repeated head CT to identify mass lesions amenable to surgical evacuation.

BIBLIOGRAPHY

A definition of irreversible coma: report of the Ad Hoc Committee of the Harvard Medical School to Examine the Definition of Brain Death. *JAMA* 1968;205:337–340.

American Academy of Pediatrics Task Force on Brain Death in Children. Report of special task force: guidelines for the determination of brain death in children. *Pediatrics* 1987;80:298–300.

American Electroencephalographic Society. Guideline III: minimum technical standards for EEG recording in suspected cerebral death. *J Clin Neurophysiol* 1994;11:10–13.

Benxel EC, Tator CH. *Contemporary management of spinal cord injury (neurosurgical topics).* Park Ridge: American Association of Neurological Surgeons; 1995.

Benzel EC. Management of acute spinal cord injury. In: Wilkins RH, Rengachary SS, eds. *Neurosurgery.* Vol. 2. New York: McGraw-Hill, 1996:2861–2865.

Bracken MB, Shepard MJ, Collins WF, et al. A randomized, controlled trial of methylprednisolone or naloxone in the treatment acute spinal-cord injury: results of the second national acute spinal cord injury study. *N Engl J Med* 1990;322:1405–1411.

Bracken MB, Shepard MJ, Holford TR, et al. Administration of methylprednisolone for 24 or 48 hours or tirilazad mesylate for 48 hours in the treatment of acute spinal cord injury: results of the third national acute spinal cord injury randomized control trial. *JAMA* 1997;277:1597–1604.

Buettner U, Zee DS. Vestibular testing in comatose patients. *Arch Neurol* 1989;46:561–563.

Coplin WM. Intracranial pressure and surgical decompression for traumatic brain injury: biological rationale and protocol for a randomized clinical trial. *Neurol Res* 2001;23:277–290.

Fehlings MG, Tator CH. An evidence-based review of decompressive surgery in acute spinal cord injury: rationale, indications, and timing based on experimental and clinical studies. *J Neurosurg* 1999;91:1–18.

Fisher C. The neurological examination of the comatose patient. *Acta Neurologica* 1969;25 (suppl 36):1–56.

Geisler FH, Dorsey FC, Coleman WP. Recovery of motor function after spinal-cord injury: a randomized placebo controlled trial with GM-1 ganglioside. *N Engl J Med* 1991;324:1829–1838.

Hadley MN. Injuries to the cervical spine. In: Rengachary SS, Wilkins RH, eds. *Principles of neurosurgery.* London: Mosby Wolfe, 1994:20.2–20.13.

Hanna JP, Frank JI. Automatic stepping in the pontomedullary stage of central herniation. *Neurology* 1995;45:985–986.

Keane J. Blindness following tentorial herniation. *Ann Neurol* 1980;8:186–190.

Lannoo E, Van Rietvelde F, Colardyn F, et al. Early predictors of mortality and morbidity after severe closed head injury. *J Neurotrauma* 2000;17:403–414.

Levy D, Plum F. Outcome prediction in comatose patients: significance of reflex eye movement analysis. *J Neurol Neurosurg Psychiatry* 1988;51:318.

Lubillo S, Bolanos J, Carreira L, et al. Prognostic value of early computerized tomography scanning following craniotomy for traumatic hematoma. *J Neurosurg* 1999;91:581–587.

Mollaret P, Goulon M. Le coma dépassé (mémoire préliminaire). *Rev Neurol (Paris)* 1959;101:3–5.

Pessin M, Adelman LS, Prager RJ, et al. "Wrong-way eyes" in supratentorial hemorrhage. *Ann Neurol* 1981;9:79–81.

Petty GW, Mohr JP, Pedley TA, et al. The role of transcranial Doppler in confirming brain death: sensitivity, specificity, and suggestions for performance and interpretation. *Neurology* 1990;40:300–303.

Prat R, Calatayud-Maldonado V. Prognostic factors in posttraumatic severe diffuse brain injury. *Acta Neurochir (Wien)* 1998;140:1257–1260.

President's Commission for the Study of Ethical Problems in Medicine and Biomedical and Behavioral Research. *Defining death: a report on the medical, legal and ethical issues in the determination of death.* Washington, DC: Government Printing Office, 1981.

Qureshi AI, Geocadin RG, Suarez JI, et al. Long-term outcome after medical reversal of transtentorial herniation in patients with supratentorial mass lesions. *Crit Care Med* 2000;28:1556–1564.

Ropper AH, Kennedy SK, Russell L. Apnea testing in the diagnosis of brain death: clinical and physiological observations. *J Neurosurg* 1981;55:942–946.

Ropper AH. Unusual spontaneous movements in brain-dead patients. *Neurology* 1984;34:1089–1092.

The Brain Trauma Foundation. The American Association of Neurological Surgeons. The Joint Section on Neurotrauma and Critical Care. Guidelines for the management of severe head injury. *J Neurotrauma* 2000;17:507–511.

The Quality Standards Subcommittee of the American Academy of Neurology. Practice parameters for determining brain death in adults (summary statement). *Neurology* 1995;45:1012–1014.

Thurman DJ, Alverson C, Dunn KA, et al. Traumatic brain injury in the United States: a public health perspective. *J Head Trauma Rehabil* 1999;14:602–615.

Uniform Determination of Death Act, 12 Uniform Laws Annotated (U.L.A.) 589 (West 1993 and West Supp. 1997).

Walsh JC, Zhuang J, Shackford SR. A comparison of hypertonic to isotonic fluid in the resuscitation of brain injury and hemorrhagic shock. *J Surg Res.* 1991;50:284–294.

Wijdicks EF. Determining brain death in adults. *Neurology* 1995;45:1003–1011.

Wijdicks EF. The diagnosis of brain death. *N Engl J Med* 2001;344:1215–1221.

Wijdicks EFM, ed. *Brain death.* Philadelphia: Lippincott Williams & Wilkins, 2001.

2. EPILEPSY

Edward B. Bromfield

EPILEPSY

BACKGROUND

History

1. From Greek word *epilepsia:* a taking hold of or seizing.
2. Ancient accounts from more than 2,500 years ago by Babylonians and Egyptians. Most detailed early description, including minor as well as major seizures: On the Sacred Disease, attributed to Hippocrates, fifth century B.C. Use of "sacred" possibly ironic, as Hippocrates is regarded as wishing to replace the earlier, supernatural explanations of epilepsy with a natural one dependent on brain function.
3. Late 19th century:
   a. H. Jackson: Model of focal seizure beginning as aura and evolving to psychomotor or convulsive seizure, and use of aura symptoms to localize seizure onset within gray matter of the brain.
   b. W. Gowers: Detailed descriptions of epileptic syndromes and related disorders; concept that "seizures beget seizures."
4. Mid 20th century:
   a. H. Berger, W.G. Walter, W. Lennox: Ability to record human electroencephalogram (EEG) from scalp and correlate with epilepsy.
   b. W. Penfield, H. Jasper: Surgical resection facilitated by identification of epileptic focus on the basis of clinical manifestations and electrocorticography (EEG recorded from the brain surface) and identification of functional cortical regions by cortical electrical stimulation.
   c. H. Merritt, T. Putnam: Identification of phenytoin as an antiepileptic drug using an animal seizure model.
   d. H. Gastaut: Advances in syndromic classification and applicability to treatment.
5. Late 20th century:
   a. Widespread use of simultaneous video–EEG recording, allowing accurate correlations of EEG and behavior.
   b. Neuroimaging revolution, allowing visualization of lesions responsible for seizure generation, facilitating surgical treatment of epilepsy.
   c. Development of new antiepileptic drugs by screening and by rational synthesis based on knowledge of seizure mechanisms.

Definitions

1. Seizure: The clinical manifestation of an abnormal, excessive, and hypersynchronous discharge of a population of cortical neurons.
2. Epilepsy: A disorder of the central nervous system (CNS) characterized by recurrent seizures unprovoked by systemic or neurologic insults.
3. Epileptic syndrome: A particular form of epilepsy, often implying specific causes, clinical manifestations, and prognosis.
4. Aura: The earliest part of a seizure, and typically the only part recalled by the patient after consciousness is lost.
5. Postictal period: Time between the end of the seizure and recovery to the baseline state.

6. Status epilepticus: 30 or more minutes of continuous or recurrent seizures without recovery to baseline function.
7. Antiepileptic drug (AED; also termed "anticonvulsant"): a medication given to prevent or suppress seizures.
8. Acute symptomatic seizure: A seizure that results directly from an acute neurologic or systemic insult.

Classification

Seizure Types

The fundamental distinction among seizure types is between partial (also termed "focal") seizures—those that are known or presumed to start in a specifiable lobe and/or hemisphere of the brain—and generalized seizures—those starting simultaneously throughout the entire cortex, or at least in widespread areas of both hemispheres. Following is a simplified version of the 1981 seizure classification system of the International League against Epilepsy (ILAE):

1. Partial seizures (seizures beginning locally)
   a. Simple partial seizures: Consciousness not impaired; all but those with motor manifestations are completely subjective. Usual duration 5 to 30 seconds; EEG pattern—focal or unilateral rhythmic discharge.
      1) Motor (localized tonic or dystonic posturing or clonic jerking)
      2) Somatosensory or special sensory (e.g., localized tingling, flashing lights, unpleasant odor)
      3) Autonomic (e.g., rising epigastric sensation)
      4) Psychic–cognitive (e.g., déjàvu, unprecipitated fear)
   b. Complex partial seizures: Consciousness impaired or lost; frequently include repetitive, automatic-appearing movements, termed "automatisms" (source of the previous term "psychomotor seizures"). Usual duration 30 to 180 seconds; EEG pattern—typically bilateral rhythmic discharge but often with an identifiable focal or unilateral onset.
      1) Beginning as simple partial seizures (see section 1.a. above)
      2) With impairment of consciousness at onset
   c. Partial seizures secondarily generalized: Partial seizure progressing to complete loss of consciousness accompanied by bilateral tonic posturing followed by clonic contractions; the latter tend to gradually slow before stopping. Usual duration 50 to 120 seconds following initial partial seizure; EEG pattern—focal or bilateral rhythmic discharge prior to generalization, then widespread polyspikes typically obscured by muscle artifact from onset of tonic phase, evolving into bursts of polyspikes and muscle artifact as clonic jerks appear.
2. Generalized seizures (bilaterally symmetric and without local onset)
   a. Typical absence (petit mal): Arrest of activity with staring and minor motor activity if any (e.g., blinking); usual duration, 5 to 10 seconds, rarely up to 30 seconds, longer absences may be accompanied by automatisms; EEG pattern of 3 Hz (rarely up to 6 Hz) generalized spike–wave complexes.
   b. Atypical absence: Compared with typical absence, often less complete but longer and more gradual behavioral arrest and recovery; EEG pattern of slow (1.5–2.5 Hz) spike–wave complexes.
   c. Myoclonic: Brief, shock-like jerking of muscles on both sides of body; duration, less than 1 second; EEG pattern of generalized polyspike–wave complex.
   d. Clonic: Series of myoclonic jerks; duration variable; EEG pattern of repeated myoclonic jerks.
   e. Tonic: Stiffening or contraction in a fixed posture, often with abduction of the shoulders and partial flexion of the elbows; usual duration 10 to 20 seconds, but often cluster; EEG pattern of rapid, diffuse polyspikes, often following a slow wave.
   f. Tonic–clonic (grand mal, convulsion): Stereotyped sequence of bilateral stiffening followed by clonic contractions; usual duration, 50 to 120 seconds; EEG pattern of low-amplitude polyspikes increasing in amplitude until obscured by muscle artifact, then in bursts corresponding to clonic jerks.

g. Atonic: Sudden loss of postural tone, usually with altered awareness; duration, 5 to 30 seconds; EEG pattern of rapid, low-voltage spikes following a slow wave, or slow-spike/polyspike–wave complexes.
3. *Unclassified* epileptic seizures (inadequate or incomplete data)

Epilepsy Syndromes

1. Epilepsy syndromes are classified along two dimensions. The first concerns whether the characteristic seizure types are partial or generalized, as discussed earlier (see Seizure Types, sections 1 and 2), and the second concerns the underlying cause of the epilepsy.
2. The cause is termed "idiopathic" if there is normal neurologic function apart from seizures, typically implying a genetic predisposition toward seizures; it is termed "symptomatic" if the seizure tendency results from another condition (e.g., brain injury, cortical malformation, or inborn error of metabolism).
3. Cryptogenic syndromes are presumed to be symptomatic, but the cause cannot be identified in an individual patient.
4. Several of the epilepsy syndromes listed in Table 2-1, in a modified version of the 1989 ILAE classification, are discussed at greater length at the end of this chapter.

Epidemiology

1. Seizure: 9% to 10% cumulative incidence (3%–4% febrile, 3% other acute symptomatic, 2%–3% epileptic)
2. Epilepsy: Incidence 30 to 50/100,000, cumulative incidence 2% to 3% by age 75, prevalence 0.5% to 0.8%
3. Bimodal peak incidence for seizures and epilepsy: Highest in first year of life and increasing after age 60

TABLE 2-1. MODIFIED INTERNATIONAL LEAGUE AGAINST EPILEPSY CLASSIFICATION OF EPILEPSY SYNDROMES

Localization related (partial, focal) epilepsies
  1. Idiopathic:
      Benign childhood epilepsy with centrotemporal spikes
      Childhood epilepsy with occipital paroxysms
  2. Symptomatic:
      Chronic progressive epilepsia partialis continua of childhood
      ("Rasmussen encephalitis")
  3. Symptomatic or cryptogenic:
      Temporal, frontal, parietal or occipital epilepsies

Generalized epilepsies
  1. Idiopathic:
      Benign neonatal familial convulsions
      Benign myoclonic epilepsy in childhood
      Childhood absence epilepsy
      Juvenile absence epilepsy
      Juvenile myoclonic epilepsy
  2. Cryptogenic or symptomatic epilepsies:
      West syndrome (infantile spasms)
      Lennox–Gastaut syndrome

Situation-related syndromes
  Febrile convulsions
  Alcohol/drug-related
  Eclampsia
  Epilepsy with specific modes of presentation (reflex epilepsies)

PATHOPHYSIOLOGY

The hypersynchronous neuronal discharge that characterizes a seizure is mediated by an imbalance between excitation and inhibition. Genetic epilepsies are likely to affect the structure and function of neurotransmitter receptors and their associated ion channels. The mechanisms by which cortical injuries produce epilepsy are unknown, but probably are related to alterations in function and connectivity of excitatory and inhibitory neurons at the margins of the injury.

Physiologic Mechanisms

1. Cellular: Alterations in distribution or function of ion channels, or in neurotransmitter synthesis, metabolism, or uptake.
2. Extracellular: Alterations in ionic environment (partially mediated by glial cells) or synaptic structure.
3. Network: Alterations in synaptic organization; alterations in number or function of inhibitory or excitatory neuronal populations. There is evidence that absence seizures result from aberration in the thalamocortical network that underlies sleep spindle generation.

Molecular Mechanisms

1. Main inhibitory neurotransmitter: γ-aminobutyric acid (GABA), which is a complex class of receptors linked to chloride channel, entry of which hyperpolarizes neurons.
2. Main excitatory transmitter: Glutamate, which has complex inotropic receptors often divided into three groups on the basis of experimental agonists [N-methyl D-aspartate (NMDA), AMPA, kainic acid]; also acts on metabotropic receptors affecting intracellular processes more slowly via G-proteins.

Genetics

1. Hypothesis: There are a collection of genes, coding mainly for neurotransmitter receptors and their associated ion channels, that determines the "seizure threshold" for a given individual.
2. Rare familial syndromes show mendelian inheritance of a critical receptor or channel mutation (e.g., autosomal dominant nocturnal frontal lobe epilepsy and the nicotinic acetylcholine receptor).
3. Common epilepsy syndromes (childhood absence or juvenile myoclonic epilepsy), likely to be oligogenic.
4. Inborn errors of metabolism or brain development may also be mendelian (tuberous sclerosis, lissencephaly syndromes).

PROGNOSIS

Natural History

1. Single unprovoked seizure: 23% to 71% 2-year recurrence rate. Risk factors include positive family history or abnormal examination, imaging, or EEG findings.
2. Recurrence 73% after second seizure; therefore two unprovoked seizures are assumed to represent epilepsy.
3. Many childhood-onset syndromes typically remit spontaneously (benign childhood epilepsy with centrotemporal spikes, childhood absence epilepsy).
4. Adolescence-onset idiopathic syndromes (e.g., juvenile myoclonic epilepsy) or symptomatic/cryptogenic cases are less likely to remit.
5. Although most cases that respond early to medical treatment remit, there is no evidence that early treatment alters the natural history.

Response to Medical Treatment

1. Approximately half (58% if idiopathic, 44% if symptomatic or cryptogenic) of all new cases respond to the first well-tolerated drug administered.
2. Patients who continue to have seizures despite adequate treatment with one appropriate drug have only a 10% to 20% chance of complete response to subsequent trials, although many can have worthwhile improvement.

Response to Nonmedical Treatment

1. Ketogenic diet
   a. A high-fat diet that produces metabolic changes mimicking starvation can produce complete or dramatic seizure reductions in 30% to 50% of children with multiple seizure types (usually cryptogenic or symptomatic generalized epilepsy syndromes).
   b. Short-term risks include weight loss, renal stones, acidosis, hemolytic anemia, lethargy, and elevated liver function tests; treatment is usually initiated in the hospital and maintained with the assistance of a dietitian.
   c. Much less information is available concerning feasibility, effectiveness, and long-term safety in adults.
2. Resective surgery
   a. Among medically refractory patients with localization-related epilepsy, a significant number, perhaps 100,000 in the United States, are candidates for resection of the epileptic focus.
   b. In appropriately selected candidates, seizure-free rates range from 60% to 80%. The best prognosis is for those with structural lesions, including especially mesial temporal sclerosis.
3. Palliative procedures
   a. For those who are not candidates for resective surgery, several procedures have been shown to produce worthwhile benefit in many patients, although complete seizure remission in only a few.
   b. These procedures include disconnection procedures such as corpus callosotomy (section of the major interhemispheric commissures, often the anterior two thirds of the corpus callosum), multiple subpial transections (shallow longitudinal cuts presumed to sever cortical–cortical connections while leaving intact the descending projection fibers needed to preserve function), or insertion of the vagus nerve stimulator (VNS).
   c. The VNS, which delivers controllable stimulations at programmable intervals to the left vagus nerve, produces a 50% decrease in seizure frequency among 25% to 45% of patients implanted. Approval is for patients 12 years of age or older with partial seizures, but younger patients and those with generalized epilepsies may respond as well or better.
4. Complementary and alternative therapies: Such activities as relaxation techniques, yoga, or exercise are under investigation, as are some herbal medicines and dietary supplements. While some of these may prove beneficial, and relaxation and related techniques appear safe, caution must be exercised, particularly with herbal preparations, since some have potentially harmful effects (including lowering the seizure threshold) or may interact with AEDs.

Medication Withdrawal

1. In general, patients who have had no seizures for at least 2 years can be considered for medication withdrawal, acknowledging a seizure recurrence risk of 20% to 40%.
2. Those who had only one seizure type that responded promptly and was controlled for many years on modest doses of one medication have the best prognosis, especially if they have normal neurologic examinations, imaging studies, and EEG. Depending on lifestyle, however, this recurrence risk may be unacceptable, and many elect to remain on medications.

3. For patients whose epilepsy can be classified into a specific syndrome, such as benign epilepsy with centrotemporal spikes or juvenile myoclonic epilepsy, the syndrome itself may imply a lower or higher recurrence risk than the overall statistics quoted in section 2 above.

DIAGNOSIS

Differential Diagnosis

1. Transient events that can mimic partial or generalized seizures include:
   a. Syncope (especially convulsive syncope)
   b. Migraine (especially migraine with aura or basilar migraine)
   c. Transient ischemic attack (TIA) (carotid or vertebrobasilar, particularly the uncommon carotid syndrome of "limb-shaking" TIA)
   d. Movement disorder (tremor, nonepileptic myoclonus, dyskinesia)
   e. Sleep disorder (especially narcolepsy–cataplexy syndrome, somnambulism)
   f. Toxic–metabolic disturbance (distinct from disturbances that can cause seizures)
   g. Psychiatric disorder (dissociative states, psychogenic nonepileptic seizures or pseudoseizures)

Evaluation

1. History: Recent or remote serious brain injury or illness; sleep deprivation or fever; presence, nature, and duration of warning, and whether either the entire event or the warning alone was ever experienced before; witness account including level of responsiveness, motor manifestations, duration of event and recovery; patient and witness assessment of functioning afterward, particularly focal symptoms, incontinence, mouth/tongue biting.
2. Physical examination: Mental status, focal features, signs of infection.
3. Laboratory studies: Electrolytes, calcium, magnesium, glucose, renal and liver function tests, toxic screen, and complete blood count (CBC).
4. Ancillary tests: Neuroimaging [magnetic resonance imaging (MRI) preferred to computed tomography (CT)], EEG (as soon as available), lumbar puncture if infection suspected.

TREATMENT

Antiepileptic Drugs

1. Principles of use:
   a. Differences among drugs in efficacy are less than differences in pharmacokinetics, interactions, likely adverse effects, and cost.
   b. There are several options for nearly every clinical situation.
   c. Unless a rapid therapeutic effect is essential, choose a low starting dose and slow titration rate. This is especially true when treating elderly or ill patients.
   d. In general, increase the dose until an adequate observation period establishes that seizures are controlled or until dose-related side effects develop; in the latter case, decrease back to the previous dose and monitor response. If seizures are not controlled, another appropriate AED should be initiated and titrated up as the patient is weaned off the first drug.
   e. Rarely, increases in dose may result in worsening of seizures. The dose should be reduced and the drug will likely need to be replaced by an alternative AED.
   f. For both ethical and logistic reasons, new AEDs are invariably tested as adjunctive therapy in adults with medically intractable partial seizures. Evidence of effectiveness in other settings is generally based on smaller studies that may or may not be well controlled, and leads to subsequent Food and Drug Administration (FDA) approval for other uses only in a minority of cases.

Therefore, off-label use is justifiable if approved AEDs are not successful or risk with the off-label alternative appears lower than that with the approved AED.

g. The most common drug interactions involving AEDs are based on induction, or, less commonly, inhibition, of the hepatic mixed-function oxidase or P450 enzyme system. As a group, the older AEDs have much stronger effects on this system than the newer drugs, although several of the latter are substrates whose metabolism is affected by addition or withdrawal of the older drugs.

h. Serum drug concentrations ("drug levels") can be useful in verifying compliance, or in providing an initial target for patients with infrequent seizures, but if used mechanically as a guide to dosing can hinder rather than help in achieving the goal of treatment: no seizures and no side effects (and ultimately, optimizing quality of life). Even for the older AEDs, published therapeutic ranges have limited scientific support, and individuals may have therapeutic responses or adverse effects either below or above this range. For the newer AEDs, therapeutic ranges are even more provisional, but are included in the following discussions for completeness.

2. Use of specific AEDs: AEDs may be categorized in several ways. Mechanistic classifications are logical but of limited clinical relevance in that several drugs work by more than one mechanism and, for many drugs, mechanisms are unknown or poorly understood. Perhaps the most useful classification concerns spectrum of action:

a. The first group of AEDs includes those that are effective against partial seizures, including simple and complex partial as well as secondarily generalized seizures. Most if not all of these also prevent primarily generalized tonic–clonic seizures; however, they are not effective against, and may worsen, other generalized seizure types, including absence and myoclonic seizures. Drugs in this class include carbamazepine (CBZ), phenytoin (PHT), phenobarbital (PHB), primidone (PRM), gabapentin (GBP), oxcarbazepine (OXC), and tiagabine (TGB).

b. The second group includes those that can be viewed as "broad-spectrum" AEDS, with activity against a variety of generalized and partial seizures. The traditional drug with this characteristic is valproate (VPA). There is evidence supporting a similar broad spectrum for the newer drugs lamotrigine (LTG), topiramate (TPM), levetiracetam (LEV), zonisamide (ZNS), felbamate (FBM), and the older drug methsuximide (MSX).

c. The third group includes drugs that do not easily fit in the above categories, including ethosuximide (ESX), a narrow-spectrum AED with established efficacy against only typical generalized absence seizures. (Interestingly, the closely related drug MSX, as noted, has a broader spectrum and is effective against partial seizures as well.) There are other, less commonly used adjunctive drugs that have different medical uses, such as acetazolamide (ACZ) and perhaps allopurinol. Finally, there are medications used in specific situations, including seizure clusters and status epilepticus, alcohol and other drug-related seizures, and specific pediatric syndromes, such infantile spasms. These include intravenous (IV), sublingual, and rectal benzodiazepines, anesthetic agents, adrenocorticotropic hormone (ACTH), and pyridoxine.

Drugs for Partial and Tonic–Clonic Seizures

Carbamazepine

1. Advantages: Considered a first-choice drug for partial and tonic–clonic seizures; familiarity; slow-release preparations allow twice a day (b.i.d.) dosing.
2. Disadvantages: Need to titrate slowly to avoid dose-related adverse effects, pharmacokinetic interactions (P450 enzyme inducer and substrate).
3. Major adverse effects:
   a. Dose related: dizziness, diplopia, nausea, sedation, mild leukopenia, hyponatremia, bradyarrhythmias (elderly)
   b. Idiosyncratic: rash [including Stevens–Johnson syndrome (SJS)], agranulocytosis, hepatic failure, pancreatitis, lupus-like syndrome
   c. Chronic: osteopenia (possibly preventable with vitamin D and calcium supplementation)

4. Teratogenicity: yes, including 0.5% to 1% neural tube defects (unclear whether extra folate prevents).
5. Initiation and titration: 100 to 200 mg at night (hs) or 100 mg b.i.d.; increase after 3 to 7 days to 200 b.i.d. Can check blood tests after 1 week on this dose: CBZ level, CBC/differential, electrolytes (Na), and perhaps albumin and aspartate aminotransferase (AST) levels. Dose should be increased at 3- to 7-day intervals to obtain a level of 4 to 12 mg/L; level should be rechecked in 4 to 6 weeks, as autoinduction may necessitate further increases. Usual maintenance doses in adults are as follows: 600 to 1,600 mg/d, up to 2,400 mg/d. In children, start at 5 to 10 mg/kg/d, maintenance 15 to 20 mg/kg/d, up to 30 mg/kg/d.
6. Pharmacokinetics: Half-life: 12 to 20 hours (shorter with enzyme-inducing drugs; autoinduction also occurs, with level falling after 2 to 6 weeks on stable dose), protein binding: 70% to 80%.
7. Usual therapeutic range: 4 to 12 mg/L
8. Preparations: Tegretol tablets 100 and 200 mg, generic 200 mg tablets, suspension 100 mg/5 mL (can solidify in tube feedings), generic 200 mg; slow-release preparations including Tegretol-XR 100-, 200-, and 400-mg caplets, and Carbatrol 200- and 300-mg capsules.

Oxcarbazepine

1. Advantages: More rapid titration than CBZ, b.i.d. dosing, minor interactions, no known hepatic or hematologic adverse effects; approved as initial monotherapy for partial seizures.
2. Disadvantages: Dose-related effects similar to those of CBZ; although only weak P450 inducer, can lower hormone (e.g., contraceptive) levels
3. Comment: Very similar chemically to CBZ but not converted to epoxide metabolite, which is thought to account for many adverse effects of CBZ
4. Major adverse effects:
   a. Dose-related: dizziness, diplopia, hyponatremia, somnolence, ataxia, gastrointestinal (GI) upset
   b. Idiosyncratic: rash (25% cross-reactivity with CBZ)
   c. Chronic: none known
5. Teratogenicity: unknown (lack of epoxide metabolite may suggest favorable relative to CBZ)
6. Initiation and titration: adults: 150 to 300 mg b.i.d., increasing by 300 to 600 mg every 1 to 2 weeks to target of 1,200 to 2,400 mg/d; children (older than 4 years): 8 to 10 mg/kg/d titrated to 20 to 40 mg/kg/d. Note: conversion from CBZ can be rapid, over 1 day to 2 weeks, at a ratio of 300 mg OXC to 200 mg CBZ.
7. Pharmacokinetics: Half-life 2 hours but converted to active monohydroxy-derivative (MHD), with half-life of 8 to 10 hours; protein binding 40%
8. Therapeutic range: 10 to 35 mg/L (MHD)
9. Preparations: Trileptal tablets 150, 300, 600 mg; syrup 300 mg/5 mL.

Phenytoin

1. Advantages: Arguably still a first-choice drug for partial and tonic–clonic seizures, although used much less in Europe than in United States; familiarity; long duration of action, especially with slow-release preparations—usually b.i.d. dosing, but can be daily (qd); parenteral loading options. May be effective against generalized tonic as well as tonic–clonic seizures, although not against absence or myoclonic seizures.
2. Disadvantages: Zero-order kinetics; pharmacokinetic interactions (strong P450 inducer); chronic cosmetic and other adverse effects
3. Major adverse effects:
   a. Dose related: dizziness, ataxia, diplopia, nausea
   b. Idiosyncratic: rash, including SJS; blood dyscrasias; hepatic failure; lupus-like syndrome
   c. Chronic: gingival hyperplasia, hirsutism, osteopenia, pseudolymphoma, ?lymphoma, ?cerebellar degeneration

4. Teratogenicity: yes
5. Initiation and titration: Adults: In nonemergent situations, can load orally; two doses of 500 mg or three doses of 300 mg can be taken 4 to 6 hours apart. Parenteral loading can be achieved IV (15 mg/kg, or 20 mg/kg for status epilepticus, not more than 50 mg/min; precursor drug fosphenytoin may be preferable for status). When loading is not needed, can initiate estimated maintenance dose of 300 to 400 mg/d, usually in two doses, checking levels in 1 to 2 weeks. Because of zero-order kinetics, increases must be proportionately less as the level rises; for example, if the steady-state level on 300 mg/d is 12mg/L, then 330 mg/d, a 10% dose increase, may be sufficient to raise the level to 18, a 50% increase. Pediatrics: 4 to 5 mg/kg/d, up to 8 mg/kg or more depending on level.
6. Pharmacokinetics: Half-life is level-dependent, 20 to 30 hours when in usual therapeutic range; protein binding: 90% (lower with renal failure or hypoalbuminemia).
7. Usual therapeutic range: 10 to 20 mg/L (arguably 5–25 mg/L)
8. Preparations: Dilantin tablets 50 mg, Dilantin and generic extended-release capsules 30 and 100 mg, and suspension 125 mg/5 mL (must be adequately mixed in bottle); Phenytek capsules 200 and 300 mg

Gabapentin
1. Advantages: Rapid titration, relatively well tolerated, no pharmacokinetic interactions, additional uses (neuropathic pain)
2. Disadvantages: Three or four times daily (t.i.d. and q.i.d., respectively) dosing recommended (although it can be given b.i.d.); perceived as less efficacious than other AEDs, although data are conflicting
3. Major adverse effects:
   a. Dose-related: sedation, dizziness, ataxia
   b. Idiosyncratic: weight gain, rash (rare), behavioral changes in children, myoclonus
   c. Chronic: none known
4. Teratogenicity: unknown
5. Initiation and titration—300 mg hs, increasing by 300 mg every 1 to 7 days to target of 1,800 to 3,600 mg/d; in elderly, 100 mg hs or b.i.d., increasing in 100- to 200-mg increments; pediatrics (older than 3 years): 10 to 20 mg/kg/d increasing to target of 30 to 60 mg/d.
6. Pharmacokinetics—Half-life: 5 to 7 hours (but brain kinetics likely slower); protein binding: none
7. Provisional therapeutic range: 4 to 16 mg/L
8. Preparations: Neurontin capsules 100, 300, 400 mg; tablets 600 and 800 mg; solution 250 mg/5 mL

Tiagabine
1. Advantages: May have antianxiety or analgesic effects; can sometimes be given b.i.d.
2. Disadvantages: Sedating; risk of nonconvulsive status epilepticus; P450 substrate
3. Major adverse effects:
   a. Dose-related—dizziness, somnolence, nausea, cognitive slowing
   b. Idiosyncratic—rash; mood changes; generalized nonconvulsive status epilepticus (doses 48 mg/d or greater)
   c. Chronic—unknown
4. Teratogenicity—unknown
5. Initiation and titration—2 to 8 mg/d, increasing by 2 to 8 mg/d at weekly intervals to target of 24 to 56 mg/d in two to four doses; pediatrics (older than 12 years): 4 mg/d, increasing by 4 mg/wk to target of 20 to 32 mg/d
6. Pharmacokinetics—Half-life: 4 to 9 hours, protein binding: 96%
7. Provisional therapeutic range: 0.1 to 0.3 mg/L
8. Preparations: Gabitril filmtabs 2, 4, 12, 16, 20 mg

Phenobarbital

1. Advantages—long half-life (daily dosing), inexpensive
2. Disadvantages—cognitive and behavioral side effects, interactions (P450 inducer)
3. Major adverse effects:
    a. Dose-related: sedation, depression, cognitive impairment
    b. Idiosyncratic: rash, hyperactivity (children), hepatic failure (rare), aplastic anemia (rare)
    c. Chronic: osteoporosis, connective tissue disorders (e.g., frozen shoulder)
4. Teratogenicity—yes
5. Initiation and titration—90 to 250 mg/d, can load IV with up to 20 mg/kg (less than 100 mg/h for status epilepticus), but sedation is universal; check steady-state levels in 2 to 3 weeks (4–5 weeks in presence of VPA); pediatrics: 2 to 7 mg/kg/d
6. Pharmacokinetics—half-life: 72 to 168 hours (less in children, more when coadministered with VPA)
7. Usual therapeutic range: 10 to 40 mg/L
8. Preparations: tablets 15, 30, 60 (or 62.5), 100 mg; suspension 15 or 20 mg/5 mL; parenteral 30, 60, 130 mg/mL.

Primidone

1. Advantages—parent compound may have efficacy beyond that of PHB metabolite, at least against myoclonic seizures; effective against tremor at low doses
2. Disadvantages—possibly more sedating than PHB alone; must be taken in divided doses, usually t.i.d. or q.i.d.; P450 inducer
3. Comment: metabolized to PHB
4. Major adverse effects:
    a. Dose-related: same as PHB
    b. Idiosyncratic: same as PHB
    c. Chronic: same as PHB
5. Teratogenicity—yes
6. Initiation and titration—100 to 125 mg hs, increasing by 125 to 250 mg every 2 to 7 days to target of 500 to 1,500 mg/d; pediatrics: 50 mg/d increasing to 10 to 25 mg/kg/d
7. Pharmacokinetics—Half-life: 6 to 22 hours (72–168 hours for PHB metabolite); P450 inducers promote conversion to PHB
8. Usual therapeutic range—5 to 12 mg/L (10–40 mg/L for PHB)
9. Preparations: Mysoline and generic tablets 50 and 250 mg; suspension 250 mg/5 mL

Drugs for Generalized Seizures

Including absence and myoclonic. These drugs also are effective against tonic–clonic partial seizures.

Valproate

1. Advantages—familiarity, best-established broad-spectrum AED; concomitant effects on migraine, bipolar illness; slow-release preparations allow b.i.d. or possibly daily dosing.
2. Disadvantages—acute and chronic adverse effects, particularly weight gain; interactions (P450 inhibitor, also competes for protein binding sites)
3. Major adverse effects:
    a. Dose-related—GI upset, anorexia, tremor, thrombocytopenia
    b. Idiosyncratic—pancreatitis (up to one in 200), hepatic failure (especially infants on polytherapy), stupor and coma, depression, rash, hyperammonemia, thrombocytopenia/thrombocytopathy
    c. Chronic—weight gain, hair loss or change in texture; ?polycystic ovarian syndrome
4. Teratogenicity—yes, including 1% to 2% incidence of neural tube defects

5. Initiation and titration—250 mg b.i.d. to t.i.d., increasing by 250 to 500 mg weekly to target of 750 to 2,000 mg/d (higher if also on enzyme-inducing drugs); pediatric: 10 to 15 mg/kg/d, increasing by 5 to 10 mg/kg/wk to 15 to 30 mg/kg/d (maximum, 60 mg/kg/d)

6. Pharmacokinetics—Half-life: 10 to 20 hours; up to 95% protein-bound, less at higher levels; partial P450 inhibitor, elevating particularly PHB and LTG

7. Usual therapeutic range: 50 to 120 mg/L

8. Preparations: Depakene or generic valproic acid capsules 250 mg, syrup 250 mg/5 mL; depakote delayed-release tablets, 125, 250, and 500 mg; depakote sprinkles slow-release capsules, 125 mg; depakote-ER extended-release capsules 250 and 500 mg; Depacon infusion 100 mg/5 mL

Lamotrigine

1. Advantages—broad-spectrum, including Lennox–Gastaut syndrome (LGS); well tolerated, relatively nonsedating; preliminary evidence suggesting safety during pregnancy; approved as monotherapy (for partial seizures) when transitioned from enzyme-inducing AED. b.i.d. dosing

2. Disadvantages—slow titration needed to minimize rash risk; susceptible to enzyme induction

3. Major adverse effects:
   a. Dose-related—dizziness, ataxia, drowsiness (or insomnia)
   b. Idiosyncratic—rash 5–10% (including 0.1% SJS, higher in children), hypersensitivity syndrome
   c. Chronic—none known

4. Teratogenicity—not established (but preliminary evidence is favorable)

5. Initiation and titration—with enzyme-inducing AEDs: 50 mg/d for 2 weeks, then 50 mg b.i.d. for 2 weeks, then increase by 50 to 100 mg weekly to target of 300 to 500 mg/d; with inducing AEDs plus VPA (or for off-label initial monotherapy or added to noninducing AEDs without VPA): 25 mg every other day (q.o.d.) for 2 weeks, then 25 mg daily for 2 weeks, then increase by 25 to 50 mg every 1 to 2 weeks to 100 to 300 mg/d; pediatric (older than 2 years): with enzyme-inducing AEDs, 2 mg/kg/d for 2 weeks, increasing by similar amount to 5 to 15 mg/kg/d; with VPA, 0.1 to 0.2 mg/kg/d for 2 weeks, increasing by 0.5 mg/kg/d to 1 to 5 mg/kg/d.

6. Pharmacokinetics—P450 substrate; half-life approximately 24 hours alone (or combination of inducing drugs and VPA, 15 hours with inducing drugs, 60 hours with VPA and no inducing drugs)

7. Therapeutic range—2 to 20 mg/L

8. Preparations: Lamictal tablets 25, 100, 150, and 200 mg; chewable dispersible tablets 5, 10, and 25 mg

Topiramate

1. Advantages—broad spectrum, including LGS; sometimes effective at low dose; weight loss; b.i.d. dosing

2. Disadvantages—slow titration needed to minimize CNS adverse effects; weight loss; at high dose can interfere with oral contraceptives

3. Major adverse effects:
   a. Dose-related—cognitive slowing, word-finding difficulties, paresthesias, dizziness
   b. Idiosyncratic—rash, GI upset, narrow-angle glaucoma; irritability
   c. Chronic—renal stones (1–2%, less in women), weight loss

4. Teratogenicity—unknown

5. Initiation and titration—25 mg/d, increasing by 25 mg/d per 1–2 wk to 200 mg/d or higher. Pediatric (>): 1–3 mg/kg/d, increasing by similar amount every 1–2 wk to 5–9 mg/kg/d.

6. Pharmacokinetics—renal and hepatic; is susceptible to enzyme induction; may elevate PHT levels slightly

7. Therapeutic range—5–20 mg/L provisionally

8. Preparations—Topamax tablets 25, 100, 200 mg; sprinkles capsules 15, 25 mg

Levetiracetam
1. Advantages—therapeutic starting dose; efficacy, lack of interactions; b.i.d. dosing
2. Disadvantages—irritability and other less common psychobehavioral effects; broad spectrum less well documented
3. Major adverse effects:
   a. Dose-related—sedation, dizziness
   b. Idiosyncratic—GI intolerance, depression, irritability
   c. Chronic—none known
4. Teratogenicity—unknown
5. Initiation and titration—250–500 mg b.i.d., increasing by 500 mg/d every 1–2 wk to target of 1,000–3,000 mg/d. Pediatric (>12): 10–20 mg/kg/d, increasing by 5–10 mg/kg every 1–2 wk to 40 mg/kg/d.
6. Pharmacokinetics—renally excreted; half-life 6–8 hours, but water soluble, suggesting brain kinetics slower
7. Therapeutic range—provisionally 10–40 mg/L
8. Preparations—Keppra tablets 250, 500, 750 mg; suspension 100 mg/5mL

Zonisamide
1. Advantages—broad spectrum, long half-life allowing qd dosing (though b.i.d. recommended).
2. Disadvantages—slow titration, sedation
3. Major adverse effects:
   a. Dose-related—fatigue, confusion, dizziness
   b. Idiosyncratic—rash (can progress to SJS; cross-reacts with sulfa drugs), hypohidrosis
   c. Chronic—renal stones
4. Teratogenicity—unknown
5. Initiation and titration—100 mg/d for 2 wk, then increase by 100 mg every 2 wks to 400 mg/d. Pediatric: 2–4 mg/kg/d, increasing by similar amount every 1–2 wk to 8 mg/kg/d.
6. Pharmacokinetics—P450 substrate; half-life 60 hours, but 25–30 with inducers
7. Therapeutic range: 20–40 mg/L provisionally
8. Preparation: Zonegran100 mg capsule

Methsuximide (MSX)
1. Advantages—broad spectrum, including partial seizures, long-half-life—dosing usually b.i.d. but can be qd.
2. Disadvantages—slow titration; CNS side effects, lack of familiarity to many clinicians
3. Major adverse effects:
   a. Dose-related—sedation, headache
   b. Idiosyncratic—rash (including SJS), psychiatric difficulties, GI upset, lupus-like syndrome, leukopenia
   c. Chronic—none known
4. Teratogenicity—unknown
5. Pharmacokinetics: Half-life of active metabolite, N,N-desmethylmethsuximide 34–80 hours in adults, 16–45 hours in children; level can be lowered by enzyme inducers; may elevate PHT, decrease CBZ
6. Initiation and titration—300 mg qhs for 1–2 wks, increasing by 300 mg every 1–2 wks to target of 900–1200 mg/d. Pediatrics: 150 mg/d increasing by 150 mg/d
7. Therapeutic range: 10–40 mg/L (N,N desmethylmethsuximide)
8. Preparations: Celontin capsules 150 and 300 mg

Felbamate (FBM)
1. Advantages: broad spectrum, including LGS; efficacious, nonsedating; approved as initial monotherapy (for partial seizures). Can be dosed b.i.d., though t.i.d. usually better tolerated.

2. Disadvantages: drug interactions; risk of potentially fatal aplastic anemia (1 in 5000) and hepatic failure (1 in 10,000)
3. Major adverse effects:
   a. Dose-related—anxiety, insomnia, fatigue, ataxia
   b. Idiosyncratic—rash, aplastic anemia, hepatic failure
   c. Chronic—weight loss
4. Teratogenicity: unknown
5. Pharmacokinetics and interactions: Half-life 15–20 hours but shortened by inducers. May act as enzyme inhibitor, elevating PHT, VPA, and PHB; however, reduces CBZ.
6. Initiation and titration: 600 b.i.d., increasing by 600 mg/d weekly to target of 2,400–4,800 mg/d. Pediatrics: 10–15 mg/kg/d, increasing to 20–40 mg/kg/d.
7. Therapeutic range: provisionally 40–100 mg/L.
8. Preparations: Felbatol tablets 400, 400 mg; suspension 600 mg/5 ml.

Drugs with Narrow Spectrum of Action or Use in Specific Situations

Ethosuximide (ESX)
1. Advantages—long half-life—usually b.i.d. dosing; effective against absence seizures
2. Disadvantages—narrow spectrum, absence only well-established target
3. Major adverse effects:
   a. Dose-related—sedation, headache
   b. Idiosyncratic—rash, psychiatric decompensation, GI upset, lupus-like syndrome
   c. Chronic—none known
4. Teratogenicity—not known
5. Initiation and titration—250 mg b.i.d., increasing by 250 mg/d at weekly intervals to 500 to 1,000 mg/d; pediatrics (older than 3 years): 250 mg/d increasing by 250 mg/wk to 15 to 20 mg/kg/d
6. Pharmacokinetics—hepatic metabolism, no protein binding; half-life 30 to 60 hours
7. Therapeutic range—40 to 100 mg/L
8. Preparations: Zarontin capsules 250 mg; solution 250 mg/5 mL

Acetazolamide
1. Advantages—well tolerated, typically used adjunctively for absence seizures, but may be used for partial seizures and intermittently for catamenial (menses-related) seizure exacerbations.
2. Disadvantages—probably low efficacy; should not be used with TPM or ZNS (renal stones).
3. Major adverse effects:
   a. Dose-related: paresthesias, weakness, hyponatremia, hypokalemia
   b. Idiosyncratic: anorexia, rash, blood dyscrasias
   c. Chronic: osteomalacia
4. Teratogenicity: yes
5. Pharmacokinetics: 2 to 13 hours halflife
6. Initiation and titration: 250 to 500 mg/d increasing to 500 to 1,000 mg/d (b.i.d. or t.i.d.); pediatrics ($\geq$4 years): 4 mg/kg/d increasing over weeks to 8 to 30 mg/kg/d.
7. Therapeutic range: none determined
8. Preparations: Diamox tablets 125 and 250 mg; slow release, 500 mg; suspension, 50 mg/mL

Benzodiazepines
These differ from each other mainly by pharmacokinetics and available routes of administration. Adverse effects include mainly sedation and slowed cognition, as well as ventilatory suppression when given IV.
1. Clonazepam—adjunctive therapy for myoclonic and atonic, less often partial, seizures; half-life 20 to 40 hours, shortened by enzyme inducers. Initial dose

0.5 mg qd or b.i.d., increasing in 0.5 mg/d intervals every 3 to 7 days to target of 1.5 to 4 mg/d. Preparations: tablets 0.5, 1, and 2 mg.

2. Clorazepate—same as clonazepam (although approved for partial seizures); half-life, 55 to 100 hours. Initial dose 3.75 mg b.i.d. to t.i.d., increasing by 3.75 to 7.5 mg every week to 15 to 45 mg/d. Preparations: tablets 3.75, 7.5, and 15 mg; slow-release tablets, 11.25 and 22.5 mg.

3. Diazepam (DZ)—rarely used orally, but widely used intravenously for status epilepticus and rectally for acute repetitive seizures. Half-life of active metabolite, desmethyldiazepam, is 20 to 40 hours, but when given IV it is redistributed out of the brain into other fatty tissues; it is also highly protein bound (99%). Therefore, when given IV, although onset of action is extremely rapid, 1 to 2 minutes, duration of action is only 15 to 20 minutes. Preparation: 5 mg/mL solution. As rectal gel (Diastat), is dosed according to age and weight and is available in rectal syringes of 2.5, 5, 10, 15, and 20 mg.

4. Lorazepam (LZ)—Used IV for status epilepticus, onset of action is slightly slower than DZ, 4 to 5 minutes, but remains in brain much longer, with duration of action of 4 to 10 hours. Protein binding is 90%. Oral lorazepam rarely used chronically, but can be given sublingually for seizure clusters, especially if the patient is too awake between seizures to tolerate rectal diazepam gel. Preparations: tablets 0.5, 1, and 2 mg; solution 0.5, 1. or 2 mg/mL.

5. Midazolam—IV for status epilepticus as alternative to DZ or LZ, and as infusion when status becomes refractory. Half-life is 1 to 2 hours. Preparation: vials 1 mg/mL or 5 mg/mL.

6. Nitrazepam and clobazam are benzodiazepines. These drugs, particularly clobazam, may have advantages in chronic therapy, but are not available in the United States.

7. Fosphenytoin (fos-PHT)—A water-soluble prodrug of phenytoin, may be given more quickly (up to 150 mg phenytoin equivalents/minute in adults) and without fear of tissue necrosis in case of extravasation; may also be given intramuscularly (IM) in nonemergent situations. Although it is not given in a propylene glycol vehicle, which has been thought to be largely responsible for the hypotensive effects of PHT, studies have not demonstrated a lower rate of this complication with fos-PHT.

OVERVIEW OF EPILEPSY PRESENTATIONS AND SYNDROMES

The following discussion consists of approaches to common clinical situations and to specific syndromes, presented when possible in order of the usual age of presentation.

NEONATAL SEIZURES

BACKGROUND

1. Neonatal seizures are usually defined as those occurring during the first month or two of life.

2. Perhaps because brain development at that stage only allows a limited repertoire of behavior, the clinical manifestations are limited, and seizures may be difficult to distinguish from normal behaviors.

3. Perhaps because of incomplete myelination, tonic–clonic seizures probably do not occur at this age.

4. Clonic and tonic seizures do occur, but typically involve different parts of the body in a migrating or asymmetric manner, even when the cause involves the brain diffusely.

5. Myoclonic jerks are more likely to occur bilaterally, but may have a nonepileptic pathophysiology in neurologically abnormal neonates, as can apnea, diffuse tonic stiffening, repetitive sucking, pedaling movements, or eye deviation.
6. In general, the EEG is much more essential to seizure diagnosis in neonates than in older children or adults.

PATHOPHYSIOLOGY

1. Seizures can occur in the neonate as the result of almost any focal or diffuse insult; depending on the insult, these can cause acute symptomatic seizures only, or result in an ongoing seizure tendency, that is, epilepsy.
   a. Electrolyte disturbances are those that increase neuronal hyperexcitability; other causes may act in a nonspecific manner causing neuronal injury, or indirectly as in deficiency of pyridoxine, a necessary cofactor in the synthesis of GABA.
   b. In about two thirds of neonates with seizures, the cause of acute seizures or epilepsy can be identified as occurring before, during, or after birth. These include congenital or postnatal infection, congenital malformation, asphyxia (most common), intracranial hemorrhage, inborn errors of metabolism (especially pyridoxine or biotinidase deficiency), hypocalcemia (either early, within the first 3 days, usually in association with other insults, or late, usually day 5 to 14, after consuming a milk formula with a high phosphate concentration), hypomagnesemia (often with hypocalcemia), hypoglycemia (often appearing within hours of birth and in association with other insults), hypo- or hypernatremia, drug withdrawal (from maternal narcotics or depressants), or drug toxicity (inadvertent injection of local anesthetics).
2. Among "idiopathic" causes of neonatal seizures are two genetic syndromes, benign familial neonatal convulsions, which has been linked to mutations in the voltage-gated potassium channel on chromosome 20 or chromosome 8, and benign neonatal convulsions, for which a genetic cause has not been identified but which, unlike neonatal seizures or status epilepticus due to an identifiable cause, is self-limited. These often begin on the fifth day of life, and are termed "fifth-day fits."

PROGNOSIS

The prognosis of neonatal seizures is strongly related to the cause. Neonates whose seizures result from congenital malformation or postnatal infection do worse than those with a transient metabolic disorder. Animal studies suggest that seizures in the neonate are both more difficult to control and less likely to produce neuronal damage than uncontrolled seizures at older ages. Apart from etiology, those with a normal EEG background and a normal examination have the best prognosis; this includes those with the diagnoses of benign familial neonatal convulsions or benign neonatal convulsions.

DIAGNOSIS

1. Diagnosis of seizures depends on distinguishing these from normal or nonepileptic causes of repetitive movements in the neonate, such as normal chewing or sucking, or benign neonatal sleep myoclonus.
   a. EEG is often critical in making this distinction. Although interictal discharges can be difficult to distinguish from nonspecific sharp transients, ictal discharges in the neonatal EEG are usually apparent because of their rhythmicity and evolution. Frequency is 0.5 to 15 Hz and most often evolves from slow to fast; spatial evolution is often less than that in adults, in that discharges can remain confined to a single electrode or, in some cases, "migrate" from one location to another.
   b. To be termed an "electrographic seizure," the minimum discharge duration is sometimes arbitrarily defined as 10 seconds.

2. Remaining metabolic and imaging tests are directed toward identifying or excluding the causes listed under Pathophysiology, section 1.b., above. If examination findings are normal and evaluation is negative, benign familial neonatal convulsions or benign neonatal convulsions may be diagnosed, depending on family history. The familial syndrome presents with seizures lasting a few days, whereas the nonfamilial syndrome may progress to status epilepticus but usually lasts less than 1 day.

TREATMENT

1. The first priority is to identify and treat any reversible infectious or metabolic cause.
2. While waiting for blood test results to return, some clinicians administer in a stepwise manner 2 to 4 mL/kg of 25% glucose, 50 to 100 mg of pyridoxine (ideally during EEG recording), 1 to 2 mL/kg of 10% calcium gluconate [over minutes during electrocardiogram (ECG) monitoring], and 0.1 to 0.2 mL/kg of 50% magnesium sulfate.
3. If ventilation and other autonomic functions are unaffected, some clinicians elect to observe or treat only with benzodiazepines. However, usually treatment is initiated with PHB or PHT.
    a. PHB is given in two 10-mg/kg boluses at 2 to 3 mg/kg/min, followed by additional boluses as needed. If this is unsuccessful, PHT may also be given in two 10-mg/kg boluses no faster than 2 mg/kg/min. PHB is maintained orally at 5 mg/kg/d, following levels frequently because of more rapid and variable metabolism than in older children.
    b. Variations in PHT absorption and metabolism in the neonate complicate its use in oral maintenance.
4. There is experimental evidence that TPM may have a neuroprotective role in neonatal seizure management, but recommendations await further research.

WEST SYNDROME (INFANTILE SPASMS)

BACKGROUND

1. West syndrome (first identified by a 19th century British pediatrician in his own child) is a generalized epilepsy syndrome, usually symptomatic or cryptogenic, that arises between 4 and 6 months of age and occurs only in the first 2 years.
2. It is defined by clusters of myoclonic–tonic seizures, sometimes termed "jackknife seizures" or "salaam attacks," and a characteristic interictal EEG finding of hypsarrhythmia, consisting of a chaotic, high-amplitude background with multifocal spikes. Each spasm lasts 2 to 3 seconds, longer than true myoclonus but shorter than most tonic seizures, and can be mainly flexor, extensor, or both. Eye deviation or nystagmus can occur; asymmetric spasms often but not always occur in infants with focal brain lesions.
3. This syndrome is relatively common, appearing in up to 40/100,000 children.

PATHOPHYSIOLOGY

1. The mechanism of generating clusters of spasms is not well understood, but the clinical manifestations and the ictal EEG showing low-amplitude fast activity or flattening, a so-called electrodecremental pattern, suggest the possibility of brainstem involvement.
2. Pathologic causes of the syndrome include nearly any kind of prenatal, perinatal, or postnatal insult, including hypoxic encephalopathy, trauma, meningitis, brain malformations, and inborn errors of metabolism.

3. Neuroectodermal disorders, particularly tuberous sclerosis, are strongly associated.

PROGNOSIS

West syndrome has a poor prognosis overall, with only 80% to 90% surviving to age 5, 70% to 90% of the survivors having developmental delay, and 50% having epilepsy. However, infants with normal neurologic development prior to onset of spasms and no known cause (idiopathic cases) may have a good outcome. Onset before 6 months is also associated with a poor prognosis, but possibly because of its relationship to symptomatic etiologies. Cryptogenic cases, that is, infants with an abnormal examination or developmental history but without a known etiology, likely have a prognosis intermediate between symptomatic and idiopathic cases. The possibility that early treatment may influence prognosis is a spur to prompt diagnosis and aggressive management.

DIAGNOSIS

1. Diagnosis depends on the occurrence of typical clinical events and a characteristic interictal and ictal EEG.
   a. Hypsarhythmia is not always present, however, and may appear only after the syndrome is established.
   b. There are also variants, termed "modified hypsarrhythmia," including EEGs with focal features, relatively few spikes, or relative synchrony between the two hemispheres.
2. Once the syndrome is diagnosed, evaluation is directed toward identifying potential causes, and includes, in addition to neurologic examination and EEG, a careful skin examination with Wood's lamp, and CT or MRI, which is abnormal in 70% to 80% of cases.
   a. Screening for inborn errors of metabolism should include urine and serum amino acids; serum organic acids, lactate, pyruvate, and ammonia levels; and liver function tests.
   b. Cerebrospinal fluid (CSF) should be examined for lactate, pyruvate, and amino acids if metabolic disease is a consideration.

TREATMENT

1. If no cause is found, pyridoxine deficiency, a very rare but dramatically treatable cause, should be considered and pyridoxine 100 to 200 mg administered IV during EEG recording; if this is the etiology, the EEG should improve within minutes.
2. The mainstay of treatment remains ACTH, which often results in seizure control and EEG improvement within days.
   a. ACTH may be given IM at 40 IU daily for 2 weeks, and if seizures continue, increased by 10 IU weekly until seizures are controlled or to a maximum of 80 IU daily.
   b. After seizures stop, the dose can be continued for a month and then tapered by 10 IU/wk. If seizures recur, the previously effective dose is resumed.
   c. Blood pressure, stool guaiac, electrolytes, calcium, phosphorus, glucose, and signs of infection must be monitored.
3. Alternatives, typically used when ACTH fails or is not tolerated, include prednisone, VPA, CZP, LTG, TPM, FBM, or TGB.
   a. VPA can be initiated at 15 mg/kg/d in three doses, and increased in 5- to 10-mg/kg/d weekly increments.
   b. Clonazepam is begun at 0.01 to 0.03 mg/kg/d in three doses, increasing by 0.25 to 0.50 mg every 3 days to 0.1 to 0.2 mg/kg/d.
   c. The AED vigabatrin, an inhibitor of GABA catabolism, is unavailable in the United States, but can be dramatically effective, especially when the spasms are due to tuberous sclerosis.

LENNOX–GASTAUT SYNDROME

BACKGROUND

1. LGS is a symptomatic or cryptogenic generalized syndrome characterized by multiple seizure types, including generalized tonic seizures, and by slow spike-wave complexes (1.5–2.5 Hz) on EEG; mental retardation is usually considered part of the syndrome, although approximately 10% of those who otherwise meet the definition have normal development. Other seizure types commonly include tonic–clonic, myoclonic, atonic, and atypical absence; "drop attacks," which may result from tonic, atonic, or myoclonic seizures that involve the postural musculature, also occur and can cause serious injury. Head drops are a fragmentary form of drop attack and may occur hundreds of times a day. Partial seizures occur less frequently but may be present, especially in older children.
2. Onset is between 6 months and 7 years, and incidence is approximately 30/100,000.
3. EEG findings include background slowing and sometimes multifocal discharges in addition to anterior predominant generalized slow spike-wave complexes; the latter are sometimes nearly continuous, except during rapid eye movement (REM) sleep. During slow-wave sleep, polyspike–wave complexes and bursts of fast spikes may occur, with or without myoclonic or tonic clinical manifestations.

PATHOPHYSIOLOGY

The same range of insults that cause infantile spasms can cause LGS, and in some cases the former can evolve into the latter. Evidence that these or other early-onset epilepsies can be caused by diphtheria-pertussis-tetanus vaccines is limited and nonconfirmatory.

PROGNOSIS

1. LGS is highly resistant to treatment, and seizures occur many times a day.
2. Mental retardation is present in approximately half at onset of seizures and the proportion increases with age, lending support to the hypothesis that poorly controlled seizures cause mental deterioration.
3. In some patients, fluctuations in cognition and behavior may vary with epileptiform activity, leading to hope that the development of more effective treatments, as has occurred to some extent over the past decade, will have a long-lasting effect on overall functioning.

DIAGNOSIS

Diagnosis is based on history, examination, and routine EEG; additional EEG techniques, such as video–EEG monitoring, may be helpful in some cases to establish which clinical behaviors have an epileptic origin.

TREATMENT

1. A variety of the "broad-spectrum" AEDs have shown efficacy in the treatment of LGS, although responses are rarely dramatic.
   a. VPA traditionally has been used, although the risk of hepatic failure is a concern in children younger than 2 years, whereas FBM also carries risk of hepatic and bone marrow toxicity; TPM and LTG are likely to be safer.
   b. Clonazepam is sometimes given adjunctively, although sedation and behavioral effects limit its use. LEV, ZNS, ACZ, and MSX are worthy of consideration, but have not been studied formally.
2. Narrow-spectrum drugs such as PHT and CBZ may be given for tonic–clonic seizures; PHT may also help control tonic and perhaps atonic seizures.
3. There is considerable evidence that the ketogenic diet can be effective in LGS,

with 30% to 50% reporting dramatic or convincing responses, and some children have been able to discontinue AEDs and show functional improvements that are maintained for a year or more, although long-term data are limited.
4. For patients with potentially injurious drop spells, corpus callosotomy is an option, and VNS has shown efficacy against LGS in retrospective studies.
5. There are anecdotal reports of immune-modulating treatments such as ACTH, IV immune globulin, or plasmapheresis having at least transient efficacy in treating this and other severe and refractory pediatric epilepsy syndromes.

FEBRILE CONVULSIONS

BACKGROUND

1. Benign febrile convulsions (FCs) constitute a situation-related syndrome usually defined as the occurrence of brief convulsions in a neurologically normal child between 6 months and 5 years, in the setting of fever noted prior to the seizure and not attributable to CNS infection. If the seizure is focal, recurs within a day, or persists beyond 15 minutes, it is termed a "complex febrile seizure." Onset is most commonly between 18 and 22 months. This is a common syndrome, occurring in 3% to 4% of the population.
2. Genetic studies have identified rare variants in which afebrile seizures later develop, or febrile seizures persist beyond the usual age limit, and have been designated "generalized epilepsy with febrile seizures plus" (GEFS+).

PATHOPHYSIOLOGY

FCs have a strong genetic component, and in GEFS+, autosomal dominant mutations of the sodium channel or GABA receptor have been found. It is likely that other channel abnormalities, perhaps with more complex inheritance, underlie the more common syndrome, and fever, which generally lowers the seizure threshold, "unmasks" the inherited tendency. The reasons for the strong relationship to age are not well understood.

PROGNOSIS

1. The prognosis of simple FC is regarded as benign, although 30% to 40% of children have a recurrence during subsequent febrile illness, especially if the index seizure occurs during the first year of life.
2. The prognosis for later development of epilepsy may be approximately four times that of the general population, but much of this risk corresponds to children who have had complex FC. An important subgroup comprises those with prolonged FC, an unknown number of whom will later develop the syndrome of mesial temporal sclerosis, usually diagnosed in the context of surgical treatment in adolescence or adulthood. At least some of these patients have accompanying anatomic abnormalities that may have predisposed them to both prolonged febrile seizures and to later development of intractable epilepsy.
3. Prognosis for neurologic development after FC is excellent, as developmental delay not apparent before the first febrile convulsion seldom occurs afterward, except in rare cases of status epilepticus.

DIAGNOSIS

1. The diagnosis depends on the child's meeting the criteria described above, and on ruling out a CNS abnormality as the cause of the seizure.
2. Lumbar puncture should be considered at initial presentation, since meningitis, especially in young children, may present with a paucity of other signs.

3. EEG is generally regarded as not useful, because nonspecific abnormalities, such as posterior slowing, have no prognostic value, and even spike-wave complexes do not strongly predict later seizures (although they may reflect the inherited low threshold underlying the syndrome). Similarly, if the examination is normal, neuroimaging is not needed.
4. Other evaluation is aimed at identifying the cause of the fever, such as viral illnesses or otitis media, which are common in the affected age group.

TREATMENT

1. Preventive treatment with standard AEDs is no longer recommended for FC.
2. Aside from acetaminophen for fever control and treatment of the underlying illness, treatment options after a first FC include diazepam given orally 0.3 mg/kg q8h at onset of subsequent fever or potential febrile illness; an alternative is rectal diazepam gel dosed according the age and weight per package insert.

BENIGN EPILEPSY WITH CENTROTEMPORAL SPIKES

BACKGROUND

1. Benign epilepsy with centrotemporal spikes (BECTS), also termed "benign rolandic epilepsy," is the most common idiopathic partial epilepsy syndrome.
2. Seizures begin between 2 and 12 years, most commonly between 5 and 10, and consist of mainly nocturnal and infrequent secondarily generalized seizures, as well as frequent diurnal or nocturnal simple partial seizures involving the oral sensorimotor cortex; this location produces the characteristic symptoms of tingling or an electrical feeling in the cheek or mouth, often progressing to twitching of the face and less commonly the hand or arm. The child cannot speak but is fully conscious.

PATHOPHYSIOLOGY

This syndrome has a genetic basis, with some families having mutations on chromosome 15; the EEG trait is more strongly penetrant than the epilepsy syndrome, which is present in only a minority of those with the characteristic EEG findings.

PROGNOSIS

Seizures stop during adolescence, typically before age 16, and patients remain neurologically normal. Similar seizures with prognoses that are less benign have been reported in patients with focal lesions in the rolandic cortex or adjacent areas.

DIAGNOSIS

Diagnosis depends on the clinical history and is established by the characteristic EEG finding of diphasic spikes and sharp waves in one or both centrotemporal regions, especially during light sleep. If the examination is normal and the history and EEG typical, neuroimaging is not necessary, though MRI should be pursued if seizures do not respond or other features are atypical.

TREATMENT

1. Because of the benign course, not all child neurologists treat patients with this syndrome, although most do once a secondarily generalized seizure occurs.
2. Any AED effective against partial seizures can be used. CBZ has been traditionally given, but GBP has been used in recent years.

3. Treatment can often be stopped after 1 to 2 years of seizure control, even if the EEG findings remain abnormal.

CHILDHOOD ABSENCE EPILEPSY

BACKGROUND

Childhood absence epilepsy (CAE) is an idiopathic, generalized epilepsy that arises between age 3 and the onset of puberty, and is characterized by very frequent (hence the previous term "pyknolepsy," from the Greek *pyknos*, meaning crowding) typical absence seizures and a characteristic EEG with normal background and 3-Hz spike–wave complexes. Absences may occur hundreds of times daily, and one third to one half of patients also have infrequent tonic–clonic seizures.

PATHOPHYSIOLOGY

Inheritance may be autosomal dominant with incomplete penetrance (higher for the EEG trait than for clinical epilepsy); the associated mutation is unknown, although it most likely affects channels associated with the thalamocortical network underlying absence seizures.

PROGNOSIS

1. Most patients respond completely to appropriate medication, and approximately two thirds remit by puberty. Positive factors for remission include lack of tonic–clonic seizures (or, if present, onset after absence seizures have begun), negative family history, and no history of nonconvulsive generalized status epilepticus.
2. If cognition, neurologic status, or EEG background are abnormal, prognosis is worse, and the possibility of an incorrect diagnosis must be considered.

DIAGNOSIS

Diagnosis is often made clinically by having the patient hyperventilate for 3 to 4 minutes, which is a potent trigger for absences, and confirmed by EEG that also includes hyperventilation. If history and EEG are characteristic and the examination is normal, neuroimaging is probably not needed.

TREATMENT

Although ESX, VPA, and LTG are equally effective against absences, for children with absences only, ESX is still the drug of choice, because of a lower risk of serious adverse effects. If tonic–clonic seizures are present, VPA or LTG is preferable, since ESX must be used with another AED, such as PHT, that will treat the tonic–clonic seizures. If ESX, VPA, or LTG does not adequately control the absences, combinations of these may be used; TPM, ZNS, and LEV may ultimately prove to be effective as well.

JUVENILE MYOCLONIC EPILEPSY AND RELATED SYNDROMES

BACKGROUND

1. Juvenile myoclonic epilepsy (JME) is an idiopathic generalized epilepsy with onset during or after puberty (usually in the teenaged years but possibly as young as 8 or as old as 30) and is characterized by myoclonic seizures, most often affecting the proximal upper extremities. It is the most common idiopathic epilepsy, accounting for perhaps 5% to 10% of all adult epilepsy cases.

   a. Myoclonic seizures usually occur within 1 to 2 hours of awakening, but may also be experienced when falling asleep in the afternoon or at other times.

   b. Approximately 90% of patients also have tonic–clonic seizures, and 10% to 30% have absences, which are much less frequent than in CAE and may also be incomplete, in that awareness may be partially preserved.

   c. EEG shows 4- to 6-Hz spike–wave and polyspike–wave complexes, less regular than those in CAE.

2. The syndrome of juvenile absence epilepsy (JAE) is similar to JME, but there are no myoclonic seizures and absences must be present. The syndrome of idiopathic epilepsy with grand mal seizures on awakening lacks the absence as well as myoclonic seizures, and that of random grand mal does not show a diurnal pattern of seizure occurrence.

3. Seizures associated with all of these syndromes are very sensitive to sleep deprivation and alcohol withdrawal, which are frequent in the age group at risk.

PATHOPHYSIOLOGY

JME and the related syndromes are genetic in origin, with a site on chromosome 6 found for JME in some ethnic groups; however, other genes may also be involved and account for some of the variability among patients with these syndromes.

PROGNOSIS

The prognosis of the adolescent-onset syndromes is not as favorable as that for CAE, as 80% to 90% require lifelong treatment. However, most seizures respond well to treatment.

DIAGNOSIS

Diagnosis depends on appropriate historic and EEG findings and may be delayed because myoclonic jerks are often ignored and their history not elicited without direct questioning. If clinical and EEG findings are typical, examination is normal, and response to medication is complete, neuroimaging is not needed; most patients, however, have had CT or MRI prior to diagnosis.

TREATMENT

1. VPA is still considered the first-choice drug, although in obese men or in women the risks of weight gain and teratogenicity may argue for an alternative. LTG is often effective, although in some patients myoclonic seizures may not respond or may even worsen. (When PHT or especially CBZ is given, worsening of absence as well as myoclonic seizures is relatively common, though these may be useful adjuncts for tonic–clonic seizures.)

2. TPM, ZNS, and LEV may be effective alternatives.

3. Finally, counseling on the need to obtain adequate sleep, avoid use of alcohol and other psychoactive substances, and maintain medication compliance is an important part of treatment.

ALCOHOL- AND DRUG-WITHDRAWAL SEIZURES

BACKGROUND

1. Alcohol-withdrawal seizures are an important situation-related syndrome, accounting for a high proportion of cases of initial seizures and status epilepticus

in susceptible populations. Seizures occur 7 to 48 hours after the last drink, most commonly between 12 and 24 hours, usually in association with other withdrawal symptoms such as autonomic arousal and agitation.
2. The timing of withdrawal seizures from other depressants, such as benzodiazepines and barbiturates, depends on the half-life of the relevant drug.

PATHOPHYSIOLOGY

Alcohol and many other depressants potentiate GABA-mediated inhibition and may block excitatory neurotransmission; the compensatory receptor changes that occur with chronic use predispose the patient to neuronal hyperexcitability and seizures in the setting of abrupt withdrawal.

PROGNOSIS

Withdrawal seizures, even in the rare cases that progress to status epilepticus, usually respond promptly to appropriate treatment, although patients may need to be observed for the later development of delirium tremens. The long-term prognosis depends on success in treating substance abuse.

DIAGNOSIS

1. Diagnosis depends on an adequate history, and is more obvious if alcohol is still present in the blood; physical examination directed toward signs of chronic alcohol abuse may be helpful.
2. The most important aspect of the evaluation is ruling out other metabolic and structural abnormalities associated with alcoholism, including hyponatremia, hypoglycemia, hypomagnesemia, and traumatic brain injury.

TREATMENT

1. Benzodiazepines are the mainstay of treatment for alcohol and benzodiazepine withdrawal, and may be used, along with phenobarbital, for barbiturate withdrawal. Lorazepam 2 to 4 mg IV or IM can be given every 2 to 4 hours as needed to minimize withdrawal symptoms without causing excessive sedation. PHT is typically not helpful unless status epilepticus develops.
2. Referral to an appropriate substance abuse program should be attempted even if the chance of success is believed to be low.

LESIONAL EPILEPSY

BACKGROUND

1. Although structural lesions account for less than half of all cases of epilepsy, this proportion is higher in patients with partial epilepsies and those with a later age of onset, especially after age 60.
   a. At younger ages, pathologic specimens suggest that microscopic structural abnormalities, often disorders of cortical development, underlie many cases of medically intractable partial epilepsy, even in those with adolescent or adult onset.
   b. Other important pathologic categories include
      1) Neoplasm, especially benign brain tumors such as gangliogliomas, oligodendrogliomas, dysembryoplastic neuroepithelial tumors, and astrocytomas
      2) Infections, particularly parasitic infections such as cysticercosis, but also long-term sequelae of bacterial and viral meningoencephalitis
      3) Traumatic brain injury, especially penetrating but also closed head injury if moderate or severe

    4) Stroke, both hemorrhagic and ischemic

    5) Congenital or acquired vascular anomalies, such as arteriovenous malformations or cavernous angiomas.

2. Clinical manifestations depend largely on the site of the lesion, although the correlation is far from perfect, since the ictal discharge may start adjacent to rather than in the lesion (depending on lesion type) and may produce no symptoms or signs until it spreads within the hemisphere or even to the contralateral hemisphere.

    a. Lesions that produce either acute symptomatic seizures or later epilepsy are typically located cortically or subcortically rather than deep.

    b. Frontoparietal lesions near primary sensorimotor cortex typically produce contralateral somatosensory and motor phenomena, while other areas of the frontal lobe produce other manifestations: bilateral posturing if near the midline supplementary motor area, or vigorous automatisms and emotional experiences with orbitofrontal and/or cingulate involvement.

    c. As a rule, frontal lobe epilepsies tend to produce frequent brief seizures that arise out of sleep.

    d. Temporal lobe epilepsies differ depending on whether the source is medial or lateral; medial temporal seizures are often characterized by a rising epigastric sensation or other autonomic disturbance, as well as emotional or olfactory auras preceding complex partial seizures that progress from motionless staring to oral automatisms. These complex partial seizures often last 2 to 3 minutes, and are followed by postictal confusion.

    e. Lateral temporal lobe seizures are associated with auditory, language, or sometimes visual phenomena.

    f. Parietal and occipital lobe epilepsies may include partial seizures characterized by elementary or formed visual hallucinations or distortions of spatial perception, including vertigo.

PATHOPHYSIOLOGY

The mechanisms by which structural lesions produce neuronal hyperexcitability are not well understood and likely vary for different types of lesions. Disorders of cortical development, for example, include neurons that may have abnormal receptors, channels, or connections, whereas foreign tissue and destructive lesions may injure specific neurons or neuronal populations to decrease inhibition or increase excitation on a neuronal or network basis. With hemorrhagic lesions, iron itself can be epileptogenic when applied to the cortex.

PROGNOSIS

Prognosis for seizure control differs with lesion type and location. For example, mesial temporal sclerosis, a hippocampal lesion often associated with prolonged FC in childhood and onset of partial seizures in adolescence or early adulthood, is frequently refractory to medical management, but amenable to surgical treatment. Among patients with neoplasms, overall prognosis depends on likelihood of growth or regrowth after resection, especially if recurrence is associated with malignant transformation, as can be seen with astrocytomas.

DIAGNOSIS

The diagnosis of structural lesions has been revolutionized by CT and especially MRI, which can reliably show not only neoplasms, abscesses, and vascular anomalies but also many disorders of cortical development and gliotic lesions such as mesial temporal sclerosis.

TREATMENT

1. Any of the drugs effective against partial and tonic–clonic seizures can be used in patients with lesional epilepsy; no drug specificity by location has been demonstrated. In the United States, CBZ and PHT are most commonly initiated, but in specific populations, VPA, LTG, TPM, GBP, and OXC may have advantages. (Of these, only VPA and OXC are FDA-approved as initial monotherapy.)

2. A significant proportion of those with lesional epilepsy will not respond to AEDs, and surgery should be strongly considered for any patient with a resectable lesion that can plausibly account for the epilepsy syndrome and whose seizures do not respond to two or more appropriate AEDs at reasonable doses. In many cases, complete resection of the lesion alone will render the patient seizure free, and many of these patients can eventually be withdrawn from medication; it is likely that in some cases the outcome is better if surrounding electrically abnormal tissue is also removed.

SPECIAL ISSUES RELATED TO EPILEPSY IN WOMEN

BACKGROUND

1. Approximately 40% of all cases of epilepsy, or almost 1,000,000 in the United States, occur in women of childbearing age. Issues that need to be considered include effects of hormones and pregnancy on epilepsy, influence of AEDs and seizures on pregnancy and pregnancy outcome, breast feeding, and other childcare issues.
2. It is important to recognize that the enzyme inducing drugs CBZ, PHT, PHB, PRM, and to a lesser extent OXC and TPM, can increase metabolism of hormones and cause failure of oral contraceptives. If there is no other effective method available, oral contraceptives can still be used, but only medium- or high-dose pills, and failure rate is still above baseline.

PATHOPHYSIOLOGY

1. Approximately one third of women with epilepsy, especially those with partial and perhaps temporal lobe seizures, report increased seizures shortly before menses or at ovulation. These so-called catamenial seizures likely reflect the important effects of hormones on neuronal excitability.
   a. In general, estrogens increase excitability and progesterones (particularly allopregnenolone) have inhibitory effects. The ratio of rising and falling levels of these two hormone classes likely accounts for the menstrual variation, and may affect seizure fluctuations during and after menopause.
   b. Occasionally, measurement of AED levels through the menstrual cycle reveals changes in absorption or metabolism that can account for the exacerbations.
2. The mechanisms by which AEDs cause teratogenicity are not well understood, and may be different for different AEDs.
   a. One hypothesis is that oxidative injury to fetal cells results from reactive AED metabolites.
   b. Folate deficiency is also associated with several AEDs and can adversely affect fetal cell division.

PROGNOSIS

1. Women with catamenial epilepsy may experience fewer seizures after menopause, though some report exacerbation during the menopause. With respect to AED teratogenicity, monotherapy with the older drugs PHT, PHB, CBZ, and VPA is associated with an approximate doubling of the rate of major congenital malformations from 2% to 3% at baseline to 4% to 7%; also, VPA and to a lesser extent CBZ elevate the risk of neural tube defects. Since major organs are formed during the first trimester, risk of major malformations is not an issue beyond that time. The possibility of effects on neurobehavioral development posed by fetal exposure later in the pregnancy is under active investigation.

2. During pregnancy, perhaps one third of women experience an increase in seizures, and it is unclear whether this proportion has declined in recent years with increased awareness of the need to increase drug doses as pregnancy progresses. Seizures can adversely affect pregnancy either by causing falls and other accidents or, at least in the case of convulsive seizures, producing fetal distress.

DIAGNOSIS

The diagnosis of catamenial seizure exacerbations is established by keeping a careful diary of seizures and menses. Close neurologic and obstetric follow-up are needed to diagnose epilepsy-related pregnancy complications.

TREATMENT

1. Catamenial seizure exacerbations can be treated by temporarily increasing the baseline AED dose, especially if fluctuations in levels have been demonstrated, by adding acetazolamide 250 to 1,000 mg/d for 10 to 14 days starting at mid cycle, or by administering natural progesterone lozenges 300 to 800 mg/d during the second half of the cycle, tapering over 2 to 3 days after onset of menses. The latter treatment is under active study; potential adverse effects include depression, breast tenderness, and hypercoagulability.

2. To minimize AED teratogenicity, an effective means of contraception must be used, and all women of childbearing age should be given supplemental folate; the optimal dose has not been determined, but at least 0.4 mg and perhaps as much as 4 mg should be given daily.

   a. Polytherapy should be avoided whenever possible, and drug withdrawal prior to conception should be considered in women who have been seizure free for at least 2 years, or in those for whom the diagnosis of epilepsy has not been established; in the latter case, video–EEG monitoring can be decisive.

   b. The most effective AED for that individual should be used at the lowest dose that controls seizures, especially the secondarily or primarily generalized tonic–clonic seizures that are most likely to put both mother and fetus at risk.

   c. Women with a family history of neural tube defects should probably not use VPA or CBZ if pregnancy is a possibility.

   d. Knowledge of potential teratogenic effects of the newer drugs will be facilitated by encouraging pregnant women taking AEDs to contact the North American AED Pregnancy Registry, as early as possible in the pregnancy, by calling the toll-free number 1-888-233-2334 (1-888-AED-AED4).

3. Treatment during pregnancy should include measurement of drug levels every 1 to 3 months, including free levels of highly protein-bound drugs. Total and, to a lesser extent, free levels tend to fall as pregnancy progresses and doses usually need to be increased.

   a. Vitamin K, 10 to 20 mg/d, is sometimes recommended during the last month of pregnancy, especially to mothers taking enzyme-inducing drugs, and vitamin K is routinely given to the baby to prevent neonatal hemorrhage.

   b. Seizures during delivery, reported to occur in 1% to 2% of women with epilepsy, may be prevented by administering AEDs parenterally when absorption is in doubt; use of parenteral or sublingual lorazepam can also be considered, though neonatal sedation is a risk.

   c. Following delivery, drug levels rise over a period of days to weeks and doses typically need to be decreased to avoid toxicity.

4. New mothers with epilepsy should be counseled to change the baby on the floor, not to bathe the baby alone, and to take other reasonable precautions consistent with the nature of the mother's seizures. Although all AEDs can be found in breast milk, especially those that are not highly protein bound, specific risks have not been identified apart from sedation with barbiturates and benzodiazepines, and the benefits of breast feeding likely outweigh the risks.

TOXEMIA OF PREGNANCY

BACKGROUND

1. Toxemia of pregnancy is a situation-related syndrome occurring in the second half of pregnancy and consisting of systemic alterations including hypertension with edema and/or proteinuria; coagulopathy and liver dysfunction are often present.
2. Cerebral involvement is similar to that associated with hypertensive encephalopathy and includes headache and cerebral edema, often causing visual phenomena and partial or tonic–clonic seizures (likely secondarily generalized).
3. Hyperreflexia is usually present.
4. The presence of coma or seizures indicates progression from preeclampsia to eclampsia.

PATHOPHYSIOLOGY

The underlying mechanism of toxemia is not known but may reflect alteration in endothelial function; effects on the brain are similar to those of hypertensive encephalopathy and likely relate to loss of autoregulation of cerebral blood flow, especially in posterior cerebral regions.

PROGNOSIS

Eclampsia has a maternal mortality rate of 1% to 2%, and there are fetal complications in one third of cases.

DIAGNOSIS

Eclampsia is diagnosed on the basis of clinical characteristics described above, typically by the obstetrician.

TREATMENT

1. The procedure essential to reversing the underlying eclamptic process is delivering the baby.
2. Seizures must still be treated, however, and in some cases preventative treatment is justified. Traditionally, obstetricians have favored use of magnesium sulfate to treat or prevent eclamptic seizures and neurologists have preferred use of traditional AEDs such as PHT. Despite some methodologic problems, recent studies have favored the obstetricians' approach.
3. Magnesium sulfate may be given IV at 20 mg of a 20% solution (4 g) over 4 minutes, with maintenance of 1 to 3 g/h, or as 5 to 10 mg IM every 4 hours, titrating to a level of 3 to 5 mmol and monitoring for arreflexia and weakness that could herald ventilatory compromise. The addition of PHT, 15 to 20 mg/kg can be considered, especially if seizures occur with adequate Mg levels; LZ 2 to 4 mg IV can also be used acutely.

SEIZURES AND EPILEPSY IN THE ELDERLY

BACKGROUND

1. The incidence of both acute symptomatic seizures and of epilepsy increase beyond age 60, and in the oldest, new seizures occur at annual rates exceeding 100/100,000.
2. The most common cause is stroke, both ischemic and hemorrhagic, but degenerative disorders including Alzheimer dementia and metastatic and primary brain tumors are important contributors.

PATHOPHYSIOLOGY

The mechanisms by which the above processes cause seizures and epilepsy depend on the type of insult and are not well understood.

PROGNOSIS

Overall, prognosis depends on the specific cause and on comorbid conditions, but in most cases, seizures respond to AED treatment at least as well as in younger individuals.

DIAGNOSIS

1. Differential diagnosis of transient neurologic dysfunction is similar to that previously outlined, but in the elderly, the likelihood of psychogenic nonepileptic seizures is lower than in younger patients, and the risk of such physiologic causes as syncope or TIA is higher.
2. Prolonged EKG or video–EEG monitoring may be required. Among sleep disorders, REM behavior disorder is a parasomnia that is much more common in the elderly, and is often associated with extrapyramidal movement disorders; polysomnography is required for diagnosis.

TREATMENT

1. Any of the traditional or newer AEDs discussed earlier may be used in the elderly population, but starting doses should be lower and doses should be increased more slowly.
2. In patients on anticoagulants or other drugs whose metabolism is altered by enzyme inducers, such AEDs as PHT and CBZ must be used with caution, particularly those with cardiac rhythm disturbances. Susceptibility to CNS adverse effects of barbiturates or benzodiazepines argues against using these agents when alternatives exist.
3. In patients taking multiple drugs for other conditions, AEDs with minimal drug-drug interactions, such as GBP, LTG, or LEV, should be strongly considered; drugs such as GBP and LEV that are principally metabolized by the kidney should be dosed according to renal function.

STATUS EPILEPTICUS

BACKGROUND

1. Status epilepticus (SE) is the most common neurologic emergency, affecting 50,000 to 200,000 in the United States annually.
2. It is usually defined as 30 or more minutes of continuous or recurrent seizures without recovery to baseline function, although some have argued for a lower cutoff of 5 to 10 minutes because most tonic–clonic seizures end within 1 to 2 minutes.
3. While any type of seizure can evolve into SE, the most important and common type is generalized convulsive SE, in which the tonic–clonic seizures can be either primarily or secondarily generalized. Other important types include complex partial SE, absence SE, myoclonic SE, and epilepsia partialis continua.

PATHOPHYSIOLOGY

1. SE reflects a failure of the usual seizure-terminating mechanisms. Why this happens only under some circumstances is not well understood.
   a. Mechanisms of neuronal injury include hypoxia–ischemia and excitotoxicity. The latter can result in neuronal death even if oxygenation and blood flow are

maintained; in animal models, a cascade of events culminating in neuronal loss occurs after 30 to 60 minutes of continuous seizures.

   b. Systemic derangements that can predispose to neurologic injury include hypotension (usually following initial hypertension), combined lactic and respiratory acidosis, cardiac arrhythmia or infarction, hyperthermia, and renal injury from rhabdomyolysis.

2. Any of the causes of acute symptomatic seizures can lead to SE. These include drug withdrawal or intoxication, metabolic derangements, head trauma, CNS infection, cardiac arrest, or stroke.

   a. SE can occur in patients with preexisting epilepsy of any cause, particularly if seizures are not well controlled or AEDs are not being taken or absorbed properly.

   b. Especially in children, SE can be the first presentation of idiopathic or cryptogenic epilepsy.

PROGNOSIS

1. The prognosis of generalized convulsive SE varies with age, etiology, and duration.

2. Mortality ranges from 2% to 3% in children to above 30% in adults, especially the elderly.

   a. Anoxic injury carries the highest mortality and alcohol or AED withdrawal the lowest.

   b. Duration of convulsive SE beyond 1 to 2 hours is associated with a mortality increase of approximately 20%.

3. Neurologic morbidity is more difficult to demonstrate than mortality but undoubtedly occurs in relation to etiology and probably duration of SE as well.

DIAGNOSIS

1. The diagnosis of generalized convulsive SE should be suspected when any patient has a witnessed convulsion and does not begin to arouse within minutes, particularly when a subsequent convulsion occurs.

   a. The condition should be distinguished from repetitive seizures, when the patient awakens between them. Although such seizure clusters may evolve into SE and need to be treated, urgency is less than with ongoing SE.

   b. As convulsive SE progresses, motor activity can become attenuated, and diagnosis is then dependent on obtaining a history of earlier convulsions, supported by ictal EEG findings.

   c. Psychogenic nonepileptic seizures, or pseudoseizures, can in some cases be prolonged and difficult to distinguish from generalized convulsive SE, but hypoxemia, rise in creatine phosphokinase level, and acidosis typically occur after convulsive seizures and their absence should raise suspicion. Avoidance behavior or other signs of awareness should be sought on examination; EEG may be required in some cases.

   d. In comatose patients, flexor or extensor posturing can occur, and paroxysmal sympathetic storm, sometimes called diencephalic seizures, also has a nonepileptic basis and responds to opiates, dopaminergic agents, or autonomic blockers but not to AEDs.

2. EEG is commonly needed to diagnose less common forms of SE, such as complex partial, absence, or postanoxic myoclonic SE.

   a. Complex partial SE typically occurs in those with a preexisting history of partial epilepsy, but it may be the initial presentation of epilepsy or of an acute neurologic insult. Clinically, there is prolonged clouding of consciousness, usually with cycling over minutes corresponding to ictal and postictal phases of discrete complex partial seizures.

   b. In absence SE, or spike–wave stupor, there is nearly continuously diminished responsiveness with bilaterally synchronous spike–wave discharges on EEG. Although the sensorium is clouded, the degree of impairment may be quite subtle. It may also present as an acute confusional state in adults or, rarely, as a psychotic disorder.

c. Myoclonic SE occurs most commonly and most ominously after a hypoxic-ischemic insult, and can present as massive or more subtle, variably rhythmic jerks; EEG typically shows a relatively flat background with polyspikes and artifact corresponding to the jerks.

d. Epilepsia partialis continua is a form of simple partial SE consisting of nearly continuous limb jerking that may be quite distal and subtle. It is associated often with structural lesions, or in the specific pediatric syndrome of Rasmussen encephalitis, with a unihemispheric progressive inflammatory disorder.

TREATMENT

1. Because of the risk of significant morbidity and mortality with prolonged SE, a preestablished time-based treatment protocol is recommended. The following incorporates elements of several published protocols:

   0–10 minutes: Assess and support cardiorespiratory function. Give nasal oxygen (O_2) and insert airway if necessary. Obtain history (especially duration of seizures, prior seizures, drugs, etc.) and perform physical and neurologic examinations. Insert IV (normal saline) and draw blood for antiepileptic blood levels, toxic screen, CBC, glucose, electrolytes including calcium and magnesium, and hepatic and renal function tests. Give thiamine 100 mg and 50 mL of 50% glucose IV. Call for EEG monitoring but do not delay treatment.

   11–30 minutes: Give LZ at 1 to 2 mg/min up to 0.1 mg/kg. Alternatively, DZ may be given at 2 to 4 mg/min up to 20 mg. (Be prepared to assist ventilation immediately when pushing benzodiazepines.) Simultaneously or immediately after, begin PHT infusion through a separate IV at 50 mg/min, or fos-PHT at 150 mg PHT equivalents/min, to 20 mg/kg. In patients known or suspected to be on AEDs, do not wait for levels before beginning infusion. Monitor ECG and blood pressure. Treat fever with antipyretics and cooling.

   31–60 min: If seizures persist, give additional 5 to 10 mg/kg PHT or fos-PHT. If ineffective, give PHB at 50 to 100 mg/min to maximum of 20 to 25 mg/kg. Alternative is IV VPA 20 to 30 mg/kg over 5 to 10 minutes. Some would skip this step and, after intubation and while recording EEG, proceed directly to:

   Above 60 minutes: Barbiturate anesthesia with pentobarbital, 5 to 15 mg/kg load given at 25 mg/min until burst-suppression appears or epileptiform activity is clearly suppressed. Maintain 0.5- to 5-mg/kg/h drip for at least several hours before tapering to look for seizure recurrence. If seizures recur, give 50-mg bolus and increase drip by 0.5 to 1.0 mg/kg/h. Alternatives include PHB in 5- to 10-mg/kg boluses given at 20-minute intervals; midazolam as a loading dose of 0.15 to 0.20 mg/kg followed by infusion of 0.05 to 0.30 mg/kg/h; or propofol given as a 1- to 3-mg/kg bolus over 5 minutes, repeated if necessary, followed by maintenance infusion of 2 to 4 mg/kg/h, which can be increased as needed after boluses up to 15 mg/kg/h as blood pressure permits.

2. The drug used to induce coma should be weaned after 1 to 2 days, while maintaining high therapeutic levels of phenytoin (18–30 mg/L) and/or phenobarbital (25–50 mg/L) and/or VPA (70–120 mg/L) during anesthesia infusion to protect against recurrent seizures during taper.

3. Hypotension during infusion of any of the above drugs should be treated by slowing or stopping the infusion and giving fluids and pressors as needed. Administration of sodium bicarbonate may be necessary to prevent circulatory collapse for severe acidosis, but overcorrection should be avoided because alkalosis renders neurons hyperexcitable and mild acidosis may be protective.

4. Thiopental has also been suggested as an alternative to pentobarbital, but may have more cardiovascular side effects and less predictable pharmacokinetics. Use of inhalation anesthetics (halothane, isoflurane) is controversial, and cannot be done without anesthesiology assistance.

5. Treatment for other forms of SE depends on the balance between risks of the specific seizure type and risks of treatment, especially if taken to the point of intubation and prolonged stay in the intensive care unit.

    a. For complex partial SE and epilepsia partialis continua, PHT, PHB, and VPA may be used, as can any of the other AEDs useful against partial seizures or the broad-spectrum AEDs; CBZ, OXC, GBP, and LEV in particular may be given orally or through a nasogastric or gastric tube and built up to therapeutic doses relatively rapidly.

    b. Drug-induced coma is typically not used unless the patient's level of consciousness continues to decline despite treatment.

    c. For true absence SE, broad-spectrum drugs, particularly VPA, should follow benzodiazepines; drugs specific for partial seizures can be tried in adults without a history of generalized epilepsy, since a similar syndrome can sometimes represent a secondarily generalized event.

    d. Epilepsia partialis continua is often refractory to the above AEDs, but may respond to FBM.

    e. In the special case of Rasmussen encephalitis, case reports have shown at least transient benefit with immune globulin or plasmapheresis, but the surgical procedure of hemispherectomy may be needed, especially if function of the contralateral upper extremity has already been lost.

    f. Postanoxic myoclonic SE may respond to benzodiazepines or VPA, and a relatively nonsedating AED such as PHT may be given to prevent tonic–clonic seizures, but there is little evidence that an already poor prognosis can be altered by AED treatment.

6. In general, proper diagnosis and treatment of SE offer both a challenge and an opportunity to avoid iatrogenic complications and improve patient outcome.

BIBLIOGRAPHY

Annegers JF, Hauser WA, Lee JR, et al. Incidence of acute symptomatic seizures in Rochester, Minnesota, 1935–1984. *Epilepsia* 1995;36:327–333.

Berg AT, Shinnar S. The risk of seizure recurrence following a first unprovoked seizure: a quantitative review. *Neurology* 1991;41:965–972.

Bromfield E, Henderson G. Seizures and cerebrovascular disease. In: Ettinger AB, Devinsky O, eds. *Managing epilepsy and co-existing disorders.* Boston: Butterworth-Heinemann, 2001:269–290.

Browne TR, Holmes GL. *Handbook of epilepsy,* 2nd ed. Philadelphia: Lippincott Williams & Wilkins, 2000.

Browne TR, Holmes GL. Epilepsy. *N Engl J Med* 2001;344:1146–1151.

Commission on Classification and Terminology of the International League Against Epilepsy. Proposal for the revised clinical and electroencephalographic classification of epileptic seizures. *Epilepsia* 1981;22:489–501.

Commission on Classification and Terminology of the International League Against Epilepsy. Proposal for the revised classification of epilepsies and epileptic syndromes. *Epilepsia* 1989;30:389–399.

Deray M, Resnick T, Alvarez L. *Complete pocket reference for the treatment of epilepsy.* Miami: C.P.R. Educational Services, 2001.

Devinsky O. Patients with refractory seizures. *N Engl J Med* 1999;340:1565–1570.

D'Onofrio G, Rathlev NK, Ulrich AS, et al. Lorazepam for the prevention of recurrent seizures related to alcohol. *N Engl J Med* 1999;340:915–919.

Engel J Jr, Pedley TA, eds. *Epilepsy: a comprehensive textbook.* Philadelphia: Lippincott-Raven, 1998.

Engel J Jr. Current concepts: surgery for seizures. *N Engl J Med* 1996;10:647–652.

First Seizure Clinical Trial Group. Randomized clinical trial on the efficacy of antiepileptic drugs in reducing the risk of relapse after a first unprovoked generalized tonic-clonic seizure. *Neurology* 1993;43:478–483.

Hauser WA, Annegers JF, Kurland LT. Incidence of epilepsy and unprovoked seizures in Rochester, Minnesota: 1935–1984. *Epilepsia* 1993;34:453–468.

Heck C, Helmers SL, DeGiorgio CM. Vagus nerve stimulation therapy, epilepsy, and device parameters: scientific basis and recommendations for use. *Neurology* 2002;59[6 Suppl 4]:S31–S37.

Kwan P, Brodie MJ. Early identification of refractory epilepsy. *N Engl J Med* 2000;342:314–319.

Leppik I. *Contemporary diagnosis and management of the patient with epilepsy,* 5th ed. Newtowne, PA; Handbooks in Health Care, 2001.

Lowenstein DH, Alldredge BK. Current concepts: status epilepticus. *N Engl J Med* 1998;338:970–976.

Medical Research Council Antiepileptic Drug Withdrawal Study Group. Randomized study of antiepileptic drug withdrawal in patients in remission. *Lancet* 1991;337:1175–1180.

Morrell MJ. Guidelines for the care of women with epilepsy. *Neurology* 1998;51[Suppl. 4]:S21–S27.

Pellock JM. Treatment of seizures and epilepsy in children and adolescents. *Neurology* 1998;51[Suppl 4]:8–14.

Schmidt D. The clinical impact of new antiepileptic drugs after a decade of use in epilepsy. *Epilepsy Res* 2002;50:21–32.

Theodore WH, Porter RJ, Albert P, et al. The secondarily generalized tonic-clonic seizure: a videotape analysis. *Neurology* 1994;44:1403–1407.

Wiebe S, Blume WT, Girvin JP, et al. A randomized, controlled trial of surgery for temporal-lobe epilepsy. *N Engl J Med* 2001;345:311–318.

Working Group on Status Epilepticus. Treatment of convulsive status epilepticus. *JAMA* 1993;270:854–859.

Wyllie E, ed. *The treatment of epilepsy: principles and practice.* Philadelphia: Lippincott, Williams, & Wilkins, 2001.

3. DIZZINESS

Robert W. Baloh

DIZZINESS

BACKGROUND

Description

1. Dizziness is a sensation of altered orientation in space.
2. Dizziness can be caused by many different pathophysiologic mechanisms.

History

1. Describe the sensation.
2. How it began.
3. How long it lasts.
4. How frequently it occurs.
5. Circumstances that induce it.
6. Associated symptoms.
7. Medications.

Classification (Common Subtypes)

1. Presyncope (near-faint dizziness): A light-headed sensation, the sensation one experiences before losing consciousness or fainting.
2. Psychophysiologic dizziness: Feeling of dissociation, as though one has left one's own body. Patients use terms such as "floating" or "swimming."
3. Disequilibrium: Patients may use the term "dizzy" to describe a sensation of imbalance that occurs only when they are standing or walking and is unrelated to an abnormal head sensation.
4. Vertigo: An illusion of movement, usually that of rotation although patients occasionally describe a sensation of linear displacement or tilt.

Epidemiology

1. Dizziness is common in all settings and patient groups.
2. Dizziness tends to be more common in women than in men.
3. The prevalence of dizziness increases with age.
4. Presyncope and vertigo represent the most common dizziness subtypes, each occurring in about a third of patients with dizziness.

PATHOPHYSIOLOGY

1. Presyncope (near-faint dizziness): The mechanism of presyncope is reduced blood flow to the entire brain. When the cerebral blood flow is partially reduced, patients experience light-headedness; when there is a greater reduction, syncope occurs.
   a. Cardiac arrhythmias produce spontaneous episodes of presyncope that can occur in any position and can be associated with other cardiac symptoms including chest pain and palpitations.
   b. Orthostatic hypotension is usually due to acute blood loss, volume depletion, and diuretics or antihypertensive medications. When the patient

stands, gravitational pooling of blood occurs in the limbs and splanchnic vasculature.

  c. Vasovagal, or neurally mediated presyncope, typically occurs when the patient is standing but, unlike orthostatic hypotension, the blood pressure is not necessarily reduced immediately upon standing. The mechanism is not fully understood but begins with an afferent signal from the arterial visceral mechanoreceptors.

  d. Hyperventilation causes presyncope by lowering the carbon dioxide content of the blood, thus producing constriction of the cerebral vasculature.

2. Psychophysiologic dizziness: The mechanism of psychophysiologic dizziness is poorly understood but it is believed to result from impaired central integration of sensory signals. Associated symptoms of acute and chronic anxiety are common.

3. Disequilibrium: Disequilibrium can result from loss of peripheral sensory input (most often vestibular, proprioceptive, or visual) or from central lesions involving the motor centers of the basal ganglia, cerebellum, and cortex.

4. Vertigo: Vertigo indicates an imbalance in vestibular tone. It can result from loss of peripheral input caused by damage to the labyrinth or vestibular nerve or it can be caused by a unilateral impairment of vestibular nuclear or vestibulocerebellar activity.

  a. Benign positional vertigo (also called "benign paroxysmal positional vertigo") is by far the most common cause of vertigo. It results from free-floating calcium carbonate crystals (normally attached to the utricular macule) that inadvertently enter the long arm of the posterior semicircular canal. With positional change, the crystals move within the endolymph and displace the cupula.

  b. Acute peripheral vestibulopathy (vestibular neuritis) occurs in epidemics, may affect several members of the same family, and more often erupts in the spring and early summer. All of these factors suggest a viral origin and pathologic studies showed atrophy of one or more of the vestibular nerve trunks, most consistent with an infectious or postinfectious process.

  c. Ménière syndrome: The principle pathologic finding is an increase in the volume of the endolymph associated with distention of the entire endolymphatic system (endolymphatic hydrops). Ruptures of the membranous labyrinth might explain the sudden episodes characteristic of the syndrome.

  d. Migraine: Vasospasm or an inherited metabolic defect could explain the commonly associated episodic vertigo.

  e. Vertebrobasilar insufficiency (VBI) is usually caused by atherosclerosis of the subclavian, vertebral, and basilar arteries. Vertigo is also common with infarction of the lateral brainstem or cerebellum.

  f. Cerebellar pontine angle tumors grow slowly, allowing the vestibular system to accommodate so that they usually produce a vague sensation of disequilibrium rather than acute vertigo.

PROGNOSIS

1. Presyncope
  a. Usually benign.
  b. Some cardiac causes may be life threatening.
  c. Orthostatic hypotension associated with degenerative neurologic diseases, such as Shy–Drager and Parkinson disease, can be severely disabling.

2. Psychophysiologic dizziness
  a. Often persists for many years.
  b. Can recur after long periods of remission.
  c. Typically is present throughout the day.
  d. Intensity varies with stress level.
  e. Associated panic and phobic symptoms can lead to agoraphobia.

3. Disequilibrium
  a. Peripheral sensory loss (vestibular, proprioceptive, or visual) tends to be mild, leading to a cautious gait, but patients remain mobile.
  b. Central causes, such as cerebellar infarction or degeneration, lead to a more profound gait disorder that is only minimally compensated over time.

4. Vertigo
   a. Benign positional vertigo (BPV) will typically have spontaneous remissions after weeks to months, but most patients will have recurrences. The incidence of BPV increases with age.
   b. Acute peripheral vestibulopathy (vestibular neuritis) is usually a monophasic illness with onset over a few hours, gradual clearing over several days, and return to baseline after a few weeks.
   c. Ménière syndrome is characterized by recurrent episodes of fluctuating hearing loss, tinnitus, and vertigo, typically lasting several hours. The natural course is for a progressive unilateral loss of hearing over several years to reach a "burnt out" stage where the episodes of vertigo subside.
   d. Migraine: Episodic vertigo occurs in about a fourth of patients. The vertigo attacks can occur during the headache, before the headache, or more often, completely independent of headache. The typical duration is from minutes to hours and the attacks will occur at irregular intervals over many years.
   e. VBI is typically abrupt in onset, usually lasting for several minutes and is usually associated with other neurologic symptoms. It can be the prodrome of infarction in the brainstem or cerebellum.
   f. Tumors in the cerebellar pontine angle are usually associated with mild dizziness and disequilibrium and are not progressive unless the tumor becomes large enough to compress the brainstem or cerebellum.

DIAGNOSIS

1. Presyncope
   a. Orthostatic hypotension: A documented drop in mean blood pressure of more than 10 to 15 mm Hg when the patient moves from a lying to standing position.
   b. Cardiac arrhythmias: Any patients with episodic presyncope of unknown cause should undergo electrocardiogram (ECG) monitoring to search for sinus pauses, sinus bradycardia, atrial fibrillation, and sustained supraventricular tachycardia.
   c. Vasodepressor presyncope: Characteristic history in a patient without neurologic or cardiovascular disease.
   d. Hyperventilation: Characteristic associated symptoms in the setting of anxiety dyspnea.
2. Psychophysiologic dizziness
   a. Associated symptoms of acute and chronic anxiety.
   b. Patients may focus on the somatic symptoms, especially the dizziness and autonomic symptoms rather than the intense anxiety associated with the attacks.
3. Disequilibrium
   a. The broad-based ataxic gait of cerebellar disorders is readily distinguished from the milder gait disorder seen with vestibular or sensory loss.
   b. Bilateral vestibular loss may or may not be associated with hearing loss. The diagnosis rests on finding decreased or absent response to caloric and rotational stimulation.
4. Vertigo
   a. BPV: A burst of torsional vertical nystagmus is induced by rapidly moving the patient from the sitting to head-hanging position (the Dix–Hallpike test). There are typically a few seconds of latency and fatigue with repeated positioning.
   b. Vestibular neuritis: Characteristic clinical profile (spontaneous prolonged vertigo that gradually resolves over days), examination findings consistent with a unilateral peripheral vestibular loss (spontaneous nystagmus and positive head thrust test), and absence of associated neurologic symptoms and signs.
   c. Ménière syndrome: Document fluctuating hearing levels (particularly in the low frequencies) in a patient with the characteristic episodes of vertigo.
   d. Migraine: Diagnosis of exclusion in the patient with long-standing recurrent attacks of vertigo, normal hearing, and headaches that meet the International Headache Society (IHS) criteria.

  e. VBI: Comes on abruptly without any apparent precipitating factor, lasts for a few minutes, then ends abruptly. There are nearly always associated symptoms such as visual loss, diplopia, dysarthria, weakness, or numbness.
  f. Brainstem infarction: Stroke syndromes involving the posterior circulation are usually easily identified on the basis of their characteristic combination of neurologic symptoms and signs.
  g. Cerebellar infarction: Can masquerade as a more benign inner ear disorder. However, profound truncal ataxia and a direction-changing, gaze-evoked nystagmus indicate a central lesion. Magnetic resonance imaging (MRI) is the procedure of choice for viewing brain structures supplied by the vertebrobasilar system.
  h. C–P angle tumors: Detailed audiometric testing followed by neuroimaging with MRI will usually lead to a definitive diagnosis. MRI with contrast is the procedure of choice because it can identify small acoustic neuromas confined to the internal auditory canal, tumors that are missed with computed tomography (CT) scanning. CT scanning may be helpful for identifying bony erosion or calcification within tumors.

TREATMENT

1. Presyncope
  a. Orthostatic hypotension
    1) Removing offending drugs or correcting the causes of blood-volume depletion will often eliminate orthostatic presyncope.
    2) In patients with autonomic insufficiency, increased salt intake can increase blood volume and elastic stockings can prevent pooling of blood in the lower extremities.
    3) In severe cases, the salt-retaining steroid fluorocortisone can expand blood volume and the α_1-adrenergic agonist midodrine can increase vascular tone.
  b. Vasovagal presyncope
    1) An explanation of the benign nature of the disorder and the mechanism is usually all that is needed to reassure the patient.
    2) Increase dietary salt and fluid intake and avoid conditions that predispose to hypotension or dehydration.
    3) A wide range of drugs including beta blockers, midodrine, serotonin reuptake inhibitors, angiotensin-converting enzyme (ACE) inhibitors, and fluorocortisone have been used but randomized placebo-controlled studies have not convincingly shown that any of these drugs are more effective than placebo. The effectiveness of placebo in controlling vasovagal presyncope and syncope in these studies indicates the importance of cortical inputs in the pathogenesis of vasovagal episodes.
  c. Cardiac disease
    1) Presyncopal dizziness associated with impaired cardiac output can be the warning sign of serious underlying cardiac disease and there is a risk for sudden death if not appropriately treated.
    2) Management of cardiac arrhythmia obviously depends on the nature of the underlying heart disease, but many patients can be helped with the insertion of a pacemaker, even if the heart disease cannot be treated.
  d. Hyperventilation
    1) Educating the patient on the vicious-cycle nature of a hyperventilation episode and reassurance regarding the benign nature of the disorder is often effective treatment.
    2) A vigorous exercise program in conjunction with supportive psychotherapy is also helpful.
    3) Pharmacologic treatment with tricyclic amines or selective serotonin reuptake inhibitors is indicated when there are associated symptoms of panic disorder. Long-term use of tranquilizers should be avoided because of the development of increased tolerance and dependency.

2. Psychophysiologic dizziness
   a. Patients with psychophysiologic dizziness need to understand that their symptoms are "real" due to physiologic changes occurring in their bodies and that the pattern of symptoms is commonly reported by other patients. They are often convinced that they have a severe neurologic disorder and that the anxiety that they have recognized is secondary to the physical disorder.
   b. Three classes of medication are commonly used in the treatment of panic disorder (tolerance and dependency can occur with aprazolam, so this drug should be used cautiously):
      1) Tricyclic amines (e.g., imipramine and desipramine)
      2) The high-potency benzodiazepines (e.g., aprazolam)
      3) The selective serotonin reuptake inhibitors (e.g., paroxetine and fluoxetine)
   c. Medications are used with supportive psychotherapy. Patients with phobic dizziness will often respond to behavioral therapy in which they are repeatedly exposed to the situations that evoke symptoms.
3. Disequilibrium
   a. Management of patients with disequilibrium due to sensory loss should improve sensory function when possible and train the brain to adjust to the sensory loss.
   b. Although most causes of peripheral neuropathy are not reversible, some are, such as those associated with autoantibodies and vitamin deficiency.
   c. Gentamicin is remarkably selective for the vestibular system so that monitoring hearing is of little use. When such drugs are used, the patient should be carefully monitored with daily examinations of gait and balance.
   d. Physical therapy programs aimed at gait-and-balance training can retrain the brain to use remaining sensory signals to compensate for the areas lost. By contrast, gait-and-balance training is of little use in patients with cerebellar lesions because the cerebellum is the key center for adapting postural reflexes.
   e. Patients with alcoholic cerebellar degeneration can stop the progression and may even show some improvement after stopping alcohol.
   f. Of the supratentorial causes of disequilibrium, Parkinson disease is often dramatically improved with L-Dopa therapy and hydrocephalus is reversed with placement of a shunt. Most can be helped by improving support with canes or a walker.
4. Vertigo
   a. Symptomatic treatment: The best therapy for acute vertigo is to eliminate the underlying cause when possible (see sections f–u below). When the pathophysiology is unknown, definitive treatment is not available, and symptoms persist, symptomatic treatment is indicated. Two general categories of drugs are used in the symptomatic treatment of vertigo—vestibular suppressants and antiemetics.
   b. Vestibular suppressants act at the level of the neurotransmitters involved in propagation of impulses from primary to secondary vestibular neurons and in the maintenance of tone in the vestibular nuclei. When taken orally, they typically take about 30 minutes to have an effect and 2 hours or more before they have a peak effect. Therefore, with severe acute vertigo, the intramuscular (IM) or even intravenous (IV) route is usually preferable. Common side effects include dryness of the mouth and sedation.
      1) Meclizine: 12.5 to 50 mg; oral, Q 8hrs as needed
      2) Dimenhydrinate: 25 to 100 mg; IM, IV, oral, suppository, Q 8hrs as needed
      3) Scopolamine: 1.5 mg; transdermal patch, Q 3 days
      4) Promethazine: 12.5 to 50 mg; IM, IV, oral, suppository, Q 8hrs as needed
      5) Lorazepam: 0.5 to 2 mg; IM, IV, oral, Q 8hrs as needed
   c. Antiemetic drugs have central dopamine and cholinergic antagonist properties and are thought to prevent nausea and vomiting by inhibiting the emetic center. Occasionally these antiemetic drugs produce serious side effects, particularly in young patients. The major reactions can be categorized symptomatically as parkinsonism, akathisia, dystonia, and dyskinesia. The latter can be acute and reversible or subacute (tardive) and prolonged or permanent.
      1) Prochlorperazine: 2.5 to 10 mg; IM, IV, oral suppository, Q 8hrs as needed
      2) Metoclopramide: 5 to 10 mg; IM, IV, oral, Q 8hrs as needed

        3) Trimethobenzamide: 100 to 200 mg; IM, IV, oral, suppository, Q 8hrs as needed

        4) Droperidol: 2.5 to 10 mg; IM, IV, Q 8hrs as needed

  d. Vestibular rehabilitation

        1) After an acute peripheral vestibular lesion, central compensation gradually evolves over several days. Even if the vestibular loss is permanent, most patients will recover.

        2) Vestibular suppressants and antiemetics may impair the compensation process so they should only be used for the first few days. As soon as vomiting ceases, the medication should be gradually withdrawn to stimulate normal compensation.

        3) Controlled studies in animals and humans have shown that an exercise program can accelerate the compensation process after an acute peripheral vestibular lesion.

  e. Sample exercises

        1) During the acute stage, when nystagmus is prominent, the patient should attempt to focus the eyes and hold them in the direction that provokes dizziness.

        2) Once the nystagmus diminishes to the point that a target can be held visually in all directions, (usually within a few days), the patient should begin eye and head coordination exercises. A useful exercise involves staring at a visual target while oscillating the head from side to side and up and down. The speed of the movement can be gradually increased, as long as the target can be kept in good focus.

        3) Target changes using combined eye and head movement to jump quickly back and forth between two widely separated visual targets.

        4) The patient should try to stand and walk while nystagmus is still present. It may be necessary to walk in contact with the wall or to use an assistant in the early stages. Slow supported turns should be made initially.

        5) As improvement occurs, head movement should be added while standing and walking. At first slow side-to-side and up-and-down movements and then fast head turns in all directions.

        6) The compensation process occurs at a variable rate, dependent on multiple factors including age, but should be nearly complete within 2 to 6 months after an acute peripheral vestibular damage. Dizziness that persists beyond this time indicates either the presence of an ongoing vestibular disorder or poor central compensation.

  f. BPV

        1) Most patients with BPV can be cured at the bedside with a simple particle-repositioning maneuver. The basic idea is to move the patient around the plane of the affected semicircular canal to allow the clot of debris to rotate around the canal and out into the utricle. The maneuver to treat the most common posterior canal variant of BPV is performed immediately after the diagnosis is confirmed with the Dix–Hallpike positioning test (Fig. 3-1).

        2) Although most patients are cured with a single particle-repositioning maneuver, the cure rate is improved by repeating the procedure until no vertigo or nystagmus occurs in any position. Occasionally, vibration applied to the mastoid region is useful, particularly if, rather than a burst of nystagmus with position change, the patient develops a slow persistent nystagmus suggesting that the debris is stuck to the wall of the semicircular canal or is attached to the cupula and not freely moving.

        3) If the patient elevates the head during the movement from one head-hanging position to the other, the particles may move back in the opposite direction, away from the utricle. It is critical that the head stays down during this phase of the positioning maneuver.

        4) When returning to the sitting position at the end of the particle-repositioning maneuver, the patient may have a brief but violent burst of vertigo as late as a few minutes after assuming the sitting position. This delayed vertigo occurs as the bolus of otolith debris drops out of the canal into the utricle.

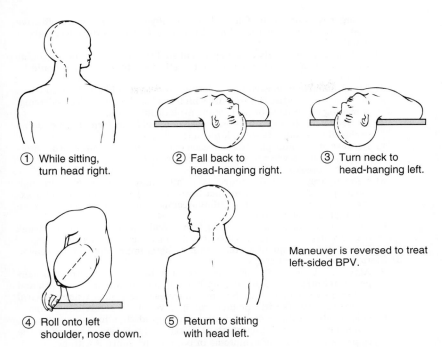

① While sitting, turn head right.

② Fall back to head-hanging right.

③ Turn neck to head-hanging left.

④ Roll onto left shoulder, nose down.

⑤ Return to sitting with head left.

Maneuver is reversed to treat left-sided BPV.

FIG. 3-1. Maneuver for treating right-sided benign positional vertigo.

g. Horizontal canal variant of BPV
  1) The patient is rolled in the plane of the horizontal semicircular canal while lying supine. The patient starts in the supine position and is rolled 90 degrees toward the normal side (the side with the lesser horizontal nystagmus), then in 90-degree steps to prone, to the abnormal side, and back to supine.
  2) Lying on the side with the healthy ear down for several hours or even overnight is also effective.
h. Home instructions
  1) Patients who have multiple recurrences of BPV can be taught to perform the particle-repositioning maneuver on their own. They can presedate themselves and often they feel more comfortable performing the maneuver in the controlled environment of their bedroom.
  2) Vibration is rarely required, but a simple neck-massage vibrator can be used if one is available.
  3) Apparently the otolithic debris cannot be cleared in some patients, explaining recurrent attacks of BPV. Such patients should be instructed to avoid extreme head-back positions (e.g., at the hairdresser or at the dentist's office), which will allow the debris to reenter the posterior semicircular canal.
i. Acute peripheral vestibulopathy (vestibular neuritis)
  1) Symptomatic treatment of the vertigo
    a) Vestibular suppressants and antiemetic drugs are effective in most patients with vestibular neuritis, but there have been few controlled studies comparing relative efficacy.
    b) Two recent randomized clinical trials comparing IV dimenhydrinate (50 mg) and lorazepam (2 mg) and IM dimenhydrinate (50 mg) and droperidol (2.5 mg) for the treatment of acute peripheral vertigo in the

emergency department found that dimenhydrinate was more effective than lorazepam and that dimenhydrinate and droperidol were about equally effective.

c) The response is clearly dose-dependent so if the initial dose of vestibular suppressant or antiemetic drug is not effective, higher doses should be tried.

d) All of the medications can be sedating, so they should not be used when performing activities that require a high level of alertness such as driving, operating machinery, or performing athletic activities.

e) Less sedating drugs such as oral meclizine and transdermal scopolamine are useful for milder vertigo later in the course.

f) Because of the multiple effects of each of these drugs, possible drug interactions should always be considered before use.

2) Vestibular exercises

a) Recovery from vestibular neuritis typically takes several weeks, although longer periods of recovery are not uncommon. The goal of vestibular exercises is to accelerate the vestibular compensation process and improve the final level of recovery.

b) In animals, compensation seems to be accelerated by stimulant drugs (e.g., amphetamine) and slowed by sedating drugs (e.g., diazepam).

c) Whether more frequent exercise leads to faster improvement is unknown.

3) Steroids and antiviral drugs

a) Acyclovir (1 g/d for 10 days) was shown to be effective in treating herpes zoster oticus (typically presenting with a combination of seventh and eighth nerve involvement), but there have been no studies using antiviral agents in patients with the more common vestibular neuritis syndrome.

b) One small placebo-controlled study suggested that high-dose steroids given for their antiinflammatory effect can significantly shorten the course and severity of symptoms in patients presenting with acute unilateral peripheral vestibulopathy.

c) Acyclovir with high-dose steroids was not better than high-dose steroids alone in managing patients with sudden deafness, the presumed auditory equivalent of vestibular neuritis. Hopefully, the results of more definitive clinical trials will be available in the near future.

j. Ménière syndrome

1) Medical management of Ménière syndrome consists of a sodium restriction diet in the range of 1 to 2 g of sodium daily with a minimum therapeutic trial of 3 months. If a good response is obtained, then the level of salt intake can be gradually increased while symptoms and signs are carefully monitored.

a) Fluid and food intake should be regularly distributed throughout the day and binges (particularly food with high sugar and/or salt content) should be avoided. Occasionally patients will notice that certain foods (e.g., alcohol, coffee, chocolate) may precipitate attacks.

b) Diuretics (hydrochlorothiazide 50 mg once or twice a day) may provide additional benefit in some patients although these drugs cannot replace a salt restriction diet. Acetazolamide (250 mg once or twice a day) has been shown to decrease the osmotic pressure of the inner ear in experimental endolymphatic hydrops in guinea pigs, but there have been no controlled studies to see how acetazolamide compares with hydrochlorothiazide or other diuretics in the treatment of Ménière syndrome.

c) Vestibular suppressants such as meclizine or promethazine are usually effective in suppressing the acute attacks of vertigo, nausea, and vomiting. The drugs should be taken as soon as possible, preferably during the prodrome if there are reliable warning symptoms. An antiemetic drug such as metoclopramide or prochlorperazine can be useful if the nausea and vomiting are severe.

d) Chronic prophylactic treatment with vestibular suppressants may be used when moderate to severe attacks recur on a frequent basis. One must balance the need to control vertigo against the need for the patient to maintain full mobility and function. In general, the stronger vestibular suppressants are more sedating and are reserved for the acute treatment of severe vertigo.

e) Vestibular exercises have a minimal role in treating patients with Ménière syndrome. This disorder is caused by a transient reversible abnormality, often with return to baseline between attacks. Although there may be a gradual progressive loss of unilateral vestibular function, it occurs slowly, typically over several years along with the central compensation process.

2) Surgery for treating Ménière syndrome

a) Shunts: Although shunting of the endolymph duct and sac are logical based on the presumed pathophysiology of Ménière syndrome, in practice these procedures have not been effective, probably because it is technically difficult to maintain an open shunt of the endolymph system.

b) Ablative surgery: Ablative procedures are most effective in patients with unilateral involvement who have no functional hearing on the damaged side. Vestibular neurectomy has the advantage of preserving hearing in a patient with residual cochlear function.

c) Gentamicin injection into the middle ear so that it enters the inner ear through the round window is a simple procedure that can be done as an outpatient and does not preclude later, more definitive surgical procedures. As noted earlier, gentamicin is remarkably selective for its vestibular ototoxicity.

k. Migraine vertigo

1) Symptomatic treatment includes analgesics, antiemetics, and antivertiginous drugs.

a) Promethazine (25 or 50 mg) is particularly effective for relief of vertigo and nausea. It has sedation as a side effect but this is usually acceptable in a patient who is eager to sleep.

b) Metoclopramide promotes normal gastric motility and may improve absorption of oral drugs.

c) Treatment of headache is dealt with in Chapter 11, Headache and Facial Pain.

2) Prophylactic treatment: The mechanism of action of these drugs in migraine is speculative; most work on an empiric basis. A trial of a migraine prophylactic agent is warranted in any patient with episodic vertigo of unknown cause who has a history of migraine headaches or a strong family history of migraine.

a) Tricyclic amines

b) Selective serotonin reuptake inhibitors

c) Beta blockers

d) Calcium channel blockers

e) Carbonic anhydrase inhibitors

l. Other peripheral cause of vertigo

m. Bacterial labyrinthitis

1) Any patient with acute or chronic bacterial ear disease associated with sudden or rapidly progressive inner ear symptoms should be hospitalized and treated with local cleansing and topical antibiotic solutions to the affected ear as well as parenteral antibiotics capable of penetrating the blood–brain barrier.

2) If the labyrinthitis is secondary to primary meningitis, it is best managed by treating the underlying meningitis. A resistant or recurrent meningitis may result from unrecognized posterior fossa epidural abscesses with dural perforation or from congenital direct communications with the cerebrospinal fluid.

3) Surgical intervention to eradicate the middle ear and mastoid infections is often required after a few days of antibiotic treatment.

n. Perilymph fistulas associated with head trauma, barotrauma, or sudden strain during heavy lifting, coughing, or sneezing

    1) Bedrest.
    2) Elevation of the head.
    3) Avoidance of straining.
    4) If symptoms persist despite bedrest, exploration of the middle ear for repair of the fistula.

o. Autoimmune inner ear disease (either in isolation or as part of a systemic autoimmune process)
    1) High-dose steroids (60 to 100 mg prednisone, 12 to 16 mg dexamethasone) maintained for 10 to 14 days and then tapered.
    2) If symptoms recur as the steroids are tapered, then more long-term immunosuppression with drugs such as methotrexate may be required.

p. Ototoxicity
    1) Prevention is the key to the management.
    2) Kidney function should be monitored when using any potentially ototoxic drug and patients in high-risk groups such as those with kidney failure should probably not be given ototoxic drugs that are excreted by the kidney.
    3) Patients should be questioned on a regular basis to identify early symptoms of vestibular loss.
    4) When the earliest effects of ototoxicity are recognized, adjustments in the dose schedule often can reduce the likelihood of developing permanent symptoms. Often other drugs can be substituted that are less ototoxic. The ototoxic effects may be reversible if the drug is stopped early enough.

q. VBI
    1) Controlling risk factors (e.g., diabetes mellitus, hypertension, hyperlipidemia)
    2) Antiplatelet drugs
    3) Anticoagulation for patients with frequent incapacitating episodes or those with symptoms and signs suggesting a stroke in evolution, particularly basilar artery thrombosis. It is also indicated in patients who continue to have recurrent transient ischemic attacks while on antiplatelet drugs.
        a) Heparin as an IV bolus of 5,000 units followed by continuous infusion of 1,000 U/h. The dosage is titrated to keep the partial thromboplastin time at approximately 2.5 times control.
        b) Warfarin is begun after 3 or 4 days with an oral dose of 5 mg/d. The daily dose is then adjusted until the international normalized ratio (INR) is between 2 and 3. Heparin is then discontinued.
        c) Intraarterial thrombolysis is an option for treatment of acute life-threatening vertebrobasilar occlusion, particularly with signs of basilar occlusion. Thrombolytics such as streptokinase, urokinase, and tissue plasminogen activator can be injected into the occluded artery after angiography reveals partial or complete occlusion. Overall reported mortality rates are still high (probably more than 50%), but dramatic recoveries are possible for a condition with an otherwise dismal prognosis.

r. Labyrinthine infarction
    1) As with other unilateral peripheral vestibulopathies, symptomatic medications can help relieve the acute vertigo and nausea.
    2) Vestibular rehabilitation exercises should be started as soon as the patient is able to cooperate.

s. Brainstem and cerebellar infarction
    1) In some select cases, intraarterial thrombolysis might be considered.
    2) Unfortunately, antivertiginous medications are less effective for controlling vertigo than for peripheral vestibular lesions, and vestibular rehabilitation exercises are usually minimally effective.

t. C–P angle tumors
    1) Observation: One might follow a patient with a small acoustic neuroma, particularly if the patient is older or has underlying medical problems. Serial MRI studies have shown that most acoustic neuromas grow slowly, if at all.

2) Surgical approaches to the C–P angle: (1) Translabyrinthine, (2) suboccipital, and (3) middle fossa. The translabyrinthine approach destroys the labyrinth but often allows complete removal of the tumor without endangering other nearby neural structures, particularly the facial nerve. The other approaches have the advantage of possibly saving residual hearing, but there is a greater risk of damage to the facial nerve.

3) Stereotactic radiosurgery using ionizing radiation provides another alternative for treating C–P angle tumors, particularly in high-risk patients. It may be ideal for managing acoustic neuromas associated with neurofibromatosis type II because eventually tumors will be bilateral in most cases.

u. Other central causes of vertigo

   1) Tumors of the cerebellum and brainstem

     a) Biopsy and surgical resection of the tumor when possible are the treatments of choice.

     b) For metastatic tumors, the primary tumor can be biopsied if it can be found.

     c) For unresectable tumors, radiation therapy is often beneficial. Prolonged survival is not uncommon with more benign astrocytomas. Medulloblastomas are very sensitive to radiation therapy.

   2) Chiari type 1 malformations, suboccipital decompression of the foramen magnum region can stop the progression and occasionally lead to improvement in neurologic symptoms and signs.

   3) Inherited ataxia

     a) Patients are encouraged to use a cane or walker to improve sensory input and to avoid falls.

     b) Regular physical therapy to maintain range of motion about all joints is critical to avoid painful contractures.

     c) A diet low in long-chain fatty acids can be effective in controlling the progression of symptoms and signs in patient with Refsum disease.

     d) Acetazolamide is often remarkably effective in relieving the episodic symptoms in patients with episodic ataxia type II and is occasionally effective in patients with episodic ataxia type I. One typically begins with a low dose (125 mg/d) and then works up to an average effective dose of between 500 and 1,000 mg/d.

BIBLIOGRAPHY

Baloh RW. *Dizziness, hearing loss and tinnitus.* New York: Oxford University Press, 1998.

Baloh RW, Honrubia V. *Clinical neurophysiology of the vestibular system,* 3rd ed. New York: Oxford University Press, 2001.

Brandt T. *Vertigo: its multisensory syndromes,* 2nd ed. London, New York: Springer-Verlag, 1999.

Hotson JR, Baloh RW. Acute vestibular syndrome. *N Engl J Med* 1998;339:680–685.

Baloh RW. Vestibular neuritis. *N Engl J Med* 2003;348:1027–1032.

Sloane PD, Coeytaux RR, Beck RS, et al. Dizziness: state of the science. *Ann Intern Med* 2001;134:823–832.

4. NECK AND BACK PAIN

Michael Ronthal

NECK PAIN

BACKGROUND

History

1. Cervical cord injury was described in ancient Egypt as "one having a disloca-tion in the vertebra of his neck while he is unconscious of his two legs and his arms and his urine dribbles—an ailment not to be treated" (Edwin Smith papyrus).
2. James Parkinson (1817) gave excellent descriptions of patients with cervical radicu-lopathy. Key in 1838 in *Guy's Hospital Reports* described a spondylotic bar at au-topsy, and 2 years later Romberg described cervical neuralgia. Victor Horsley per-formed the first successful surgery for cervical spondylosis in 1892 and in the same year, Gowers described exostoses growing from the vertebral bodies into the spinal canal that might compress cord or nerve.
3. With the development of x-ray technology, Bailey and Casamajor (1911) discussed osteoarthritis of the spine and described five patients with cervical radiculopathy. In 1932, Peet and Echols reported that the "chondroma" of previous authors was really a protrusion of the intravertebral disc. Bull correlated the radiology of osteo-phytes at the neurocentral joints of Luschka with radicular symptoms but pointed out that the absence of osteophytes cannot exclude pressure on the root due to periarticular soft tissue swelling invisible on radiographs.
4. In 1951, Frykholm distinguished nuclear herniation from annular protrusion and suggested that root sleeve fibrosis might cause root compression. In 1953, Taylor pointed out that the cord could also be compressed by hypertrophy or buckling of the ligamentum flavum.

Description

Pain in the neck and associated brachalgia is secondary to pathology or irritation of pain-sensitive structures. These are the muscles surrounding the cervical spine, bone, disc, dura, apophyseal joints, and nerve roots. On rare occasions, pain is generated within the substance of spinal cord itself. Pain generated by neck muscle spasm is often referred diffusely as a headache.

Cervical Spondylosis
1. The most common neck pathology is cervical spondylosis. Fifty percent of people older than 50 years and 75% of people older than 65 years have typical radiologic changes of spondylosis—disc space narrowing and reactive osteophytes.
2. Limitation of neck rotation is the cardinal sign and this may be seen in association with any combination of radiculopathic or myelopathic signs.

Trauma
1. Trauma can result in a variety of painful conditions. Minor injuries result in short-lived episodes of spasm and pain in the neck, but more significant injuries can cause fractures, dislocations, acute disc herniation, and soft-tissue injuries to the nerve roots and the cord itself.

2. After an acute flexion–extension injury the cord damage may be due to an intramedullary contusion or hematoma (hematomyelia) rather than extrinsic compression by disc or bone.

Inflammatory Conditions
Ankylosing spondylitis and rheumatoid arthritis may cause pain, spondylitis is a risk factor for fracture whereas rheumatoid may cause C-1 to C-2 subluxation.

Neoplasia
Mass lesions in neck structures may trigger pain by irritating pain sensitive structures.

Infection
Although rare, acute or chronic bacterial infection may cause cord compression and is both dangerous and treatable.

CERVICAL SPONDYLOSIS

PATHOPHYSIOLOGY

1. Cervical spondylosis is a disorder of the cervical spine characterized by disc degeneration, reactive osteophyte formation and spondylotic ridges, facet and uncovertebral joint arthritis, thickening of the ligamentum flavum, and sometimes ossification of the anterior longitudinal ligament as well as ligamentum flavum. There may be subluxation of the vertebral bodies due to lax ligaments.
2. The initial disc prolapse or rupture may result in an acute painful syndrome characterized by neck pain and brachalgia. This is sometimes called a "soft" disc as opposed to a "hard" disc, which refers to the chronic bony change and osteophyte formation.

Physiologic Mechanisms

1. Simple compression of nerve roots in the exit foramina by bony structures cannot be the entire pathology in that patients with radiculopathy tend to fluctuate over time. Moreover, the degree of bony change seen on imaging studies does not always correlate with the severity of the signs and symptoms.
2. There must be reversible soft-tissue pathology in the exit foramina and it is this soft tissue inflammatory reaction that responds to immobilization and allows for improvement in 80% to 90% of patients with adequate conservative treatment or perhaps just the passage of time.
3. Fixed and persistent root signs, which denote irreversible injury, may be due to local demyelination, root sleeve fibrosis, or axonal injury.

Symptoms

1. Neck pain: Irritation of nerve roots leads to reflex posterior cervical spasm resulting in local muscle tenderness and local neck pain.
2. Headache: Because of confluence of afferents (spinothalamic and quintothalamic pathways) pain may be referred to the back of the head (C-2) and more anteriorly to trigeminal innervated areas.
3. Root Pain: Pain radiates down the arm.

Dysfunction

1. Radiculopathy: The finding of clinical signs of radiculopathy is an indicator of the segmental level of pathology and the examiner should have an excellent knowledge

TABLE 4-1. CERVICAL MYOTOMES

Segmental Level	Main Testable Muscles	Muscle Action
C-4	Infraspinatus	External rotation of the shoulder
C-5	Deltoid	Shoulder abduction
	Biceps/brachioradialis	Elbow flexion
C6-7	Triceps (+lower fibers of pectoralis)	Elbow extension
C-6	Extensor carpi radialis	Radial wrist extension
C-7	Extensor digitorum	Finger extension
C-8	Flexor digitorum	Finger flexion
T-1	Interossei	Finger abduction
	Abductor digiti minimi	Little finger abduction

Note: This is a simplified schema designed to help with root localization. Muscles by and large have innervation from multiple segments and this table, while being clinically useful, is not meant to be strictly anatomically correct.

of the various dermatomes, myotomes, and the segmental levels of the tendon reflexes in the upper limbs (Table 4-1).

2. Myelopathy: A good practical approach to cord pathology is to consider it in terms of treatment:
   a. The appellation "medical myelopathy" refers to pathology in the cord that does not require surgical intervention.
   b. "Surgical myelopathy" refers to cord dysfunction on a mechanical basis for which surgical intervention is helpful or curative. The individual pathology plays a major role in decision making and the rapidity with which treatment is offered is of great importance. The presence of bladder dysfunction lends a sense of urgency, and prolonged urinary retention without adequate treatment is a poor prognostic sign.

Cord Compression

Extrinsic cord compression is the most common cause of central cord dysfunction.
1. Acute cord compression: Compression of the spinal cord can cause dysfunction of any component of the cord at that level. Thus, any combination of partial or complete long-tract dysfunction may be seen, the segmental level is signaled by the root dysfunction.
2. Chronic cord compression:
   a. Although it is easy to understand deficits of function in the presence of acute large disc herniations, myelopathy in chronic cervical spondylosis is more difficult to explain. It is seen particularly in those individuals with a congenitally narrow spinal canal. A posteroanterior diameter of 14 to 15 mm as measured by radiograph predisposes to myelopathy and spinal dimensions measured in patients with a spondylotic myelopathy range from 7 to 17 mm. Osteophytic ridging anteriorly and hypertrophy of the ligamentum flavum posteriorly results in a pincer effect on the cord, particularly with flexion–extension movements. Massive osteophytes and ligamentous hypertrophy will sometimes compress the cord even in the absence of congenital spinal stenosis.
   The degree of cord compression as seen on imaging studies does not necessarily correlate with the clinical signs of myelopathy. Myelopathic signs wax and wane in the absence of observable changes on the imaging studies. Decompression of the spinal cord does not always halt progression of spondylotic cervical myelopathy. Simple mechanical compression cannot therefore be the whole story.
   b. Various explanations have been offered including vascular compromise, intermittent subluxation, impingement of the spinal cord on anterior ridges with

flexion movements, and friction as the cord moves, albeit slightly, cranially and caudally with head flexion–extension movements. Lastly, it has been posited that a tight spinal canal and its contents may interfere with venous return from the cord (drainage is upward) and resultant venous congestion and stagnant hypoxia may play a role in myelopathy and, in particular, may be a factor causing wasting and weakness of the intrinsic muscles of the hands indicating dysfunction a few segments below the usual levels of mechanical compression.

PROGNOSIS

Although spondylosis is very common, there are no reliable data about the natural history that could be used to assess treatment for any grade of severity or complication, either conservative or invasive. In general, it is thought that a spondylotic myelopathy is a disease with a lengthy clinical course marked by long periods of nonprogressive disability. Neck pain waxes and wanes. In spondylotic radiculopathy, longitudinal studies suggest that the symptoms resolve in time and in one study, 90.5% of patients with cervical radiculopathy were asymptomatic or only mildly affected after a mean follow-up period of almost 6 years.

DIAGNOSIS

Symptoms

1. Local pain:
   a. Pain is usually felt at the back of the neck and is often worse in the morning on arising, whatever the pathology. The pain may be referred diffusely to the head including the frontal region, even the orbits and occasionally the face. It is variously described as constant, aching, a feeling of pressure or weight on top of the head, or as a tight constricting band around the head. It is aggravated by head and neck twisting, flexion, or extension. Patients often report that they awaken with pain, heat helps, and the pain dissipates in the warm shower.
   b. Referred pain from muscle spasm does not throb.
   c. Brachalgia precipitated by or aggravated by shoulder movements reflects local pathology in the shoulder rather than the neck, although neck and shoulder pathology may coincide.
2. Radicular pain: Radicular involvement causes referred pain in the distribution of the root and pain may radiate down the arm and even into the fingers. Radiation to the thumb and index finger suggests C-6 origin. The pain is usually described as deep and aching, but can be sharp and lancinating and sharp episodes may be triggered by neck movement. There may be tingling or numbness in the arm.
3. Myelopathic symptoms: Involvement of the spinal cord may result in a complaint of gait disorder or the patient may be aware of weakness in the lower limbs. Urgency of micturition and urgency with incontinence signals the development of upper motor neuron bladder dysfunction and indicates the presence of a small contracted spastic bladder.

Signs

1. Local neck signs: The clinical diagnosis of cervical spondylosis is made on the finding of restricted neck movement. Normal neck movement will allow for rotation such that the chin approximates the point of the shoulder, less than that is due to osteoarthritis of the cervical spine. There may be associated palpable posterior cervical muscle spasm and local tenderness of the muscles to even light palpation.
2. Radicular signs: Radicular signs include myotomal weakness (Table 4-1), dermatomal sensory loss for pinprick temperature or light touch, and perhaps a dropped reflex. In cervical spondylosis, the biceps or triceps reflexes may be increased in the face of root (lower motor neuron) weakness because of associated cord involvement.

3. Myelopathic signs: Extrinsic cord compression can result in any combination of central cord or long-tract dysfunction.
4. Central cord syndrome: The most common cause of dissociated sensory loss (loss of pinprick and temperature sensation with preserved touch, vibration sense, and position sense) in the upper limbs is cervical spondylosis, although occasional patients will have primary central cord pathology.
5. Motor only syndrome: In the lower limbs, there may be spasticity, weakness, or hyperreflexia with or without extensor plantar responses.
6. Sensory syndrome
   a. On the sensory side, pinprick loss may involve any distribution in the lower limbs; occasionally, there is a pseudoradicular band pattern on the abdomen. Vibration sense is frequently absent from the costal margins distally. Loss of position sense is as significant for gait disorder as weakness or spasticity.
   b. In myelopathy, only the finding of clear pointers to a root level indicates the segmental level of dysfunction.
7. Bladder syndrome: Bladder symptoms may present early or late. Frequency, urgency, and urgency incontinence indicate a small spastic contracted bladder secondary to upper motor neuron dysfunction.
8. Mixed syndrome: Any combination of the above.

Diagnostic Tests

1. Magnetic resonance imaging (MRI)
   a. Imaging is done not only to prove the diagnosis but also to exclude other pathology. MRI is the best modality. The degree of change seen on imaging does not necessarily correlate exactly with the severity of the clinical presentation and a good deal of degenerative change may be silent. Conversely, the physical signs may reflect relatively mild changes on MRI. In patients with severe pain and radiculopathy, even in the absence of myelopathy imaging is indicated to define the pathology. In patients with mild or even moderate but controllable pain without myelopathy, it is reasonable to delay imaging for a few weeks to see if the situation resolves itself, which it often does. Most patients will have spondylosis or an acute disc prolapse compressing a nerve root. An occasional mass lesion other than disc will require surgical intervention in its own right, and negative scan findings suggest a "medical" radiculopathy—if zoster is suspected, an antiviral agent is indicated.
   b. Myelopathy: In cervical spondylosis the finding of signs of myelopathy indicates imaging of the cervical spine.
   c. Pain: In patients with severe pain in the neck with or without radiculopathy in whom the diagnosis of cervical spondylosis seems unlikely either because of age or associated systemic signs, MRI is imperative.
2. Radiographs
   a. When the MRI findings are relatively mild as compared to the physical signs related to cord dysfunction, flexion–extension radiographs of the cervical spine should be done to exclude subluxation. No more than 3-mm shift should be seen in so-called stress views.
   b. When the clinical picture is very much that of spondylosis and radiculopathy without associated complicating systemic disease, it is reasonable to treat and image in a few weeks if there is no response to conservative management.
3. Computed tomography (CT): If MRI is not available or contraindicated, CT scanning and plain radiographs for bony pathology may help with the diagnosis.
4. Myelography: Myelography is seldom necessary but is still done in the occasional patient with a cardiac pacemaker in whom MRI is contraindicated. It may be combined with CT.
5. Spinal tap: In cases of myelopathy where the imaging findings are negative, the spinal fluid should be examined for infection, inflammation, or a neoplastic process, and blood studies should be pursued to exclude systemic disease.
6. Electromyogram (EMG) and nerve conduction (NC) studies: EMG and NC studies

may confirm muscle denervation, localize the problem to root, or reveal peripheral entrapment as a complicating pathology (double crush).

Differential Diagnosis

Although cervical spondylosis is the most common cause of neck and arm pain, one should be aware of other causes of radiculopathy and myelopathy. Again, division into "medical" and "surgical" pathologies guides rational thinking.

1. Medical pathology: On the medical side, one should consider inflammatory processes causing myelitis including demyelination, viral infection such a zoster, granulomatous disease such as tuberculosis or sarcoidosis, and Luetic disease. Carcinomatous meningitis is an occasional cause. Today one always includes human immunodeficiency virus (HIV) and its complications as a possible cause of unusual neurologic presentations.

2. Surgical pathology: Surgical disease in the spine may compress the roots or the cord itself and although the most common cause of mechanical compression of these structures is cervical spondylosis or cervical disc prolapse, the differential diagnosis includes benign or malignant tumors, either primary or secondary compressing the cord, and bacterial infections—epidural abscess. Primary intramedullary pathology is rare but dissociated sensory loss suggests syringomyelia, which may be amenable to surgical intervention. Primary intramedullary gliomas are rare in adults, but an occasional lymphoma causes myelopathy.

TREATMENT

The various modalities of treatment for cervical spondylosis have not been validated in controlled trials so that it is impossible to practice evidence-based medicine (Table 4-2). There is no evidence, and in the absence of evidence, we rely on experience and clinical intuition.

Local Symptoms

1. Pillows: Neck pain may respond to simple analgesics but is often severe and recalcitrant. During sleep, tossing and turning in the absence of support exacerbates

---

TABLE 4-2. MANAGEMENT ALGORITHM FOR NECK SYNDROME

Neck Pain Alone
1. Sleep on hard pillows
2. Sleep in a collar
3. Try local heat
4. Analgesic: acetaminophen or NSAID
5. Chronic pain: Add an antidepressant
   If no response in 2 wk: Muscle relaxant: Metaxolone 400 mg t.i.d. or diazepam 2 mg t.i.d.
   No response in a further 2 wk: imaging

Radiculopathy
   As above, but start treatment with a cervical collar at diagnosis.

Myelopathy
   Imaging: Best modality is MRI unless contraindicated.
   1. Significant cord compression—neurosurgical opinion.
   2. Mild compression and/or medical contraindication to surgery—persist with collar day and night for 2–3 wk and then long-term night use.
   3. No cord compression at all—spinal tap.

NSAID, nonsteroidal antiinflammatory drug; MRI, magnetic resonance imaging; t.i.d., three times a day.

spasm. The patient should sleep on two very firm pillows. A buckwheat husk pillow laid on a cheap feather (not down) pillow should be tried. The patient should sleep using whatever pillow and position are most comfortable. Local heat of any sort is comforting.

2. Collar: A soft cervical collar used only at night is frequently of symptomatic value, and if the pain is severe, it can be worn during the day as well. It is frequently stated by the cognoscenti that the use of the collar causes weakness of neck muscles. There is no basis for this statement, and the benefits of resting the neck far outweigh any theoretic and perhaps magical contraindications.

3. Drugs: If the above first steps fail, a muscle relaxant can be tried. An old standby is a small dose of diazepam, say 2 to 4 mg p.o. daily, but tailor-made muscle relaxant drugs are popular. Among these, metaxalone 400 mg, one to two tablets three times a day, is a little less sedating than some of the others on the market. Because the pain can be chronic, a reactive depression is common and an antidepressant is worth considering both for its psychiatric effect and for the benefits seen in all cases of chronic pain. Amitriptyline has been validated as a treatment for chronic pain, but some patients cannot tolerate the drug because of sedation and anticholinergic effects. Any of the selective serotonin reuptake inhibitor (SSRI) drugs, say citalopram 20 mg p.o. daily, often works just as well although support for its use is not documented in the literature. Narcotic analgesics are almost never necessary for neck spasm–related pain.

4. Physical therapy: Physical therapy is often prescribed. As long as the therapist restricts treatment to local heat and gentle massage, no harm will ensue. More vigorous treatment, manipulation, and exercises usually exacerbate the problem.

5. Chiropractic: Chiropractic manipulation is mentioned only to condemn it. It may be of temporary symptomatic benefit in many patients, but although rare, the complication of vertebral artery injury can be a disaster. Manipulation runs counter to the theme of rest and nonaggravation, which given time are almost always successful.

6. Pain clinics: Patients with persistent pain may benefit from a visit to the pain clinic for a cervical epidural steroid injection. Local botulinum toxin type A (Botox) injection treatment is currently being evaluated as a means of breaking the pain/muscle spasm/pain cycle.

Radiculopathy

1. Analgesia: Radiculopathic pain can be extremely severe so that the first order of business is analgesia. In general, the principle is to "use what it takes" to block the pain; if mild analgesics fail, escalate to more potent preparations and occasionally resort to narcotics. Propoxyphene preparations, tramadol, codeine, and oxycodone should be tried in succession for rapid relief. More powerful narcotics should not be withheld for severe resistant pain but if the patient becomes sedated, one has overstepped the mark.

2. Collar: The neck should be immobilized in a soft cervical collar, which minimizes irritation to the nerve root.

3. Steroids: A short burst of steroid (prednisone 60 mg daily for 4–5 days) is favored by some, but is unproven.

4. Surgery
   a. Most patients with radicular pain will improve within a week or two, but if the pain is severe and without resolution or if analgesics fail, surgery is an option. Removal of a herniated disc by anterior approach, with or without fusion) almost always cures the radicular component of the pain fairly dramatically.
   b. A recent Cochrane review records that the available small randomized trials of surgery do not provide reliable evidence on the effects of surgical intervention for cervical spondylotic radiculopathy. It is not clear whether the short-term risks of surgery are offset by any long-term benefit. In one study of 81 patients, surgically treated patients with radiculopathy experienced faster control of pain, but the long-term results were similar for conservatively treated patients.

c. In the long term, neurologic deficits due to cervical radiculopathy tend to recover spontaneously, but exercise of the limbs may hasten the process and strengthen weak muscles.

Myelopathy

There is no good epidemiologic data on the natural history of spondylotic myelopathy. Progressive disability is not inevitable; the disease can remain static for long periods, and even severe disability can improve spontaneously with time.
1. Surgery
   a. The role of surgery in spondylotic myelopathy is still unproven. There is some suggestion that it is of value in severe myelopathy (12 of 49 patients randomly allocated to surgery or conservative treatment in one study only).
   b. Rowland reviewed the literature in 1992 and reported as follows: Of 261 patients subjected to cervical laminectomy, 60% improved, 34% were unchanged, and 6% worsened. Of 385 patients subjected to anterior surgery, 52% improved, 24% were unchanged, and 23% worsened. Of 136 patients treated conservatively, 44% improved, 34% were unchanged, and 23% worsened. Perioperative morbidity varies from surgeon to surgeon, but in general death or disability can be expected in 4% to 5% of the surgical group.
   c. Since 1992, two further studies were published that do not make a case either for or against conservative versus surgical management. (Table 4-3).
2. Suggested paradigm of management: What follows is a practical guide to management based on experience, it usually "works."
   a. Image: MRI is indicated in all patients with clinical signs of myelopathy. This will define the pathology, exclude nonspondylotic patients, and guide management. If MRI is contraindicated, CT or "spiral" CT is usually sufficient for diagnosis. Very occasionally, myelography and CT/myelography will be necessary.
   b. Assess "whole patient":
      1) Take into account the age and general condition of the patient—if there is a major contraindication to surgical treatment, there is no real issue to discuss provided the diagnosis is indeed cervical spondylosis—the best management is neck immobilization with a cervical collar.
      2) Anticholinergics may be useful to control bladder symptoms.
   c. Mild to moderate cervical stenosis:
      1) For patients with mild to moderate myelopathy whose images reveal only mild cervical stenosis, advise the patient to wear a soft cervical collar during the day and at night.
      2) Resolution of the signs of myelopathy after 2 to 3 weeks indicates a more conservative approach, and the patient should continue to sleep in a cervical collar long term. Alternatively, failure of resolution would suggest a neurosurgical opinion.

TABLE 4-3. RECENT CONTRIBUTIONS: SURGICAL VERSUS CONSERVATIVE TREATMENT OF SPONDYLOTIC MYELOPATHY

Author	N and Study Description	Result
Kadanka et al. (2000)	48 patients; "mild/moderate" myelopathy; randomized	No difference
Sampath et al. (2000)	62 patients; severity not detailed; not randomized	Small benefit from surgery

From Kadanka Z, Bednarik J, Vohanka S, et al. Conservative treatment versus surgery in spondylotic cervical myelopathy: a prospective randomized study. *Eur Spine J* 2000;9:538–544, with permission. Sampath P, Bendebba M, Davis JD, et al. Outcome of patients treated for cervical myelopathy: a multicenter study with independent clinical review, *Spine* 2000;25:670–676, with permission.

   d. Severe cervical stenosis: The presence of severe cervical stenosis and cord compression on imaging together with significant clinical signs of myelopathy suggests an early surgical opinion. Severe imaging abnormalities of cervical spondylosis but with only minor clinical signs of myelopathy should be managed conservatively.

BACK PAIN

BACKGROUND

The literature on neck and arm pain is relatively sparse; papers on back pain, however, are legion. Ninety percent of the population will have, at one time or another, an episode of low back pain with or without radiation down the lower limb. Major risk factors for low back pain include lifting heavy objects (25 lb or more), driving motor vehicles, and for unknown reasons, cigarette smoking. Possible risk factors include frequent stretching, reaching, pulling, and pushing on the job. Sedentary occupations, jobs in which workers stay in one position for long periods of time, jobs requiring frequent twisting without lifting, lack of physical fitness, psychologic symptoms, and frequent participation in bowling are often quoted as risk factors, but the evidence is weak or inconsistent.

HISTORY

At the New England Surgical Society meeting in Boston in September of 1933, Mixter and Barr described surgery as a treatment for lumbar disk disease demonstrated by myelography.

PATHOPHYSIOLOGY

Lumbar Disc Degeneration

1. Anatomy: The outer ring–like circumference of the disc is called the annulus fibrosis, which is composed of concentric layers of intertwined annular collagenous bands. The central part of the disc is soft and contains cells derived from the primitive notochord. Collagen crosslinks contribute to the mechanical stability of the disc and are altered with age. The anterior and posterior longitudinal ligaments further strengthen the disc space; the posterior ligament is strongly attached to the annulus fibrosis and is frequently torn in cases of free-fragment disc herniation. The outer annulus and the posterior longitudinal ligament are innervated by the sinuvertebral nerve, which is recurrent from each dorsal root ganglion. Degenerated human lumbar discs contain more nerve tissue and are more vascular than normal discs.
2. Disc hydration: The nucleus pulposus contains proteoglycan (chondroitin and collagen) that draws water into the nucleus by osmosis. The proteoglycan and water content of the nucleus pulposus decline with age, and degenerated discs have less chondroitin sulfate, particularly in the posterior part of the disc. Disc dehydration is part of disc degeneration.
3. Disc vascularity: The disc has a low metabolic rate and receives its nutrients by diffusion from capillary beds of the cartilaginous vertebral body end plate. In disc degeneration, normal anastomotic vessels on the anterolateral surface of the disc are replaced by small tortuous vessels in the annulus. Macrophages and blood vessels are prominent in surgical specimens of herniated disc fragments. Despite its low metabolic rate, the disc matrix may be biologically active and its cells may undergo apoptosis as part of degeneration.

4. Mechanical stress: Disc degeneration is related to mechanical stress. Vertebral column stress is normally transmitted to the disc from the central part of the end-plates but in degenerative states, stress is transmitted more to the periphery, likely because of dehydration in the nucleus pulposus that accompanies aging. When intradisc pressure is increased, degenerated discs herniate at lower pressures than normal discs. Annulus elasticity is lowest in the posterolateral part of the disc.
   a. Biochemical effects of disc stress: Degenerated disc have higher levels of fibronectin, which may lead to increased proteolysis. Increases in nitrous oxide (NO), prostaglandin E2 (PGE2), and interleukin-6 (IL-6) are seen in herniated discs as well as cathepsin G.
   b. Inflammatory component: The nucleus pulposus induces an inflammatory reaction with release of cytokines. Macrophages are the most commonly found cell type in both acute and chronic disc herniation, but macrophage inflammation does not correlate with clinical outcomes in humans. Radicular pain may be, in part at least, due to an inflammatory response to the portion of the nucleus that has been extruded.

Disc Herniation

1. Definitions:
   a. Disc bulge: A symmetric extension of the disc beyond the end plate.
   b. Disc protrusion: A focal area of extension still attached to the disc. Disc herniations may be lateral, to impinge on the nerve roots as they pass through the intervertebral foramina, or central, to impinge on the cauda equina with resultant risk to bladder function.
   c. Extruded fragment: An extruded fragment of disc that is no longer attached to its source.
   d. Spondylolisthesis: A congenital defect in the pars interarticularis predisposes to spondylolisthesis usually at L-5 to S-1, which is often associated with degeneration of the disc at that interspace.
   e. Spinal stenosis: Exuberant overgrowth of osteophytes and facet joint osteoarthritis may result in narrowing of the neural canal—lumbar spinal stenosis.
   f. Lateral recess stenosis: Narrowing of the intervertebral exit foramina caused by osteoarthritis of the facet joints results in narrowing of the exit foramina—lateral recess stenosis.
2. Pain-sensitive structures: As with neck pain, we should consider the origin of pain in terms of pathology affecting the pain sensitive structures. Local pain in the back may result from irritation of bone, dura, disc, and facet joints and from resultant muscle spasm in paraspinal muscles and glutei. Impingement or irritation of nerve roots, which extend from their origin in the conus to their exit foramina, causes referred pain radiating down the lower limb.

Paraspinal Muscle Trauma/Spasm

1. Many patients give a history of back pain secondary to lifting a heavy weight or other unaccustomed strain and imaging findings, at least early on, may be negative. In patients with negative imaging results, pain often originates in the paraspinal muscles, which may be traumatized locally.
2. While primary neoplasia in the lumbar spine is rare, metastatic disease (often from the prostate) is relatively common. Occasional patients will have subacute and chronic infections in the epidural space or intrathecally, and intrathecal neoplasms causing cauda equina syndromes occasionally present.

PROGNOSIS

1. Disc degeneration can occur in the absence of pain.
2. Of patients with back pain presenting to a primary care practice setting, at least a third will persist with pain at 3 months and about 10% will still be symptomatic after a year, although 95% of patients return to their previous occupation within a

year. Failure to return to work at 3 months is a poor prognostic sign. Psychosocial factors such as level of education, job satisfaction, being a "breadwinner," and lower age have a significant impact on return to work in these patients.

Radiculopathy

1. Most patients improve spontaneously and only about 10% come to surgery.
2. Unfavorable outcome with conservative therapy is more likely in patients with disease duration of more than 30 days, increased pain on sitting, and more pain on coughing, sneezing, or straining. A positive straight leg-raising test is associated with a poor outcome. Surgery for large relatively acute discs is of immediate symptomatic value. However, even in patients with weakness, it is difficult to prove that surgical intervention is beneficial in the long term. Five years after disc herniation 50% to 60% of patients have complete relief of pain.

DIAGNOSIS

Symptoms

1. Local pain: Pain in the low back may be severe and knife-like or dull and aching. It is aggravated by movement, coughing, stooping, and straining.
2. Radicular pain
   a. When a lumbar root is irritated, the pain refers down the leg. Because the most common roots afflicted by disc herniation are L4-5 and L-5 to S-1 the pain will radiate down the lower limb in sciatic distribution from buttock to posterior thigh to calf.
   b. For L-5 radiculopathy the pain classically radiates to the big toe and for S-1 radiculopathy it radiates to the little toe. It may be felt more diffusely as a muscle ache in the calf and never gets as far as the toes. The pain is often aggravated by coughing, stooping, or straining, but in any particular patient aggravating and relieving features may be unique.
   c. High radicular pain is referred to the anterior thigh.
3. Bladder retention: Pressure on the cauda can interfere with bladder function and cause retention. On occasion severe pain can do the same, as can anticholinergic drugs. Retention of urine lends a sense of urgency to the workup and treatment and indicates immediate imaging.
4. Spinal neurogenic claudication: In patients with severe spinal stenosis, a claudication history may be the clue. Uni- or bilateral sciatica after walking a set distance with recovery on resting or stooping is suggestive. Pedal pulses should be palpated to exclude vascular claudication.

Signs

1. Mechanical: The paraspinal lumbar muscles may be in spasm and are firm and tender to palpation. There may be a "sway back" deformity. On flexion ("touch your toes"), there is loss of normal mobility and the lumbar segment is held relatively rigidly. Passive straight leg raising may be reduced on the side of the radiculopathy. Normally, it is possible to elevate the outstretched lower limb to 90 degrees above the horizontal plain. Severe limitation correlates with severe root compression. Pain in sciatic distribution on the contralateral side (crossed straight leg–raising test) suggests a more central disc protrusion. In patients with even large central disc herniations, the straight leg-raising test may be normal.
2. Neurologic
   a. Wasting: On inspection, there may be atrophy of extensor digiti minimi (EDB) on the dorsolateral aspect of the foot just distal to the ankle. It is often difficult to evaluate atrophy of the small muscles of the sole, but the calf itself may be smaller as compared to the unaffected side.
   b. Weakness: The distribution of weakness will depend on the particular root that is dysfunctional; it may be subtle or severe, even to the extent of causing foot

TABLE 4-4. LUMBAR MYOTOMES

Segmental Level	Main Testable Muscles	Muscle Action
L1-2	Iliopsoas	Hip flexion
L-3	Adductor longus	Hip adduction
	Brevis	
	Magnus	
	Minimus	
L3-4	Quadriceps	Knee extension
L-4	Tibialis anterior	Ankle extension
L-5	Extensor hallucis longus	Toe extension
	Hallucis brevis	
	Digitorum longus	
	Digitorum brevis	
	Gluteus medius	Hip abduction
L-5 to S-1	Hamstrings	Knee flexion
S-1	Gastrocnemius	
	Soleus	Ankle flexion
	Flexor digitorum brevis	Toe flexion

Note: This is a simplified schema designed to help with root localization. Muscles by and large have innervation from multiple segments and this table, while being clinically useful, is not meant to be strictly anatomically correct.

drop (Table 4-4). In patients with L-5 radiculopathy, the weakness shares the pattern of "upper motor neuron weakness" and the best clue to lower motor neuron origin is atrophy of EDB, which occurs fairly early. There is no good tendon reflex to test for L-5, but the ankle jerk is a good marker for S-1. An extensor plantar reflex clearly indicates pyramidal tract involvement, but the patient could have mixed upper and lower motor neuron signs.

c. Sensory loss: Sensory loss is usually subtle but, if present, will follow the relevant dermatomes. Sensory loss on the lateral thigh is not likely radicular, but suggests more the diagnosis of meralgia. Saddle sensory loss suggests cauda pathology. Paraspinal sensory loss is a hard marker of root dysfunction and sensation for pinprick in the paraspinal region should always be tested.

d. Sphincter dysfunction: No evaluation of back pain and sciatica is complete without a rectal examination. Assess for anal sphincter tone, the ability to contract down on command and for rectal sensation. In addition, the pelvis itself should be digitally explored.

Diagnostic Tests

1. MRI: MRI is the best study to demonstrate disc pathology and, perhaps more important, to exclude other pathologies. It should be done immediately in patients with sphincter disturbance, in patients with severe pain and a markedly reduced straight leg–raising test, and in patients with bilateral signs and symptoms. In others, the imaging can be delayed for a week or two in the hope of spontaneous recovery, which would obviate the necessity of imaging.
2. CT: Indicated if for some reason MRI is not available or is contraindicated.
3. EMG: Favored by some, this test may help to localize root dysfunction and exclude peripheral disease, but is not essential in the diagnostic armamentarium of the astute bedside clinician. Normal findings on NC studies with distal denervation signs on EMG suggest an axonal neuropathy, one cause of which could be radiculopathy. Dysfunction may be localized to a particular root by the distribution of the electric changes of nerve injury on EMG. Delayed F and H waves help with localization, an abnormal H wave supports S-1 radiculopathy, and a delayed F wave in the common peroneal nerve supports localization to L-5. Paraspinal denervation signs on EMG

indicate the root as the likely site of pathology, and is the electric counterpart of testing for paraspinal sensory loss at the bedside.

4. Lumbar puncture: In patients with significant signs and symptoms but in whom the imaging study findings do not offer an explanation, a spinal tap is indicated to search for infection and/or malignancy.

5. Myelography: An unsatisfactory invasive test that may miss far-lateral discs. It is rarely used, but can be combined with CT.

6. Discography can prove that the disc is the source of low back pain by reproducing the patient's symptoms when the disc is injected with contrast medium under fluoroscopy. The test is almost never used except in some specialized centers.

Red Flags: Emergency Imaging

1. While most back and referred root pain encountered in clinical practice are likely to be mechanical based on disc degeneration and facet joint pathology, the treating physician should be sensitized to signs and symptoms that may be secondary to disc or other pathology compressing the *cauda equina:*
   a. Night pain
   b. Bilateral referred pain down the lower limbs
   c. Bladder dysfunction
   d. Bilateral signs in the lower limbs
   e. Poor sphincter tone
   f. Boney tenderness of the spine to percussion

2. Background disease. In patients with known malignancy, diabetics, intravenous drug abusers, and in patients infected with HIV, special caution should be exercised.

Differential Diagnosis

The differential diagnosis of multiple lumbar nerve root lesions apart from disc degeneration or spinal stenosis includes congenital anomalies, primary and secondary tumors, and infections.

1. Congenital anomalies
   a. Dysraphism: Tethered cord, meningocele and intrasacral cysts, filum lipomas. The clue may be a tuft of hair in the midline.
   b. Vascular anomalies.
   c. Enterogenous cyst.

2. Primary tumors
   a. Consider chordoma, ependymoma, particularly the pseudomucinous variety, neurofibroma.
   b. Meningiomas are uncommon in this area.

3. Secondary tumors: These may arise in bone or be seeded in the subarachnoid space presenting as meningeal carcinomatosis with multiple discrete nodule in the cauda or simply thickening of the cauda.

4. Infection
   a. Bacterial infection (acute, subacute, or chronic) initially seeds the disc space, which may be destroyed by the infection, before it invades bone. An epidural abscess or granuloma may present as a cauda equina syndrome with bilateral lower limb signs and symptoms, saddle sensory loss, and sphincter disturbance.
   b. Herpes simplex and cytomegalic inclusion body virus infections can also present as cauda syndromes.

5. Look-alikes for sciatica and lower limb pain:
   a. Trochanteric bursitis: This may be the primary cause of pain even in the presence of disc degeneration and is diagnosed by the finding of point tenderness and "cured" on injecting steroid in local anesthetic into the tender area—as the anesthetic takes, the pain settles within minutes only to return within a few hours.
   b. Meralgia: Entrapment of the lateral femoral cutaneous nerve as it passes over the anterior superior iliac spine causes pain radiating to the lateral thigh, often

to the anterior thigh and sometimes to the groin. There is local tenderness at the iliac spine and a patch of decreased pinprick sensation of variable size over the lateral thigh.

TREATMENT

Evidence-based Treatment: The Cochrane Database

Over the years, various treatments have come and gone and, even now, if we are to practice evidenced-based medicine it is hard to be dogmatic that any particular form of treatment for back pain and sciatica due to disc degeneration is more effective than another or is better than supportive therapy only (Table 4-5). Current recommendations from the Cochrane database:

1. Bed rest: There is little if any difference in the effects of bed rest as compared to exercise as measured at 3 weeks in the management of sciatica. Two days of bed rest helps as much as a week of rest.
2. Exercise therapy: Exercises may be helpful for patients with chronic low back pain. No specific exercises are effective for the treatment of acute low back pain. Advise to stay active as a single treatment for back pain and sciatica. There may be a small benefit for patients with acute simple low back pain.

TABLE 4-5. MANAGEMENT ALGORITHM FOR BACK SYNDROME

Back Pain Alone or with Unilateral Root Signs and Symptoms
1. If severe: bed rest 2 d only
2. Firm mattress to sleep on
3. Analgesic: NSAID or acetaminophen; escalate to more potent preparations as needed.
    Gabapentin in escalating doses, start at 100 mg t.i.d.
4. Muscle relaxant: Metaxolone 400 mg t.i.d. or diazepam 2 mg t.i.d.
    No response after 3 wk—image
    a. If major pathology—neurosurgical opinion
    b. If minior pathology—epidural steroid injection

Bilateral Root Signs or Symptoms or Bladder Dysfunction
Image immediately with MRI (CT if MRI contraindicated)
1. MRI shows large disc herniation—neurosurgical opinion
2. MRI shows minor pathology—epidural steroid injection
3. MRI negative—spinal tap

Chronic Pain Syndrome with No Indication for Surgery after workup
1. Add antidepressant
2. If no response, refer to multidisciplinary treatment program

Indications for urgent imaging in lumbar disc syndromes
1. Bilateral signs/symptoms
2. Sphincter dysfunction
3. Unremitting pain, worse at night
4. Weight loss, history of known cancer
5. Immunosuppressed
6. IV drug abuser

Indications for back surgery in lumbar disc syndromes
1. Severe unremitting pain
2. Severe and/or progressive neurologic deficit
3. Sphincter disturbance
4. Spinal stenosis with disabling neurogenic claudication

NSAID, nonsteroidal antiinflammatory drug; t.i.d., three times a day; MRI, magnetic resonance imaging; CT, computed tomography; IV, intravenous.

3. Massage for low back pain might be beneficial for subacute and chronic nonspecific low back pain if combined with exercises and education.
4. There is no hard evidence that lumbar supports are beneficial.
5. Back schools may be effective for patients with recurrent and chronic low back pain in occupational settings.
6. Behavioral therapy may be beneficial for patients with chronic low back pain.
7. There is no evidence to support the use of transcutaneous electrical nerve stimulation (TENS) in the treatment of chronic low back pain.
8. There is no convincing evidence for injection therapy.
9. Nonsteroidal antiinflammatory drugs are effective for short-term symptomatic relief in patients with acute low back pain. No specific drug is better than another. No proof of efficacy for chronic low back pain.

Suggested Paradigm

General Measures
1. For patients with severe pain, 2 days of bed rest is worthwhile.
2. As part of rehabilitation, patients should be taught how to lift weights (with bent knees and a straight back). At a minimum, MacKenzie back exercises keep the patient aware of the possibility of injury in an unguarded moment and may provide some measure of prophylaxis. Back school is intended to help the patient to cope, to avoid excessive therapy, and to decrease the costs both for the patient and for society but does not reduce the time to return to work.

Pain Control
1. Nonsteroidals are good analgesics and may be slightly better than acetaminophen.
2. Stronger analgesia should be provided as needed in a fashion similar to that described for neck and arm pain.
3. Very occasionally narcotics may be necessary. Propoxyphene, tramadol, codeine, and codeine derivatives should be tried in succession. Gabapentin sometimes is of benefit.
4. Patients with chronic pain should be tried on antidepressant

Muscle Relaxants
Muscle relaxants are of some limited benefit for low back pain. Metaxalone 400 mg three times a day (t.i.d.) is a good start.

Steroids
For acute disc herniations, some favor a short course of high-dose prednisone (60 mg daily for 5 days), which is safe, if unproven.

Injection Treatment
1. Epidural steroid and intraarticular facet injections are unproven, but experience suggests that they are of at least temporary symptomatic value in more than 50% of patients, particularly in those with acute onset of symptoms.
2. Injection therapy should be used only when the diagnosis has been confirmed by imaging, and should be done by experienced physicians in the setting of a pain clinic. Absence of proof is not proof of absence.

Manipulation
1. Osteopathic or chiropractic spinal manipulation for acute back pain may be of some short-term symptomatic value in some patients, but is unproven in chronic low back pain. When compared with standard treatment for acute pain, it produces similar results.
2. It is not cost-effective compared to conventional supportive care, possibly because of repeated visits to the chiropractor for "adjustments."
3. Complications include fractures and precipitation of a cauda equine syndrome.

Surgery

1. Definite indications:
   a. Cauda equina syndrome with sphincter disturbance.
   b. Progressive weakness.
   c. Severe intractable pain.
   d. Spinal stenosis with neurogenic claudication may respond to epidural steroid injections for a while, but in the end decompressive surgery offers the only cure.
2. Relative indications: The treatment of patients in whom there are no definite indications for surgery is controversial. There is no scientific evidence to support the long-term effectiveness of any form of surgical decompression or fusion for degenerative lumbar spondylosis compared with natural history, placebo, or conservative treatment. The literature suggests that microdiscectomy is as good as formal laminectomy. Relook surgery carries a poor prognosis. In patients with a short history, severe pain, prominent focal signs, and a large disc herniation on imaging studies, surgery offers good immediate relief. The pain of spondylolisthesis is likely to respond to fusion.

BIBLIOGRAPHY

Cervical Spine

Adams CBT, Logue V. Studies in cervical spondylotic myelopathy. *Brain* 1971;94:587–594.

Arnasson O, Carlsson CA, Pellettieri L. Surgical and conservative treatment of cervical spondylotic radiculopathy and myelopathy. *Acta Neurochir (Wien)* 1987;84:48–53.

Bednarik J, Kadanka Z, Vohanka S, et al. The value of somatosensory- and motor evoked potentials in predicting and monitoring the effects of therapy in spondylotic cervical myelopathy: Prospective randomized study. *Spine* 1999;24:1593–1598.

Brain WR, Wilkinson M. *Cervical spondylosis and other disorders of the cervical spine.* Philadelphia: Saunders, 1967.

Fouyas IP, Statham PFX, Sandercock PAG. Cochrane review on the role of surgery in cervical spondylotic radiculomyelopathy. *Spine* 2002;27:736–747.

Kandanka Z, Bednarik J, Vohanka S, et al. Conservative treatment versus surgery in spondylotic myelopathy: a prospective randomized study. *Eur Spine J* 2000;9:538–544.

Nurick S. The natural history and the results of surgical treatment of the spinal cord disorder associated with cervical spondylosis. *Brain* 1972;95:101–108.

Ronthal M. *Neck complaints: the most common complaints series.* Boston: Butterworth-Heinemann, 2000.

Rowland LP. Surgical treatment of cervical spondylotic myelopathy: time for a controlled trial. *Neurology* 1992;42:5–13.

Sampath P, Bendebba M, Davis JD, et al. Outcome of patients treated for cervical myelopathy: a multicenter study with independent clinical review. *Spine* 2000;25:670–676.

Lumbar Spine

Akerlind I, Hornquist JO, Bjurulf P. Psychological factors in the long-term prognosis of chronic low back pain. *J Clin Psychol* 1992;48:596–605.

Andersson GB, Lucente T, Davis AM, et al. A comparison of osteopathic spinal manipulation with standard care for patients with low back pain. *N Engl J Med* 1999;341:1426–1431.

Boos N, Semmer N, Elfering A, et al. Natural history of individuals with asymptomatic disc abnormalities in magnetic resonance imaging: predictors of low back pain-related medical consultation and work incapacity. *Spine* 2000;25:1484–1492.

Carey TS, Garett JM, Jackman AM. Beyond the good prognosis. Examination of an inception cohort of patients with chronic low back pain. *Spine* 2000;25:115–120.

Cavanaugh JM, Ozaktay AC, Yamashita HT. Lumbar facet pain: biomechanics, neuroanatomy and neurophysiology. *J Biomech* 1996;29:1117–1119.

Cochrane Database of Systematic Reviews. 2002; Issue 4.

Falco FJ. Lumbar spine injection procedures in the management of low back pain. *Occup Med* 1998;13:121–141.

Nachemson A, Zdeblick TA, O'Brien JP. Lumbar disc disease with discogenic pain: what surgical treatment is most effective? *Spine* 1996;21:1835–1838.

Saal JA. Natural history and nonoperative treatment of lumbar disc herniations. *Spine* 1996;21[Suppl 24]:2S–9S.

Vucetic N, Astrand P, Guntner P, et al. Diagnosis and prognosis in lumbar disc herniations. *Clin Orthop* 1999;361:116–122.

Wheeler AH, Murrey DB. Chronic lumbar spine and radicular pain: pathophysiology and treatment. *Curr Pain Headache Rep* 2002;6:97–105.

5. SLEEP DISORDERS

John W. Winkelman and Robert B. Fogel

DISORDERS OF EXCESSIVE SOMNOLENCE

OVERVIEW

BACKGROUND

1. Disorders of excessive somnolence (DOES) are extremely common with approximately 10% of the general population reporting this symptom chronically.
2. In a recent poll from the National Sleep Foundation, 22% reported experiencing daytime sleepiness at least several times a week.
3. Sleepiness (an increased propensity to fall asleep) must be distinguished from fatigue or lack of energy.
4. Sleepiness can be quantified subjectively using the Epworth Sleepiness Scale (Table 5-1) or objectively via the Multiple Sleep Latency Test (MSLT) or Maintenance of Wakefulness Test (MWT).

PATHOPHYSIOLOGY

1. Sleep drive is contributed to by both homeostatic (duration of prior wakefulness) and circadian (internal clock) processes.
2. The causes of sleepiness can be grouped into three major categories:
   a. Inadequate sleep time
   b. Fragmentation of sleep
   c. Excessive sleep drive

PROGNOSIS

1. Depends on underlying cause.
2. Sleepiness of any cause is associated with an increased risk of motor vehicle collisions and industrial accidents.

DIAGNOSIS

1. Distinguish sleepiness from fatigue.
2. Fatigue is a nonspecific symptom that can be caused by many medical and/or psychiatric illnesses.
3. General algorithm (Fig. 5-1).

TREATMENT

Depends on underlying cause.

INSUFFICIENT SLEEP

BACKGROUND

1. Most common cause of excessive daytime sleepiness.
2. Chronic, partial sleep restriction much more common than total sleep deprivation.
3. Chronic sleep restriction is a prevalent problem in today's society, exacerbated by social, occupational, and environmental factors.

TABLE 5-1. EPWORTH SLEEPINESS SCALE

In the last 30 days, how likely were you to dose off or fall asleep in the following situations (in contrast to just feeling tired)?	High Chance (3)	Moderate Chance (2)	Slight Chance (1)	Never Doze (0)
1. Sitting and reading	?	?	?	?
2. Watching TV	?	?	?	?
3. Sitting inactive in a public place (e.g., theater, church)	?	?	?	?
4. As a passenger in a car for an hour without a break	?	?	?	?
5. Lying down to rest in the afternoon when circumstances permit	?	?	?	?
6. Sitting and talking to someone	?	?	?	?
7. Sitting quietly after lunch without alcohol	?	?	?	?
8. In a car while stopped for a few minutes in traffic	?	?	?	?

Total score of >12 indicates clinically important daytime sleepiness.

PATHOPHYSIOLOGY

1. While individual variability likely exists in terms of total sleep need, most adults require at least 7 hours of sleep each night.
2. Subjective measures of sleepiness tend to stop rising whereas objective measures of sleep drive (MSLT) and performance rise continuously as the duration of sleep restriction continues.
3. Short-term (less than 2 weeks), chronic partial sleep restriction (4–6 hours per night) is associated with changes in mood and psychomotor performance testing as well as endocrinologic changes such as increased cortisol level and mild insulin resistance.

PROGNOSIS

1. Symptoms of daytime sleepiness should be completely reversible with increased total sleep time.
2. Preliminary data from the Nurses Health Study suggest increased cardiac morbidity and overall mortality associated with chronic partial sleep restriction (less than 6 hours per night).

DIAGNOSIS

1. This should be obvious from the history and suspected as contributing to excessive daytime sleepiness (EDS) in anyone obtaining less than 7.5 hours of sleep on a regular basis.
2. Sleep diaries (logs kept by the patient) can be useful in documenting total sleep time.
3. In rare instances further testing, such as actigraphy (wrist-worn motion sensitive device that can be used to estimate sleep and wake) can be used to objectively quantify total sleep time for long periods.
4. Polysomnography rarely required.

TREATMENT

1. Increasing total sleep to 8 hours or greater on a regular basis.
2. May require lifestyle or occupational change to accomplish this goal.

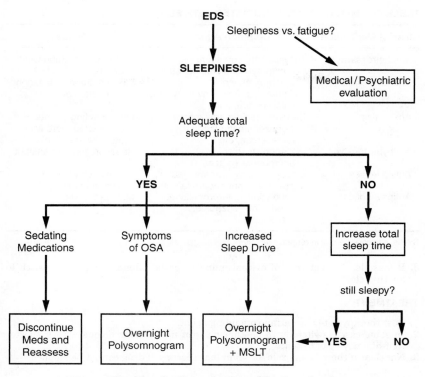

FIG. 5-1. Algorithm for the evaluation of daytime sleepiness.

MEDICATIONS

BACKGROUND

1. An often overlooked, but important contributor to symptoms of daytime sleepiness.
2. A wide variety of agents have been associated with increased sleepiness.

PATHOPHYSIOLOGY

1. Depends on mechanism of action of drug.
2. Can be a desired action of the drug that becomes undesirable if it carries over into daytime or an unwanted side effect not related to the drug's primary action.
3. Must be able to cross blood–brain barrier and act within the central nervous system (CNS).

PROGNOSIS

1. EDS secondary to medication effect should be readily reversible if drug can be discontinued.

DIAGNOSIS

1. Careful review of all medications (Table 5-2) including nonprescription drugs.
2. Rule out other causes of EDS.

TABLE 5-2. MEDICATIONS ASSOCIATED WITH EDS

Class of Medication	Common Agents	Notes
Antidepressant	Tricyclic antidepressants (amitriptyline, doxepine, etc.)	Much less common with SSRIs
Antihistamines	Brompheniramine, diphenhydramine, hydroxyzine, chlorpheniramine	Less common with second-generation agents
Anxiolytics	Benzodiazepines (diazepam, clonazepam flurazepam, temazepam, etc.)	Longer acting agents associated more with daytime sedation
Antihypertensives	α-2 agonists (clonidine), α-1 antagonists (prazosin)	Sedation can be transient
Antiepileptics	Gabapentin, topiramate, gabitril, phenytoin, phenobarbital	Rates have varied in different studies
Antipsychotics	Thioridazine, chlorpromazine, quetiapine, clozapine, olanzapine	May be transient

SSRIs, selective serotonin reuptake inhibitors.

3. If feasible, attempt trial of discontinuing potential offending agent or switch to another class.

TREATMENT

1. Best therapy is to discontinue offending agent.
2. In some cases, switching to another class of medications or one with a shorter half-life may be of benefit.
3. Not clear if there is any role for stimulant therapy, if drug cannot be stopped.

NARCOLEPSY

BACKGROUND

1. A disorder characterized by abnormal sleepiness, disturbed nocturnal sleep, and pathologic manifestations of rapid eye movement (REM) sleep during wakefulness.
2. Classic tetrad of daytime sleepiness, cataplexy, sleep paralysis, and hypnagogic hallucinations.
3. Other associated symptoms can include "sleep attacks" and automatic behavior.
4. Relatively rare disorder (25–50/100,000), with substantial ethnic variation.
5. Strongly associated with specific HLA haplotype—DQB1-0602 (present in more than 90% of those with narcolepsy–cataplexy)—although no clear autoimmune process has been identified.

PATHOPHYSIOLOGY

1. Recent data have identified a new peptide—orexin (or hypocretin)—produced only in the lateral hypothalamus and projecting widely throughout the brain.
2. A dog model of narcolepsy has been shown to be due to a defect in the orexin-2 receptor, and an orexin peptide knockout mouse has features of classic narcolepsy.
3. Most patients with narcolepsy and cataplexy have a specific loss of orexin neurons located in the lateral hypothalamus, and cerebrospinal fluid (CSF) levels of this peptide are low in patients with narcolepsy and cataplexy.
4. Orexin normally increases wakefulness and inhibits REM sleep by acting on specific brainstem centers including the locus coerulus and the dorsal raphe.

5. Absence of orexin causes symptoms of daytime sleepiness and allows partial manifestations of REM sleep (such as muscle paralysis) to occur during wakefulness.

PROGNOSIS

1. The disease is lifelong and typically unremitting.
2. In some studies, the severity and number of cataplectic attacks may decrease over time.
3. Narcolepsy has been associated with an increased incidence of other sleep disorders including obstructive sleep apnea, periodic leg movements of sleep, and REM sleep behavior disorder.

DIAGNOSIS

1. Symptoms typically begin in the second decade, although they can rarely occur before the age of 10 or after age 50.
2. Diagnosis is typically delayed for as much as 10 years.
3. EDS is the primary symptom, which is often briefly relieved by short (30 minutes) naps, only to quickly return.
4. Cataplexy is a sudden, transient loss of (or reduction in) muscle tone. Typically occurs in conjunction with strong emotion (laughter or anger). It may be complete or partial and the episodes are typically brief (seconds to minutes). It is seen in approximately 70% of narcoleptics and is pathognomonic for the disorder.
5. Other symptoms include sleep paralysis (episodes characterized by an inability to move that occurs at sleep onset or upon awakening) and hypnagogic hallucinations (visual or auditory hallucinations that appear to represent dream mentation occurring right at sleep onset).
6. Polysomnography typically demonstrates shortening of sleep-onset and REM latency and disruption of sleep architecture with frequent brief awakenings. Polysomnography is necessary to exclude sleep disorders that could account for excess daytime sleepiness.
7. MSLT results usually demonstrate mean sleep latencies less than 5 minutes and classically show the occurrence of sleep-onset REM periods (SOREMPs) in at least two of five nap opportunities.

TREATMENT

1. Typically required for life.
2. General supportive measures include the avoidance of sleep deprivation and the use of short naps during the daytime to improve functioning.
3. Medications used for the treatment of EDS include stimulant or wakefulness-promoting agents (Table 5-3).
   a. Stimulant medications include the amphetamines methylphenidate and pemoline. Efficacy appears to be related to the ability to release and prevent reuptake of dopamine.

TABLE 5-3. STIMULANT MEDICATIONS

Medication	Daily Dose Range (mg)
Methylphenidate (Ritalin)	5–80 (divided doses)
Methylphenidate (Ritalin-SR)	20–60 daily
Methylphenidate (Concerta, Metadate, Focalin)	18–54 daily
Dextroamphetamine (Adderall)	5–60 (divided doses)
Dextroamphetamine (Adderal-XR)	20–60
Pemoline (Cylert)	75–150
Modafinil (Provigil)	100–400 (daily or twice a day)

TABLE 5-4. MEDICATIONS FOR CATAPLEXY

Medication	Daily Dose Range
Clomipramine (Anafranil)	25–75 mg
Imipramine (Tofranil)	75–150 mg
Protriptyline (Vivactil)	15–20 mg
Fluoxetine (Prozac)	20–40 mg
Paroxetine (Paxil)	20–40 mg
Sertraline (Zoloft)	50–200 mg
Venlafaxine (Effexor)	75–150 mg
Sodium oxybate (Xyrem)	3–9 g (given in two evenly divided doses at night)

    b. Common side effects of these medications include nervousness, irritability, tremors, palpitations, weight loss, and nocturnal sleep disruption. More severe side effects (tachycardia, hypertension) are rare.

    c. Pemoline is rarely used anymore because of potential hepatotoxicity.

    d. Modafinil is a new wakefulness-promoting agent that may affect CNS dopamine levels, but the mechanism of action is incompletely understood.

    e. Modafinil is somewhat less potent than other stimulants but tends to be better tolerated. Headache is the most common side effect (10%).

    f. Treatment typically includes modafinil as first line, with stimulants added if this does not completely reverse EDS.

    g. Often combine long-acting medications with immediate-release medications for maximum benefit.

4. Medications used for the treatment of cataplexy include the tricyclic antidepressants, selective serotonin reuptake inhibitors (SSRIs), and sodium oxybate (Table 5-4).

    a. Efficacy of these medications appears to be due to their ability to inhibit norepinephrine reuptake.

    b. Tricyclic antidepressants (e.g., imipramine, clomipramine, and protriptyline) are all effective in relatively low doses. Their use is limited because of prominent anticholinergic side effects.

    c. SSRIs have become initial treatment of choice for cataplexy (fluoxetine, paroxetine, venlafaxine, etc.) and have fewer side effects. Required doses are often higher than with tricyclic antidepressants (TCAs).

    d. Sodium oxybate is an endogenous hypnotic that can consolidate sleep. Recent studies have shown it to be effective in improving cataplexy and EDS.

        1) Use is restricted because of reports of abuse of this agent.

        2) It is administered in a dose immediately before bedtime, which is then repeated 2 to 5 hours later.

        3) The most common side effect is nausea.

5. Occasional patients will require sedative medications to help consolidate nocturnal sleep. Use of agents with the shortest effective half-life is recommended.

6. Extremely important to encourage adequate sleep time and to evaluate and treat any other concurrent sleep disorders that may be contributing to symptoms.

IDIOPATHIC CENTRAL NERVOUS SYSTEM HYPERSOMNOLENCE

BACKGROUND

1. Less well defined and understood than narcolepsy.

2. Characterized by EDS, often prolonged nocturnal sleep episodes, naps that are unrefreshing, and difficulty arising from sleep.

3. No manifestations of abnormal REM phenomenon.

PATHOPHYSIOLOGY

1. Not well understood.
2. Thought to be of CNS origin, but no obvious structural or functional abnormality has been discovered. No clear genetic predisposition.
3. May represent a heterogenous group of disorders, including sequelae of prior viral illness, neurodegenerative disease, and idiopathic cause.

PROGNOSIS

Tends to be lifelong and unremitting.

DIAGNOSIS

1. Strict diagnostic criteria do not exist.
2. Of utmost importance to rule out other known causes of EDS, including medication use (prescribed or illicit), sleep-disordered breathing, and so forth.
3. Polysomnography classically demonstrates prolonged sleep with high sleep efficiency and normal proportions of each sleep stage.
4. MSLTs reveal shortened sleep latency (less than 8 minutes, but often longer than in classic narcolepsy) without evidence of SOREMPs.
5. Can be difficult to distinguish from narcolepsy without cataplexy, although treatment is identical.

TREATMENT

1. Often difficult to treat satisfactorily.
2. Lifestyle and behavior modification to avoid sleep deprivation and good sleep hygiene are of some help.
3. Naps usually not helpful (unlike narcolepsy).
4. Major mode of therapy is stimulant medications (Table 5-4).
   a. Modafinil (see above) is initial treatment of choice because of its safety and side-effect profile.
   b. Amphetamines or methylphenidate can be added if needed.
   c. The combined use of long- and short-acting medications often provides the best effect.

SLEEP-DISORDERED BREATHING

BACKGROUND

1. Most common etiology of EDS evaluated in clinical sleep medicine.
2. Major subtypes include:
   a. Obstructive sleep apnea (OSA): Characterized by repetitive episodes of pharyngeal collapse during sleep.
   b. Central sleep apnea (CSA): Characterized by periods of absent respiratory effort that may occur sporadically or in a cyclic pattern such as in Cheyne–Stokes respiration.
   c. Sleep-related hypoventilation: Periods of decreased ventilation with profound hypercapnia, most commonly associated with neuromuscular weakness or chest wall abnormalities.
3. Causes EDS secondary to fragmentation of sleep and recurrent arousals.
4. Associated with recurrent hypoxemia, hypercapnia, and sympathetic nervous system activation.

PATHOPHYSIOLOGY

1. OSA associated with a small and collapsible pharyngeal airway behind the uvula, tongue, or both in conjunction with sleep-related changes in pharyngeal dilator muscle activation.

2. Risk factors for OSA include obesity, middle age, gender (twice as common in males), as well as abnormalities of the upper airway such as retrognathia or macroglossia.
3. CSA usually due to alterations in respiratory drive with increased drive and decreased drive predisposing.
4. CSA of the Cheyne–Stokes type is most commonly seen in patients with systolic congestive heart failure (CHF) but periodic breathing also seen with brainstem abnormalities.
5. Sleep-related hypoventilation in patients with neuromuscular weakness is exacerbated by sleep-related changes in muscle activation especially during REM sleep when ventilation is primarily maintained by diaphragm activation.

PROGNOSIS

1. OSA has been associated with an increased risk of systemic hypertension, motor vehicle collision, and decreased quality of life.
2. Increasing data suggest OSA also independently associated with cardiovascular diseases such as myocardial infarction, CHF, and stroke.
3. Prognosis for idiopathic CSA is less well defined.
4. Cheyne–Stokes respirations in patients with CHF are an independent predictor of mortality.
5. Sleep-related hypoventilation in neuromuscular disease is a precursor to daytime respiratory failure.

DIAGNOSIS

1. Polysomnography is the gold standard for diagnosis of sleep-related breathing abnormalities.
2. The presence or absence of respiratory effort can be determined using mechanical bands around the chest and abdomen or intercostal electromyogram (EMG).
3. Severity of disease quantified by the apnea–hypopnea index (number of abnormal respiratory events per hour of sleep) with less than five to ten an hour being normal.
4. Severity also influenced by degree of oxygen desaturation.
5. Other diagnostic modalities include limited-sleep studies and overnight oximetry.

TREATMENT

Obstructive Sleep Apnea

1. Conservative measures may improve OSA including weight loss and avoidance of alcohol and sedative medications.
2. In some patients whose apnea occurs primarily while sleeping supine, the use of an uncomfortable object in the nightshirt/gown can be used to limit sleep in this position.
3. Positive airway pressure therapy applied via a nasal mask is the primary modality of therapy. Continuous positive airway pressure (CPAP) works as a pneumatic splint, preventing airway collapse.
4. CPAP has been demonstrated to decrease daytime sleepiness, improve overall function and quality of life, and in some studies lower blood pressure in comparison to placebo.
5. Long-term compliance is the major limitation to CPAP use, with some data suggesting 65% of patients continue to use it for 12 months or longer.
6. Required CPAP pressure is determined during a "titration" study that can usually be performed during the same night as the diagnostic polysomnogram (split-night study).
7. Modifications of traditional CPAP include the use of "auto-titrating" devices that can modify the pressure over the night and bilevel positive airway pressure, which provides a lower pressure on expiration from inspiration. Neither has clearly been demonstrated to be superior to traditional CPAP but may be useful in certain patients.

8. Oral appliances are custom-made mouthpieces that function by advancing the mandible and tongue, thus enlarging the pharyngeal airway.
9. Overall efficacy of oral appliances is approximately 50% in OSA, but many patients prefer these devices to CPAP.
10. Surgical therapy of OSA includes minimally invasive procedures (such as radiofrequency ablation) and more invasive procedures such as uvulopalatopharyngoplasty (UPPP).
11. Success rates for surgery vary depending on the procedure but for UPPP are approximately 40% to 50%.
12. In a minority of patients whose apnea is adequately treated, EDS remains a significant problem. In these patients the addition of modafinil has been shown to improve symptoms while not substantially reducing CPAP compliance.

Central Sleep Apnea

1. Treatment of idiopathic central sleep apnea is difficult.
2. Options include the use of respiratory stimulants such as medroxyprogesterone and noninvasive ventilation provided via a nasal mask (bilevel positive pressure).
3. In patients with Cheyne–Stokes respiration associated with CHF, optimizing therapy for heart failure is the primary therapy (afterload reduction, diuretics, beta-blockers, etc.).
4. Both supplemental oxygen and nasal CPAP have been shown to be effective for long-term therapy of Cheyne–Stokes ventilation.
5. Emerging data suggest that CPAP therapy in patients with Cheyne–Stokes associated with CHF may be associated with an increase in transplant-free survival.

Sleep-related Hypoventilation

1. Noninvasive ventilation (NPPV) usually applied using bilevel positive airway pressure via a nasal or oronasal mask is first-line therapy.
2. This therapy has been associated with improved sleep quality, decreased daytime and nighttime Pco_2, and improved daytime functioning.
3. In slowly progressive diseases (such as postpolio syndrome, some muscular dystrophies) NPPV has been associated with prolonged survival without the need for tracheostomy and mechanical ventilation.
4. In rapidly progressive diseases [such as amyotrophic lateral sclerosis (ALS)] the effect on survival is less clear, but there does appear to be a benefit based on uncontrolled studies.
5. For those who cannot tolerate NPPV (e.g., severe bulbar symptoms in ALS) or those who require ventilatory support during the day, tracheostomy and long-term ventilation remain the only options.
6. Supplemental oxygen may relieve dyspnea in these patients, but should be used with caution as it can markedly worsen hypercapnia.

BRAIN INJURY

BACKGROUND

1. Described as a cause of EDS since 1941, although in most early cases other causes (such as sleep apnea) were not adequately excluded.
2. Overall prevalence not known, but is thought to be relatively low.
3. Sleepiness usually seen in conjunction with other posttraumatic brain injury complaints such as intellectual difficulties, headaches, and memory problems.

PATHOPHYSIOLOGY

1. Etiology not well understood.
2. Sleepiness appears to be more common with injuries of the hypothalamus.

3. One study suggested a correlation between the severity of initial injury (duration of comatose state) and the severity of persistent EDS.
4. Tend to have prolonged nocturnal sleep along with frequent naps, such that total sleep time over 24 hours can be 12 to 15 hours.
5. Although posttraumatic narcolepsy has been reported, most patients do not have evidence of REM sleep dysregulation (such as cataplexy).

PROGNOSIS

1. No long-term follow-up studies exist.
2. Appears to be a lifelong symptom, although some improvement may occur with time.

DIAGNOSIS

1. Must carefully rule out other disorders associated with EDS, including sleep-disordered breathing.
2. Medications often contribute to EDS.
3. History and appropriate testing important to rule out a seizure disorder presenting as hypersomnolence.
4. Nocturnal polysomnography indicated to rule out coexisting sleep disorders.
5. MSLT is used to quantify the degree of daytime sleepiness.

TREATMENT

1. General measures include limitation of medications that can exacerbate symptoms of daytime sleepiness, avoidance of sleep deprivation, and the use of occasional naps.
2. Treatment of any coexisting sleep disorder (such as sleep apnea or periodic limb movement disorder) essential.
3. Symptomatic relief may require the use of stimulant or wake-promoting agents (Table 5-4)
4. Modafinil would be considered the initial agent of choice, given its safety profile, although no well conducted trials of this agent or any other stimulant have been performed in patients with traumatic brain injury.
5. Headache may be a limiting factor in the use of modafinil.
6. Some success has been reported with the use of other stimulants as well.

SLEEPINESS IN NEUROLOGIC DISORDERS

BACKGROUND

1. Sleepiness (as well as sleep disturbance) has been reported in a number of neurologic disorders, including Parkinson disease, cerebrovascular diseases and certain muscular dystrophies, most prominently myotonic dystrophy.
2. Unfortunately, the prevalence of this symptom has not been well defined for most of these disorders.

PATHOPHYSIOLOGY

1. In general not well understood.
2. In patients with Parkinson disease, daytime sleepiness appears to be most commonly caused by disturbed sleep, secondary to coexisting sleep-disordered breathing, periodic limb movements, or medications.
3. Patients with cerebrovascular disease have a high incidence of sleep apnea. Primary sleepiness in patients after stroke is most commonly seen as a result of bilateral damage to the paramedian hypothalamus. It has also been reported with infarcts of the pons and medial medulla.

4. Patients with myotonic dystrophy have an increased prevalence of sleepiness, even in the absence of sleep-disordered breathing. The etiology is unknown.

PROGNOSIS

1. Depends on the underlying disease, but little long-term data are available.
2. Symptoms tend to be lifelong.

DIAGNOSIS

1. As with head trauma, consideration of a seizure disorder is important.
2. Polysomnography (often followed by MSLT) is indicated to exclude sleep-disordered breathing, periodic limb movements and other causes of sleep disruption.
3. Careful review of medications is indicated.

TREATMENT

1. General measures include limitation of medications that can exacerbate symptoms of daytime sleepiness, avoidance of sleep deprivation, and the use of occasional naps.
2. Treatment of any coexisting sleep disorder (such as sleep apnea or periodic limb movement disorder) is essential.
3. Symptomatic relief may require the use of stimulant or wakefulness-promoting agents (Table 5-4).
4. Modafinil would be considered the initial agent of choice, given its safety profile, although no well-conducted trials of this agent or any other stimulant have been performed in patients with neurologic disorders.
5. Headache may be a limiting factor in the use of modafinil.
6. Some success has been reported with the use of other stimulants.

INSOMNIA

OVERVIEW

BACKGROUND

1. Insomnia is the description given to the complaints of difficulty falling asleep, staying asleep, or nonrestorative sleep. It is extremely common, with approximately one third of individuals having at least short-term difficulties in any given year, and 10% to 15% of adults reporting consistent or serious insomnia.
2. The subtype of insomnia complaint (difficulty falling asleep, staying asleep, or non-restorative sleep) is not consistent over time, and thus the diagnostic value of these subtypes is not substantial.
3. More common with advancing age and in women.
4. Most individuals with chronic insomnia do not seek assistance from a health care professional.

PATHOPHYSIOLOGY

1. The timing and duration of sleep are determined by underlying "homeostatic" sleep drive (duration of prior wakefulness) and circadian (internal clock) processes.
2. Chronic insomnia is best considered a symptom of an underlying problem rather than a disorder itself. On the other hand, acute insomnia is usually produced by a defined precipitating event.

PROGNOSIS

1. Depends upon the underlying cause (see below).
2. Insomnia has been associated with poor cognitive and psychomotor performance, poor quality of life, increased health care utilization, increased absenteeism, and increased risk of developing mood or anxiety disorders or substance abuse.

DIAGNOSIS

Based on history; polysomnography usually not indicated.

TREATMENT

Depends on underlying cause (see below) (Fig. 5-2).

ACUTE INSOMNIA

BACKGROUND

Usually 1 day to 3 weeks in duration.

PATHOPHYSIOLOGY

Associated with unfamiliar sleep environment, situational stress, acute medical illness or pain, shift work, or caffeine or alcohol use.

PROGNOSIS

Generally time-limited, unless insomnia itself produces a cycle of worsening insomnia due to maladaptive behaviors and anxiety regarding sleep ("conditioned insomnia," see below).

DIAGNOSIS

Available from history.

TREATMENT

1. If insomnia is limited to 1 or 2 days, treatment is usually unnecessary.
2. Relief from the underlying cause of the insomnia should be sought.
3. Insomnia beyond a few days should be treated with hypnotic medication (see Table 5-5).
   a. Benzodiazepine receptor agonists (BzRAs) are first-line agents for short-term use given their efficacy, tolerability, and the wide range of half-lives available.
   b. Alternative agents to BzRAs should be prescribed to individuals with a history of substance or alcohol abuse or dependence.
4. If indicated, stress-reduction techniques should be recommended.

INSOMNIA SECONDARY TO PSYCHIATRIC DISORDERS

BACKGROUND

1. Most common causes of chronic insomnia, accounting for up to 50% of all insomnias.
2. Anxiety disorders, depressive disorders, substance abuse, schizophrenia, and bipolar disorder all produce substantial insomnia.

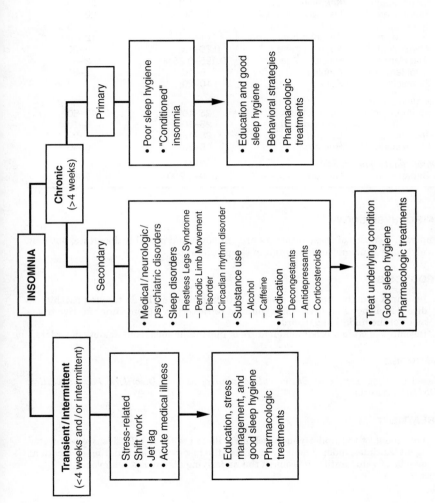

FIG. 5-2. Algorithm for the management of insomnia.

TABLE 5-5. COMMONLY USED PHARMACOLOGIC TREATMENTS FOR INSOMNIA

Generic Name	Trade Name	Common Dose Range (mg)	Half-life, Including Active Metabolites (h)
Benzodiazepine receptor agonists			
Clonazepam	Klonopin; others	0.5–1.0	30–60
Flurazepam	Dalmane; others	15–30	20–60
Temazepam	Restoril; others	7.5–30	6–18
Lorazepam	Ativan; others	1–2	12–18
Alprazolam	Xanax; others	0.25–1.0	6–20
Triazolam	Halcion; others	0.125–0.25	2–3
Zolpidem	Ambien	5–10	2–3
Zaleplon	Sonata	10–20	1–1.5
Sedating antidepressants			
Amitriptyline	Elavil; others	25–100	10–50
Doxepin	Sinequan; others	25–100	6–10
Trazodone	Desyrel	25–150	5–9
Mirtazapine	Remeron	7.5–30	20–40
Other sedating agents			
Gabapentin	Neurontin	300–1,200	5–9

PATHOPHYSIOLOGY

Underlying causes of these disorders are unknown and probably disparate, but may involve neurotransmitters essential in sleep regulation.

PROGNOSIS

1. Insomnia usually improves or remits with treatment of the underlying psychiatric disorder, although it is the most common refractory symptom after effective treatment of the underlying disorder.
2. Insomnia is often a prodromal feature of impending mood and anxiety disorders.

DIAGNOSIS

Based on *Diagnostic and Statistical Manual of Mental Disorders, Fourth Edition (DSM-IV)* criteria.

TREATMENT

1. Treatment of the underlying psychiatric illness with an effective, well-tolerated agent. At times, independent treatment of the insomnia with sedating medications may be of value until remission of the underlying disorder is achieved.

PRIMARY INSOMNIA

BACKGROUND

1. Composed on three subtypes
   a. Conditioned or "psychophysiologic insomnia"
   b. Sleep-state misperception
   c. Idiopathic insomnia
2. May account for 10% to 20% of all chronic insomnias.

PATHOPHYSIOLOGY

1. All subtypes are considered to be caused by cognitive and physiologic hyperarousal.
2. Conditioned insomnia is actually an anxiety disorder, caused by fear of insomnia and its consequences. Usually begins with insomnia from another cause, but then develops into chronic condition, as a negative vicious cycle of worsening anxiety regarding sleeplessness produces worsening insomnia.
3. Idiopathic insomnia is usually lifelong and is usually a diagnosis of exclusion.
4. Sleep-state misperception is a disparity between polysomnographic recorded sleep and patient perception of sleep.

PROGNOSIS

1. Often produces chronic insomnia with severe anxiety regarding sleeplessness.
2. May develop into anxiety/mood/substance use disorders.

DIAGNOSIS

1. Based on history, although the original cause of insomnia is usually remote and cannot be identified.
2. Polysomnography usually not of diagnostic value.

TREATMENT

1. Cognitive–behavioral techniques have demonstrated the best long-term efficacy.
   a. Relaxation procedures: Progressive muscle relaxation, biofeedback, yoga, and meditation. Mastery of technique and daily use are essential.
   b. Sleep restriction therapy: Restricts time in bed to the amount the patient reports sleeping (usually 5–6 hours). Produces short-term sleep deprivation, promoting easier time falling and staying asleep, and subsequent increased confidence and reduced anxiety regarding sleep. Once sleep improves, expansion of time in bed by 30 minutes/night/wk, achieves more normal total sleep duration. Sleep diaries and regular appointments are valuable.
   c. Stimulus control: Get out of bed when not asleep. Limits negative association of bed and sleep-onset period. Is counterintuitive to many with insomnia.
2. Sleep hygiene measures are essential for all individuals with insomnia.
   a. Keep stable bedtime and wake times 7 d/wk.
   b. Avoid stressful activities in the evening (physical and emotional).
   c. Avoid caffeine after noon and alcohol after 5 PM.
   d. Avoid daytime napping.
   e. Sleeping environment should be quiet, safe, and relaxing.
   f. Regular exercise.
3. Hypnotic and anxiolytic medications may be of value when used on a nightly or intermittent basis.
   a. Always use the shortest half-life agent that will produce good-quality sleep to avoid daytime side effects (sedation, cognitive dysfunction, psychomotor impairment, anticholinergic effects).
   b. Initially, individuals may require long-acting BzRAs to treat daytime anxiety regarding sleeplessness. These can be tapered after 1 to 4 weeks as cognitive–behavioral measures become effective.

RESTLESS LEGS SYNDROME/PERIODIC LEG MOVEMENTS OF SLEEP

BACKGROUND

1. Restless legs syndrome (RLS) is divided into primary and secondary forms on the basis of the underlying etiology although the phenotypes are indistinguishable.

2. Prevalence is 1% to 3% of those under age 50, rising to 10% to 15% of individuals over the age of 70. Women are affected twice as often as men.
3. Periodic leg movements of sleep (PLMS) are present in approximately 80% of those with RLS. PLMS has a 10% to 50% prevalence in the general population, depending on age. Most with PLMS do not have RLS.

PATHOPHYSIOLOGY

1. Underlying biochemistry and anatomic pathology are unknown.
2. Approximately one third of primary RLS is familial, with early-onset (before age 30) cases possibly having an autosomal dominant mechanism.
3. Serum and/or CSF ferritin levels may be low, indicating a possible role of iron (through its involvement in dopamine production) in pathophysiology of RLS.
4. Secondary RLS is seen with chronic renal failure, iron deficiency, rheumatoid arthritis, antidepressant use, and pregnancy.
5. PLMSs are more common in those with dopaminergic disorders.

PROGNOSIS

1. Can have a waxing-and-waning course, but most cases that come to medical attention are chronic and unremitting.
2. RLS and PLMS may predict mortality in patients with end-stage renal disease.

DIAGNOSIS

1. Clinical features
   a. Based exclusively on clinical history.
   b. Dysesthesia and restlessness in the legs (or arms) that are relieved by movement.
   c. Symptoms are exclusively present or worse in the evening or at night compared to the daytime.
   d. Symptoms are exacerbated by sleep deprivation.
2. Polysomnography: 80% have PLMS on polysomnography—dorsiflexion of big toe, foot, and at times, flexion of the knee and hip in a rhythmic (every 15–30 seconds) pattern.
3. Laboratory evaluation to assess ferritin level (keeping levels greater than 40 μg/L).

TREATMENT

1. Dopaminergic agents, the first-line therapy, are extremely effective in relieving symptoms of RLS and decreasing PLMS.
   a. Pramipexole (0.25 mg starting dose, increase by 0.25 mg every 3 days to effective dose, usually 0.25–1.0 mg) or ropinirole (0.25–2.0 mg) 2 hours before symptom onset; if needed before 6 to 8 PM may also need to be given before bed to relieve symptoms all night.
   b. L-Dopa/carbidopa (25/100–100/400 mg) given 1 hour before symptom onset, although dosing every 4 to 6 hours is necessary even with sustained-release (SR) formulation.
   c. Most serious complication is of "augmentation": earlier appearance of symptoms during the day, which can then occur earlier and earlier with earlier dosing of medication, leading to refractory symptoms. More common with L-Dopa than with dopamine agonists.
   d. Side effects include nausea, insomnia, peripheral edema, orthostasis, fatigue, and muscle or joint pain.
   e. Need for coadministered sedating medication (e.g., gabapentin, BzRA, trazodone) is common due to dopaminergic-induced or other causes of insomnia.
   f. Avoid in individuals with history of or current psychosis.
2. Opioids are second-line agents, as they are less effective than dopaminergic agents and have the potential for misuse.

    a. Oxycodone or codeine in small doses are very effective in relieving RLS symptoms, particularly in those with painful dysesthesia.

    b. Dose escalation of these compounds in these patients is unusual.

3. Gabapentin is also a second-line agent. Although it is generally not as effective as an opioid, there are less concerns with its use.

    a. Dose of 1,800 mg, usually in divided doses in the evening and before bed.

    b. To be used cautiously in those with renal insufficiency or failure.

4. BzRAs are third-line agents.

    a. Generally only useful if other medications are contraindicated or as hypnotic agents.

    b. Avoid use of long-acting BzRAs (e.g., clonazepam, diazepam, flurazepam) due to daytime side-effects unless there is coexistent anxiety disorder.

CIRCADIAN RHYTHM DISORDERS

BACKGROUND

1. Heterogeneous group of disorders in which the body's internal clock is not synchronized with external clock time, producing difficulty sleeping at environmentally appropriate times and/or inappropriate daytime sleepiness.

2. Common disorders given the numbers of individuals who work rotating or night shifts or travel across time zones.

3. Age-related forms are seen, with delayed sleep-phase syndrome (DSPS) observed in up to 10% of adolescents and advanced sleep-phase syndrome (ASPS) commonly observed in the elderly.

PATHOPHYSIOLOGY

1. Shift-work sleep disorder and jet lag develop as a result of a lag in the body's internal clock and the resultant disparity between internal and external clocks.

2. Age-related forms are thought to be due to a combination of physiologic and behavioral processes. For example, going to sleep later produces later wake times, which produce later initial daytime exposure to light, producing a shift in clock time (equivalent to westward travel).

PROGNOSIS

1. Adjustment to desynchrony of internal and external clocks is relatively rapid when light is received at the appropriate times. However, symptoms may be chronic due to lack of appropriately timed light or behavioral factors.

2. Health status may be poorer and work-related accidents may be more common in those working nocturnal or rotating shifts.

DIAGNOSIS

1. DSPS is most often observed in adolescents, who have difficulty with sleep-onset insomnia and difficulty awakening in the morning, although these are normal when allowed to go to bed and awaken late.

2. ASPS is usually observed in the elderly, who report early sleep onset and awakenings, although sleep may be of normal duration and quality.

TREATMENT

1. DSPS is best treated with slow (e.g., half-hour every 1–2 days) advance (earlier) of morning awakenings to get bright (e.g., 2,500 lux) morning light, combined with earlier bedtimes at the same rate. Use of nocturnal sedatives (Table 5-5) or use of

melatonin (1–3 mg) may assist with earlier bedtime and wake time. Use of sleep logs is strongly encouraged.
2. ASPS is treated with evening (8 PM to midnight) bright (2500–4000 lux) light.

INSOMNIA SECONDARY TO MEDICATIONS OR MEDICAL/NEUROLOGIC DISORDERS

BACKGROUND

1. Medical/neurologic illnesses are common causes of chronic insomnia and may account for more variance in predicting insomnia than all other predictive variables.
2. Apparent influence of advanced age on insomnia may be mediated by health status, not age.

PATHOPHYSIOLOGY

1. Pain, shortness of breath, and nocturia are the most common symptoms predicting insomnia.
2. Some neurologic disorders may produce insomnia through involvement of sleep centers (e.g., Parkinson disease, stroke, Alzheimer disease, multiinfarct dementia, etc.).
3. Many medications may contribute to insomnia (serotonergic and noradrenergic antidepressants, corticosteroids, decongestants).

PROGNOSIS

Depends on the underlying disease state.

DIAGNOSIS

1. Any subtype (initial, maintenance, or nonrestorative sleep) of insomnia may be present.
2. Polysomnography may be of value in ruling out sleep-disordered breathing or PLMS given the high prevalence of these sleep disorders in many neurologic diseases.

TREATMENT

1. Treatment of the underlying symptoms (e.g., pain, shortness of breath, nocturia).
2. Adherence to good sleep hygiene.
3. Use of empiric pharmacotherapy (Table 5-5) if cannot treat underlying symptoms/disorder.

PARASOMNIAS

OVERVIEW

BACKGROUND

1. Parasomnias are abnormal, complex, motor events, or sensory experiences arising from sleep.
2. Much more common in children (5%–15%) than adults (1%).
3. Usually are benign, but may be associated with traumatic injury, embarrassment, or rarely, legal consequences.

PATHOPHYSIOLOGY

1. Divided into non-REM and REM parasomnias on the basis of the sleep state from which they arise.
2. REM parasomnias are usually related to dream content with absence of motor atonia (REM behavior disorder) or excessively emotional dreams (nightmares).

PROGNOSIS

Depends on the specific parasomnia.

DIAGNOSIS

Polysomnography is often indicated to distinguish between the different parasomnias and between parasomnias and other sleep disorders (e.g., movement disorders during sleep, nocturnal seizures, sleep apnea).

TREATMENT

Specific to the parasomnia.

SLEEPWALKING AND NIGHT TERRORS

BACKGROUND

1. Approximately 2% of adults report these parasomnias, but they are more common in children and adolescents.
2. New-onset, frequent episodes in adults require evaluation and polysomnography.
3. Clinical evaluation usually not necessary in children.

PATHOPHYSIOLOGY

1. These non-REM parasomnias are considered "disorders of arousal" in which an internal or external stimulus leads to partial arousal from sleep in a predisposed individual.
2. RLS, sleep apnea, stress, environmental noise, and medications may all precipitate events.
3. Family history may be present in up to 50% of individuals.
4. Association with psychiatric illness is controversial.

PROGNOSIS

1. Usually intermittent, benign, and time-limited in children.
2. Events in adults occasionally lead to sexual or violent behavior or injury.

DIAGNOSIS

1. Clinical features:
   a. Episodes usually occur within first third of the night (often within the first hour), usually arising from slow-wave sleep.
   b. Individual is relatively unresponsive to the environment.
   c. Fear and autonomic arousal are the affective hallmarks of night terrors.
   d. Amnesia is usually present for the event.
   e. Stereotyped events suggest need for full-montage electroencephalogram (EEG) to assess for frontal lobe seizures.
2. Polysomnography often does not document parasomnia events, although frequent brief arousals from slow-wave sleep may be observed.

TREATMENT

1. In children, regular bed- and wake times, avoidance of sleep deprivation, reassurance of parents, and safety of sleep environment are usually sufficient.
2. In adults, the above behavioral measures are essential. In addition, use of benzodiazepines (triazolam, lorazepam) is indicated if events are frequent and associated with adverse consequences.

RAPID EYE MOVEMENT BEHAVIOR DISORDER

BACKGROUND

1. Rapid eye movement behavior disorder (RBD) is predominantly a disorder of older men.
2. Evaluation and treatment are always indicated.

PATHOPHYSIOLOGY

1. Damage to brainstem areas (substantia nigra, pedunculopontine nucleus) has been documented by autopsy. Loss of striatal dopamine transporters has been shown by functional MRI (fMRI) and single photon emission computed tomography (SPECT).
2. RBD may be produced by serotonergic antidepressants.

PROGNOSIS

May presage the emergence of Parkinson disease by 4 to 10 years in up to 50% of cases.

DIAGNOSIS

1. Clinical features
   a. Enactment of dreams, usually of a vivid, fearful, violent content.
   b. Sleep-related injury to spouse or patient is common.
   c. Disrupted sleep.
2. Polysomnographic features include increased phasic EMG activity and loss of EMG atonia during REM sleep.

TREATMENT

1. Safety of the sleeping environment.
2. Use of benzodiazepines: clonazepam [0.5–2.0 mg at bedtime (qhs)] or lorazepam (1.0–3.0 mg qhs).
3. Possible benefit of melatonin (3 mg qhs) for those whom benzodiazepines are contraindicated.

BIBLIOGRAPHY

Aldrich MS. The clinical spectrum of narcolepsy and idiopathic hypersomnia. *Neurology* 1996;46:393–401.

Allen RP, Barker, Wehrl F, et al. MRI measurement of brain iron in patients with restless legs syndrome. *Neurology* 2001;56:263–265.

Anonymous. A randomized, double blind, placebo-controlled multicenter trial comparing the effects of three doses of orally administered sodium oxybate with placebo for the treatment of narcolepsy. *Sleep* 2002;25:42–49.

Ayas ND, White J, Manson M, et al. A prospective study of sleep duration and coronary artery disease in women. *Arch Int Med* 2002 (*in press*).

Barthlen GM. Nocturnal respiratory failure as an indication of noninvasive ventilation in the patient with neuromuscular disease. *Respiration* 1997;64[Suppl 1]:35–38.

Broughton R. Sleep disorders: disorders of arousal? *Science* 1968;159:1070–1080.

Cerveri IF, Fanfulla M, Zoia C, et al. Sleep disorders in neuromuscular diseases. *Monaldi Arch Chest Dis* 1993;48:318–321.

Chemlli RM, Willie JT, Sinton CM, et al. Narcolepsy in orexin knockout mice: molecular genetics of sleep regulation. *Cell* 1999;98:409–412.

Chokroverty S, Jankovic J. Restless legs syndrome: a disease in search of identity. *Neurology* 1999;52:907–910.

Dinges DF, Pack F, Williams K, et al. Cumulative sleepiness, mood disturbance, and psychomotor vigilance performance decrements during a week of sleep restricted to 4-5 hours per night. *Sleep* 1997;20:267–267.

Earley C, Connor JR, Beard JL, et al. Abnormalities in CSF concentrations of ferreting and transferring in restless legs syndrome. *Neurology* 2000;54:1698–1700.

Fleetham JA, Ferguson KA, Lowe AA, et al. Oral appliance therapy for the treatment of obstructive sleep apnea. *Sleep* 1996;19[Suppl 10]:S288–S290.

Francisco GE, Ivanhoe CB. Successful treatment of post-traumatic narcolepsy with methylphenidate: a case report. *Am J Phys Med Rehabil* 1996;75:63–65.

Good JL, Barry E, Fishman PS. Posttraumatic narcolepsy: the complete syndrome with tissue typing. Case report. *J Neurosurg* 1989;71[5 Pt 1]:765–767.

Heckmatt JZ, Loh L, Dubowitz V. Night-time nasal ventilation in neuromuscular disease. *Lancet* 1990;335:579–582.

Javaheri S. Treatment of central sleep apnea in heart failure. *Sleep* 2000;3:S224–S227.

Jenkinson C, Davies RJ, Mullins R, et al. Comparison of therapeutic and subtherapeutic nasal continuous positive airway pressure for obstructive sleep apnoea: a randomised prospective parallel trial. *Lancet* 1999;353:2100–2105.

Langdon N, Shindler J, Parkes JD, et al. Fluoxetine in the treatment of cataplexy. *Sleep* 1986;9:371–373.

Larsen JP. Sleep disorders in Parkinson's disease. *Advances in Neurology* 2003;91:329–334.

Lin L, Faraco J, Li K, et al. The sleep disorder canine narcolepsy is caused by a mutation in the hypocretin (orexin) receptor 2 gene. *Cell* 1999;98:365–376.

Lyall RA, Donaldson N, Fleming T, et al. A prospective study of quality of life in ALS patients treated with noninvasive ventilation. *Neurology* 2001;57:153–156.

Maccario M, Ruggles KH, Meriwether MW. Post-traumatic narcolepsy. *Mil Med* 1987;152:370–371.

Mendelson W. A 96-year-old woman with insomnia. *JAMA* 1997;277:990–996.

Mitler MM, Hajdukovic R. Relative efficacy of drugs for the treatment of sleepiness in narcolepsy. *Sleep* 1991;14:218–220.

Mitler MM, Hajdukovic R, Erman MK. Treatment of narcolepsy with methamphetamine. *Sleep* 1993;16:306–317.

Mitler MM, Erman M, Hajdukovic R. The treatment of excessive somnolence with stimulant drugs. *Sleep* 1993;16:203–206.

Mitler MM, Aldrich MS, Koob GF, et al. Narcolepsy and its treatment with stimulants: ASDA standards of practice. *Sleep* 1994;17:352–371.

Montgomery P, Dennis J. Bright light therapy for sleep problems in adults ages 60+ (Cochrane Review). *The Cochrane Library* 2003;1:CD003403.

Montplaisir J, Nicolas A, Denesle R, et al. Restless legs syndrome improved by pramipexole. *Neurology* 1999;52:938–943.

Morin CM, Daley M, Ouellet MC. Insomnia in adults. *Curr Treat Options Neurol* 2001;3:9–18.

Nishino S, Ripley B, Overeem S, et al. Hypocretin (orexin) deficiency in human narcolepsy. *Lancet* 2000;355:39–40.

Novak M, Shapiro CM. Drug-induced sleep disturbances: focus on nonpsychotropic medications. *Drug Safety* 1997;16:133–149.

Ohayon MM, Guilleminault C, Priest RG. Night terrors, sleepwalking, and confusional arousals in the general population: their frequency and relationship to other sleep and mental disorders. *J Clin Psychiatry* 1999;60:268–277.

Peppard P, Young T, Palta M, et al. Prospective study of the association between sleep disordered breathing and hypertension. *N Engl J Med* 2000;342:1378–1384.

Remmers JE, deGroot WJ, Sauerland EK, et al. Pathogenesis of upper airway occlusion during sleep. *J Appl Physiol* 1978;44:931–938.

Roth T, Roehrs TA. Etiologies and sequelae of excessive daytime sleepiness. *Clin Ther* 1996;18:562–576; discussion 561.

Rothdach AJ, Trenkwalkder C, Haberstock J, et al. Prevalence and risk factors of RLS in an elderly population: the MEMO study—Memory and Morbidity in Augsburg Elderly. *Neurology* 2000;54:1064–1068.

Schenck CH, Mahowald MW. REM sleep parasomnias. *Neurol Clin* 1996;14:697–720.

Sher AE, Schechtman KB, Piccirillo JF. The efficacy of surgical modifications of the upper airway in adults with obstructive sleep apnea syndrome. *Sleep* 1996;19:156–177.

Simonds AK. Nasal ventilation in progressive neuromuscular disease: experience in adults and adolescents. *Monaldi Arch Chest Dis* 2000;55:237–241.

Sin D, Fitzgerald F, Parker J. Risk factors for central and obstructive sleep apnea in 450 men and women with congestive heart failure. *Am J Respir Crit Care Med* 1999;160:1101–1106.

Sin D, Logan A, Fitzgerald F, et al. Effects of continuous positive airway pressure on cardiovascular outcomes in heart failure patients with and without Cheyne-Stokes respiration. *Circulation* 2000;102:61–66.

Smith MT, Perlis ML, Park A, et al. Comparative meta-analysis of pharmacotherapy and behavior therapy for persistent insomnia. *Am J Psychiatry* 2002;159:5–11.

Spiegel KLR, Van Cauter E. Impact of sleep debt on metabolic and endocrine function. *Lancet* 1999;1435–1439.

Thannikal TC, Moore RY, Nienheus R, et al. Reduced number of hypocretin neurons in human narcolepsy. *Neuron* 2000;27:469–474.

Thorpy MJ, Wagner DR, Spielman AJ, et al. Objective assessment of narcolepsy. *Arch Neurol* 1983;40:126–127.

Zucconi M, Oldani A, Ferini-Strambi L, et al. Nocturnal paroxysmal arousals with motor behavior during sleep: frontal lobe epilepsy or parasomnia? *J Clin Neurophysiol* 1997;14:513–522.

6. NEUROONCOLOGY

Santosh Kesari and Patrick Y. Wen

PRIMARY BRAIN TUMORS

BACKGROUND

Primary brain tumors (PBTs) are a heterogeneous group of neoplasms with varied outcomes and management strategies.

Epidemiology

1. Approximately 35,000 PBTs are diagnosed annually in the United States; 18,000 are malignant and result in 13,000 deaths each year.
2. There has been a steady rise in incidence of PBTs during the last two decades, in part due to increased sensitivity of imaging modalities.
3. Incidence of PBTs is 11 to 19/100,000 persons/year. There is an early peak between ages 0 and 4 years (incidence of 3.1/100,000), a trough between 15 and 24 years (1.8/100,000), and then a gradual rise in incidence to reach a plateau between 65 and 79 years (18/100,000).
4. Central nervous system (CNS) tumors account for 1.5% of all new cancers and 2.4% of all cancer deaths annually.
5. PBTs are the most common type of solid tumor in children, the second leading cause of cancer death under the age of 15 years, and the third leading cause of death under age 30.
6. In adults, the most common tumor types (in decreasing order of frequency) are glioblastoma multiforme (GBM), meningioma, astrocytoma, pituitary adenoma, vestibular schwannoma, oligodendroglioma, ependymoma, and medulloblastoma.
7. In children, the most common tumor types in decreasing frequency are medulloblastoma, astrocytoma, GBM, ependymoma, craniopharyngioma, neuroblastoma, and hemangioma.

Genetic Factors

One percent to 5% of patients with brain tumors have an underlying genetic syndrome that increases their risk of developing a brain tumor (Table 6-1).

Environmental Factors

There are only two unequivocal risk factors for PBTs:
1. Cranial irradiation is associated with an increased risk for meningiomas (tenfold risk) and gliomas (three- to sevenfold risk) with a latency period of 10 to 20 years after exposure.
2. Immunosuppression is associated with an increased risk for CNS lymphoma.

PATHOPHYSIOLOGY

1. Most PBTs arise from cells of glial origin.
2. Cell of origin of astrocytomas is debatable, but both astrocytes and precursor cells can form astrocytomas.
3. Angiogenesis plays a major role in tumor growth and survival.

TABLE 6-1. GENETIC SYNDROMES ASSOCIATED WITH BRAIN TUMORS

Neurofibromatosis type 1: Autosomal dominant (loss of gene encoding neurofibromin on chromosome 17.
Associated with: Schwannomas
Astrocytomas (including optic nerve gliomas)
Meningiomas
Neurofibromas
Neurofibrosarcomas

Neurofibromatosis type 2: Autosomal dominant (mutation of *NF2* gene on chromosome 22)
Associated with: Bilateral vestibular schwannomas
Astrocytomas
Multiple meningiomas
Ependymomas

Von Hippel–Lindau syndrome: Autosomal dominant (mutation of *VHL* gene on chromosome 3)
Associated with: Hemangioblastomas
Pancreatic cysts, retinal angiomas, renal carcinoma, pheochromocytoma

Li–Fraumeni syndrome: Autosomal recessive (germline mutation of *p53*)
Associated with: Gliomas
Sarcomas, breast cancer, and leukemias

Turcot syndrome: Autosomal dominant (mutation to the adenomatous polyposis coli gene on chromosome 5 or germline mutations in one of several enzymes involved in DNA nucleotide mismatch repair)
Associated with: Gliomas
Medulloblastomas
Poliposis coli

Basal cell nevus syndrome (Gorlin syndrome, nevoid basal cell cancer syndrome): germline mutations of the patched (*PTCH*) gene
Associated with: Medulloblastoma

Familial meningiomas
Familial gliomas

Molecular Genetics

1. Familial syndromes account for less than 5% of CNS tumors. The genetic syndromes associated with brain tumors are listed in Table 6-1.
2. Brain tumors result from a multistep process driven by the sequential acquisition of genetic alterations. These include loss of tumor suppressor genes (e.g., *p53* and *PTEN*) and amplification and overexpression of protooncogenes such as the epidermal growth factor receptor (EGFR) and the platelet derived growth factors (PDGF) and their receptors (PDGFR). The accumulation of these genetic abnormalities results in uncontrolled cell growth and tumor formation.
3. Glioma: The molecular genetics of glioblastomas evolving from low-grade astrocytomas (secondary glioblastomas) are different from that of de novo glioblastomas (primary glioblastomas). This may have implications in the selection of targeted molecular therapies for these tumors.
   a. Genetic changes in secondary glioblastomas
      1) Low-grade astrocytoma
         a) *p53* mutations (more than 65%)
         b) PDGF-A, PDGFR-α overexpression (60%)
      2) Anaplastic astrocytoma
         a) Loss of heterozygosity (LOH) 19q (50%)
         b) Retinoblastoma gene (*Rb*) alteration (25%)

    3) Secondary glioblastomas
      a) LOH 10q (DMBT1 deletion)
      b) *PTEN* mutations (5%)
      c) PDGFR-α amplification (less than 10%)
      d) Deleted colon cancer (DCC) loss of expression (50%)
  b. Genetic changes in primary (de novo) glioblastomas
    1) Epidermal growth factor (EGFR) amplification or overexpression (40%–60%)
    2) *PTEN* mutation (30%)
    3) *MDM2* amplification or overexpression (50%)
    4) P16 deletion (30%–40%)
    5) LOH 10p and 10q
    6) *Rb* alteration
4. Oligodendroglioma: Loss of chromosomes 1p and 19q, EGFR and PDGF/PDGFR overexpression.
5. Medulloblastoma: Amplification of myc, LOH 17p, 10q, 9 (sonic hedgehog/patched signaling pathway).

PROGNOSIS

1. The prognosis of brain tumors is determined by tumor type, grade, and location and by patient age and functional status [Karnofsky performance status (KPS)].
2. As a result of this marked heterogeneity, the prognostic features and treatment options must be carefully reviewed for each patient.
3. Resectability is a key determinant of prognosis and depends on the location and the invasiveness of the neoplasm.
4. Histologic grade of the tumor is important and clearly dictates the survival but care must be taken as sampling errors may underestimate the grade. Furthermore low-grade neoplasms can transform to higher grade neoplasms.
5. Advances in surgery, radiation therapy, and chemotherapy have led to improvement in prognosis for some low-grade gliomas and anaplastic oligodendrogliomas (AOs), but not for GBMs.

DIAGNOSIS

Location

1. The frequency of tumors at a location depends on age and type of tumor.
2. In adults, 70% of tumors occur in cerebral hemispheres and in children, 70% of tumors occur in posterior fossa.

Clinical Presentation

1. Symptoms are due to variety of effects caused by brain tumors including pressure against adjacent structures, elevated intracranial pressure (ICP), and seizures.
2. Symptoms can be acute or subacute but generally are progressive and depend on the size, location, and growth rate of tumor and peritumor edema.
3. Acute symptoms can result from seizures, intratumoral hemorrhage, or rapid growth or edema in eloquent areas.
4. Among patients with new-onset seizures, 5% are found to have a brain tumor.
5. Generalized and focal seizures occur in 15% to 95% of patients with supratentorial tumors and are more common in low-grade tumors and meningiomas.
6. Can present with generalized or focal signs.
7. Increased ICP symptoms include change in mental status, headache, nausea, vomiting, drowsiness, and papilledema.
8. Headache is the presenting feature in 35% of patients and develops in up to 70% during course of disease. It is usually bilateral, diffuse, and typically worsened with Valsalva maneuvers and lying down.
9. Focal signs include hemiparesis, sensory loss, ataxia, aphasia, memory loss, neglect, and visual loss.

Diagnostic Tests

1. Magnetic resonance imaging (MRI) enhanced with gadolinium is the test of choice for diagnosis of brain tumors.
2. Sometimes computed tomography (CT) with contrast is the only choice in patients with pacemakers or metallic implants.
3. Tumor cells have been found in the peritumoral edema, which corresponds to the T_2-weighted MRI abnormalities.
4. Other modalities such as magnetic resonance spectroscopy (MRS), positron emission tomography (PET), and single photon emission tomography (SPECT) are helpful in distinguishing tumor from radiation necrosis or inflammation.
5. Functional MRI can be used to define eloquent areas to assess risk of surgery.
6. The presence of multiple lesions on a contrast-enhanced study favors a metastatic process, but metastases can present as a solitary lesion in up to 50% of patients.
7. Lumbar puncture (LP) for routine cerebrospinal fluid (CSF) studies, cytology, and flow cytometry is useful to rule out leptomeningeal involvement of tumors, especially in the case of lymphoma, medulloblastoma, pineal tumors, and germ cell tumors. LP is generally contraindicated if elevated ICP is suspected or if there are large mass lesions.
8. In cases of suspected metastatic disease, a full workup to search for a primary tumor should be undertaken and includes ocular, testicular, breast (mammogram in females), and prostate examinations (males) and urinalysis, complete blood count, peripheral smear, stool guaiac testing, body CT, bone scan, and occasionally PET scan.
9. Stereotactic biopsy or craniotomy with resection of the mass allows histologic diagnosis and should be performed in most patients.

Pathology

1. The classification, prognosis, and treatment of brain tumors is ultimately dependent on the histopathologic features of the surgical specimen in the clinical context.
2. Classification of tumor is based on presumed cell of origin: Of primary CNS tumors, 60% arise from glial cells (astrocytes, oligodendroglial cells, and ependymal cells), 20% from the meninges, and 20% from neurons, Schwann cells, lymphocytes, and cells of the pituitary gland.
3. Glial tumors are graded on the basis of cellularity, nuclear atypia, mitoses, microvascular proliferation, and necrosis according to the World Health Organization (WHO) system or the St. Anne–Mayo system.
4. Errors can occur when a small sample is taken for biopsy in a heterogeneous tumor such that it is not reflective of the biology of the entire tumor.
5. Grading for astrocytomas:
   a. WHO grade I (pilocytic astrocytoma) is very slow growing.
   b. WHO grade II (low-grade astrocytoma) shows relatively homogenous appearance, hypercellularity, nuclear atypia, and ill-defined tumor margins. Pleomorphic xanthoastrocytoma is a more benign variant.
   c. WHO grade III (anaplastic astrocytoma) shows high cellularity, mitosis, and pleomorphism.
   d. WHO grade IV (GBM) shows features of grade III but also has necrosis and vascular proliferation.

Differential Diagnosis

1. A wide differential must be kept in mind during the initial evaluation of a brain mass as many treatable conditions can mimic brain tumors.
2. The differential should always include other PBTs, lymphoma, metastases, abscesses, viral infections, encephalomyelitis, demyelination, stroke, vascular anomaly, vasculitis, and granulomatous and inflammatory disease.

TREATMENT

Treatment of patients with brain tumors require close cooperation of a multidisciplinary team of physicians including neurologists, neurosurgeons, radiation therapists, oncologists, neuroradiologists, neuropathologists, and psychiatrists.

Supportive Care

1. Corticosteroids:
   a. Used to reduce symptomatic vasogenic edema surrounding tumors, which lowers ICP and mass effect. Clinically improvement begins within 24 to 48 hours with maximum improvement by fifth day.
   b. Response independent of type of corticosteroid used (dexamethasone, methylprednisolone, prednisone, hydrocortisone) when given in equivalent doses.
   c. Dexamethasone used widely due to low mineralocorticoid (salt-retaining) side effects.
   d. Dexamethasone usually given as bolus of 10 mg and then 16 mg/d by mouth (p.o.) or intravenous (IV) in divided doses.
      1) Oral absorption is excellent.
      2) Half-life is long enough for it to be given twice daily.
   e. Higher doses (up to 40 mg) can be given to critically ill patients until definitive treatment (surgery, radiation) is undertaken.
   f. Side effects include glucose intolerance, oral candidiasis, opportunistic infections including *Pneumocystis carinii* pneumonitis (PCP), gastric irritation, adrenal suppression, steroid myopathy, osteoporosis, and psychiatric problems.
   g. Patients may need glucose monitoring and H_2 blockers or proton pump inhibitors to reduce gastric irritation.
   h. Patients who are likely to remain on steroids for prolonged periods should have PCP prophylaxis [e.g., 160 mg of trimethoprim plus 800 mg of sulfamethoxazole (Bactrim DS) daily or 3 d/wk].
   i. Steroids should be tapered to the lowest dose possible to avoid complications.
   j. Patients who are on steroids for prolonged periods may need adjustments to control edema perioperatively, during chemotherapy, and radiation treatments.
2. Anticonvulsants:
   a. Prophylactic anticonvulsants are not recommended for patients unless they have history of seizures. There is no evidence that patients with brain tumors who have never had a seizure benefit from prophylactic anticonvulsants.
   b. Prophylactic anticonvulsants should be given to patients undergoing craniotomies, but can be tapered off 2 to 4 weeks after the procedure.
   c. Commonly used anticonvulsants include phenytoin, carbamazepine, and valproate.
   d. More than 20% of patients receiving phenytoin or carbamazepine develop drug rashes.
   e. The newer anticonvulsants, such as levetiracetam, have less drug interactions and are better tolerated.
   f. Cytochrome P450 enzyme-inducing antiepileptic drugs (EIAED), such as phenytoin, may increase the metabolism of many chemotherapeutic agents and reduce their efficacy.

Prevention of Venous Thromboembolism
Patients with brain tumors have an increased risk of developing venous thromboembolism (VTE) (30% lifetime risk in patients with GBM). Extra care must be taken to prevent VTE in the perioperative period. When a patient develops VTE, anticoagulation is usually safe after the perioperative period and more effective than inferior vena cava filtration devices.

Additional Supportive Care
Many patients with brain tumors benefit from physical and occupational therapy, psychiatric consultation, visiting nurses, social services, patient support groups, and brain

tumor organizations [American Brain Tumor Association (2720 River Rd, Des Plaines, IL 60018; tel. (847) 827-9910 or patient line: (800) 886-2282; e-mail: info@abta.org), the Brain Tumor Society (124 Watertown St, Ste 3-H, Watertown, MA 02472; tel. (800) 770-TBTS (8287); e-mail: info@tbts.org), and the National Brain Tumor Foundation (414 Thirteenth St, Ste 700, Oakland, CA 94612-2603; tel. (510) 839-9777 or information line: (800) 934-CURE (2873); e-mail: nbtf@braintumor.org)].

Definitive Therapy

Surgery

1. Decisions regarding aggressiveness of surgery for a PBT are complex and depend on the age and performance status of the patient; the feasibility of decreasing the mass effect with aggressive surgery; the resectability of the tumor (including the number and location of lesions), and, in patients with recurrent disease, the time since the last surgery.
2. Biopsy or surgical resection is performed on most patients to obtain histologic confirmation of the type and grade of tumor and provide information on prognosis and treatment.
3. Biopsy is performed using stereotactic devices or intraoperative MRI. Biopsies are performed for tumors that are deep or in eloquent areas where surgical resection is contraindicated.
4. Due to heterogeneity in the tumor, a small biopsy sample may be nondiagnostic or not representative of the whole tumor.
5. Appropriate localization of biopsy to obtain the highest grade area is important.
6. Extensive tumor resection is the surgical procedure of choice for most tumors and improves neurologic function and survival. This can be achieved for many extraaxial tumors, but very few intraaxial tumors can be resected completely.
7. Partial resection can be palliative by improving neurologic function and improving survival when total resection is not possible.
8. Repeated partial resections may be beneficial, especially for benign tumors.
9. Patients who develop hydrocephalus (usually due to tumors that obstruct the third or fourth ventricles) require a ventriculoperitoneal (VP) shunt to reduce ICP.
10. Some tumors such as brainstem gliomas have characteristic imaging features. Biopsy is usually not done due to high risk of neurologic deficits. Patients are treated without tissue diagnosis.
11. Intraoperative MRI can help in clarifying normal and abnormal tissue thereby allowing for more complete resection.
12. A postoperative MRI, with and without contrast, should be performed within 24 to 72 hours after surgery to document the extent of disease following surgical intervention.

Complications of Surgery

1. The standard risks of anesthesia and neurosurgery include hemorrhage, stroke, increased edema, direct injury to normal brain, infection, and venous thromboembolism.
2. Postoperative hemorrhage may require evacuation if producing focal deficits.
3. Cerebral edema is usually present preoperatively and may be exacerbated during surgery by mechanical retraction, venous compression, brain manipulation, and overhydration. Generally steroids are given for several days prior to craniotomy.
4. Risk of infection is increased with length of operation and introduction of foreign materials (shunt tubing, clips, chemotherapy polymers) and most infections are due to cutaneous and airborne pathogens. Most patients are given perioperative prophylactic antibiotics.
5. Communicating hydrocephalus can occur transiently postoperatively.
6. Neuroendocrine disturbances such as syndrome of inappropriate secretion of antidiuretic hormone (SIADH) can occur after surgery and electrolytes and fluid balance should be carefully monitored to prevent hyponatremia and cerebral edema.
7. Surgery of the hypothalamic–pituitary axis can result in various degrees of panhypopituitarism and diabetes insipidus.

Radiation Therapy

1. Radiation therapy (RT) for patients with PBTs usually involves a limited field encompassing the tumor volume (commonly defined as the region showing T_2-weighted abnormalities on an MRI scan plus a 1- to 2-cm margin).
2. Usual dose is 6,000 cGy for high-grade PBT, 5,400 cGy for low-grade PBT, and 3,600 cGy for spinal tumors in 180- to 200-cGy fractions over approximately 6 weeks. The dose is 3,000 cGy in 10 fractions for brain metastases.
3. Several different treatment approaches are used including conformal external beam (most common), stereotactic brachytherapy, stereotactic radiosurgery (SRS), and stereotactic radiotherapy (SRT).
4. Increasingly sophisticated techniques are available to administer conformal irradiation, including intensity-modulated radiation therapy (IMRT), which allows variation of radiation dose in different parts of the radiation field.
5. Brachytherapy, which involves surgical implantation of radioactive isotopes, is now rarely performed. Replaced by SRS, which is noninvasive.
6. SRS involves the treatment of small intracranial targets using a large, single fraction of ionizing radiation in stereotactically directed narrow beams. It allows a high dose of radiation to be delivered to the tumor while relatively sparing surrounding brain. SRS can be administered using x-rays from stereotactic linear accelerators, gamma irradiation from cobalt sources in gamma knives, and protons from cyclotrons (proton beam therapy). Radiation necrosis is relatively common. Risk increases with dose and volume treated; 5% to 10% of patients require surgical resection of necrotic area for symptomatic relief.
7. SRT is stereotactic radiation administered in multiple fractions to reduce risk of radiation injury to surrounding structures.

Chemotherapy

1. The blood–brain barrier (BBB) provides the CNS with a privileged environment and consists of the cerebrovascular–capillary endothelium. Only physiologically small, lipid-soluble drugs or actively transported drugs can cross the BBB.
2. Chemotherapy useful for primary central nervous system lymphoma (PCNSL), anaplastic oligodendrogliomas, oligodendrogliomas, anaplastic astrocytomas, and medulloblastoma. Only modest efficacy in glioblastoma.

NEUROEPITHELIAL TUMORS

PILOCYTIC ASTROCYTOMA

BACKGROUND

1. The most common noninfiltrative, focal astrocytoma in childhood.
2. Mainly in children and adolescents but 25% in patients older than 18.
3. Also seen in individuals with neurofibromatosis type I (NF1).

PATHOPHYSIOLOGY

Mostly sporadic, but deletions of 17q (NF1) associated with 15% of optic gliomas in patients with NF1.

PROGNOSIS

1. Indolent course, often surgically resectable, and rarely transforms.
2. Greater than 90% 10-year survival for supratentorial lesions after total resection.

3. A 95% 25-year disease-free survival for cerebellar astrocytoma after total resection.
4. A 74% to 84% 10-year survival for subtotal resection.
5. In children, 75% stable at 4-year follow-up after surgery and chemotherapy (vincristine and actinomycin D) when too young to receive radiation.

DIAGNOSIS

Location

1. In children, it arises in the cerebellum, optic pathway, and hypothalamus.
2. In young adults, it arises in cerebrum, brainstem, optic nerve, thalamus, and hypothalamus.

Clinical Presentation

Clinical features depend on location. Cerebellar lesions produce symptoms secondary to obstruction of CSF flow or pressure on cerebellum leading to headaches and ataxia.

Diagnostic Tests

MRI shows a cyst with mural nodule that enhances.

Pathology

1. WHO grade I, grossly well-circumscribed, and gelatinous appearance.
2. Two microscopic patterns: a tightly packed parallel array of well-differentiated astrocytes with Rosenthal fibers (globular, refractile, homogenous, eosinophilic bodies) and a loose matrix of astrocytes, long slender piloid "hair-like" cells, and amphophilic granular bodies.

Differential Diagnosis

Low-grade diffuse astrocytoma, ependymoma, and ganglioglioma.

TREATMENT

1. Some tumors in surgically inaccessible areas (e.g., optic nerve glioma) grow very slowly and may be observed for many years before definitive therapy is required.
2. Surgically curable if complete resection possible.
3. Conformal radiation or SRT helpful if resection not possible or for recurrent tumor.
4. Chemotherapy with agents such as carboplatin and vincristine useful in young children.

LOW-GRADE DIFFUSE ASTROCYTOMA

BACKGROUND

1. Low-grade diffuse astrocytomas are slow-growing tumors.
2. Although referred to as "low-grade," these tumors grow and gradually evolve to higher grade astrocytomas, ultimately causing morbidity and reduced survival.
3. Early diagnosis difficult due to nonfocal findings with these tumors.

Epidemiology

1. Low-grade astrocytomas comprise 10% of all adult PBTs and 25 to 30% of all cerebral gliomas; 1,500 new cases diagnosed in United States each year.
2. Incidence 1.3 to 2.2/100,000 and peaks in third and fourth decades.

3. In adults, most arise in the cerebral hemispheres and in children most arise in the posterior fossa.

PATHOPHYSIOLOGY

Most tumors have *p53* mutations and overexpression of *PDGF*.

PROGNOSIS

1. Highly variable and depends on age and amount of residual tumor.
2. Positive prognostic factors include long duration of symptoms, excellent postoperative neurologic status, and low MIB-1 proliferation index (less than 3%–5%).
3. Low-grade glioma has median survival of 5 to 7 years with gross total resection, 35% at 5 years with biopsy or subtotal resection, and 46% at 5 years with subtotal resection and radiation.

DIAGNOSIS

Clinical Presentation

Usually present with new-onset seizures (50%–70%). Less commonly with headaches, focal deficits, or subtle neurobehavioral changes.

Diagnostic Tests

1. CT shows a low-density mass or occasionally a partially calcified mass that does not show enhancement.
2. MRI typically shows a nonenhancing white matter mass, hypointense T_1, hyperintense T_2, and fluid-enhanced inversion recovery (FLAIR) with ill-defined borders and little or no edema.
3. PET shows glucose hypometabolism.

Pathology

1. WHO grade II, low-grade tumor.
2. Hypercellular, well-differentiated astrocytes; may be cystic, infiltrative.
3. Diffuse variants include fibrillary, protoplasmic, and gemistocytic.
4. Biopsy results can be misleading, as gliomas often have varying degrees of cellularity, mitoses, or necrosis from one region to another.

Differential Diagnosis

Includes high-grade tumor, oligodendroglioma, ganglioglioma, dysembryoplastic neuroepithelioma (DNT), infarction, demyelination, progressive multifocal leukoencephalopathy (PML), and vasculitis.

TREATMENT

1. Maximal resection associated with improved survival. Advances in neurosurgery, including intraoperative mapping and intraoperative MRI, have allowed more aggressive resection of these tumors with preservation of neurologic function.
2. Standard radiation dose for low-grade astrocytomas is 4,500 to 5,400 cGy, given at a rate of 180 to 200 cGy/d.
3. Radiation usually administered to T_2-weighted MRI abnormality together with a 1- to 2-cm margin. Increasingly more conformal therapy with SRT and IMRT. Whole-brain irradiation is associated with increased neurotoxicity and no longer used.
4. Adjuvant irradiation (following surgery) prolongs survival in patients who have only subtotal resection.

5. Timing of irradiation controversial. Adjuvant irradiation delays recurrence but overall survival similar to patients who do not receive irradiation until there is evidence of recurrent disease.
6. Chemotherapy with agents such as temozolomide or procarbazine, CCNU (lomustine), vincristine (PCV) has a limited role in patients with diffuse infiltrating tumors.

PLEOMORPHIC XANTHOASTROCYTOMA

BACKGROUND

1. Rare focal astrocytoma with characteristic clinical, imaging, and pathologic features.
2. Most common in second and third decade of life.

PATHOPHYSIOLOGY

1. Believed to originate from subpial astrocytes due to its superficial location with attachment to the leptomeninges.
2. *p53* mutations found in a small portion of patients.

PROGNOSIS

1. Indolent lesions.
2. Good with resection, 76% 10-year survival.
3. Rare anaplasia associated with poor prognosis.

DIAGNOSIS

Location

Predilection for superficial temporal and parietal lobes involving the leptomeninges and, rarely, the dura.

Clinical Presentation

Usually have a long history of seizures before diagnosis. Occasionally causes headaches and focal deficits.

Diagnostic Tests

MRI shows a heterogenous, superficial meningocerebral nodule, often associated with a cyst. Iso- to hypointense on T_1-weighted images and enhancing.

Pathology

WHO grade II; enlarged, lipid-laden astrocytes; inflammation; extreme pleomorphism; cellular atypia; and spindle and multinucleated giant cells. No necrosis or vascular hyperplasia.

Differential Diagnosis

Can be mistaken histologically for fibrous histiocytoma of the meninges, giant cell astrocytoma with histiocytic infiltration, and lipidized giant cell glioblastoma multiforme. Must also be differentiated from other forms of gliomas and DNT.

TREATMENT

1. Surgical resection
2. RT and chemotherapy for recurrent tumor

SUBEPENDYMAL GIANT CELL ASTROCYTOMA

BACKGROUND

1. Subependymal giant cell astrocytoma (SEGA) is a slow-growing focal astrocytoma.
2. Found in children and young adults.
3. Mostly associated with tuberous sclerosis (TS) and present in 15% of patients with TS.

PATHOPHYSIOLOGY

1. Associated with neurocutaneous disorders such as TS and nevus sebaceous syndrome.
2. Partial loss of chromosome 22q.

PROGNOSIS

1. Slow growing and benign
2. Rarely malignant degeneration

DIAGNOSIS

Location

Arises in the wall of the lateral ventricle, attached to caudate head.

Clinical Presentation

May obstruct CSF flow at the foramen of Monro and cause obstructive hydrocephalus producing headache and visual disturbance.

Diagnostic Tests

MRI shows an intraventricular enhancing mass.

Pathology

1. WHO grade I, giant astrocytes with glassy, eosinophilic cytoplasm, without significant anaplasia. May express neuronal markers.
2. Lesion represents neoplastic transformation of "candle guttering" subependymal nodules in TS.

Differential Diagnosis

Choroid plexus tumors, ependymoma, subependymoma, and astrocytoma.

TREATMENT

1. Surgical debulking for obstructive symptoms.
2. Occasional role for SRS or SRT.
3. No role for chemotherapy.

HIGH-GRADE ASTROCYTOMAS

BACKGROUND

1. In adults, high-grade astrocytomas (HGAs) are the most common PBT (60%–70%) and includes anaplastic astrocytoma (AA), anaplastic mixed oligoastrocytoma (AOA) and glioblastoma multiforme (GBM).
2. Approximately 12,000 new cases of HGA are diagnosed each year and account for 2.3% of all cancer-related deaths. Incidence of GBM is 3 to 4/100,000.
3. AA has a bimodal peak in first and third decades (peak age, 35–50 years).
4. GBM peak age 50 to 60 years.
5. Male to female ratio is 3 to 2.

PATHOPHYSIOLOGY

1. Usually sporadic. HGA often arise from low-grade astrocytomas.
2. Difficult to treat because they diffusely infiltrate surrounding tissues and frequently cross the midline to involve the contralateral brain.
3. Associated with EGFR and PDGF overexpression, and *p16*, *PTEN*, and *p53* mutations (see Primary Brain Tumors, Pathophysiology, Molecular Genetics, above).

PROGNOSIS

1. Uniformly fatal despite aggressive therapy. Occasional long-term survivors.
2. Factors that portend a poor prognosis: age older than 50, subtotal resection, poor functional status (KPS less than 70), abnormal mental status.
3. For GBM, the median survival is 10 to 12 months despite maximal therapy.
4. For AA, the median survival is 2 to 3 years with maximal therapy.
5. For AOA, the median survival is 3 to 5 years with maximal therapy.

DIAGNOSIS

Location

Cerebral hemispheres, especially frontal (40%) and temporal (30%) lobes, and rarely in brainstem, cerebellum, and spinal cord in adults.

Clinical Presentation

1. Patients often present with symptoms of increased ICP (headache, nausea, vomiting), seizures, or focal neurologic findings related to the size and location of the tumor and associated peritumoral edema.
2. Can have symptoms up to 2 years before diagnosis in AA and for several months with GBM.

Diagnostic Tests

1. Both AA and GBM on CT and MRI can show heterogeneous enhancing lesions with vasogenic edema, mass effect, and frequently, tracks along white matter paths including the corpus callosum ("butterfly glioma"). Occasionally have associated hemorrhage or calcification. GBM usually also has ring enhancement and central necrosis.
2. MRS shows elevated choline peaks (reflecting active membrane synthesis) and decreased *N*-acetyl aspartate peaks (reflecting neuronal loss).
3. In recurrent glioma, PET, thallium/technetium SPECT, or MRS can help distinguish radiation necrosis (hypometabolic) from tumor (hypermetabolic).
4. Histologic diagnosis ultimately depends on obtaining tissue via biopsy or craniotomy.

Pathology

1. AA (WHO grade III): Endothelial proliferation, mitoses, nuclear atypia, hyperchromatic nuclei.
2. GBM (WHO grade IV): Pseudopalisading areas of necrosis, endothelial vascular proliferation, pleomorphism, and mitosis. Variants include giant cell glioblastoma (large bizarre cells), small cell glioblastoma, and gliosarcoma (spindle cell component).

Differential Diagnosis

Includes other PBTs, metastases, lymphoma, and abscess.

TREATMENT

Surgery

1. Craniotomy with maximal safe resection of tumor improves neurologic deficits and quality of life and results in modest prolongation of survival.
2. The extent of tumor debulking should be documented with an immediate postoperative MRI scan performed with and without contrast.
3. If resection is not possible because tumor is in eloquent area, it should be biopsied to obtain histologic diagnosis. Every effort should be made to obtain tissue from area of actively growing tumor (usually enhancing area). PET and perfusion MRI may help direct biopsy.

Radiation Therapy

1. RT is standard treatment. Ameliorates symptoms and improves survival by 50% to 100%.
2. Usually 6,000 cGy in 30 to 32 180- to 200-cGy fractions given to localized field surrounding the area of the tumor (T_2 abnormality plus 2-cm margin) plus coned-down radiation to the tumor bed.
3. Patients should be followed up closely with serial MRI scans after the completion of RT.
4. Because RT can produce additional BBB dysfunction, corticosteroid requirements may increase and scans may look worse during the first 1 to 2 months after completion of RT, even though there is no actual tumor progression.
5. Despite RT, 80% of tumor recur within primary site of disease.
6. Other radiotherapy methods such as brachytherapy, hyperfractionation, radiosurgery, and radiosensitizers have not significantly improved survival.

Chemotherapy

1. Adjuvant chemotherapy is marginally beneficial in prolonging survival and improving quality of life. Overall, it produces an approximately 10% increase in median survival and a small increase in long-term survivors. Benefit greater for young patients and those with AA and AOA.
2. Alkylating agents are the most active chemotherapeutic agents for HGA.
3. Carmustine (BCNU), PCV [procarbazine, CCNU (lomustine), and vincristine], and temozolomide all have equal efficacy.
4. BCNU (carmustine) is administered IV in doses of 200 mg/m^2 as a single dose or 80 mg/m^2 for 3 days every 6 to 8 weeks. Usually six cycles administered. Dose-limiting toxicities include marrow suppression, pulmonary hepatic, and nausea.
5. PCV [procarbazine (60mg/m^2) p.o. on days 8 to 21 every 6 weeks], CCNU (110mg/m^2 p.o. every 6 weeks), vincristine [1.4mg/m^2 (maximum, 2 mg) on days 8 and 29] every 6 weeks for six cycles. Toxicity similar to that of BCNU. Vincristine may produce neuropathy.

6. Temozolomide 150 to 200mg/m^2 p.o. days 1 through 5 every 28 days for 6 to 12 months. Toxicities include nausea and marrow suppression. May have radiosensitizing activity when given with RT (75 mg/m^2 daily for 6 weeks with RT, followed by 4 weeks off treatment, and then six cycles of standard-dose temozolomide produced 16-month median survival in one study). Use of prolonged low-dose temozolomide increases risk of PCP. Patients receiving this regimen require PCP prophylaxis.
7. Irinotecan (CPT-11), a topoisomerase inhibitor, also has modest activity (350 mg/m^2 IV every 3 weeks for patients on non-EIAED; 750 mg/m^2 IV every 3 weeks for patients on EIAED).
8. Carboplatin, etoposide, tamoxifen, and *cis*-retinoic acid have minimal activity.
9. Slow-release polymer wafers impregnated with BCNU (Gliadel wafers) placed in the wall of the surgical cavity at time of debulking improves survival in newly diagnosed and recurrent GBM by approximately 2 months.

Experimental Therapies

Targeted molecular therapy (e.g., inhibitors of EGFR and PDFGR), inhibitors of angiogenesis (e.g., thalidomide), viral gene therapy, tumor vaccines (dendritic and telomerase), immunotoxins, monoclonal antibodies, and inhibitors of tumor invasion are being evaluated in clinical trials.

GLIOMATOSIS CEREBRI

BACKGROUND

1. Gliomatosis cerebri is characterized by widespread dissemination of neoplastic astrocytes, often involving an entire cerebral hemisphere with or without discrete mass lesions.
2. These tumors are rare. Peak incidence is 40 to 50 years of age.

PATHOPHYSIOLOGY

Molecular genetic alterations in gliomatosis cerebri resemble those in diffuse astrocytomas.

PROGNOSIS

Prognosis is variable but often worse than that for GBM.

DIAGNOSIS

Location

Diffuse infiltration without discrete tumor masses, usually deep in thalamus and basal ganglia.

Clinical Presentation

Cognitive/neurobehavioral changes, headaches, seizures, and papilledema.

Diagnostic Tests

MRI shows homogenous hypodense areas, loss of gray–white junction, swollen hemispheres, diffuse increase in T_2 and FLAIR signal, and minimal to no enhancement.

Pathology

1. Grossly diffuse enlarged brain, microscopically extensive gray–white matter infiltration of tumor cells.
2. Graded from low grade to high grade (WHO grades II–III).
3. Rarely an oligodendroglioma.

DIFFERENTIAL DIAGNOSIS

Inflammatory, infectious, or demyelinating process in the appropriate clinical context.

TREATMENT

1. Stereotactic biopsy needed for diagnosis, usually not resectable.
2. Some patients respond temporarily to radiotherapy.
3. Occasional response to temozolomide, PCV, or BCNU.

BRAINSTEM GLIOMA

BACKGROUND

1. In children, brainstem gliomas account for 15% of PBTs and include diffuse pontine glioma (80%), cervicomedullary glioma, dorsally exophytic glioma, tectal glioma, and focal glioma.
2. In adults, brainstem gliomas are uncommon and account for less than 3% of gliomas.

PATHOPHYSIOLOGY

Usually astrocytic in origin. Its prognosis is generally worse than the pathology would suggest because of its location.

PROGNOSIS

Diffuse pontine glioma has a poor prognosis with a median survival of only 1 year despite aggressive therapy. Intrinsic focal low-grade brainstem gliomas have a better prognosis: 80% 5-year survival.

DIAGNOSIS

Clinical Presentation

Brainstem gliomas present with cranial nerve (CN) palsies, ataxia, weakness, and numbness.

Pathology

Diffuse brainstem gliomas are not usually biopsied. Diagnosis is based on characteristic imaging findings. Focal lesions, especially if they are exophytic, sometimes can be biopsied.

Differential Diagnosis

Includes ependymoma, medulloblastoma, vascular malformation, cysticercosis, encephalitis, tuberculoma, multiple sclerosis, postinfectious encephalomyelitis, or gliosis.

TREATMENT

1. Surgery may be indicated for cervicomedullary, focal, cystic, or exophytic tumors.
2. Biopsy (open or CT-guided stereotactic) is indicated when the diagnosis of brainstem glioma is in doubt.
3. Treatment for diffuse brainstem glioma is RT (54–56 Gy in daily fractions of 1.8–2.0 Gy).
4. VP shunt may be necessary for obstructive hydrocephalus.
5. Chemotherapy with PCV, temozolomide, carboplatin of limited benefit.

OLIGODENDROGLIOMA

BACKGROUND

1. Comprise up to 20% to 30% of gliomas (increasingly diagnosed as criteria expanded).
2. Most occur at ages 30 to 50, men more often than women.
3. Most common primary tumor to hemorrhage.

PATHOPHYSIOLOGY

1. Arise from oligodendrocytes or glial precursor cells.
2. Mixed oligoastrocytomas probably develop from a common glial stem cell.
3. Many have deletions in chromosome 1p and 19q and *EGFR* and *PDGF* overexpression.
4. Anaplastic oligodendrogliomas (AOs) also have deletions in chromosomes 9p and 10q and overexpression of *CDK4*.

PROGNOSIS

1. Deletions in 1p and 19q are favorable prognostic factors as they are sensitive to chemotherapy and radiotherapy.
2. Oligodendroglioma: Median survival is 8 to 15 years.
3. Anaplastic oligodendroglioma: Median survival is 3.9 years but chemosensitive subset with 1p and 19q deletions may have median survival more than 10 years.
4. Mixed oligoastrocytomas tend to have a prognosis intermediate between AO and AA.

DIAGNOSIS

Location

Frontal and temporal lobes most common.

Clinical Presentation

Usually present with seizures; occasionally headaches, focal deficits, or personality changes.

Diagnostic Tests

CT and MRI show calcification in 50% to 90%; well demarcated, usually no enhancement; located near cortical surface, with little or no edema; cystic (20%); hemorrhage (10%). AOs usually enhance.

Pathology

1. Oligodendroglioma, WHO grade II; AO, WHO grade III.

2. Grossly soft, grayish-pink tumors frequently with calcifications, hemorrhages, cysts, delicate vessels.
3. Microscopically round nuclei with perinuclear halo ("fried-egg" appearance in paraffin), delicate branching vessels ("chicken wire" vasculature), calcification, perineuronal satellitosis (secondary structures of Scherer).
4. Mixed oligoastrocytoma contains both oligodendroglial and astrocytic components.
5. Anaplastic variant has high cellularity, increased mitotic rate, pleomorphism, microvascular proliferation, and occasional necrosis.

Differential Diagnosis

1. Oligodendroglioma must be differentiated from astrocytoma, ganglioglioma, DNT.
2. AO can be confused with AA and GBM.

TREATMENT

1. Complete surgical resection preferred and improves survival.
2. RT improves symptoms and survival in patients with partial resection. Patients with 1p deletion have increased response to RT. Trend toward deferring RT because many patients have chemosensitive tumors.
3. Approximately 65% of AOs are sensitive to PCV chemotherapy and radiation. Complete responses are seen in 30% of patients. Most tumors with loss of both chromosomes 1p and 19q are sensitive to chemotherapy. Tumors with intact 1p and no *p53* mutations very unlikely to respond to chemotherapy. Tumors with 1p deletions are usually treated with four to six cycles of PCV followed by RT. Temozolomide also active in AO. Tumors with intact 1p treated with RT.
4. Increasing evidence that grade II oligodendrogliomas are also sensitive to PCV and temozolomide.

EPENDYMAL TUMORS

BACKGROUND

1. Ependymomas are tumors derived from ependymal cells that line the ventricular surface.
2. Subependymomas are slow-growing benign lesions that often do not require treatment.
3. Ependymoblastoma is a primitive neuroectodermal tumor (PNET) that occurs in the first 5 years of life.

Epidemiology

1. Mostly in childhood in the first decade and is the most common intraventricular tumor in children.
2. In adults, usually occurs in spinal cord.
3. Slight male preponderance.
4. Comprises 2% to 8% of all PBTs, 6% to 12% of intracranial gliomas in children (much less common in adults), and 60% of spinal cord gliomas (most common spinal cord glioma).
5. Median age of onset for posterior fossa tumor is 6.5 years. Second peak at 30 to 40 years for spinal cord tumor.

PATHOPHYSIOLOGY

1. *NF2* gene inactivation on chromosome 22 and mutations on chromosome 11q13.
2. Amplification of *mdm2* gene in 35% of cases.
3. A 50% incidence of allelic loss of 17p in pediatric cases.

PROGNOSIS

1. Poor prognostic factors: age younger than 2 years, incomplete resection, supratentorial location, duration of symptoms less than 1 month, and anaplastic histology.
2. The 5-year survival after complete resection and radiotherapy is 70% to 87% compared to 30% to 40% for partially resection; overall 10-year survival of 50%.
3. In children, fourth-ventricle tumors clinically more aggressive.
4. Anaplastic ependymoma has a 12% 5-year survival.
5. Subependymoma is indolent and often does not require treatment.
6. The prognosis for ependymoblastoma is poor with death within 1 year of surgery.

DIAGNOSIS

Location

1. Infratentorial in 60% of cases.
2. Most frequently in fourth ventricle (70%), lateral ventricles (20%), and cauda equina (10%).
3. In adults, commonly occurs in lumbosacral spinal cord and filum terminale (myxopapillary ependymoma).
4. May spread via CSF and seed other locations (12%).
5. Ependymoblastoma usually in cerebrum with frequent craniospinal metastasis.

Clinical Presentation

1. Intracranial tumors produce symptoms due to obstruction of CSF flow (headaches, nausea, vomiting, visual disturbance), ataxia, dizziness, hemiparesis, and brainstem symptoms.
2. Spinal cord tumors present as a chronic, progressive myelopathy or cauda equina syndrome (see section on Spinal Cord Tumor).

Diagnostic Tests

1. MRI shows a well-demarcated, heterogenous, enhancing intraventricular mass, with frequent calcifications. Obstructive hydrocephalus and hemorrhage may be present.
2. Spinal MRI should be done to rule out neuraxis dissemination.

Pathology

1. Grossly well circumscribed, tan, and soft tissue.
2. Microscopically densely cellular with ependymal rosettes, blepharoplasts, and perivascular pseudorosettes.
3. In cauda equina, the myxopapillary form common.
4. Anaplastic ependymomas have malignant features such as mitotic activity, pleomorphism, and necrosis.
5. Ependymoblastoma has ependymoblastic rosettes in fields of undifferentiated cells.
6. Subependymoma is a benign lesion located within ventricles. Has both ependymal and astrocytic features.

Differential Diagnosis

Subependymoma, anaplastic ependymoma, ependymoblastoma, astrocytomas, medulloblastoma.

TREATMENT

1. Surgical resection is treatment of choice but many tumors recur regardless of completeness of resection.

2. For ependymoma and anaplastic ependymoma, postoperative local radiation (4,500–6,000 cGy) improves survival.
3. Craniospinal radiation reserved for tumors with CSF spread.
4. Chemotherapy is used in children younger than 3 years to delay onset of RT.
5. Results of chemotherapy are generally poor.

CHOROID PLEXUS TUMORS

BACKGROUND

1. Choroid plexus tumors are derived from the choroid plexus epithelium.
2. Peak incidence in first two decades of life. It is the most common intracranial tumor in the first year of life.
3. Accounts for less than 1% of all intracranial tumors.

PATHOPHYSIOLOGY

1. Possible role for simian virus 40 (SV40) in pathogenesis.
2. Choroid plexus papilloma (CPP) (WHO grade I) histologically resembles normal choroid plexus and probably represents local hamartomatous overgrowths.
3. Choroid plexus carcinoma (CPC) (WHO grades III–IV) account for 10% of choroid plexus tumors. They are aggressive tumors with dense cellularity, mitoses, nuclear pleomorphism, focal necrosis, loss of papillary architecture, and invasion of neural tissue. They frequently seed CSF pathways. Usually occurs in children younger than 8 years.

PROGNOSIS

1. Good with CPP. With complete resection, 80% 5-year survival; 4.3% recurrence rate overall.
2. Poor with CPC.

DIAGNOSIS

Location

1. In adults, common in fourth ventricle, lateral ventricle, and third ventricle.
2. In children, most common in lateral ventricles and cerebellopontine angle (CPA).

Clinical Presentation

Present with symptoms secondary to CSF obstruction or CSF overproduction, headaches, nausea, vomiting, ataxia.

Diagnostic Tests

MRI shows homogenous, enhancing mass with prominent flow voids due to rich vascularization, frequent calcification.

Differential Diagnosis

Ependymoma, astrocytoma, metastases.

TREATMENT

1. Surgical resection.
2. Postoperative RT for CPC; RT at recurrence for CPP.

NEURONAL AND MIXED NEURONAL–GLIAL TUMORS

BACKGROUND

1. Initially thought to be hamartomas, but these are ganglion cell tumors that form a continuum between those with mixed ganglion and glial cell components (gangliogliomas) and some that are relatively pure ganglion cell tumor.
2. Include ganglioglioma, gangliocytoma, DNT, neurocytoma, and dysplastic gangliocytoma of the cerebellum (Lhermitte–Duclos disease).

Epidemiology

1. Occur in children and young adults in first three decades of life.
2. Account for less than 1% of glial neoplasms.
3. Neurocytomas occur in patients aged 20 to 40.

PATHOPHYSIOLOGY

1. Uncertain.
2. Gain of chromosome 7 in neurocytomas.
3. Gangliogliomas associated with Down syndrome, callosal dysgenesis, and neuronal migration disorders.
4. Lhermitte–Duclos disease may occur as part of Cowden disease (mucosal neuromas and breast cancer), an autosomal dominant disorder caused by germline mutation of *PTEN* gene.

PROGNOSIS

1. Ganglioglioma: Indolent, cured with surgery. If subtotal resection, 41% progress. Rare malignant transformation from glial component; 89% 5-year and 84% 10-year survival.
2. Neurocytoma: Good with resection, recurrence and CSF spread are rare.
3. DNTs are indolent.
4. Lhermitte–Duclos disease: Good with resection.

DIAGNOSIS

Location

1. Gangliogliomas have a predilection for temporal lobe but also occur in the basal ganglia, optic pathway, brainstem, pineal gland, cerebellum and spinal cord.
2. Neurocytomas are intraventricular, usually in body of lateral ventricle, attached to septum pellucidum. Rarely in pons, cerebellum, spinal cord, or brain parenchyma.
3. DNTs involve predominantly the cerebral cortex, especially temporal lobes.
4. Lhermitte–Duclos disease occurs in cerebellum.

Clinical Presentation

1. Gangliogliomas usually present with seizures and, less often, headaches and focal deficits.
2. Neurocytomas present with symptoms of hydrocephalus.
3. DNTs usually have chronic complex partial seizures.
4. Lhermitte–Duclos disease presents with ataxia and hydrocephalus.

Diagnostic Tests

1. Ganglioglioma: MRI is nonspecific and shows a well-demarcated, superficial, nonenhancing mass with increased T_2 and FLAIR signal. Can have cysts or calcification.

2. Neurocytoma: MRI shows a heterogenous mass with multiple cysts, calcification, occasional hemorrhage, variable enhancement; some have a "honeycomb" appearance on T_1-weighted images.
3. DNT: MRI shows a multicystic mass with gyrus-like configurations, cortical dysplasia.
4. Lhermitte–Duclos disease: MRI shows increased T_2 and FLAIR abnormality in cerebellum.

Pathology

1. Gangliogliomas (WHO grades I–II) have neuronal and astrocytic neoplastic cells, granular bodies, Rosenthal fibers, large irregular ganglion cells, and perivascular infiltrates.
2. Neurocytomas (WHO grade I) have small uniform, well-differentiated neuronal cells, frequently misdiagnosed as oligodendrogliomas.
3. DNTs (WHO grade I) have a glioneuronal element, nodular component, and cortical dysplasia.
4. Gangliocytomas (WHO grade I) are well-differentiated neoplastic cells with neuronal characteristics, no malignant transformation.
5. Lhermitte–Duclos (WHO grade I) disease has a dysplastic gangliocytoma confined to cerebellum, Purkinje cell layer is absent.

TREATMENT

1. Surgical resection; complete resection is curative for all these conditions.
2. RT may have limited role for recurrent gangliogliomas.
3. Anaplastic gangliogliomas may respond to chemotherapy with temozolomide or PCV.

PINEAL PARENCHYMAL TUMOR

BACKGROUND

1. Rare tumors that account for fewer than 1% of all intracranial tumors; 14% to 30% of pineal region tumors.
2. Pineocytoma most common between 25 and 35 years; pineoblastoma most common in first two decades.

PATHOPHYSIOLOGY

Arise from pinocyte in pineal gland.

PROGNOSIS

1. Pineocytoma is slow growing and has favorable prognosis following resection; 86% 5-year survival.
2. Pineoblastoma has poorer prognosis; less than 50% 5-year survival.
3. Pineal parenchymal tumors of intermediate differentiation (PPTIDs) have an intermediate prognosis.

DIAGNOSIS

Location

Pineal gland; pineoblastoma has relatively frequent leptomeningeal metastases.

Clinical Presentation

1. Most commonly presents with noncommunicating hydrocephalus from obstruction of aqueduct of Sylvius and Parinaud syndrome (paralysis of upgaze, convergence–retraction nystagmus, light–near dissociation) due to compression of midbrain tectum. Ophthalmoplegia, ataxia, weakness, numbness, and memory loss may also occur.
2. Hypothalamic dysfunction (diabetes insipidus, precocious puberty) when tumors encroach anteriorly; sleep disturbance due to abnormal melatonin regulation.

Diagnostic Tests

1. MRI shows a variably enhancing pineal region mass with or without leptomeningeal enhancement.
2. Serum and CSF alpha fetoprotein (AFP) (yolk sac tumors) and β-human chorionic gonadotropin (β-hCG) (choriocarcinoma) are negative and help to exclude germ cell tumors.
3. Check CSF cytology and contrast-enhanced MRI of spine to rule out leptomeningeal metastases if not contraindicated.

Pathology

1. Grossly displaces surrounding structures; does not invade; can seed leptomeninges.
2. Pineocytoma: Well-differentiated with small, uniform, mature cells resembling pinocytes.
3. PPTID, as name implies, has intermediate histologic appearance.
4. Pineoblastoma is high grade and histologically identical to PNETs. Composed of highly cellular sheets of small cells with round/irregular nuclei and scant cytoplasm. Occasional Homer–Wright or Flexner–Wintersteiner rosettes.

Differential Diagnosis

Germ cell tumors [germinoma, teratoma, dermoid, choriocarcinoma, embryonal carcinoma, endodermal sinus (yolk sac) tumor], astrocytoma, ependymoma, choroid plexus papilloma, meningioma, metastases and nonneoplastic lesions including pineal cyst, arachnoid cyst, arteriovenous malformation, Vein of Galen aneurysm, and cavernous malformation.

TREATMENT

1. Surgical exploration and complete resection.
2. Ventricular shunting for hydrocephalus.
3. Local irradiation for incompletely resected or recurrent pineocytoma.
4. Craniospinal RT for pineoblastoma and PPTID.
5. Role of chemotherapy unclear but usually given for pineoblastoma and often given for PPTID.
6. Chemotherapeutic agents include cisplatin, carboplatin, etoposide, cyclophosphamide, and vincristine.

MEDULLOBLASTOMA

BACKGROUND

1. Medulloblastomas are the most common (20%) malignant tumor of childhood.
2. Comprise more than one third of all pediatric posterior fossa tumors.
3. Incidence 0.5/100,000.
4. Male to female ratio 2 to 1.

5. Occurs in first decade of life (ages 5–9 years), 70% diagnosed before age 20. Second peak in the 20's to 30's (30% of cases).

PATHOPHYSIOLOGY

Ninety percent are sporadic but can occur in Gorlin syndrome (basal cell carcinomas, congenital anomalies) caused by germline mutation of gene encoding the sonic hedgehog receptor PTCH. May also arise in Turcot syndrome caused by germline mutation of the adenomatous polyposis coli (*APC*) gene. Rarely, they occur in patients with ataxia–telangiectasia, xeroderma pigmentosum, or Li–Fraumeni syndrome.

PROGNOSIS

1. Patients generally classified into poor-risk and standard-risk groups.
2. Poor-risk factors include residual disease greater than 1.5 cm³, metastases detected by contrast-enhanced MRI, and malignant cells in CSF obtained by LP.
3. The 5-year survival rate for standard-risk patients is approximately 70% to 80%. The 10-year survival rate is above 50%.
4. The 5-year survival rate for poor-risk patients is 40% to 50%.
5. Infants tend to have worse prognosis than older age groups.
6. Desmoplastic variant associated with better prognosis.
7. Tumors expressing neurotrophin-3 receptor, TrkC, have better prognosis; increased expression of neuroregulin receptors erbB2 and erbB4 and *c-myc* associated with worst prognosis.

DIAGNOSIS

Location

1. Midline cerebellum, inferior vermis (85%), and fourth ventricle.
2. Tends to infiltrate the cerebellar hemispheres and frequently (25%–30% of cases) have leptomeningeal metastases ("drop metastases"). Systemic metastases rare (bone and lung).
3. Desmoplastic variant (15%) more lateral in cerebellar hemisphere.

Clinical Presentation

1. Most tumors present with signs of increased ICP (headache, nausea, and vomiting) due to obstruction of CSF flow. Patients may also have ataxia and diplopia.
2. In older age groups, tumor more often occurs in cerebellar hemispheres, resulting in truncal ataxia and cerebellar dysfunction.

Diagnostic Tests

1. MRI or CT shows a high-density, enhancing tumor, usually midline, often distorting or obliterating the fourth ventricle, and producing hydrocephalus. Calcification may be present.
2. High tendency to metastasize to other parts of the CNS; therefore, entire neuraxis should be imaged.
3. May also metastasize outside of CNS to bone; therefore, a bone scan and bone marrow aspirate should also be performed.

Pathology

1. Grossly soft, pinkish-gray mass, granular with necrosis.
2. Microscopically highly cellular tumors with abundant dark staining round or oval nuclei and scant, undifferentiated cytoplasm typical of "small round blue cell tumors." Mitoses and apoptotic cells are abundant. Homer–Wright rosettes (sheets

of cells forming rosettes around a central area filled with neuritic processes) in up to 40% of cases.
3. Have both neuronal and glial differentiation and some with mesenchymal differentiation.
4. Desmoplastic variant has abundant reticulin and collagen.

Differential Diagnosis

Astrocytomas, ependymomas, ependymoblastoma, large cell PNET (aggressive course), medullomyoblastoma (contains immature muscle cells, malignant), melanotic PNET, and embryonal tumors (atypical teratoid or rhabdoid tumors, highly malignant and therapy-resistant).

TREATMENT

1. Surgical resection needed to relieve mass effect and some may require a VP shunt for decompression.
2. Goal is maximal surgical resection because residual tumor greater than 1.5 cm is associated with increased risk of relapse.
3. Surgery occasionally complicated by "cerebellar mutism" (mutism and emotional lability).
4. Craniospinal RT indicated in all patients after surgery.
5. RT comprising 5,000 to 5,500 cGy usually administered to the posterior fossa and 3,600 cGy applied to the remainder of the cranium and the spine of all high-risk patients.
6. Craniospinal RT of 2,400 cGy for standard-risk patients, especially those younger than 5 years.
7. Craniospinal RT frequently produces neurocognitive complications in children.
8. Current studies are evaluating lower doses of craniospinal RT in conjunction with chemotherapy in children to reduce long-term complications of RT.
9. SRS boost often administered to any residual nodules of tumor.
10. Sensitive to chemotherapy: adjuvant therapy with agents such as cisplatin and etoposide, and cyclophosphamide and vincristine. Other active agents include lomustine, procarbazine, and carboplatin. Adjuvant chemotherapy improves survival in patients with high-risk disease and possibly also for patients with standard-risk disease.
11. Controversy regarding use of chemotherapy before or after RT. No evidence that preradiation chemotherapy is more effective.
12. In infants and young children, chemotherapy is sometimes used alone and RT deferred until they are 3 years old.

CRANIAL AND SPINAL NERVE TUMORS

SCHWANNOMA

BACKGROUND

1. Schwannomas are benign tumors that originate from the Schwann cell at the glial–Schwann cell junction (Obersteiner–Redlich zone) of the peripheral nerves.
2. Vestibular schwannomas (acoustic neuroma) arise from the vestibular portion of the eighth nerve.
3. In periphery, arise from paraspinal dorsal nerve roots and cutaneous nerves.

Epidemiology

1. Incidence 1/100,000, female-to-male ratio (1.5:1).
2. Occurs in middle adult life and rare in childhood.
3. Most commonly arises from vestibular nerve (usually solitary; frequently bilateral in NF2).
4. Vestibular schwannomas account for 8% of all intracranial tumors and 80% of CPA tumors in adults.

PATHOPHYSIOLOGY

1. Increased incidence in NF2. Patients often have bilateral acoustic schwannomas and multiple cranial and spinal schwannomas, meningiomas, and gliomas.
2. Inactivating mutations of NF2 gene also frequent in spontaneous schwannomas.

PROGNOSIS

1. Slow-growing tumors usually cured by surgery.
2. Malignant degeneration rare in the CNS but more common in the PNS.

DIAGNOSIS

Location

Most common CN VIII in the CPA but may occur wherever Schwann cells are present (other CNs, spinal nerves, and peripheral nerve trunks).

Clinical Presentation

1. Most common include unilateral hearing loss, tinnitus, and unsteadiness from acoustic nerve dysfunction evolving over months to years.
2. Dysfunction of other CNs and brainstem occurs if it becomes large enough [trigeminal dysfunction (loss of corneal reflex, facial numbness), facial weakness, ataxia, vertigo].
3. Isolated vertigo uncommon as initial symptom.

Diagnostic Tests

1. Audiometry is helpful for detecting unilateral sensorineural hearing loss.
2. Brainstem auditory evoked potentials abnormal in more than 90% of patients (prolongation of waves I–III and I–V latency).
3. MRI with gadolinium is the most sensitive imaging modality and shows intradural, extraaxial, enhancing mass.
4. In the spine, tumor may extend through the intervertebral foramen, resulting in an hourglass appearance.
5. CT scan useful to delineate the anatomy of the bones involved.

Pathology

1. Two types of distinct histology: Antoni A (compact, elongated cells with occasional nuclear palisading) and Antoni B (loose, reticulated tissue).
2. Arise at the periphery of nerve; usually encapsulated and compress but do not invade adjacent neural tissue.

Differential Diagnosis

1. Most common CPA tumor. Differential includes meningioma, cholesteatoma, epidermoid, metastatic disease, glioma.

2. Schwannomas arising from spinal roots may resemble meningiomas and neurofibromas.

TREATMENT

1. Small asymptomatic lesions can often be observed and treated only if they increase in size.
2. Surgical resection can be complete for tumors smaller than 2 cm and can preserve hearing in 75% of patients.
3. Surgical morbidity is related to size of tumor (lower than 5% for tumors smaller than 2 cm, 20% for tumors larger than 4 cm) and includes facial paralysis, hearing loss, CSF leak, imbalance, and headache.
4. If hearing is good, then one should also consider early treatment as delay may result in hearing impairment.
5. SRS probably equally effective, especially in older patients and those at high risk for surgery. Fractionated SRT associated with less morbidity.

NEUROFIBROMA

BACKGROUND

1. Arise from cells with features of Schwann cells, fibroblasts, and perineural cells and are usually benign.
2. Almost always associated with NF1 and usually multiple.
3. Malignant peripheral nerve tumors (MPNTs) occur in 1/10,000 and arise de novo or from sarcomatous degeneration of a preexisting plexiform neurofibroma.

PATHOPHYSIOLOGY

Associated with NF1.

PROGNOSIS

Additional lesions tend to arise and in NF1, malignant degeneration may occur.

DIAGNOSIS

Location

Most involve dorsal spinal nerve roots, major nerve trunks, or peripheral nerves. CN involvement very rare.

Clinical Presentation

Cutaneous neurofibromas present as small painless masses. Nerve root neurofibromas may present with pain and sensorimotor disturbance.

Diagnostic Tests

MRI shows widening of the neural foramina with pedicle erosion in neurofibromas arising from spinal roots.

Pathology

1. Hyperplasia of Schwann cells and fibrous elements of the nerve. Elongated wavy interlacing hyperchromatic cells with spindle-shaped nuclei in a disorderly loose mucoid background with collagen fibrils. Nerve fibers are intertwined in the tumor.

2. Plexiform neurofibroma associated with NF1, which has an increased incidence of malignant transformation.
3. Malignant peripheral nerve sheath tumors (MPNSTs) are highly malignant sarcomas, many occur in NF1 with preexisting plexiform neurofibroma.

Differential Diagnosis

Perineuriomas arise from pericytes.

TREATMENT

1. Palliative surgical decompression as needed.
2. RT occasionally useful in malignant tumors.

MENINGEAL TUMORS

MENINGIOMA

BACKGROUND

1. Arise from cells that form the outer layer of the arachnoid granulations of the brain (arachnoid cap cells).
2. Meningioma is the most common benign tumor and the second most common PBT in adults.
3. Represents approximately 20% of all intracranial neoplasms and 25% of intraspinal tumors.
4. Rare in first two decades and increases progressively thereafter.
5. Peak incidence in fourth to fifth decades, strong female predominance (3:2).
6. Higher incidence in patients with breast cancer.
7. Pregnancy may be associated with tumor progression (strong hormonal influence).

PATHOPHYSIOLOGY

1. Proven risk factors are female gender, increasing age, NF2, and history of cranial irradiation.
2. Meningiomas have partial or complete deletions of chromosome 22.
3. Patients with NF2 may have multiple meningiomas.
4. Progesterone receptors are present in 70% of tumors and play a role in tumor growth.
5. PDGF, EGFR, vascular endothelial growth factor (VEGF), and their receptors are expressed in meningiomas.

PROGNOSIS

1. Excellent for most patients. Median survival more than 10 years.
2. Most are slow-growing lesions that remain stable for many years.
3. Of meningiomas, 4.7% to 7.2% have atypical features and 1% to 2.8% have anaplastic features and much worse prognosis. Median survival for malignant meningiomas is less than 2 years.
4. Recurrence is related to completeness of the resection and location.
5. Poor prognostic factors include papillary histologic characteristics, large number of mitotic figures, necrosis, and invasion of cortical tissue by tumor cells.

DIAGNOSIS

Location

1. Mostly extraaxial and intracranial.
2. Ninety percent are supratentorial involving the cerebral convexities (50%, parasagittal, falx, or lateral convexity), skull base (40%, sphenoid wing, olfactory groove, or suprasellar), posterior fossa, foramen magnum, periorbital region, temporal fossa, and ventricular system.
3. Intraspinal tumors account for 25% of primary spinal tumors and are usually in thoracic segment.

Clinical Presentation

1. Present with seizures, headaches, and focal deficits.
2. Twenty percent are asymptomatic and are an incidental finding.
3. Spinal meningiomas present with pain, weakness, numbness, and gait unsteadiness.

Diagnostic Tests

1. MRI or CT with contrast shows a well-defined, homogenously enhancing extraaxial mass that may be calcified. If edema present usually indicates a higher grade tumor or a secretory meningioma.
2. On T_1- and T_2-weighted sequences, meningiomas can be easily missed as they are isointense to slightly hypointense compared with brain or spinal cord.
3. "Dural tail" sign at the margin of tumor is characteristic.
4. MR venography or CT angiography may be useful to determine patency of adjacent venous sinuses.

Pathology

1. Gross examination shows well-circumscribed, rubbery to hard masses that indent brain with no invasion. On sphenoid ridge may be en plaque.
2. Microscopically shows whorls, psammoma bodies, intranuclear pseudoinclusions; epithelial membrane antigen is positive.
3. Benign variants (WHO grade I): meningothelial, fibrous, transitional, psammomatous, secretory, microcystic, chordoid, lymphoplasmacytic-rich, metaplastic, and clear cell.
4. Atypical meningiomas (WHO grade II): increased mitotic activity (four mitoses per ten high-power fields) and increased cellularity, small cells with high nucleus/cytoplasm ratio, prominent nucleoli, patternless growth and spontaneous necrosis.
5. Anaplastic (malignant) meningioma (WHO grade III) variants: papillary, rhabdoid, and malignant meningioma are more aggressive with high rates of metastases.

Differential Diagnosis

Dural metastases, hemangiopericytoma, hemangioblastoma, melanocytoma, meningioangiomatosis, sarcoma, solitary fibrous tumor, and melanoma.

TREATMENT

1. Asymptomatic lesions (smaller than 2 cm without edema) are frequently seen on routine imaging for unrelated problems and can be followed up clinically and with serial imaging.
2. Asymptomatic lesions near vital structures should be considered for resection due to increased operative morbidity later.
3. Symptomatic or enlarging lesions should be resected.

4. Complete surgical removal of a meningioma confers long-term disease-free survival: 95% at 5 years, 70% to 90% at 10 years, and less than 70% at 15 years. Subtotal resection confers a lower disease-free survival of 63% at 5 years, 45% at 10 years, and 8% at 15 years.
5. RT may be indicated in patients with progressive symptoms due to recurrent meningioma in whom surgery is subtotal or contraindicated. Disease-free survival at 10 years is approximately 70% and approaches that of patients undergoing a complete surgical resection.
6. Patients with atypical or anaplastic meningiomas should have RT after surgery. Control rates at 10 years after RT for atypical meningioma and malignant meningioma are 13% and 0%, respectively.
7. SRS is an option for tumors smaller than 3 cm and not adjacent to vital structures. Fractionated SRT may be used for larger tumors and those near vital structures.
8. Although meningiomas express estrogen and progesterone receptors, antiestrogens and antiprogesterone (RU486) have not been effective in clinical studies.
9. Anecdotal reports of efficacy with chemotherapy (hydroxyurea, interferon alpha).
10. Clinical trials using inhibitors of PDGFR (Imatinib) and EGFR (Erlotinib) are ongoing.

HEMANGIOPERICYTOMA

1. Considered to be a different entity from meningiomas.
2. Densely cellular and vascular tumor arising from dura.
3. Clinical presentation, diagnosis, and treatment (surgery and RT) similar to those for atypical meningioma.
4. Sixty percent survival at 15 years.

HEMANGIOBLASTOMA

BACKGROUND

Account for 7% of posterior fossa tumors. Most common cause of intraaxial posterior fossa tumor in adults.

PATHOPHYSIOLOGY

Twenty-five percent of hemangioblastomas are associated with von Hippel–Lindau (VHL) syndrome. Autosomal dominant disorder caused by germline mutation of *VHL* gene, causing constitutive overexpression of VEGF. Associated with retinal angiomas, renal cell carcinoma, pheochromocytoma, and pancreatic and liver cysts.

PROGNOSIS

Good for isolated hemangioblastomas; cured if completely resected. Prognosis of patients with VHL poorer. Dependent on extent and location of hemangioblastomas and other tumors.

DIAGNOSIS

Clinical Presentation

1. Age, 30 to 65 years.
2. Headaches, ataxia, and focal neurologic deficits. Some patients may have symptoms from associated lesions as part of VHL syndrome (visual symptoms from retinal angiomas and symptoms from renal carcinomas and pheochromocytomas).

Diagnostic Test

MRI typically shows enhancing cystic lesion with mural nodule.

Pathology

Hemangioblastomas are grossly well-circumscribed, vascular, often cystic tumors containing yellowish lipid, and nodule on the cyst wall. Microscopically there are three cell types (stromal, endothelial, pericyte). Cyst wall may contain Rosenthal fibers (difficult to distinguish from pilocytic astrocytoma). Clusters of foamy cells separated by blood-filled vascular spores.

Differential Diagnosis

Pilocytic astrocytoma, metastases, ependymoma, medulloblastoma, vascular malformation.

TREATMENT

1. Small, asymptomatic lesions can be observed.
2. Surgical excision is treatment of choice. Tumors often very vascular.
3. RT and SRS may be of benefit for recurrent or inoperable tumors.
4. Clinical trials using inhibitors of VEGF under way.

PRIMARY CENTRAL NERVOUS SYSTEM LYMPHOMA

BACKGROUND

1. Primary central nervous system lymphoma (PCNSL) is a diffuse non-Hodgkin lymphoma (NHL) that is confined to CNS.
2. Most (90%) are B cell lymphomas, diffuse and large cell type, and classified as a stage I_E NHL.

Epidemiology

1. Four percent of all CNS tumors; 1% of NHL. Incidence is 0.43/100,000. Slightly greater in males.
2. Increasing incidence in immunocompromised patients [patients with acquired immunodeficiency syndrome (AIDS), organ transplant recipients], in part due to better detection.
3. Three percent of patients with AIDS develop PCNSL during the course of their disease.
4. Incidence has increased among immunocompetent hosts and elderly males for unclear reasons by approximately threefold.
5. Frequently disseminates to the leptomeninges (25%) and vitreous humor (20%).
6. In immunocompetent hosts, mean age is 50 to 60 years and in immunocompromised patients the mean age is 30 years.

PATHOPHYSIOLOGY

1. Controversy surrounding its site of origin in immunocompetent patients. No known risk factors.
2. In immunocompromised patients, related to uncontrolled proliferation of B cells latently infected with Epstein–Barr virus (EBV).

PROGNOSIS

1. Highly malignant, mean survival of 3.3 months with supportive care only.
2. RT alone prolongs median survival to 12 to 18 months.
3. In immunocompetent patients, median survival 19 to 42 months with maximal treatment.
4. In immunocompromised patients median survival 6 to 16 months with maximal treatment.
5. Neuraxis dissemination (60%) and systemic lymphoma (10%) in patients who survive 1 year after radiation.

DIAGNOSIS

Location

1. Periventricular, subcortical, and usually multifocal in 40% of cases (90% in patients with AIDS).
2. Retinal or vitreous infiltration (20%), sometimes restricted to the eye only.
3. Diffuse meningeal infiltration (40%).
4. Spinal cord involvement occasionally.

Clinical Presentation

1. Frequently present with cognitive and behavioral changes. Some patients may have headache, seizures, and focal deficits.
2. Multifocal symptoms nearly 50% of the time.
3. Symptoms maybe present for 1 to 2 months before diagnosis.

Diagnostic Tests

1. MRI hypodense on T_1-weighted images, isodense or hypodense on T_2-weighted images. Usually homogenously enhancing. In immunocompromised patients, lesions can be ring-enhancing. Usually periventricular and may involve deep structures such as basal ganglia.
2. SPECT scanning using gallium 67 and thallium 201 and PET show increased uptake in PCNSLs and help differentiate them from infections.
3. Ophthalmologic evaluation is essential to rule out ocular involvement (20% of PCNSL) by slit-lamp exam.
4. Staging to rule out systemic lymphoma with bone marrow biopsy and body CT (3% of patients are identified with extraneural disease). Value of systemic staging controversial.
5. Biopsy (usually stereotactic) or CSF analysis needed for diagnosis.
6. LP for CSF analysis shows lymphocytic pleocytosis in over 50% of cases, increased protein 85%, up to 90% positive cytology with three LPs. PCR for *IgH* gene rearrangement may be more sensitive but not yet in wide use.
7. Use of steroids before tissue sampling can decrease the yield. Should hold steroids until after biopsy if possible.
8. HIV testing should be done on all patients.

Pathology

1. Grossly better demarcated then diffuse gliomas, granular light tan appearance.
2. WHO grade IV. Microscopically perivascular orientation of cells ("angiocentric"), often expanding a vessel wall with reticulin deposition. Necrosis common. Noncohesive, large, irregular nuclei, prominent nucleoli, scant cytoplasm, usually large B-cell, but occasionally T-cell.

Differential diagnoses

1. Infections—especially in HIV positive patients and includes opportunistic infections such as toxoplasmosis (most common), cryptococcal abscesses, tuberculoma, nocardia abscesses, syphilitic gummas, and Candida abscesses.
2. Metastases from occult non-CNS neoplasms, gliomas, intravascular or systemic lymphoma, and vasculitis.

TREATMENT

1. Biopsy for histologic diagnosis usually required. No benefit from resection.
2. 90% responds to RT (usually 4,000 cGy whole brain RT +/− 1,400–2,000 cGy boost to tumor) but recurs in 1–2 years.
3. Corticosteroids: 40% have a partial or complete response but tumor rapidly recurs.
4. Chemotherapy is increasingly first treatment of choice.
5. High-dose IV methotrexate (HDMTX) ($>1g/m^2$) has a 50–80% response rate.
6. Other active agents include procarbazine, high-dose cytarabine, lomustine, vincristine, rituximab, and temozolomide.
7. No standard regimen but most patients treated with chemotherapy (which should include HDMTX), followed by RT. Median survival improved to >40 months.
8. CSF penetration of HDMTX good. Probably no need for additional intrathecal chemotherapy to treat leptomeningeal disease.
9. Use of MTX before RT reduces risk of leukoencephalopathy. However, RT in patients above 60 years still associated with significant leukoencephalopathy. Trend towards deferring RT in these patients and treating them only with chemotherapy.

GERM CELL TUMORS

BACKGROUND

1. Most common tumor of pineal gland (60%) and most are malignant.
2. Peak incidence second decade, predominantly males (3:1); 95% occur before age 33.
3. Germinomas account for 60% of germ cell tumors. Teratoma and mixed germ cell tumors (20%–30%). Embryonal carcinoma, endodermal sinus (yolk sac) tumor, and choriocarcinoma rare.

PATHOPHYSIOLOGY

Arise from primitive midline germ cells in the pineal or hypothalamic regions. Indistinguishable histologically from those tumors that occur in the gonads of young adults.

PROGNOSIS

1. Benign teratomas have a 100% 5-year survival.
2. Germinomas have an 80% to 90% 5-year survival following surgery and RT. Some patients cured.
3. Malignant nongerminomatous germ cell tumors have a poor prognosis. Survival rarely more than 2 years.

DIAGNOSIS

Location

Midline in pineal, sellar and suprasellar regions, posterior fossa and sacrococcygeal area.

Clinical Presentation

1. Parinaud syndrome (paralysis of upgaze, convergence-retraction nystagmus, light-near dissociation) secondary to compression of the tectum of the midbrain.
2. Obstructive hydrocephalus.
3. Suprasellar tumors may present with visual symptoms and hypothalamic and endocrine dysfunction.
4. Teratoma associated with spina bifida if located in sacrococcygeal area.

Diagnostic Tests

1. MRI or CT scan of brain: Most tumors show calcification. Usually enhances significantly with contrast. Teratomas have heterogenous appearance with solid and cystic areas, and frequently areas of fat and calcification.
2. Spine MRI and CSF examination necessary to determine extent of CSF seeding.
3. Serum and CSF tumor markers can be helpful. These include AFP (endodermal sinus tumor, embryonal carcinoma, and malignant teratoma) and β-hCG (germinoma, teratoma, choriocarcinoma, embryonal carcinoma, malignant teratoma, and undifferentiated germ cell tumor). Germinomas rarely secrete markers (fewer than 10% secrete β-hCG).
4. Endocrine evaluation and visual field examination (suprasellar lesions).

Pathology

1. Germinoma composed of large malignant germ cells and small reactive lymphocytes.
2. Teratoma has all three germ cell layers present (epidermal, dermal, vascular, glandular, muscular, neural, cartilaginous).
3. Yolk sac tumor composed of primitive-appearing epithelial cells.
4. Embryonal carcinoma is composed of large cells that proliferate in sheets that form papillae.
5. Choriocarcinoma contains cytotrophoblasts and syncytiotrophoblastic giant cells.

Differential Diagnosis

Same as that for pineal parenchymal tumors and pituitary adenomas, depending on location.

TREATMENT

1. Stereotactic biopsy for tumors with evidence of CSF dissemination and elevated AFP.
2. Open biopsy allows for more accurate tissue sampling.
3. Resection appropriate for more benign pathologies such as teratoma.
4. Ventricular shunting for hydrocephalus.
5. Germinomas highly radiosensitive (focal irradiation of 5,000 to 5,500 cGy).
6. Cranial irradiation for all other germ cell tumors.
7. Craniospinal RT reserved for patients with evidence of CSF seeding.
8. SRS used to treat residual areas of tumor after conventional RT.
9. Chemotherapy used for nongerminomatous malignant germ cells tumors. A wide variety of regimens have been tried including those derived from treatments for testicular cancer such as cisplatin, vinblastine, and bleomycin or cisplatin, etoposide, and ifosfamide.

CYSTS AND TUMOR-LIKE LESIONS

BACKGROUND

1. There are several nonneoplastic lesions that can be found incidentally and include epidermoid and dermoid cysts, lipoma, and hamartomas.
2. Epidermoids and dermoids represent approximately 2% of intracranial tumors.
3. Colloid cyst affects young to middle-aged adult.
4. Hypothalamic hamartoma is a dysplastic lesion usually occurring in first decade of life.

PATHOPHYSIOLOGY

Usually incidental lesions due to rests of embryonal tissue remaining in nervous system.

PROGNOSIS

These are benign lesions that can usually be resected. Epidermoid and dermoid cysts may recur.

DIAGNOSIS

Location

1. Epidermoid cyst usually in CPA, intrasellar and suprasellar regions, and intraspinal.
2. Dermoid cyst usually midline, related to fontanel, fourth ventricle, or spinal cord.
3. Colloid cyst is usually in the third ventricle at foramen of Monro.
4. Lipomas are found in corpus callosum, hypothalamus, sella, and spinal cord.
5. Hypothalamic hamartoma is in the hypothalamus.

Clinical Presentation

1. Epidermoid cyst presents with cranial abnormalities, seizures, hydrocephalus, and aseptic meningitis.
2. Dermoid cyst presents with symptoms of hydrocephalus, focal deficits, and occasionally repeated bacterial meningitis due to association with dermal sinus tract.
3. Colloid cyst presents with headaches, drop attacks, and rarely sudden death due to obstruction of foramen of Monro.
4. Lipomas are usually incidental and frequently associated with other congenital anomalies, such as agenesis of corpus callosum. Occasionally they cause symptoms from mass effect.
5. Hypothalamic hamartoma presents with gelastic seizures and endocrine abnormalities (precocious puberty).

Diagnostic Tests

1. Epidermoid cyst on CT is a low-density cyst with irregular enhancing rim; on MRI, it has variable signal depending on lipid content.
2. Dermoid cyst on MRI has heterogenous signal due to hair and sebaceous content.
3. Colloid cyst on MRI is a spheric, thin-walled lesion and hyperintense on T_1-weighted lesion.
4. Lipoma is low density on all imaging modalities.
5. Hypothalamic hamartoma on MRI usually is a small discrete mass near floor of third ventricle, which does not enhance. Hypothalamic–pituitary hormones may be abnormal.

Pathology

1. Epidermoid cyst contains squamous epithelium surrounding a keratin-filled cyst.
2. Dermoid cyst contains both epidermal and dermal structures (hair follicles, sweat glands, sebaceous glands).
3. Colloid cyst contains goblet and ciliated columnar epithelial cells surrounding a cystic cavity.
4. Lipoma contains mature adipose tissue.
5. Hypothalamic hamartoma consists of a well-differentiated but disorganized neuroglial tissue.

Differential Diagnosis

Pilocytic astrocytoma, glioma, metastases. CPA epidermoids should be differentiated from vestibular schwannomas, meningiomas, and arachnoid cysts.

TREATMENT

1. Epidermoid, dermoid, and colloid cysts can be surgically resected.
2. Lipomas should be followed clinically and excision is usually not necessary.
3. Hypothalamic hamartoma should undergo resection if possible. Long-acting gonadotrophin- releasing hormone analogs may also be helpful. Some patients need endocrine replacement.

TUMORS OF THE SELLAR REGION

PITUITARY ADENOMA

BACKGROUND

1. Pituitary adenoma is the most common sellar tumor and may grow up into suprasellar space and laterally to invade cavernous sinus (primary suprasellar masses usually do not grow down through the diaphragm).
2. Arise from cells of the adenohypophysis, predominantly corticotrophs, somatotrophs, lactotrophs, gonadotrophs, and rarely, thyrotrophs.
3. Classified anatomically as microadenomas (less than 10-mm diameter) and macroadenomas (greater than 10-mm diameter).
4. Classified functionally according to secreted products.
5. Prolactinoma is the most common (27%), usually a microadenoma. Symptoms are from primary hypersecretion or stalk effect (flow of dopamine impeded). Presents with amenorrhea and galactorrhea in females, and decreased libido and impotence in males.
6. Growth hormone (GH) (21%) secretion causes gigantism and acromegaly.
7. Corticotropin-secreting adenomas (8%) produce Cushing disease.
8. Follicle stimulating hormone/luteinizing hormone (FSH/LH) (6%) secreting adenomas.
9. Thyrotropin-secreting adenomas (1%) are rare and are usually secondary to primary thyroid myxedema.
10. Nonsecreting adenomas (35%) usually present with compressive symptoms.

Epidemiology

1. Ten percent to 15% of all intracranial neoplasms, male-to-female ratio 1 to 2, and third most common primary intracranial neoplasm.

2. Incidence 1 to 14/100.000 and found in 6% to 22% of unselected autopsies.
3. Present from late adolescence through adulthood.
4. Frequency in decreasing order is prolactinoma, nonsecreting adenoma, GH-secreting adenoma, corticotropin-secreting adenoma, glycoprotein-secreting adenoma.

PATHOPHYSIOLOGY

1. Cause symptoms by disrupting hypothalamic–pituitary–adrenal axis or by direct compression of adjacent structures.
2. Multiple endocrine neoplasia type 1 (MEN1) is an autosomal dominant syndrome due to allelic loss of tumor suppressor gene menin on chromosome 11q13. Patients develop tumors of the pituitary gland, pancreatic islets, and parathyroid glands.
3. Expression on *c-myc* correlates with clinical aggressiveness and *ras* mutations mark an invasive tumor.

PROGNOSIS

1. Related to size and cell type of tumor.
2. Seventy percent to 90% remission rate 1 year after resection.
3. Visual recovery best when impairment has been brief.
4. Endocrine status improves after surgery (fertility may return in 70% of patients).
5. Pregnancy can precipitate symptomatic tumor growth of prolactinomas in 25% of macroadenomas but only 1% of microadenomas.
6. Prolactinomas can be controlled in 95% patients with dopamine agonists, surgery, and RT.
7. Cushing disease can be controlled with surgery in 93% of microadenomas and 50% of macroadenomas.
8. Acromegaly can be controlled with surgery in 85% of microadenomas and 40% of macroadenomas.

DIAGNOSIS

Location

1. Sella and parasellar.
2. Can invade the cavernous sinus, third ventricle, hypothalamus, or temporal lobe.

Clinical Presentation

1. Present with insidious neurologic symptoms late including headaches and visual disturbance due to compression of optic chiasm located above the sella.
   a. Usually bitemporal superior quadrantanopia, then bitemporal hemianopia.
2. Present with insidious endocrine manifestations early if hormonally active and include hypofunction or hyperfunction.
   a. Hypopituitarism especially of gonadotropin and GH systems.
   b. Prolactin excess causes galactorrhea or amenorrhea in women (one fourth of all women with secondary amenorrhea and galactorrhea have prolactin-secreting tumors). Men present with impotence and loss of libido.
   c. GH excess causes acromegaly or gigantism (rarely due to ectopic tumor).
   d. Corticotropin excess causes Cushing disease.
3. Hemorrhage or infarct of tumor may produce pituitary apoplexy (abrupt headache, visual loss, diplopia, drowsiness, confusion, coma).
4. Pregnancy, head trauma, acute hypertension, and anticoagulation predispose to apoplexy.

Diagnostic Tests

1. MRI with sagittal and coronal views with contrast may reveal microadenoma or larger compressive lesions and demonstrate the relationship between tumor and

surrounding vital structures (optic chiasm, cavernous and sphenoid sinuses, hypothalamus).
2. Serum studies:
   a. Prolactin [normal less than 15 ng/mL, greater than 200 ng/mL usually tumor, level of 15–200 ng/mL can be due to adenoma or caused by medications (phenothiazines, antidepressants, estrogens, metoclopramide) or by disorders that interfere with normal hypothalamic inhibition of prolactin secretion (hypothyroidism, renal and hepatic disease, hypothalamic disease)].
   b. Insulin-like growth factor 1 (IGF1), GH, thyroid function tests (TFTs), FSH, LH, testosterone (male), estrogen (female), cortisol, corticotropin, electrolytes, and glucose.
   c. Urine electrolytes, 24-hour urine free cortisol, and dexamethasone suppression test for Cushing disease.
   d. With pituitary source, cortisol does not suppress with low-dose dexamethasone (0.5 mg q6h for eight doses) but does suppress with higher dose (2 mg q6h for eight doses).
   e. Adrenal or ectopic sources do not suppress with either dose.
   f. Elevated IGF and decreased GH response to oral glucose load for GH excess.
3. If MRI does not show a tumor, petrosal sinus sampling can provide evidence for a pituitary origin of corticotropin. Body CT also needed to search for lung or adrenal tumors.

Pathology

Classified according to hormonal products.

Differential Diagnosis

Craniopharyngioma, germinomas, teratomas, meningiomas, pituitary carcinoma, dermoids, epidermoids, metastatic tumors, hypothalamic/optic nerve glioma, hypothalamic hamartoma, nasopharyngeal tumors, posterior pituitary tumors (granular cell tumor and astrocytomas), metastases, chordoma and nonneoplastic lesions such Rathke cleft cyst, lymphocytic hypophysitis, abscess, histiocytosis X, sarcoidosis, and aneurysms.

TREATMENT

1. Surgery is treatment of choice for most pituitary tumors (except prolactinomas), especially if there is visual compromise. Tumors within the pituitary sella and those with limited extrasellar extension can usually be approached via the transsphenoidal route with substantially reduced operative morbidity. Extension beyond the sella laterally or superior extension with invasion or entrapment of the optic chiasm typically necessitates a superior surgical approach through a transfrontal craniotomy.
2. Patients undergoing surgery are usually treated with corticosteroids as prophylaxis against adrenal insufficiency.
3. Diabetes insipidus (DI) can occur after surgery but is usually transient.
4. Adjuvant postoperative RT (including SRT) reduces the rate of recurrence for functioning adenomas (one series reports from 42% to 13%). Usually 5,000 cGy given over 5 to 6 weeks.
5. Subtotally resected nonfunctioning tumors and functioning tumors with normal hormone levels often watched with serial MRI and hormone levels. RT used only if there is evidence of tumor growth.
6. Prolactinoma responds well to medical therapy (bromocriptine: a dopamine agonist that shrinks tumor by reducing prolactin) and seldom requires surgery. In symptomatic women, 80% success with medical therapy. Bromocriptine is safer in pregnancy. Initial dosage of bromocriptine is 1.25 to 2.5 mg/d, increasing by 2.5 mg/d every 3 to 7 days, up to 15 mg/d.

7. Cabergoline (0.25 mg p.o. twice weekly; maximum, 1 mg twice weekly) and quinagolide (0.03–0.5 mg daily) are dopamine agonists that have longer half-lives, greater potency, and fewer side effects than bromocriptine.
8. GH-secreting adenoma: Transsphenoidal resection with or without the somatostatin analogs octreotide [50 μg subcutaneously (s.c.) three times daily (t.i.d.)] and lanreotide [30–60 mg intramuscularly (IM) every 10–14 days]. Bromocriptine, cabergoline, and quinaolide have also been used.
9. Others symptomatic tumors need transsphenoidal resection.

CRANIOPHARYNGIOMA

BACKGROUND

1. Slow-growing tumor that originates from remnants of embryonic squamous cell rests (Rathke pouch) in the region of the pituitary stalk.
2. Incidence 0.5 to 2 cases/million/y.
3. Account for 1% of adult intracranial tumors and 6% to 10% of childhood intracranial neoplasms.
4. Bimodal age distribution (first peak, 5–10 years; second peak, 50–60 years).
5. Most common supratentorial tumor in childhood and second most common parasellar tumor.

PATHOPHYSIOLOGY

Sporadic, no genetic association known.

PROGNOSIS

1. Usually benign.
2. Sixty percent to 93% 10-year recurrence-free survival; 64% to 96% 10-year overall survival.
3. Recurrence rate worse for tumors larger than 5 cm and incompletely resected tumors.

DIAGNOSIS

Location

Above sella, but some in sella.

Clinical Presentation

1. Due to slow growth, diagnosed 1 to 2 years after onset of symptoms.
2. Hypopituitarism and DI secondary to compression of pituitary gland and hypothalamus.
3. Visual abnormalities (bitemporal hemianopsia) secondary to compression of optic chiasm/tracts.
4. Headache and vomiting due to elevated ICP.

Diagnostic Tests

Strongly enhancing, cystic, and calcified mass (80% in children and 40% in adults) in the suprasellar region with frequent intrasellar component.

Pathology

1. Grossly multicystic, well-delineated lesions that contain dark, viscous liquid within cystic spaces.

2. Microscopically variable types of epithelium, some resembling "adamantinoma-tous" (more common) and others papillary and squamous. May have calcification, keratin debris, cholesterol clefts, macrophages, and hemosiderin. Rosenthal fibers in adjacent brain.

Differential Diagnosis

Pituitary adenoma, hypothalamic/optic system glioma, Rathke cleft cyst, dermoid, epidermoid, hypothalamic hamartoma, germinoma, giant aneurysm, sarcoidosis, histiocytosis X, and lymphocytic hypophysitis.

TREATMENT

1. Surgical resection treatment of choice. Complete resection possible in 50% to 90% of cases but often associated with significant morbidity due to relation to vital neural and neuroendocrine structures. Even with complete resection only 65% of patients free of recurrence at 10 years.
2. RT, especially SRT, is assuming an increasing role, particularly for patients with incomplete resection and recurrent disease. Ninety percent 10-year survival when surgery combined with RT.
3. Radioisotopes such as phosphorus 32 (^{32}P) are occasionally administered into cysts to prevent recurrence.
4. Ventriculostomy needed for hydrocephalus.
5. Cyst material can cause chemical meningitis.
6. Endocrine dysfunction and learning disabilities common and require therapy.

SPINAL CORD TUMORS

BACKGROUND

1. Spinal cord tumors account for 10% of all primary CNS tumors.
2. Spinal cord tumors can be divided into three groups on the basis of their location: intradural/intramedullary, intradural/extramedullary, and extradural.
3. Intradural/intramedullary account for 4% to 10% of spinal cord tumors, 80% of which are gliomas and ependymoma. Myxopapillary ependymomas predominate in the cauda equina and lumbar region, astrocytomas predominate in the cervical region. They are slow growing and usually cause symptoms for many years. Other tumors include hemangioblastoma, paraganglioma, dermoid, epidermoid, and lipoma.
4. Intradural/extramedullary tumors are mostly benign. In adults, schwannomas are the most common intraspinal tumor. They are slow-growing tumors that usually arise from posterior nerve roots. Meningiomas are the second most common primary intraspinal tumor. Most (80%) occur at the level of the thoracic spinal cord. Together, schwannomas and meningiomas account for 80% of intradural/extramedullary tumors. Others tumors include neurofibroma, ependymoma, lipoma, epidermoid, and dermoid.
5. Extradural benign tumors include osteoid osteoma, osteoblastoma, osteochondroma, giant cell tumor, aneurysmal bone cyst, hemangioma, and eosinophilic granuloma.
6. Extradural malignant tumors include metastatic disease, plasmacytoma, myeloma, chordoma, osteosarcoma, Ewing sarcoma, chondrosarcoma, lymphoma, and malignant fibrous histiocytoma.

PATHOPHYSIOLOGY

Cause dysfunction by compression and edema.

PROGNOSIS

1. Complete resection of nerve sheath tumors and meningiomas is curative.
2. Intramedullary tumors such as ependymomas can often be resected. Recurrence-free survival is greater than 75% at 10 years. Myxopapillary ependymomas of the cauda equina have a particularly good prognosis. Astrocytomas are more difficult to resect and a minority have high-grade histology and a poor prognosis.
3. Patients with NF1 or NF2 have an increased risk of developing secondary tumors and patients with NF1 with spinal neurofibromas have an increased risk of long-term mortality (60% 10-year survival).

DIAGNOSIS

Clinical Presentation

1. Pain is the most common symptom.
2. Extramedullary tumors produce symptoms by compression of nerve roots before cord.
3. Intramedullary tumors present with symptoms for 6 months to 3 years, commonly with axial spinal pain, radicular pain, and sensorimotor deficits.
4. For schwannomas, the most common symptom initially is pain in a radicular distribution. They grow slowly so patients may have symptoms for months to years before diagnosis.
5. Extradural tumors produce unremitting back pain that may be radicular in nature. Initially there are no neurologic deficits, but advanced tumors produce myelopathy.

Diagnostic Tests

1. Imaging may show bone erosion of the pedicles and intervertebral foramina (e.g., schwannoma) or bony destruction (metastases, lymphoma).
2. Contrast-enhanced MRI shows much better anatomic soft-tissue detail then CT.
3. MRI shows expansive lesion; gliomas frequently associated with syringomyelia.
4. CT myelography may be useful if MRI cannot be done.

Pathology

Depends on the tumor type.

Differential Diagnosis

1. Intramedullary: demyelination, amyotrophic lateral sclerosis (ALS), dural arteriovenous fistula, atriovenous malformation (AVM), hemangioblastoma, lipoma, and epidermoid.
2. Extramedullary: cervical spondylosis, epidermoid, dermoid, sarcoma, metastasis, myeloma, and extramedullary hematopoiesis.

TREATMENT

1. Surgical resection is usually the treatment of choice for most spinal cord tumors. Preoperative embolization may be helpful for vascular tumors such as hemangioblastoma. Complete resection often feasible for schwannomas, meningiomas, and ependymomas.
2. Intraoperative neurophysiologic monitoring helpful in decreasing morbidity.
3. Astrocytomas are more infiltrating and complete resection possible only in 20% of cases, but can be decompressed by laminectomy, partial resection, and repair of syringomyelia.

4. Postoperative results are generally related to preoperative neurologic condition. Where there are maximal deficits before surgery, significant recovery is unlikely. Where there are mild or modest deficits, excellent functional recovery may be expected.
5. Patients with subtotal resection may be treated with RT or observed closely and treated with further surgery or RT when recurrent disease is documented.
6. Postoperative radiation can delay recurrence or progression of symptoms. Patients usually receive 3,500 to 4,500 cGy.
7. Chemotherapy has a very limited role for high-grade gliomas and recurrent tumors.

NEUROLOGIC COMPLICATIONS OF SYSTEMIC CANCER

BRAIN METASTASES

BACKGROUND

1. Brain metastases (BMs) are present at autopsy in 10% to 30% of patients who die of cancer.
2. Incidence 100,000 to 170,000 new cases per year in the United States.
3. Frequency in decreasing order are lung, breast, melanoma, unknown primary, colon/rectum, renal cell, testicular, and thyroid.
4. Fifty percent to 80% have multiple metastases in CNS (especially melanoma and lung cancer).
5. Most common primary in men is lung and in women, breast.
6. Melanoma has a strong propensity for CNS.
7. Prostate cancer commonly metastasizes to skull but rarely to brain parenchyma.
8. Hematologic cancers such as Hodgkin disease and chronic lymphocytic leukemia (CLL) rarely cause parenchymal metastases.
9. Hemorrhagic metastases include melanoma, choriocarcinoma, renal, thyroid and lung.

PATHOPHYSIOLOGY

1. Metastases reach the brain by hematogenous or direct spread from adjacent structures such as leptomeninges and dura.
2. Eighty percent of metastases are supratentorial at gray–white junction due to tumor emboli lodging at small vessels.
3. Frequency of structures is proportional to blood flow [cerebral hemisphere (80% to 85%), cerebellum (10 to 15%), brainstem (5%)].
4. Exceptions to this are tumors arising from the pelvis [prostate, uterine, gastrointestinal (GI) tract], which have a predilection for the posterior fossa for unclear reasons.
5. Symptoms caused by mass effect, edema, destruction of brain structures, increased ICP, cerebral irritation resulting in seizures, and intratumoral hemorrhage.
6. Patients with BM may also have leptomeningeal metastasis (LM) (especially posterior fossa BM).

PROGNOSIS

1. Generally poor, but most patients die of systemic disease.
2. If treated with steroids alone, the median survival is 1 month; RT extends mean survival to 3 to 6 months.
3. Single brain metastases treated with surgery or SRS and whole-brain RT (WBRT) have a median survival of 8 to 16 months.

4. The Radiation Therapy Oncology Group (RTOG) classified patients into three recursive partitioning analysis classes:

Class I: KPS above 70%; age, younger than 65 years; controlled primary disease, metastases only to brain; median survival, 7.1 months.
Class II: Patients who do not fall into class I or III; median survival, 4.2 months.
Class III: KPS lower than 70%; median survival, 2.3 months.

DIAGNOSIS

Clinical Presentation

Most patients present with headaches, behavioral change, and focal neurologic deficits such as weakness, numbness, gait unsteadiness, and visual symptoms; 10% to 20% present with seizures; 5% present with intracranial hemorrhage.

Diagnostic Tests

1. On CT scan, 40% of patients have solitary lesions, 60% have multiple lesions.
2. Contrast-enhanced MRI is more sensitive and shows a higher percentage with multiple lesions (70%–80%). Triple-dose–contrast MRI and magnetization-transfer MRI may increase the sensitivity of the test but are not performed routinely.
3. For patients with known primary tumor, restaging studies to determine the extent of systemic disease should be performed (chest, abdomen, pelvic CT, bone scan, serum tumor markers, possible spine MRI).
4. For patients without a known primary tumor, a systemic evaluation to find the primary tumor is required as it is generally easier to biopsy a non-CNS site. The focus of the search should be the lung.
  a. Evaluation may include chest, abdomen, and pelvic CT; peripheral blood smear; breast examination; stool guaiac; liver function tests; and urinalysis.
  b. Blood tumor markers and PET scan may occasionally be helpful.

Pathology

1. Depends on primary and generally has the same features as the primary neoplasm.
2. Grossly most are spheroid and well-demarcated, but on microscopic examination have a somewhat infiltrative appearance.

Differential Diagnosis

PBTs, especially gliomas and lymphomas, demyelination, abscess, emboli.

TREATMENT

Supportive Care

1. Patients with symptomatic edema should receive treatment with corticosteroids [10-mg dexamethasone loading dose and then 8 mg twice a day (b.i.d. or 4 mg four times a day (q.i.d.)].
  a. Oral absorption of dexamethasone is excellent; IV administration is necessary only if the patient cannot take oral medications.
  b. There is some evidence that 4 mg b.i.d. may be as useful as 8 mg b.i.d. The minimum dose of steroids necessary to prevent symptoms from peritumoral edema should be used.
  c. Patients who are likely to require prolonged treatment with corticosteroids should also receive PCP prophylaxis [e.g., sulfamethoxazole 800 mg/trimethoprim 160 mg (Bactrim DS) daily or three times weekly].

2. Patients with seizures should be treated with standard antiepileptic drugs (AEDs). Patients who have never had seizures usually do not require AEDs (possible exception are patients with melanoma metastases, which have a predilection for the cortex, and patients with both brain metastases and LMs).

Surgery

1. High-dose steroids (4–6 mg q6h) are useful in decreasing cerebral edema and should be started when diagnosis is made before surgery. If lymphoma is in the differential, steroids should be avoided.
2. Surgery is recommended with a single metastasis in an accessible location and controlled systemic disease. It provides symptomatic relief and improves survival, local tumor control, and quality of life.
3. Surgery may also be considered in some patients with:
   a. Multiple metastases in which there is a large symptomatic lesion
   b. Symptomatic recurrent brain metastasis in patients with controlled systemic disease
   c. Symptomatic radiation necrosis from SRS

Whole-brain Radiation

1. WBRT (3,000–4,000 cGy, given in 10–20 fractions) should be the treatment of choice for patients with multiple metastases, patients with a single metastasis who are not surgical candidates, or patients with progressive systemic disease.
2. WBRT following surgery or focal RT decreases local recurrence and risk of neurologic death but does not improve overall survival.
3. WBRT may occasionally be useful in patients who have received prior WBRT and develop recurrent BM. Reirradiation in selected patients may prolong survival by 3 to 4 months.
4. Ongoing studies evaluating radiosensitizers such as RSR13, motexafin gadolinium, and chemotherapeutic agents such as temozolomide are under way.

Stereotactic Radiosurgery

1. SRS is used to treat tumors 3 cm in diameter or less. Larger lesions can be treated with SRT in which the focused radiation is given in several fractions to reduce the incidence of neurotoxicity and radiation necrosis.
2. Advantages of SRS:
   a. Noninvasive
   b. Outpatient procedure
   c. Cost-effective compared with surgery
3. Produces good local tumor control (range, 65%–95%; median, 81%) in radiosensitive tumors such as breast cancer and radioresistant tumors such as melanoma, renal cancer, and sarcoma.
4. Overall median survival of approximately 11 months, but this is dependent on patient selection.
5. Indications:
   a. One to three recurrent BMs in patients with prior RT.
   b. As an alternative to surgery in patients with small single BM without significant mass effect.
   c. Findings from RTOG trial 9508 suggest that SRS plus WBRT is better than WBRT alone for single BM, one to three BMs in patients with KPS above 70%, age younger than 50 years, and in those with non–small cell lung cancer (NSCLC).
6. SRS can be used alone (without WBRT) in selected patients with newly diagnosed BM with radioresistant pathology such as sarcoma and renal cell cancer.

7. Complications of SRS:
   a. Acute: (fewer than 10%) seizures, headache, edema, nausea, and rarely, hemorrhage.
   b. Subacute: alopecia, edema, and necrosis.
   c. Chronic (8%–16%): seizures, headache, neurologic deterioration (edema/necrosis). Surgery to remove necrosis required in 5% to 20% of patients.

Chemotherapy

1. Systemic chemotherapy is generally not thought to be useful due to:
   a. Inability of many drugs to cross BBB.
   b. Tumors causing BM are relatively insensitive to chemotherapy.
   c. Patients with BM have been treated with chemotherapy for their systemic disease and the BM represents chemoresistant clones.
   d. Tendency in prior studies to use drugs that cross the BBB rather than drugs that are most effective for the particular histology being evaluated.
2. BMs from chemosensitive tumors often respond to chemotherapy [choriocarcinoma, germ cell tumors, ovarian cancer, and small cell lung carcinoma (SCLC)]. Some patients with breast cancer and NSCLC may also respond to chemotherapy.

CALVARIAL AND SKULL BASE METASTASES

BACKGROUND

1. Fifteen percent to 25% of all patients with cancer, usually in the setting of bony metastases elsewhere in the body.
2. More than 50% are asymptomatic.
3. Most common tumors are from the breast, lung and prostate, renal, thyroid, and melanoma.

PATHOPHYSIOLOGY

1. Hematogenous spread or invasion from skull base tumor.
2. May cause venous sinus thrombosis.

PROGNOSIS

Prognosis is generally good. Most dural metastases can be effectively treated with RT and surgery.

DIAGNOSIS

Clinical Presentation

Local mass, pain, headache, seizures, focal deficits.

Diagnostic Tests

Contrast-enhanced MRI.

Differential Diagnosis

Meningioma.

TREATMENT

1. RT.
2. Large symptomatic lesions may require surgical resection.

SPINAL/VERTEBRAL METASTASES

BACKGROUND

1. Epidural spinal cord compression (SCC) is a neurologic emergency.
2. Should be suspected in any patient with cancer with back pain, leg weakness, or numbness.

Epidemiology

1. Epidural SCC occurs in 5% of all patients with cancer (more than 25,000 cases each year in the United States).
2. In 10% to 20% of cases, SCC is the initial manifestation of cancer (especially lung cancer).
3. Most common tumors in adults associated with SCC include lung (15%–20%), breast (15%–20%), prostate (15%–20%), multiple myeloma (5%–10%), NHL (5%–10%), renal cell carcinoma (5%–10%), colorectal carcinoma, and sarcoma.
4. In children, the most common associated tumors are sarcomas (especially Ewing), germ cell tumors, and Hodgkin disease (HD).
5. Sixty percent of symptomatic metastases occur in thoracic spine, 30% in lumbosacral spine, and 10% in cervical spine.
6. Ten percent to 30% of patients will have multiple SCC sites; therefore, imaging of the entire spine is crucial.

PATHOPHYSIOLOGY

1. Epidural location account for only 5% to 10%; most occur in vertebral body (60%) or posterior elements (30%).
2. Tumor usually reaches the vertebral column by hematogenous spread. Less commonly. tumor may reach the spinal cord by through an intervertebral foramen from a paraspinal mass (especially lymphoma), by direct hematogenous spread to the extradural fat or bone marrow, or by retrograde spread via communication with Batson venous plexus.
3. Compression of spinal cord from tumor and peritumoral edema.

PROGNOSIS

1. Depends on the primary tumor, extent of systemic disease, and severity of symptoms at presentation.
2. Ninety percent to 100% of patients who are ambulatory at onset of treatment remain so at the end of treatment.
3. Only 13% to 30% of patients who are nonambulatory at presentation regain the ability to ambulate following treatment.
4. Early diagnosis and treatment of SCC is therefore crucial for good outcome.
5. Seventy percent to 90% of patients have significant pain relief with treatment.
6. Median survival of patients presenting with SCC is 6 to 10 months and depends on degree of disability, extent of extraspinal metastases, clinical status, and sensitivity of underlying malignancy to RT and chemotherapy.

DIAGNOSIS

Clinical Presentation

1. At presentation, 95% of patients with SCC have back pain.
2. Pain precedes SCC by weeks to months.
3. Unlike pain from osteoarthritis, pain from SCC tends to be worse with recumbency, possibly as a result of distention of the epidural venous plexus.
4. Seventy-five percent have neurogenic weakness, sensory level may be present. In general, sensory complaints and findings are less prominent than motor complaints and findings.

5. SCC involving the spinal cord (which usually ends at the level of L-1) produces upper motor neuron weakness, hyperreflexia, extensor plantar responses, and sensory loss. The sensory level is usually several spinal segments lower than the true level of SCC. Radicular sensory loss or loss of reflexes tends to be a more reliable indicator of the level of SCC.

6. SCC involving the cauda equina (below L-1) causes pain, weakness and sensory loss in a radicular distribution, decreased reflexes, and flexor plantar responses.

7. Patients with advanced SCC develop urinary retention with overflow and progress to paraplegia.

8. Patients with cervical cord lesions may have Lhermitte sign, which is an electric sensation in the back and extremities produced by flexion of the neck.

Diagnostic Tests

1. Spinal radiographs show evidence of metastasis in 80% to 90% of patients. Plain films were falsely negative in 10% to 17% of patients.

2. Bone scan is more sensitive than plain radiographs and is occasionally used.

3. MRI with gadolinium is the imaging modality of choice to diagnose epidural SCC. Because 10% to 30% of patients have more than one SCC site, the entire spine must be imaged.

4. CT myelography may be helpful in patients who cannot have MRI. Myelography carries a small risk of exacerbating a neurologic deficit due to pressure shifts in the event of complete spinal subarachnoid block ("spinal coning").

Differential Diagnosis

1. Benign disorders: Degenerative spine disorders, osteomyelitis, epidural abscess, hematomas, transverse myelitis, granulomatous disorders, vascular malformation, epidural lipomatosis, extramedullary hematopoiesis.

2. Cancer-related disorders: LMs, spinal cord metastases [often cause hemicord syndrome (Brown–Sequard syndrome)], radiation myelopathy, chemotherapy-related myelopathy, paraneoplastic myelopathy, and neoplastic or radiation plexopathy.

TREATMENT

Supportive Care

1. Corticosteroids: Controversy regarding the dose of corticosteroids. No definite evidence that an initial bolus of 100 mg of dexamethasone is more effective than 10 mg. Higher doses associated with greater frequency of side effects. For most patients, 10-mg bolus of dexamethasone and then 16-mg/d maintenance in divided doses is adequate. A 100-mg bolus and 96-mg/d maintenance may be reasonable for patients who are paraplegic. Patients receiving high doses of dexamethasone should receive H_2-blockers or proton pump inhibitors.

2. Nonsteroidal antiinflammatory medications and opiates for pain control.

3. Stool softeners and laxatives to prevent constipation.

4. Deep vein thrombosis prophylaxis in patients who are not ambulatory.

Radiation Therapy

1. RT is preferred treatment and should be started as soon as possible after SCC is diagnosed. No evidence that laminectomy is more effective than RT.

2. Usually give ten fractions of 300 cGy to involved area with a margin of one to two vertebral bodies.

3. For patients who have received prior irradiation for SCC with good results, reirradiation for recurrent SCC may provide useful palliation.

Surgery

1. Role of surgery for SCC is limited.
2. Laminectomy and RT produce equivalent results.
3. Surgery is indicated if there is spinal instability, tissue diagnosis is needed, or tumor is radioresistant or for patients who have received prior RT.
4. Anterior decompression is used to resect tumor and stabilize the spine but is associated with greater morbidity. Recent studies suggest anterior decompression and RT may be more effective than RT alone.

Chemotherapy

Can be given for chemosensitive tumors such as lymphoma and SCLC.

Hormonal Therapy

May occasionally be useful in hormone-responsive tumors such as prostate and breast cancer, although RT remains the treatment of choice for these tumors.

LEPTOMENINGEAL METASTASES

BACKGROUND

1. LM is defined as infiltration of the leptomeninges by systemic cancer. It is also referred to as carcinomatous/neoplastic meningitis, or leptomeningeal carcinomatosis.
2. Should be considered in any patient with multifocal symptoms and signs in the neuraxis.

Epidemiology

1. LM is an increasingly common complication of cancer and occurs in 5% of patients with solid tumors and more than 10% of leukemias and lymphomas.
2. One third have concomitant parenchymal brain metastases.
3. Most common causes are breast cancer, lung cancer, NHL, malignant melanoma, gastrointestinal neoplasms, and acute leukemias.
4. LM is very common in acute lymphoblastic leukemia (ALL) and some types of lymphomas (Burkitt lymphoma). Prophylactic CNS treatment is generally given in these conditions.

PATHOPHYSIOLOGY

1. Tumor cells travel to CSF space via hematogenous route, direct extension from brain metastases, venous route (from bone marrow), and perineural spread.
2. Once these cells reach the CSF, they are disseminated throughout the neuraxis by the constant flow of CSF.
3. Cause symptoms by direct invasion of neural structures, alternation of metabolism in CSF, and obstruction of CSF flow.

PROGNOSIS

1. Generally poor response to treatment. Many patients also have uncontrolled systemic disease.

2. In untreated patients, disease is progressive and leads to death within 6 to 8 weeks due to progressive neurologic dysfunction.
3. Early, aggressive treatment can occasionally improve neurologic symptoms and improve quality of life, especially in patients with lymphoma/leukemia (80%) and breast cancer (50%).
4. Melanoma and lung cancer tend to have a poor response.
5. With optimal treatment median survival is 3 to 6 months and patients often die of systemic disease.

DIAGNOSIS

Clinical Presentation

1. Usually multifocal symptoms and signs in the neuroaxis, including subacute altered mental status, headaches, seizures, papilledema, cranial neuropathies (especially CNs III, VI, and VII), polyradiculopathies, and occasionally bladder and bowel dysfunction.
2. Can be fulminant in acute lymphoblastic leukemia.

Diagnostic Tests

1. MRI of the brain and spine with gadolinium may show nodular or diffuse enhancement of the leptomeninges, dura or nerve roots, and hydrocephalus.
2. LP for CSF cytology can confirm the diagnosis; however, several LPs may be needed (85% sensitive after three LPs).
3. An abnormal CSF profile (elevated CSF protein, decreased glucose, and lymphocytic pleocytosis) is present in 95% of patients and may be sufficient in the appropriate clinical context in the absence of positive CSF cytology.
4. Reactive processes can sometimes be mistaken for malignant lymphocytes.
5. Polymerase chain reaction (PCR) for immunoglobulin gene rearrangement studies for lymphoma may be helpful.
6. Leptomeningeal biopsy maybe needed if CSF is nondiagnostic and no primary tumor is identified.
7. CSF tumor markers usually not very sensitive or specific. Carcinoembryonic antigen (CEA) may be useful for carcinomas, cancer antigen 125 (CA-125) for ovarian cancer, cancer antigen 15-3 (CA 15-3) for breast cancer, melanin for melanoma, βhCG for choriocarcinoma and germ cell tumors, AFP for teratoma and yolk sac tumors.

Differential Diagnosis

Inflammatory (vasculitis, paraneoplastic), demyelinating (multiple sclerosis), granulomatous (Wegener, sarcoidosis), infectious (bacterial, viral, Lyme disease, tuberculosis, cryptococcus, cysticercosis), primary leptomeningeal neoplasms, and intracranial hypotension following LP.

TREATMENT

1. Goals of treatment in patients with LMs are to improve or stabilize the neurologic status of the patient and to prolong survival.
2. Corticosteroids occasionally relieve symptoms transiently until definitive treatment.
3. Standard therapy involves RT to symptomatic sites of the neuraxis and to disease visible on neuroimaging studies. Intrathecal chemotherapy may have a role in some patients.
4. Treatment should be determined on the basis of the patient's functional status (KPS) and patients stratified into "poor-risk" and "good-risk" groups.

a. The poor-risk group includes patients with a low KPS; multiple, serious, fixed neurologic deficits; and extensive systemic disease with few treatment options.
b. The good-risk group includes patients with a high KPS, no fixed neurologic deficits, minimal systemic disease, and reasonable systemic treatment options.
5. Patients in the poor-risk group are usually offered supportive care measures including analgesics for pain, increased ICP, or leptomeningeal irritation. RT may occasionally be administered to symptomatic sites.
6. Good-risk patients should also receive appropriate supportive care measures as described above, along with radiation to symptomatic sites and to areas of bulk disease identified on neuroimaging studies. In addition, intrathecal or intraventricular [using a surgically implanted subcutaneous reservoir and ventricular catheter (SRVC)] chemotherapy is administered. Initially, intrathecal chemotherapy is usually given by LP, and the SRVC is placed later to administer the drugs more conveniently.
7. Due to CSF flow abnormalities in these patients, a CSF flow study (e.g., ^{111}I-DTPA) allows detection of flow abnormalities, which may predict impaired targeting of areas and increased toxicity (leukoencephalopathy).
8. Methotrexate, the drug most frequently used, is administered twice weekly at a dose of 10 to 12 mg. Oral leucovorin (10 mg every 12 hours for six doses) is sometimes administered to prevent myelosuppression and mucositis. Once the CSF clears, the drug is administered less frequently.
9. Intrathecal thiotepa (10 mg twice a week) can be effective in solid tumors.
10. Cytarabine (AraC, 50 mg twice a week) is effective for lymphomatous and leukemic meningitis.
   a. A liposomal encapsulated formulation of cytarabine (DepoCyt) (50 mg every two weeks) allows patients with lymphomatous meningitis to be treated every 2 weeks rather than twice weekly and appears to be more effective than AraC.
   b. High-dose systemic cytarabine (3 g/m^2 q12h) penetrates well into the CNS and is sometimes used in patients with leukemia or lymphoma who have both systemic and CNS disease.
11. High-dose methotrexate is used in patients with LM from solid tumors.
12. Treatment duration is dependent on response. Should follow clinically and with CSF cytology.
13. Steroids recommended during treatment to reduce headaches caused by the chemical meningitis.

PARANEOPLASTIC SYNDROMES

BACKGROUND

1. In patients with cancer, paraneoplastic syndromes of the nervous system are disorders that are not caused by the direct effects of the cancer itself or its metastases or by indirect effects such as infections, metabolic disturbances, nutritional deficiencies, or cerebrovascular disorders, or by the effects of antineoplastic therapies.
2. Although neurologic complications are common in patients with cancer, most are due to metabolic disarray, nutritional deficiencies, and complications related to cancer treatment. True paraneoplastic syndromes are rare. They occur in fewer than 1% of patients with cancer.

PATHOPHYSIOLOGY

1. Autoimmune-mediated injury to the nervous system accounts for most cases.
2. Antibodies and cellular immunity directed against tumor antigens also react with

similar antigens in neuronal tissues in the CNS and peripheral nervous system, resulting in neurologic injury.

3. Autoimmune pathophysiology well documented only for a few paraneoplastic syndromes: Lambert–Eaton myasthenic syndrome (LEMS), myasthenia gravis, neuromyotonia.
4. Autoantibodies detected in serum and CSF. Most react with both tumor and neurons.
5. Affected tissues usually have inflammatory infiltrate, cell loss, microglial proliferation, and gliosis present.

Significance

1. Paraneoplastic neurologic syndromes account for a high percentage of certain disorders (70% of LEMS, 50% of subacute cerebellar degeneration, 50% of opsoclonus–myoclonus in children, 20% of opsoclonus–myoclonus in adults, 20% of subacute sensory neuronopathy).
2. Frequently occur before diagnosis of the underlying cancer. Recognition of these syndromes syndrome may lead to the diagnosis of the underlying tumor at an early stage.
3. Usually produce significant neurologic disability.
4. Often mistaken for metastatic disease.
5. Provide information concerning autoimmune disorders and tumor immunology.

PROGNOSIS

1. Most patients develop profound neurologic disability. Response of neurologic deficits to treatment is often poor.
2. Course of underlying neoplasm often indolent, possibly because of antitumor immunologic response.

DIAGNOSIS

Clinical Presentation

Presents as subacute disorder (over several weeks) affecting nervous system. Can occur from months to years before discovery of the malignancy. See below for specific features of individual paraneoplastic disorders.

Diagnostic Tests

1. Appropriate antibody testing should be performed depending on the clinical presentation. Antibodies present in both serum and CSF, but titers are higher in the CSF.
2. CSF can show lymphocytic pleocytosis, elevated protein level, elevated IgG level, and oligoclonal bands.
3. MRI of affected area usually normal but may show abnormal T_2-signal in the affected areas and allows metastatic disease to be excluded.
4. Body CT scans and occasionally PET scans may help locate primary tumor.

Differential Diagnosis

Direct infiltration by primary tumor, metastatic disease, reversible nutritional deficiencies, drug toxicity, cerebrovascular disease, and infections.

TREATMENT

Usually not effectively treatable. Some respond to treating the underlying cancer. Most do not respond to steroids, IV immunoglobulins (IVIGs), protein A immunoadsorption column, plasmapheresis, or vitamins.

TABLE 6-2. PARANEOPLASTIC SYNDROMES AFFECTING THE NERVOUS SYSTEM

Paraneoplastic syndromes of the brain and cerebellum
  Paraneoplastic cerebellar degeneration
  Paraneoplastic encephalomyelitis (limbic encephalitis, brainstem encephalitis, myelitis)
  Paraneoplastic opsoclonus–myoclonus

Visual paraneoplastic syndromes
  Cancer-associated retinopathy
  Melanoma-associated retinopathy
  Optic neuritis

Paraneoplastic syndromes of the spinal cord
  Paraneoplastic stiff man syndrome
  Paraneoplastic necrotizing myelopathy
  Motor neuron syndromes amyotrophic lateral sclerosis, subacute motor neuronopathy)

Paraneoplastic syndromes of the peripheral nervous system
  Paraneoplastic sensory neuronopathy
  Acute polyradiculoneuropathy (Guillain–Barré syndrome)
  Brachial neuritis
  Vasculitis of the nerve and muscle
  Subacute or chronic sensorimotor peripheral neuropathy
  Sensorimotor neuropathies associated with plasma cell dyscrasias
  Autonomic neuropathy
  Neuromyotonia

Paraneoplastic syndromes of the neuromuscular junction
  Lambert–Eaton myasthenic syndrome
  Myasthenia gravis

Paraneoplastic syndromes of muscle
  Polymyositis/dermatomyositis
  Acute necrotizing myopathy
  Carcinoid myopathy
  Cachectic myopathy

PARANEOPLASTIC SYNDROMES OF THE BRAIN AND CEREBELLUM

CEREBELLAR DEGENERATION

1. Subacute cerebellar syndrome with truncal and appendicular ataxia progressing over weeks or months. Dysarthria, diplopia, vertigo, nystagmus (Tables 6-2 and 6-3).
2. Usually associated with SCLC, HD, breast cancer, and gynecologic malignancies.
3. Autoantibodies: anti-Yo (breast and gynecologic malignancies), anti-Tr (HD), anti-Hu (SCLC), anti-Ri (breast cancer), anti–voltage gated calcium channel (SCLC).
4. Poor response to antitumor therapy, immunosuppression with IVIG, or plasmapheresis.

PARANEOPLASTIC ENCEPHALOMYELITIS

1. Paraneoplastic encephalomyelitis (PEM) is a specific neurologic syndrome dependent on predominant site of inflammation (cortical encephalitis, limbic encephalitis, brainstem encephalitis, cerebellitis).

TABLE 6-3. ANTIBODIES ASSOCIATED WITH PARANEOPLASTIC NEUROLOGIC SYNDROMES

Antibody	Associated Cancer	Syndrome
Anti-Hu	SCLC, other	Focal encephalitis, myelitis, encephalomyelitis, sensory neuronopathy, peripheral neuropathy
Anti-Yo	Gynecologic, breast	Cerebellar degeneration
Anti-Ri	Breast, gynecologic, SCLC	Cerebellar ataxia, opsoclonus, brainstem encephalitis
Anti-Tr	Hodgkin lymphoma	Cerebellar degeneration
Anti-CV2 or anti-CRMP1-5	SCLC, other	Focal encephalitis, myelitis, encephalomyelitis, cerebellar degeneration, peripheral neuropathy
Anti-Ma proteins[a]	Testicular germ cell tumors and other cancers	Limbic, brainstem encephalitis, cerebellar degeneration
Antiamphiphysin	Breast, SCLC	Stiff man syndrome, encephalomyelitis
Anti-VGKC[b]	Thymoma, others	Neuromyotonia, limbic encephalitis
Anti-VGCC[b]	SCLC	LEMS, cerebellar degeneration
Antiacetylcholine receptor[b]	Thymoma	Myasthenia gravis

SCLC, small cell lung cancer; LEMS, Lambert–Eaton myasthenic syndrome.
[a]Antibodies Ma2 (also called anti-Ta antibodies) usually associated with limbic and brainstem encephalitis and germ cell tumors. Antibodies directed at Ma1 usually associate with brainstem encephalitis, cerebellar degeneration and several types of cancer (lung, breast, ovary, etc.)
[b]These antibodies are also identified in the nonparaneoplastic form of the syndrome.

2. Frequently associated with subacute sensory neuronopathy, myelitis, and autonomic dysfunction.
3. Limbic encephalitis characterized by subacute confusion, memory loss, psychiatric symptoms, and seizures.
4. Pathology characterized by perivascular inflammatory infiltrate and neuronal loss.
5. MRI may occasionally show increased T_2 signal in affected area.
6. Usually associated with SCLC (anti-Hu, anti-CV2, anti-CRMP 5), testicular cancer (anti-Ma2), and a variety of tumors (anti-Ma1).
7. Some patients respond to treatment of cancer. Rare responses to immunosuppression.

OPSOCLONUS–MYOCLONUS

1. Subacute opsoclonus, myoclonus, ataxia.
2. Usually associated with neuroblastoma in children; breast cancer, SCLC in adults.
3. Anti-Ri (breast and gynecologic cancer), anti-Hu, anti-Yo, Anti-Ma2.
4. May respond to treatment of tumor, steroids, and IVIG. Prognosis better in children.

PARANEOPLASTIC SYNDROMES OF THE EYE

CARCINOMA-ASSOCIATED RETINOPATHY

1. Carcinoma-associated retinopathy (CAR) is subacute onset of episodic visual obscuration, photosensitivity, night blindness, impaired color vision, and light-induced glare.
2. Examination shows decreased visual acuity, impaired color vision, scotomas, attenuated retinal arterioles.
3. Electroretinogram (ERG) demonstrates reduced or flat photopic and scotopic responses, consistent with dysfunction of the cone and rod photoreceptors.
4. Usually precedes diagnosis of underlying cancer (SCLC).
5. Serum may have antibodies against retinal photoreceptor antigens such as recoverin.
6. Prognosis poor. Anecdotal reports of improvement with steroids, plasmapheresis, and IVIG.

MELANOMA-ASSOCIATED RETINOPATHY

1. Melanoma-associated retinopathy (MAR) affects patients with melanoma.
2. Patients present with photopsias and progressive visual loss.
3. ERG reveals a markedly reduced B wave in the presence of a normal dark-adapted A wave.
4. Serum contains antibody against bipolar cells of retina.
5. Response to treatment is usually poor.

OPTIC NEURITIS

Usually associated with PEM, but occasionally may be only finding.

PARANEOPLASTIC SYNDROMES OF THE SPINAL CORD

STIFF MAN SYNDROME

1. Characterized by rigidity and stiffness of axial musculature and painful spasms.
2. EMG shows continuous motor unit activity, improved with diazepam.
3. Associated with antibodies to γ-aminobutyric acid (GABA)–glycine synapses; presynaptic (anti-GABA, antiamphiphysin); postsynaptic (antigephyrin).
4. Most commonly associated with breast, lung, and colon cancer and HD.
5. May respond to treatment of the underlying tumor, steroids, diazepam, and other drugs that enhance GABA-ergic transmission (baclofen, sodium valproate, and vigabatrin). Role of IVIG and plasmapheresis unclear.

MYELITIS (USUALLY PART OF PARANEOPLASTIC ENCEPHALOMYELITIS)

1. Acute necrotizing myelopathy.
   a. Acute or subacute myelopathy resulting in death.

   b. Associated with lymphoma and lung cancer.
   c. No known therapy.
2. Amyotrophic lateral sclerosis (AML).
   a. Association with cancer controversial.
   b. Possibly associated with lymphoma, breast cancer, SCLC.
3. Subacute motor neuronopathy.
   a. Subacute lower motor neuron weakness, usually affecting lower extremities.
   b. Associated with HD and NHL.
   c. Improves spontaneously.
   d. No specific treatment except for physical therapy.

PARANEOPLASTIC SYNDROMES OF THE DORSAL ROOT GANGLIA AND NERVE

SUBACUTE SENSORY NEURONOPATHY

1. Subacute sensory loss, often associated with painful paresthesias and dysesthesias.
2. All sensory modalities affected. May be asymmetric.
3. Patients frequently have sensory ataxia and pseudoathetosis.
4. Nerve conduction studies show small amplitude or absent sensory nerve action potentials with normal motor potentials and F waves.
5. Often associated with encephalomyelitis and autonomic dysfunction.
6. Associated with SCLC and anti-Hu antibody.
7. Pathologically there is inflammation of dorsal root ganglion and neuronal loss.
8. Occasional response to steroids and treatment of underlying tumor. Response to other forms of immunosuppression poor.

PERIPHERAL NEUROPATHIES

SUBACUTE AXONAL OR DEMYELINATING NEUROPATHIES

1. Difficult to differentiate from neuropathies caused by nutritional and metabolic causes and by chemotherapy.
2. Some neuropathies develop before or at the time of diagnosis of the cancer.
3. May respond to steroids or IVIG.

VASCULITIS OF THE NERVE AND MUSCLE

1. Painful, asymmetric, or symmetric sensorimotor polyneuropathy or mononeuritis multiplex.
2. Associated with SCLC and NHL.
3. Erythrocyte sedimentation rate (ESR) and CSF protein levels are usually elevated.
4. Nerve biopsy shows intramural and perivascular inflammatory infiltrate, usually without necrotizing vasculitis. Muscle biopsy may also show vasculitis.
5. May respond to treatment of tumor and immunosuppression (steroids, cyclophosphamide).

PERIPHERAL NEUROPATHIES OF MONOCLONAL GAMMOPATHIES

Associated with multiple myeloma, osteosclerotic myeloma, Waldenström macroglobulinemia, B-cell NHL, chronic lymphocytic leukemia (see Neuromuscular Chapter).

Multiple Myeloma

1. Five percent to 10% of patients with multiple myeloma have symptomatic neuropathy; one third have electrophysiologic evidence of neuropathy.
2. Patients may develop mild sensorimotor axonal neuropathy, pure sensory neuropathy, subacute or chronic demyelinating neuropathy, or amyloid neuropathy.
3. Treatment of myeloma often does not improve neuropathy.

Osteosclerotic Myeloma

1. More than 50% of patient have chronic demyelinating polyneuropathy with motor predominance.
2. May be part of POEMS syndrome (*p*olyneuropathy, *o*rganomegaly, *e*ndocrinopathy, *M* component, and *s*kin changes).
3. Treatment of sclerotic lesions often leads to improvement in neuropathy.

Waldenström Macroglobulinemia

1. Five percent to 10% of patients have neuropathy resulting from IgM M-protein against myelin-associated glycoprotein (MAG) or various gangliosides.
2. Symmetric sensorimotor polyneuropathy; predominant involvement of large sensory fibers.
3. Nerve conduction studies show slow conduction velocities and prolonged distal motor and sensory latencies consistent with demyelinating neuropathy.
4. Treatment includes therapy for underlying Waldenström macroglobulinemia (chlorambucil, cyclophosphamide, fludarabine) and IVIG or plasmapheresis.

GUILLAIN–BARRÉ SYNDROME AND BRACHIAL PLEXOPATHY

1. Associated with HD and NHL.
2. Identical clinically to Guillain–Barré Syndrome (GBS) and brachial plexopathy from nonneoplastic causes.
3. Responds to standard treatments for GBS (IVIG, plasmapheresis) and brachial plexopathy (steroids).

NEUROMYOTONIA (ISAAC SYNDROME)

1. Caused by autoantibodies to voltage-gated potassium channels that increase the release of acetylcholine and prolong the action potential, resulting in spontaneous, continuous muscle fiber activity.
2. Patients experience cramps, muscle weakness, hypertrophic muscles, excessive sweating.
3. EMG show fibrillations, fasiculations, continuous discharges.
4. Associated with thymoma, HD, SCLC, plasmacytoma.
5. Phenytoin, carbamazepine and plasmapheresis produces symptomatic relief.

AUTONOMIC NEUROPATHY

1. Usually associated with PEM.
2. Associated with SCLC (anti-Hu antibodies), HD, NHL, carcinoid tumor of the lung, pancreatic and testicular cancer.
3. Orthostatic hypotension, dry mouth, erectile dysfunction, sphincter dysfunction, esophageal and gastrointestinal dysmotility, and cardiac dysrhythmia.

PARANEOPLASTIC SYNDROMES OF THE NEUROMUSCULAR JUNCTION

LAMBERT–EATON MYASTHENIC SYNDROME

1. Caused by antibodies to presynaptic voltage-gated calcium channels (VGCCs) impairing acetylcholine release from presynaptic motor terminal.
2. Fifty percent to 70% of patients have underlying cancer, usually SCLC.
3. Neurologic symptoms usually precede or coincide with diagnosis of cancer.
4. Symptoms include fatigue, leg weakness, muscle aches, vague paresthesias.
5. Dry mouth and other autonomic symptoms common.
6. CN symptoms usually mild and transient (usually diplopia).
7. Examination shows proximal muscle weakness, absent reflexes, sluggishly reactive pupils, and occasionally, ptosis.
8. Brief exercise may potentiate reflexes and improve strength transiently.
9. Nerve conduction studies show small-amplitude compound muscle action potential (CMAP).
   a. At slow rates of repetitive nerve stimulation (2–5 Hz) decremental response more than 10% is seen.
   b. At fast rates (20 Hz or greater) facilitation occurs (more than 100%).
   c. Maximal muscle contraction also results in increase in the amplitude of CMAP.
   d. Facilitation of more than 100% in multiple muscles or more than 400% in a single muscle diagnostic of LEMS.
   e. Presence of antibodies to P/Q-type VGCC in serum is also diagnostic of LEMS.
   f. Treatment involves therapy for underlying cancer; 3,4-diaminopyridine, pyridostigmine, and immunosuppression with IVIG, plasmapheresis, prednisone, or azothioprine may also be helpful.

MYASTHENIA GRAVIS

1. Ten percent of patients with myasthenia gravis have thymoma; one third of patients with thymoma develop myasthenia.
2. Patients have antitintin and acetylcholine receptor antibodies.
3. Treatment consists of removal of thymoma, anticholinesterases, and immunosuppression.

PARANEOPLASTIC SYNDROMES OF THE MUSCLE

POLYMYOSITIS/DERMATOMYOSITIS

1. Polymyositis is caused by cell-mediated cytotoxic mechanisms; dermatomyositis is caused by humoral-mediated vasculopathy.
2. Polymyositis may be associated with graft versus host disease (GVHD).
3. Association of cancer with polymyositis controversial.
4. Approximately 10% of patients with dermatomyositis have an underlying cancer.
5. Ovarian and breast cancer in women; lung and gastrointestinal cancer in men.
6. Patients present with subacute proximal muscle weakness (especially neck flexors, pharyngeal, and respiratory muscles). In dermatomyositis, there may be purplish discoloration of eyelids (heliotrope rash) with edema, and erythematous, scaly lesions over knuckles.
7. Serum creatine kinase level is elevated. EMG shows myopathic changes.
8. Course of myositis independent of underlying cancer.
9. Treatment of tumor may or may not improve neurologic syndrome. Steroids, immunosuppressants, and IVIG may be helpful.

ACUTE NECROTIZING MYOPATHY

1. Rapidly progressive myopathy leading to death in weeks.
2. Associated with many cancers, especially SCLC.

NEUROLOGIC COMPLICATIONS OF CANCER TREATMENT

CHEMOTHERAPY

BACKGROUND

1. Neurologic complications of chemotherapy can affect the CNS and peripheral nervous system.
2. Can be the dose-limiting factor in many cases.
3. Neurotoxicity often is increased when combined with RT.
4. Very common in patients undergoing treatment.

PATHOPHYSIOLOGY

Cause symptoms by a variety of mechanisms but mostly due to direct nervous system damage.

PROGNOSIS

Usually good, most symptoms stabilize or improve after stopping drug.

DIAGNOSIS

Location

Injury anywhere along neuraxis depending on drug.

Clinical Presentation

1. Neurologic symptoms depending on agent and route of administration.
2. Acute encephalopathy: Ifosfamide, procarbazine, 5-fluorouracil (5-FU), methotrexate (high dose), cisplatin, cytarabine, interferons, interleukin-2, corticosteroids.
3. Seizures: Busulphan (high dose), ifosfamide, interferon.
4. Vasculopathy and strokes: High-dose methotrexate, asparaginase.
5. Chronic encephalopathy: Methotrexate, cytarabine, interferon.
6. Methotrexate and cytarabine increase risk of leukoencephalopathy when given with RT.
7. Cerebellar dysfunction: Cytarabine (high dose), 5-FU, ifosfamide.
8. Cranial neuropathies: Cisplatin, vincristine.
9. Myelopathy/meningitis: Intrathecal methotrexate, cytarabine, and thiotepa.
10. Peripheral neuropathy: Cisplatin, oxaliplatin, vinca alkaloids, paclitaxel, docetaxel, thalidomide, bortezomib.
11. Myopathy: Corticosteroids.

Diagnostic Tests

MRI, EMG/NCS (nerve conduction studies), electroencephalogram (EEG), and routine blood work may be needed depending on symptomatology.

Pathology

Depends on agent and symptoms but usually diagnosed on clinical grounds.

Differential Diagnosis

Paraneoplastic disorders, metastases, metabolic encephalopathy, radiation toxicity.

TREATMENT

1. Usually need to discontinue chemotherapy.
2. Supportive care.
3. Gabapentin and tricyclic antidepressants for neuropathic pain.
4. Vitamin supplementation may help.

RADIATION THERAPY

BACKGROUND

1. RT may affect the nervous system by (a) direct injury to neural structures included in the radiation portal or (b) indirectly by damaging blood vessels or endocrine organs necessary for functioning of the nervous system or by producing tumors.
2. RT complications typically divided into acute (hours or days), early delayed (2 weeks to 4 months), and late delayed (4 months to several years) reactions.
3. Very common in treated patients and increases with increasing survival.

PATHOPHYSIOLOGY

1. Injury to glia, neurons, blood vessels, and stem cells.
2. Neurotoxicity is dependent on the total dose, fraction size, length of treatment, and the total volume of the involved nervous system in addition to length of survival, comorbid factors (diabetes, hypertension, older age), and concomitant chemotherapy.

PROGNOSIS

Generally poor as these are irreversible processes.

DIAGNOSIS

Usually clear from history but must repeat imaging studies to rule out recurrent tumor and in the case of radiation necrosis, a biopsy or resection may be needed.

TREATMENT

1. Supportive care with steroids.
2. May require surgery in case of radiation necrosis and tumors.
3. Anecdotal reports of benefit with anticoagulation.

Sequelae of Radiation Therapy to the Brain

1. Acute reactions.
   a. May occur when large fractions of radiation (usually more than 300 cGy) are given to patients with cerebral edema and increased ICP.
   b. Within hours of RT, the patients develop evidence of increased ICP with headache, nausea, vomiting, somnolence, and exacerbation of signs and symptoms caused by the lesion. Rarely, cerebral herniation and death may occur.
   c. Usually respond to corticosteroids, and if necessary, mannitol and diuretics.
   d. Can often be avoided by starting patients on steroids before beginning RT and initiating RT with fractions of 200 cGy or less if patients have large amounts of edema.
2. Early delayed reactions
   a. Several weeks to several months following radiation.
   b. Possibly related to transient demyelination resulting from injury to oligodendrocytes.
   c. Characterized by somnolence, headache, nausea, vomiting, fever, exacerbation of neurologic deficits, and transient deterioration in cognitive function.
   d. When the posterior fossa is irradiated, ataxia, dysarthria, diplopia and nystagmus may occur.
   e. MRI and CT scan findings are usually normal.
   f. Corticosteroids can be helpful, but most patients recover spontaneously within 6 to 8 weeks. Very rarely, the condition can be progressive and result in death.
   g. Recognition of the early delayed reaction is important because it is usually transient and the appearance of new symptoms at this time does not necessarily indicate treatment failure or the need for a change in therapy.
3. Late delayed reaction
   a. Develops months to years after radiation and affects white matter more than gray matter.
   b. Etiology is unknown but hypothesis include
      1) Injury to small and medium vessels and tissue necrosis from ischemia
      2) Radiation injury to glial cells, especially oligodendrocytes, leading to demyelination
      3) Injury to neural stem cells
      4) Autoimmune damage
   c. Several syndromes are recognized.

4. Leukoencephalopathy
   a. Delayed encephalopathy (leukoencephalopathy) presents with progressive dementia, apathy, gait disturbance, and incontinence of urine. MRI shows cerebral atrophy and white matter changes without recurrent tumor or radiation necrosis.
   b. Symptoms occur 6 to 36 months or more after treatment. Large daily fractions increases risk.
   c. Communicating hydrocephalus may be due to radiation-induced obliteration of the arachnoid granulations. Some patients improve after ventricular shunting.
5. Radiation necrosis
   a. Related to radiation dose, fraction size, and duration of therapy; usually occurs in radiation field.
   b. Delayed by 6 months to several years (peak, 18 months) after RT.
   c. Interstitial brachytherapy and radiosurgery associated with high risk for radiation necrosis.
   d. May also occur if brain is included in radiation field of head and neck neoplasm.
   e. Symptoms are similar to those of an expanding recurrent tumor.
   f. MRI/CT usually not able to distinguish recurrent tumor from radiation necrosis.
   g. PET, thallium/technetium SPECT, and MRS may help distinguish recurrent tumor from radiation necrosis.
   h. High-dose steroids can temporarily palliate the symptoms.
   i. Surgical resection of necrotic mass maybe needed.
   j. Anecdotal report of benefit from anticoagulation.

Secondary Involvement of the Brain By Irradiation

1. Vascular effects:
   a. Stenosis of both intra- and extracranial vessels may occur months or years after RT, resulting in transient ischemic attacks and strokes. Pathology is similar to that of atherosclerosis. In general, the larger the diameter of the vessel involved, the longer the latency between the RT and the vasculopathy. Treatment is identical to that for cerebrovascular disease from typical atherosclerosis. When extracranial vessels are involved, endarterectomy may occasionally be of benefit, but the surgery may be technically difficult.
   b. Small-vessel disease may also complicate RT.
   c. Vascular abnormalities are especially common in children and have a predilection for the supraclinoid portion of the internal carotid artery. Occlusion of the vessel is sometimes associated with Moyamoya changes.
   d. Radiation-induced telangiectasia, cavernomas, angiomatous malformations, and aneurysms occur rarely and may lead to delayed hemorrhage in the brain.
   e. Cervical RT may rarely lead to carotid rupture.
2. Radiation-induced tumors:
   a. Uncommon. More frequent in patients who have been exposed to radiation in childhood.
   b. Usually appear years or decades after RT. Mean latent interval is 17.6 years.
   c. Meningiomas and sarcomas are the most common tumors occurring in the nervous system, but gliomas and malignant schwannomas may also develop.
   d. Relative risk for developing brain tumors was 9.5 for meningiomas, 2.6 for gliomas, 18.8 for nerve sheath tumors, and 3.4 for other tumors.
   e. Clinical features and treatment of these tumors are similar to those of tumors that arise without prior RT, but the tumors are often more aggressive.
3. Endocrinopathies:
   a. Endocrine disorders can be the consequence of direct irradiation of an endocrine gland (e.g., thyroid irradiation in patients with HD) or as a result of hypothalamic–pituitary dysfunction secondary to cranial irradiation.
   b. In children, the most common endocrinopathy is GH deficiency. Gonadotrophin deficiency and secondary and tertiary hypothyroidism occur less frequently.
   c. In adults, GH deficiency is common, but rarely symptomatic. Sixty-seven percent of adult males experience sexual difficulties, usually decreased libido and

impotence, within 2 years of RT. These problems are thought to result from gonadotrophin deficiency from hypothalamic damage. Hypothyroidism and hypoadrenalism occur less commonly and may require hormonal replacement. Hyperprolactinemia may also occur.

Myelopathy

1. Spinal cord more sensitive than brain to radiation.
2. Early delayed radiation myelopathy results in Lhermitte sign, a sudden "electric shock" sensation with neck flexion; begins several weeks to 6 months after treatment to neck or upper respiratory tract tumors and slowly improves within several months.
3. Late delayed radiation myelopathy occurs in two forms:
   a. Most common form. Occurs 6 months to 10 years or more after exposure to RT
      1) Incidence ranges from 0.2% to 5% of patients receiving spinal cord doses of 45 Gy in 180- to 200-cGy fractions.
      2) Characterized by an asymmetric myelopathy progressing over weeks, months, or rarely years to paraparesis or quadriparesis.
      3) Initially hemicord (Brown–Sequard) syndrome, eventually symmetric myelopathy develops.
      4) Occasionally the myelopathy stabilizes, leaving the patient moderately to severely weak.
      5) Imaging studies are usually normal, although swelling and enhancement may be seen in the acute stages and atrophy may occur at a later stage.
      6) Differential diagnosis includes epidural spinal cord compression, intramedullary metastases, and the rare paraneoplastic necrotic myelopathy.
      7) There is no effective treatment, although there are anecdotal reports of benefit from steroids, anticoagulation, and hyperbaric oxygen.
   b. A second form of delayed radiation myelopathy involves injury to lower motor neurons and occurs especially after pelvic irradiation
      1) Etiology is unclear. It was originally thought to result from injury to anterior horn cells, but involvement of proximal nerve roots is also a possibility.
      2) Three months to 14 years after irradiation, a flaccid asymmetric paraparesis develops, affecting both distal and proximal muscles, and associated with atrophy, fasiculations, and loss of reflexes. Sensory loss and sphincter disturbance are usually absent but may occasionally be a late complication. The syndrome usually stabilizes after a few months.
      3) Sensory and motor nerve conduction studies are normal, but EMG shows denervation. The CSF protein is often elevated.
      4) Imaging studies of the spine are usually normal but nerve roots may show enhancement.
      5) Differential diagnosis include radiation plexopathy, LMs, GBS, AML, and paraneoplastic subacute motor neuronopathy.
      6) There is no effective treatment.

Cranial Neuropathy

1. Generally rare (fewer than 1% of patients).
2. Visual loss may follow irradiation of the eye or the brain. Caused by a radiation-induced "dry eye syndrome," glaucoma, cataracts, retinopathy, or optic neuropathy.
3. Optic neuropathy typically occurs months to years after irradiation, with a peak at 12 to 18 months. Two clinical syndromes are seen:
   a. Painless, progressive monocular or bilateral visual loss with mild papilledema or optic atrophy, which may at times lead to complete blindness.
   b. Sudden visual loss as a result of central retinal artery or vein thrombosis.
4. Risk of optic neuropathy may be increased with concomitant administration of chemotherapy.

5. Deafness may result from an otitis media and rarely from vascular damage to the cochlear or vestibular nerves.
6. Radiation damage to other CNs is usually associated with large doses of irradiation (6,500 cGy or more) and are uncommon.

Brachial Plexopathy

1. Brachial plexopathy occurs after radiation for breast cancer or lymphoma.
2. Early delayed brachial plexus reaction may develop several months after irradiation. Described mainly in patients with breast cancer. Characterized by paresthesias in the forearm and hand, and occasionally pain, weakness, and atrophy in C-6 to T-1 muscles. Symptoms usually improve over several weeks or months. Nerve conduction studies show segmental slowing.
3. Late delayed radiation plexopathy involving the brachial plexus occurs 1 year or more (median, 40 months) after RT with doses of 6,000 cGy or more.
4. Clinically: tingling and numbness of fingers, weakness in hand or arm.
5. Signs usually referable to the upper brachial plexus (C5-6 dermatomes).
6. Pain later in the course.
7. Differential diagnosis includes infiltrating tumor of the brachial plexus (usually painful) with involvement predominantly of the lower brachial plexus (C7-T1 dermatomes).
8. EMG shows myokymic discharges in more than 50% of cases of radiation plexopathy and none in cancerous cases.
9. Contrast MRI may help distinguish radiation fibrosis from tumor infiltration.
10. Surgical exploration of brachial plexus occasionally necessary for diagnosis.
11. No specific treatment; anecdotal reports of improvement with anticoagulation.

Lumbosacral Plexopathy

1. Early delayed, generally transient lumbosacral plexopathy rare. Usually develops several months (median, 4 months) after RT. Presents with distal bilateral paresthesias of the lower limbs. Neurologic examination is usually normal. Improvement in 3 to 6 months.
2. Clinical features of late delayed lumbosacral plexopathy are similar to those of brachial plexopathy. This condition develops 1 to 30 years (median, 5 years) after irradiation. The patient may stabilize after several months or years. There is usually asymmetric weakness of one or both legs, with less-marked sensory loss. The foot is frequently involved. Pain is usually mild or absent. Myokymic changes may be seen on EMG. The usual course of the disease is usually one of gradual progression, although some patients may stabilize after several months or years.
3. No specific treatment; anecdotal reports of improvement with anticoagulation.

HEMATOPOIETIC STEM CELL TRANSPLANTATION

BACKGROUND

1. Hematopoietic stem cell transplantation (HSCT) used with increasing frequency to treat patients with cancer.
2. In allogeneic HSCT, the replacement marrow or peripheral blood stem cells are obtained from HLA-compatible donors and infused into the patient after high doses of chemotherapy and RT administered to treat the underlying neoplasm.
3. In autologous HSCT, the replacement marrow or peripheral blood stem cells are harvested from the patient and then reinfused into the patient after high-dose chemotherapy and RT.
4. Neurologic complications common, especially encephalopathy, CNS infections, and cerebrovascular disorders. More frequent with allogeneic HSCT.

PATHOPHYSIOLOGY

1. High-dose chemotherapy and radiation results in
   a. immunosuppression and infection
   b. organ damage and metabolic encephalopathy
   c. vascular injury and cerebrovascular complications
   d. direct neurotoxicity
2. GVHD in allogeneic HSCT results in autoimmune disorders such as myasthenia gravis, polymyositis, and chronic inflammatory demyelinating neuropathy (CIDP).

PROGNOSIS

Patients who undergo HSCT and develop neurologic complications tend to have worse prognosis.

DIAGNOSIS

Clinical Presentation

1. Toxic/metabolic encephalopathy
2. CNS infections
3. Seizures
4. Cerebrovascular complications (hemorrhages from thrombocytopenia, thrombosis from hypercoagulable state)
5. Complications of chemotherapy, RT, immunosuppressive agents
6. GVHD-associated myasthenia gravis, polymyositis, CIDP

Diagnostic Tests

Blood work, neuroimaging studies, LP, EEG, and NCS depending on the symptoms.

Differential Diagnosis

Frequently complex and varies depending on specific complication.

TREATMENT

1. Varies depending on the specific complication.
2. Complications associated with GVHD treated with immunosuppression.

BIBLIOGRAPHY

Bateller L, Dalmau J. Paraneoplastic neurologic syndromes. *Neurol Clin* 2003;21:221–248.

Behin A, Delattre J-Y. Neurologic sequelae of radiation therapy in the nervous system. In: Schiff D, Wen PY, eds. *Cancer neurology in clinical practice.* Totowa, NJ: Humana Press, 2003:173–192.

Bernstein M, Berger MS, eds, *Neuro-oncology: the essentials.* New York: Thieme Medical Publishers, 2000.

DeAngelis LM. Brain tumors. *N Engl J Med* 2001;344:114–123.

Glantz MJ, Cole BF, Forsyth PA, et al. Practice parameters: anticonvulsant prophylaxis in patients with newly diagnosed brain tumors. *Neurology* 2000;54:1886–1893.

Kaye AH, Laws ER, eds. *Brain tumors: an encyclopedic approach,* 2nd ed. London: Churchill Livingstone, 2001.

Kesari S, Batchelor T, Leptomeningeal metastasis. *Neurol Clin* 2003;21:25–66.

Kleihues P, Cavenee WK, eds. *Pathology and genetics of tumours of the nervous system.* Oxford: Oxford University Press, 2000.

Krouwer HGJ, Widjicks EFM. Neurologic complications of bone marrow transplantation. *Neurol Clin* 2003;21:319–352.

Lassman AB, DeAngelis LM. Brain metastases. *Neurol Clin* 2003;21:1–24.

Levin VA, ed, *Cancer in the nervous system.* New York: Churchill Livingstone, 2002.

Plotkin SR, Wen PY. Neurologic complications of cancer therapy. *Neurol Clin* 2003;21:279–318.

Posner JB, *Neurological complications of cancer: contemporary neurology series no. 45,* Philadelphia: FA Davis, 1995.

Rifenberger G, Louis DN. Oligodendroglioma: toward molecular definitions in diagnostic neuro-oncology. *J Neuropath Exp Neurol* 2003;62:111–126.

Schiff D. Spinal metastases. In: Schiff D, Wen PY, eds. *Cancer neurology in clinical practice.* Totowa, NJ: Humana Press, 2003:93–106.

Schiff D, Wen PY, eds. *Cancer neurology in clinical practice.* Totowa, NJ: Humana Press, 2003.

Wen PY, Marks PW. Medical management of patients with brain tumors. *Curr Opin Oncol* 2002;14:299–307.

7. MULTIPLE SCLEROSIS AND OTHER DEMYELINATING DISEASES

David M. Dawson

MULTIPLE SCLEROSIS

BACKGROUND

1. Multiple sclerosis (MS) is the most common disabling neurologic condition of young adults, at least in European and North American populations. It was first recognized as a disease entity in the latter part of the 19th century. Charcot, in Paris, described the ataxia and oculomotor abnormalities that are often observed in younger patients. The pathologic features at autopsy, described in the first few decades of the 20th century, are now well known.
2. Theories of the cause of MS have reflected concepts that were popular in different eras. Lesions of MS are often found close to small venules, and thrombosis of these veins was at one time thought to be important. Stress is believed by some to play a role, reflecting ideas of the psychosomatic movement of several decades ago. A search for viruses, as intact infective agents or as DNA fragments, has continued for many decades. Authorities now classify MS as an inflammatory autoimmune disease with a strong genetic background, and current research focuses on the deviations of the immune system that must explain its pathophysiology.
3. In most patients, MS is a chronic disease. It begins with a focal inflammatory lesion of the nervous system, developing over days and recovering after months, in 85% of patients. Further lesions develop and cause clinical relapses, usually at a rate of one or two relapses per year. Magnetic resonance imaging (MRI) data have shown us that in actuality lesions occur in the brain and spinal cord at a far more rapid pace, often ten times as frequently as relapses that are clinically recognized. After a number of years, or even decades, most patients enter a slowly progressive phase of the illness, with increasing disability. Impairment of gait, reduced visual acuity, paresthesias and pain, loss of bladder control, and cognitive deficits dominate the clinical picture after the progressive phase has advanced further. In large registries of patients, for example from France and from Denmark, it is found that reduction in life span due to MS is not common, but that most—75% to 80%—of patients are disabled and unable to work by age 65.
4. Other variants of MS occur. About 10% of patients have primary progressive MS (PPMS) (i.e., no relapses are recognized and the patient steadily worsens from the onset). Another 10% have so-called benign MS, with few relapses and no disability even though they have been known to have the disease for many decades. A small number of patients have acute MS, with frequent and large lesions and poor recovery, and it is among this group that a fatal outcome is seen.
5. Most of the data regarding treatment of MS are derived from studies that exclude variant forms of MS and instead use the commoner version of the disease, with relapses followed after time by a secondary progressive phase. Since the variant forms have not been tested, it is often difficult clinically to decide whether a form of treatment is appropriate for an individual patient. Wide variations in the course of the disease make it imperative that carefully designed clinical trials furnish the evidence for treatment.

Epidemiology

1. Onset of MS is typically in the mid 20's, although the diagnosis may be delayed for several years.
2. The ratio of females to males is 1.77 to 1.0.
3. There are zones of high incidence and medium incidence and there are places in the world where the disease is almost unknown.
4. High incidence includes all of Europe, North America, New Zealand, and southern Australia. In these areas, more than 60 persons of 100,000 have MS. In Minnesota and many of the Northeastern states, one person of every 500 has MS.
    a. Race plays a much larger role than does geography. For example, U.S. residents of Japanese or Native American inheritance have a much lower incidence of MS than do their neighbors of European ancestry. A north–south gradient of MS prevalence is discernible, for example in the United States, where the disease is more than twice as common in the northern tier of states than in the south.
    b. However, there are many exceptions. The latitude of Japan is comparable to that of the United States, yet Japanese, even those residing in the United States or Hawaii, are far less likely to develop MS (and if they do, the disease may be quite atypical). MS is common in Italy, including southern Italy and Sicily, while rare in parts of the Middle East of identical latitude.
5. High incidence of MS correlates best with a genetic background that includes ancestry in Scandinavia, the British Isles, Scotland, or the remainder of the European continent. A clinician should be cautious about making a diagnosis of MS in a patient of Southeast Asian, sub-Saharan African, or Native American ancestry.
    a. The incidence of MS in blacks residing in the United States is about 25% that of whites.
    b. The striking data regarding the familial incidence of MS are discussed under Genetics.

PATHOPHYSIOLOGY

1. The typical lesion of MS is a few millimeters to a centimeter in size. Viewed three-dimensionally, a lesion is often ovoid or linear rather than circular. (This is a feature of the MRI appearance.) Activated T cells and macrophages are present. The cells express T helper 1 (T_H1) kinds of cytokines such as interferon gamma (IFN-γ), tumor necrosis factor (TNF), and interleukin-2 (IL-2). B cells are present but seem to play a lesser role, and antibodies, such as antimyelin antibodies, are not of great importance. Cytokines of the T_H2 series such as IL-4, IL-10, and IL-13 are reduced. Many kinds of proinflammatory molecules, such as integrins and other adhesion molecules, are up-regulated.
2. The tissue in which this inflammatory reaction occurs is variably damaged. Myelin is often stripped away and removed by macrophages; nerve fibers may or may not survive. In some patients the destruction of myelin-producing cells (oligodendrocytes) is marked, and the cells seem not to be able to recover and remyelinate. In other patients, many oligodendrocyte precursors can be found, some remyelination occurs, and a lesion may evolve to a "shadow plaque." Chronic lesions with poor recovery have the appearance on biopsy, at autopsy, or on MRI of an empty astroglial scar. The term *multiple sclerosis* refers to these late-stage discolored plaques or scars. Through demyelinated areas, transmission of nerve impulses is blocked and signals fail to arrive at their destination.

Genetics

1. In general in the United States, the prevalence of MS is about 0.1%.
2. If a mother has MS, her children have a 3% to 5% chance of also having MS—at least a 20-fold increase.
3. If a father has MS, his son has a 1% chance, and his daughter a 2% chance, of having MS.
4. A sibling of an affected person has a 3% to 4% chance of having MS. This applies also to nonidentical twins.

5. An identical twin has a 30% chance of having MS—especially if one counts twins with only abnormal MRI or spinal fluid findings.
6. Full-scale genome screens have shown no convincing locus for an "MS gene." It is likely that a number of genes contribute liability by increasing immune reactivity to common viruses or to antigenic components of myelin to which other persons are nonreactive.

DIAGNOSIS

1. Typical relapses come on over a few days, last for weeks or months, and then clear. Over 80% of patients begin with relapses, and the history of these events is vital in arriving at the correct diagnosis. Three typical relapses:
   a. Optic neuritis: Clouding or blurring of central vision in one eye, with loss of measured acuity to 20/50 or less and impaired pupillary response in that eye. Some local pain, made worse by eye movement. Usually full recovery.
   b. Myelopathy: Often sensory only; numbness and tingling from a certain level on the trunk on down through the rest of the body. If marked, some weakness of gait or unsteadiness.
   c. Brainstem attack: Double vision, dizziness, ataxia, facial numbness.
2. Each of these relapses may leave some residual. After several attacks of various types, a patient may present common mid-stage deficits.
   a. Mild reduction in vision in one eye
   b. Nonconjugate eye movements, with diplopia
   c. Extensor plantar responses and inability to walk heel-and-toe
   d. Reduced vibration sense in the legs
   e. Urgency of bladder function
3. Late-stage deficits include dementia, inability to stand or walk, slurred speech, ataxia, incontinence, and marked sensory loss in hands and in legs.

Diagnostic Testing

Magnetic Resonance Imaging

1. MRI is now the dominant laboratory method of diagnosis in MS. MS lesions are usually easily detected and often are characteristic. By scan, the lesions are:
   a. Bright on T_2-weighted and fluid-attenuation inversion recovery (FLAIR) images, indicating a higher than normal water content.
   b. Usually invisible on T_1-weighted images, indicating that the tissue itself is intact.
   c. Fresh lesions—weeks old—will enhance with gadolinium.
   d. Present in many areas of brain, but characteristically found adjacent to the lateral ventricles, in the corpus callosum (best seen on midline sagittal images), and in the connections of the cerebellum. The periventricular lesions actually touch the ventricular wall, because that is where the small veins are—unlike small vascular lesions, which are several millimeters away from the ventricular wall.
   e. Often ovoid or linear in shape.
   f. Size varies—some may be huge, 10 cm or more in diameter. A centimeter or half a centimeter is a common size.
   g. Lesions are common in the spinal cord, especially the cervical cord opposite C-2 or C-3 vertebra. Cord lesions are usually ovoid or linear, small, and do not enhance.
2. About half the patients with MS have scan findings that are *characteristic* of MS. Another 40% or more have visible lesions, but the pattern is nonspecific. Only a few have normal scan findings; such patients present great diagnostic difficulty and repeated scanning and other examinations may be required.
3. The newly published official diagnostic criteria for MS are referred to in the Bibliography (McDonald WI, Compston A, Edan G, et al. Recommended diagnostic criteria for multiple sclerosis: guidelines from the International Panel on the Diagnosis of Multiple Sclerosis. *Ann Neurol* 2001;50:121–127). These criteria delete the terms *possible, probable,* and *definite* MS, and they rely heavily on MRI.

Other Tests

1. Lumbar puncture is needed in some patients with MS. Characteristic findings in the cerebrospinal fluid (CSF) in MS are a modest number of lymphocytes (less than $50/mm^3$), total protein less than 0.8 g/L, elevated immunoglobulin G (IgG) levels, and oligoclonal banding on electrophoresis. The last is the most sensitive of the CSF tests, being present in 75% to 80% of patients with established MS.

2. Evoked potential testing—especially testing of visual potentials—will occasionally help. It is of value mainly in those few patients with normal findings on brain MRI and spinal cord types of deficit.

Differential Diagnosis

Many other neurologic conditions can be confused with MS. They fall into two categories:

1. Diseases that look like MS clinically, including other central nervous system (CNS) inflammatory diseases such as lupus, sarcoidosis, and chronic meningitis, and degenerative processes such as hereditary ataxia, adrenoleukodystrophy, and motor neuron disease.

2. Diseases that look like MS by MRI findings, including other causes of "white spots."

   a. Vascular disease: Small-vessel disease in hypertension, migraine, CADASIL (cerebral autosomal dominant anteriopathy).

   b. Infections: Lyme disease, human immunodeficiency virus (HIV).

   c. Granulomatous disease: Sarcoid, Behçet disease.

   d. Monosymptomatic demyelinating disease: Transverse myelitis and acute disseminated encephalomyelitis (ADEM), in other words multifocal demyelination, often postviral, nonrecurring, and seen mainly in children.

   In some circumstances, these disorders are indistinguishable from MS. They are many hundreds of times less common.

TREATMENT

Treating Symptoms

Depression

Approximately half the patients with MS at some time undergo an episode of clinical depression. Symptoms of irritability, altered sleep pattern, and low self-esteem occur. Women are twice as likely as men to become depressed. There is little correlation with disability, in fact depression may be more common in the earlier stages, with less disability. Some authorities believe there is a causative connection in that some of the frontal lobe and limbic connections may be damaged by MS lesions; this point is hard to prove.

1. Selective serotonin reuptake inhibitors (SSRIs) are the mainstay of treatment of depression: Prozac, Zoloft, Paxil, or second-generation drugs such as Wellbutrin or Celexa (Table 7-1).Care should be taken that the dose is sufficient. Most SSRIs reduce libido.

2. In addition to drug therapy, counseling or some other form of supportive psychotherapy has a proven benefit. Ideal treatment is a combination of the two.

TABLE 7-1. MEDICATIONS FOR DEPRESSION IN MULTIPLE SELEROSIS

Medication	Initial Dose	Final Dose Range
Fluoxetine (Prozac)	10 mg	10–80 mg
Paroxetine (Paxil)	10 mg	10–50 mg
Sertraline (Zoloft)	25 mg	25–200 mg
Citalopram (Celexa)	10 mg	20–60 mg
Venlafaxine (Effexor)	37.5 mg	75–300, given twice a day

3. Tricyclic antidepressants are helpful but have many side effects, such as dry mouth and drowsiness. On the other hand, they may help insomnia or urinary urgency. Examples are amitriptyline 25 to 75 mg/d or nortriptyline 50 to 150 mg/d.
4. Fatigue can be a compounding issue and may be hard to distinguish from depression. Use of an energizing agent such as modafinil or methylphenidate on a trial basis may be helpful (see section on Fatigue).
5. If there is a history of manic disorder, psychiatric consultation is advisable, because bipolar disease requires a separate set of long-term preventive drugs such as lithium carbonate, carbamazepine, or valproate.
6. Depressed patients need to be followed, the success of treatment assessed, and risk of suicide should be considered at all times. In apathetic patients, thyroid deficiency, sleep apnea, and adverse effects of other medications should be considered.

Fatigue

The fatigue of MS, experienced by many patients, is no different from ordinary fatigue—it is inappropriately pervasive and not relieved by rest. Careful planning, avoidance of exhausting exercise, short rest periods, and other coping strategies may help. The following medications are in use:
1. Amantadine (Symmetrel) 100 mg, two or three times a day. This medication has been in use for more than 20 years for MS. About a third of patients find it useful. Hallucinations, ankle swelling, and skin mottling may be seen, especially in older patients.
2. Modafinil (Provigil), 100 or 200 mg twice a day. This agent was approved for producing wakefulness in patients with narcolepsy. Some insurance plans will cover its cost only for this approved use. Data supporting its use for MS fatigue are scant, but promising.
3. Pemoline (Cylert), starting at 18.75 mg/d, up to 37.5 mg twice a day, has some useful effects. Reports of abnormal liver chemistries have limited its use, and it is advisable to check routine chemistries every 3 months.
4. Methylphenidate (Ritalin) 5 to 10 mg/d, up to a maximum of 40 mg/d. A long-acting version (Concerta), at a dose of 18 mg once or twice a day, may be preferable.

Cognitive or Memory Problems

In some patients with MS, the lesions of the central white matter destroy nerve fibers and their coverings. The results of this axon loss are gradual atrophy of the white matter, enlargement of the ventricular system, and behavioral and cognitive deficits. In minor form, this process may be common, and many patients with MS will note memory and recall problems, difficulty handling complex or multiple stimuli, or inability to concentrate well. In a more severe form, emotional lability, poor judgment, and personality change may occur.
1. Structuring of the environment may help: avoidance of complexity, doing "one thing at a time," asking for help.
2. Search for fatigue or depression (see above) may provide a therapeutic option.

Spasticity

1. Several kinds of symptoms are a consequence of an increase in spinal cord reflexes leading to spasticity of the extremities. Walking may become slower and labored, with adduction of the hips and trouble lifting the toes and ankles ("foot drop"). Spontaneous spasms may occur, especially at night, and may be painful; usually these are flexor spasms of both legs. Spasticity is accompanied by varying degrees of weakness and clumsiness.
   a. Physiotherapy and exercise have a limited but important role. Maintenance of joint flexibility by stretching and range of motion can be accomplished by many techniques. Aerobic training may be detrimental.
   b. Baclofen blocks γ-aminobutyric acid (GABA), one of the major spinal cord inhibitory transmitters. The dose varies from 20 to 100 mg/d. Side effects include drowsiness and hypotonicity with reduced reflexes at large doses. The drug has its best effects on flexor spasms and often affects walking speed only slightly.

    c. Tizanidine (Zanaflex) is used for the same indications. Its mode of action is different, and some patients may prefer it. The drug is available as a 4 mg tablet; it must be increased very slowly from a starting dose of 2 mg at bedtime, to a maximum of 16 to 20 mg/d. It can produce drowsiness, but not hypotonicity.

    d. Benzodiazepines, such as clonazepam (Klonopin) 0.5 to 2.0 mg at bedtime, have some usefulness but tachyphylaxis and dependency limit their value.

    e. Dantrolene (Dantrium) is used only rarely because of liver toxicity. However, it has a role for acute spasticity or muscle contracture.

    f. Gabapentin (Neurontin) has been tried at doses of 900 to 1,800 mg/d, but the data supporting its use for spasticity are fragmentary.

2. For severe spasticity, an intrathecal pump system is available, consisting of a subcutaneous programmable reservoir and a tiny catheter into the spinal subarachnoid space, which delivers baclofen. There is good clinical trial evidence supporting the use of these devices, and they have very few complications.

Urinary Urgency

Many patients with MS have impairment of reflex bladder function. The most common pattern is one of a small-capacity bladder, with urgent and involuntary contractions but incomplete emptying. Less commonly, a hypotonic bladder, with difficulty initiating urination and a large postvoiding urinary residual, are found.

1. Oxybutynin (Detrol) may be used empirically. It is effective in patients with hypertonic bladders in whom involuntary contractions and dyssynergy of sphincter function are the main problems. Dosages range from 2.5 mg to 10 to 15 mg/d; a long-acting version may be more convenient. Dry mouth and constipation are encountered at high dose levels. If it is not helpful, it should be stopped.

2. Tolterodine (Detrol) is used in the same manner, and may be substituted for oxybutynin. Dry mouth is less of a problem. Dosage is 2 mg, once or twice a day.

3. Other anticholinergic drugs, including tricyclic antidepressants, are sometimes useful.

4. For severe hypotonicity with retention, and especially with frequent urinary tract infections (UTIs), self-catheterization is indicated. For men, external drainage systems may be used, but they will not empty the bladder well. Referral to a urologist for assessment and training is usually required.

Pain

1. Pain is a common component of MS, particularly in mid-stage disease. Pain may be dull or burning and is often located in a large region, such as an arm, a leg, one side of the body, a bandlike sensation over the trunk, or in the face. Sharp lancinating pain in the face may be identical to idiopathic trigeminal neuralgia.

2. Consideration should always be given to the possibility of non-MS pain, including various forms of nerve root compression, visceral pain, and psychogenic causes including depression. Various medications may be helpful:

    a. Gabapentin (Neurontin) may be used at dosages up to 3,600 mg/d. Beyond that dose level, little further medication is absorbed by active intestinal transport. Some patients are drowsy or lethargic at dosages of 600 to 900 mg/d and are unlikely to achieve much benefit.

    b. Tricyclic antidepressants, such as amitriptyline 50 to 75 mg/d or nortriptyline at 100 to 150 mg/d, are helpful, but dry mouth, urinary retention, and other symptoms due to anticholinergic side effects may occur.

    c. Carbamazepine (Tegretol) at dosages of 400 to 1,000 mg/d is helpful. The long-acting form of the medication is preferable. Other anticonvulsants can be tried as well, including valproate (500–1,500 mg/d) or topiramate (Topamax) (50–150 mg/d).

Alternative or Complementary Medicine

1. In the United States about half the patients with MS are involved in some type of nontraditional treatment in addition to conventional medical therapies. These nontraditional treatments may be classified as follows:

a. Biologically based therapies, such as herbs, diet, bee venom, or bee stings
b. Non-Western medical systems, such as Chinese, Tibetan, or homeopathic approaches
c. Mind–body intervention, including meditation, yoga, and prayer
d. Manipulative or body-based treatments including chiropractic or massage
e. Energy therapies, such as magnets, Reiki, and therapeutic touch
2. Most of these treatments are complementary with standard conventional approaches and can be used with them. A nonconfrontational approach can lessen the risk that patients will abandon or avoid important avenues of treatment. Some of these treatments are helpful, a few may be promising, and most are unproven.

Treatments That Alter the Course of the Disease

1. The six principles of treatment are listed in Table 7-2 and discussed in detail below. Drugs, safety during pregnancy is considered in Table 7-3.
2. Five drugs are now approved for use in patients with MS to affect the course of the disease. Four of them are specifically for relapsing patients and reduce the number of relapses and the activity of the disease as visualized on MRI scans. All four are incomplete treatments in the sense that there continue to be relapses, although at a reduced rate. Three of these four are beta-interferons, and the other is a synthetic polypeptide designed to resemble myelin basic protein.
3. One drug is approved for secondary progressive MS. That drug, mitoxantrone, is a chemotherapy agent administered at relatively low dose.
4. None of the five agents is particularly toxic or difficult to use, although there are side effects. Decisions about which to use and when are not easy and normally will be carried out by a practitioner with some knowledge and experience in the field. Practice patterns are changing rapidly as further data are made available about these agents.
    a. Relapses with significant impairment of function should be treated with high-dose intravenous (IV) corticosteroids.
        1) This principle is based on 30-year-old data, when adrenocorticotropic hormone (ACTH) was the preferred form of steroid therapy, and more recently, on data from the Optic Neuritis Treatment Trial. Disability is shortened, and in some instances the residual from an attack is lessened.
        2) Commonly used protocols now use methylprednisolone 1,000 mg/d administered IV over 1 to 2 hours for 3 to 5 days. Dexamethasone, orally or IV, can also be used. Most authorities do not use an oral taper of prednisone after the IV steroids.

TABLE 7-2. SIX PRINCIPLES OF MANAGEMENT IN MULTIPLE SCLEROSIS

1. Relapses with significant impairment of function should be treated with high-dose intravenous corticosteroids.
2. All relapsing–remitting patients should be receiving long-term immunomodulatory treatment.
3. Secondary progressive patients need aggressive treatment early. Late treatment (more than a few years after the onset of the progressive phase) accomplishes little.
4. Primary progressive patients cannot be expected to respond to any disease-altering treatment.
5. Multiple sclerosis is a lifelong illness, and there is no current paradigm for discontinuation of therapy once started. If one treatment is not tolerated, or fails, another should be sought.
6. Patients need to be watched for signs of disease activity by clinical and/or magnetic resonance imaging monitoring. Changes or additions in treatment need to be started before there is irreversible loss of function.

TABLE 7-3. SAFETY OF MULTIPLE SCLEROSIS DRUGS WHEN USED DURING PREGNANCY

Category B: Animal data show no fetal harm; no human data available
 Glatirimir (Copaxone)
 Pemoline
 Oxybutinin (Ditropan)
 Antidepressants such as SSRIs

Category C: Animal data show fetal harm; no human data available
 Corticosteroids
 Interferon beta Ia
 Interferon beta Ib
 Baclofen
 Amantadine (Symmetrel)
 Tizanidine (Zanaflex)
 Carbemazepine (Tegretol) and other antiepileptic drugs

Category C: Known to cause fetal harm when administered to humans
 Mitoxantrone (Novantrone)
 Cyclophosphamide (Cytoxan)
 Methotrexate

SSRIs, selective serotonin reuptake inhibitors.
From Damke EM, Shuster EA. Pregnancy and multiple sclerosis, *Mayo Clin Proc* 1997;72:977–989, with permission.

   b. All relapsing–remitting patients should be on treatment. This principle is based on data from longitudinal studies of patients followed up clinically and with serial MRI studies. Such studies, mainly from Canada and Britain, have shown the following facts:
     1) Most relapsing patients will eventually develop disability. Put another way, only 10% of MS patients have benign MS.
     2) After a single attack of demyelinating disease, the likelihood of a second attack is accurately predicted by the MRI findings. A patient with optic neuritis and more than two demyelinating lesions on an initial scan has five times the risk of a second neurologic event (thus acquiring a diagnosis of MS) as does a patient with negative scan findings.
     3) While patients with short-lived, limited, or spontaneously clearing attacks have a less severe course, these clinical predictors are highly unreliable in predicting eventual outcome.
     4) Also, while patients with less activity on their MRI scans (as measured by enhancement with gadolinium or increasing numbers of lesions) have a less severe course, these predictors are equally unreliable.
   c. Therefore, since it cannot be known if there are patients who could forgo treatment, the current recommendation is for all to be treated.
 5. Which of the four approved drugs for relapsing MS to use?
   a. The four drugs are known by the abbreviation *ABCR* and by their trade names:
     1) Avonex (IFN-β1a, intramuscular)
     2) Betaseron (IFN-β1b)
     3) Copaxone (glatiramer)
     4) Rebif [IFN-β1a, subcutaneously(s.c.)]
   b. All four of the approved drugs for relapsing MS produce approximately the same 30% reduction in annual attack rate. There is no valid way to choose between them based only on effectiveness. All are available only as injectable drugs.

c. The clinical trials to establish effectiveness have varied in their inclusion criteria, follow-up details, duration of treatment, and other parameters and cannot be easily compared. Only one published trial has been a head-to-head trial; this favored the higher dose IFN (Rebif) over the lower dose (Avonex) measured over a short trial lasting 12 months.

d. Frequency, mode of injection, dose, and side effects vary. Convenient prefilled syringes and automatic injection devices are increasingly available.

e. Some IFN preparations seem to be more likely to produce abnormalities of liver chemistries or have been detected to produce neutralizing anti-IFN antibodies. The higher dose IFNs—Betaseron and Rebif—cause these problems more than does Avonex.

f. Most patients and doctors choose between drugs on the basis of ease of administration and side-effect profile. If side effects from one drug are limiting, a change easily can be made to another.

g. Some details of the choice between the four approved drugs:

   1) Depression can be induced by IFNs, especially by higher dose IFNs. In a depressed patient, Copaxone might be preferred.

   2) Widespread urticaria can occur with Copaxone, either early or late in treatment, and requires discontinuation.

   3) Neutralizing antibodies (NAbs) are more likely to occur with higher dose IFNs. Their presence may be suggested if a patient again begins to have relapses after a period of stability. There is a commercially available test for NAbs but its frequent use is precluded by its high cost and by apparently meaningless variations in antibody levels. In large studies, the group of patients with NAbs had more relapses than the antibody-free patients.

   4) Injection-site reactions can occur with any of the drugs administered s.c. They are most marked with Betaseron. Copaxone may cause areas of dimpling owing to adipose damage.

   5) There appears to be a delay in onset of action of several months with Copaxone. In a patient with a very active scan containing multiple areas of enhancement or in a patient with more than three relapses in the last 6 months, most neurologists would use a high-dose IFN, such as Rebif.

   6) Details of the prescriptions:

   a) Avonex: 30 μg intramuscularly (IM) weekly. Dispensed as a kit for each month, containing medication and syringes.

   b) Betaseron: 250 μg s.c. every other day (q.o.d.). Dispensed as a kit. Usually begun at half-dose to reduce the flu-like symptoms at onset of therapy.

   c) Copaxone: 20 mg s.c. daily. Dispensed as a kit containing prefilled syringes; may be used with or without an auto-injection device.

   d) Rebif: 44 μg s.c. three times a week. Usually begun with a schedule of escalating dose over 1 month. Dispensed as a kit with auto-injection device.

6. Patients with secondary progressive disease need aggressive treatment early. As part of the natural history of most patients with MS, relapses slowly decline in number. In two IFN trials that contained a placebo arm lasting more than 2 years, the relapse rate in the placebo patients declined by about two thirds. (Of course, with successful treatment the relapse rate goes even lower.) The natural history of MS, unfortunately, also is that most relapsing patients will enter the secondary progressive phase of the illness, and disability will steadily increase from that point on. Therefore, at any one time, about half the patients with MS in a given group will be in the secondary progressive phase. It is likely that there has been some change or evolution in the basic pathology in these patients. The change cannot be recognized on MRI scans, except by the fact that atrophy of white matter structures and enlargement of the ventricular system are found as its consequence.

Once disability due to secondary progressive MS is well established and present for more than a few years, it is very unlikely to be reversible. For this reason, if aggressive therapy is decided upon, it should be used relatively early. For a patient who has been wheelchair-dependent for 3 years, it is probably too late.

Treatment for Secondary Progressive Multiple Sclerosis

1. IFNs: A number of trials of IFN-β for secondary progressive MS have been reported. One trial in Europe seemed to show a positive effect, but these patients were having relapses in addition to steady progression, and the major effect seen was on the relapse rate. A trial organized in the United States probably contained fewer patients with "transitional" MS who were still having relapses; it showed no effect of IFN-β on disability. Accumulation of disability due to incomplete recovery from relapses can certainly occur, and this aspect of secondary progressive MS is preventable with IFN therapy.
2. Long-term IV steroids, usually given as a monthly bolus of 1,000 mg of methylprednisolone, are in use in many MS clinics. There has not been an adequate trial of such usage in either relapsing or secondarily progressive MS. A more common usage is to give the steroid as a 3- to 5-day course, administered several times per year when apparent relapses are detected. If steroids are given frequently, bone density needs to be followed and appropriate therapy instituted when osteoporosis occurs.
3. Low-dose oral chemotherapy agents.
   a. Azathioprine has been in use for decades, especially in Europe. Meta-analysis of a large amount of data, typically of dosage ranges of 100 to 200 mg/d, shows a very small positive effect. It is not often used.
   b. Methotrexate has been used in dosages of 7.5 to 20 mg orally once a week. A sensitive assay of hand function in wheelchair patients showed a detectable minor effect of the drug. It is often used as an "add-on" in combination with Copaxone or an IFN. No class I or II data are available to support this usage.
   c. Mycophenolate, in doses typically used for transplantation recipients, has been reported only in pilot studies.
4. IV chemotherapy agents: The rationale behind the use of these agents is that intense nonspecific immunosuppression will arrest the progressive phase of axon and myelin destruction. Two agents are now in widespread use, cyclophosphamide and mitoxantrone. They share the potential problems of infection, marrow failure, or other common difficulties with chemotherapy, and both have a lifetime total dose limitation. This means that even if effective, another strategy has to be available for the time when that limit is reached.
   a. Mitoxantrone, commonly prescribed for myelogenous leukemia, is a member of the anthracenedione group. It inhibits DNA repair and causes crosslinks and scissions in nucleic acids. In patients with MS, it has a striking suppression of enhancement in lesions seen on MRI. Because a 1998 trial of two dose levels of the drug compared with placebo showed a statistically significant effect on disability, mitoxantrone (Novantrone) has been approved by the Food and Drug Administration for use in secondary progressive MS. The drug is given IV once every 3 months at a dose of 12 mg/m^2 to a maximum dose of 140 mg/m^2. The maximum dose is usually reached in about 2 years. It is well tolerated. Cardiac toxicity can occur and must be watched for.
   b. Cyclophosphamide has been in use for nearly 20 years for progressive forms of MS. The drug is an alkylating agent with powerful cytotoxic and immunosuppressive effects. No adequately controlled study has been carried out, although there are extensive class II data. The drug is usually given as a monthly bolus infusion of 800 mg/m^2 or increased from that level to obtain a nadir in total white blood cells (WBCs). Each infusion produces some nausea, anorexia, and modest alopecia. One obvious long-term risk of the drug is that of metaplasia and eventual malignancy of bladder mucosa. Long-term oral cyclophosphamide carries a significant risk of induction of other neoplasms, which has not been observed with the IV bolus program. Ovarian and testicular function are impaired; women in their 30's who are treated commonly enter the menopause.
   c. Both these drugs, if used, should be given by an oncologist or specialist familiar with their use and the potential complications of the treatment. Unfortunately, their records of success are only modest. Even if there is a response, one is

faced with the problem of subsequent therapy after the maximum has been reached.

General Treatment Comments

1. Patients with PPMS cannot be expected to respond to any disease-altering treatment.
    a. PPMS, although certainly demyelinating, may not be the same disease as relapsing or secondarily progressive MS. There is a preponderance of males, the lesions and clinical deficits are often located mainly in the spinal cord, and the lesions seen on MRI scans are often unimpressive. To make a firm diagnosis, additional evidence from evoked potentials testing or CSF examination is often required.
    b. Many observations of the effects of IFNs, Copaxone, chemotherapy agents, and high-dose bolus steroids and the results of a number of clinical trials make it clear that PPMS does not reliably respond to any of these treatments. Symptomatic treatment should be emphasized, and in this arena, some progress can often be made in the individual patient.
2. MS is a lifelong illness and there is no current paradigm for discontinuation of treatment. The entity of benign MS does exist, and in every MS clinic there are patients who have had several relapses years or decades ago, who have no disability, who have MRI scans showing inactive disease, and who do not need any form of treatment. Unfortunately, the current estimates are that 90% of patients with MS are not like that. If a patient is doing well on long-term IFN or Copaxone, the drug needs to be continued without interruption indefinitely. Nearly all of the clinical trials can be criticized for their short duration and for measuring endpoints that are not important. In the end, a significant treatment effect will be seen if the drugs prevent disability.
3. Patients need to be observed for signs of disease activity by clinical and/or MRI monitoring. Since the therapies for relapsing MS are only partially effective, some patients will respond and others will not. It may be a matter of careful judgment to decide if a patient's disease has come under control or not. Patients should be encouraged to report with new symptoms. Periodic examinations should be performed. The role of periodic MRI scanning is less clear. A routine annual MRI scan probably is of little value. During that year, new enhancing lesions may have come and gone. Alternatively, a false impression of major disease activity may be furnished by a scan that happens to detect a small enhancing lesion of little import. Centers with access to frequent MRI scanning have shown that new lesions detected by MRI are about ten times as frequent as clinically detected lesions.
4. When to switch or change?
    a. A patient with little or no disability and no relapses on treatment should remain on treatment even if MRI shows a few enhancing lesions.
    b. A patient with some disability and still working or able to work, but abnormal gait or balance, needs to be watched carefully. In this patient, the risk is of progressive disease. An MRI scan may be beneficial. A scan that reveals enhancement indicates that a change of therapy is needed. A patient beginning to use a cane is one at high risk for further progression.
    c. A patient with major side effects from IFN—persisting flu-like symptoms after injection, depression, or headache—can be switched directly to Copaxone.
    d. A patient with major side effects from Copaxone—urticaria or syncope after injection—can be switched to IFN.
    e. A patient with relapses on Avonex can be switched to high-dose IFN, Betaseron or Rebif.
    f. A patient who has two or three relapses in 6 months or four relapses a year on treatment should be classified as a treatment failure. Alternate or additional therapy must be sought. Consultation or a second opinion is desirable. Neutralizing antibodies may have formed, or the patient may have entered the progressive phase or may simply be a nonresponder. In any case, a change is needed.

BIBLIOGRAPHY

Barkhof F, Filippi M, Miller D, et al. Comparison of MRI criteria at first presentation to predict conversion to clinically definite multiple sclerosis. *Brain* 1997;12:2059–2069.

Beck RW, Cleary PA, Anderson MM, et al. A randomized controlled trial of corticosteroids in the treatment of acute optic neuritis (Optic Neuritis Treatment Trial or ONTT). *N Engl J Med* 1992;326:581–588, and 1993;239:1764–1769.

Brex PA, Ciccarelli O, O'Riordan JI. A longitudinal study of abnormalities on MRI and disability from multiple sclerosis. *N Engl J Med* 2002;346:158–164.

Fazekas F, Deisenhammer F, Strasser-Fuchs S, et al. Randomized placebo-controlled trial of monthly IV immunoglobulin therapy in relapsing-remitting MS *Lancet* 1997;349:589–593.

Goodin DS, Frohman EM, Garmany GP, et al. Disease modifying therapies in MS: Subcommittee of the American Academy of Neurology and the MS Council for Clinical Practice Guidelines. *Neurology* 2002;58:169–178.

Hartung HP, Gonsette RE and the MIMS Study Group. Mitoxantrone in progressive MS: a placebo-controlled, randomized, observer-blind European phase III study, *Mult Scler* 1999;4:325.

Hohol M, Olek MJ, Orav EJ, et al. Treatment of progressive MS with pulse cyclophosphamide/methylprednisolone: response to therapy is linked to the duration of progressive disease. *Mult Scler* 1999:5:403–409.

IFNB Multiple Sclerosis Study Group. Interferon beta 1b is effective in relapsing-remitting multiple sclerosis. *Neurology* 1993;43:655–661.

Jacobs LD, Beck RW, Simon JH, et al. Intramuscular interferon beta-1a therapy initiated during a first demyelinating event in multiple sclerosis (the CHAMPS study Group). *N Engl J Med* 2000;343:898–904.

Johnson KP, Brooks BB, Ford CC, et al. Sustained clinical benefits of glatiramer acetate in relapsing remitting multiple sclerosis patients observed for 6 years. *Mult Scler* 2000;6:255–266.

McDonald WI, Compston A, Edan G, et al. Recommended diagnostic criteria for multiple sclerosis: guidelines from the International Panel on the diagnosis of multiple sclerosis. *Ann Neurol* 2001;50:121–127.

Miller D, et al. Natulizumab in multiple sclerosis. *Mult Scler* 2001;7[Suppl 1]:1.

Noseworth JH, Lucchinetti C, Rodriquez M, et al. Medical progress: multiple sclerosis. *N Engl J Med* 2000;343:938–952.

Panitch HS, Goodin DS, Francis G, et al. The EVIDENCE study. Comparison of Rebif (Serono) vs. Avonex (Biogen) in relapsing-remitting MS. *Neurology* 2002;59:1496–1506.

PRISMS Study Group. Randomised double-blind placebo-controlled study of interferon beta 1a in relapsing/remitting multiple sclerosis [erratum appears in *Lancet* 1999;353:678]. *Lancet* 1998;352:1498–1504.

8. MOTOR NEUROPATHIES AND PERIPHERAL NEUROPATHIES

Anthony A. Amato

SPINAL MUSCULAR ATROPHIES

BACKGROUND

A number of spinal muscular atrophies (SMAs) have been identified on the basis of age of onset, degree of physical impairment, life expectancy, mode of inheritance, and genetic localization.

PATHOPHYSIOLOGY

1. SMA types 1 through 3 are allelic and caused by mutations in the spinal motor neuron gene (*SMN* gene) located on chromosome 5q13.
2. Kennedy disease or X-linked bulbospinal neuronopathy is caused by mutations (expanded CAG repeats) in the androgen receptor gene.

PROGNOSIS

1. There are three major subtypes of autosomal recessive SMA:
   a. SMA type I (SMA-1), commonly known as Werdnig–Hoffmann disease, manifests within the first 6 months of life and most affected children do not survive past the second year of life.
   b. SMA type II (SMA-2), the chronic infantile subtype, presents between the ages of 6 and 18 months and is associated with survival into the second or third decade.
   c. SMA type III (SMA-3), more frequently referred to as Kugelberg–Welander disease, manifests after the age of 18 months and can be associated with a normal life expectancy.
2. Kennedy disease is another progressive form of SMA that may present in early or adult life (dependent on size of the mutation).

DIAGNOSIS

Clinical Features

1. The age of onset and severity of weakness is variable in the different forms of SMA.
2. Most are characterized by generalized, symmetric proximal greater than distal weakness and atrophy, although there are rare forms associated with mainly distal extremity weakness.
3. Fasciculations are often evident in extremity and bulbar muscles.
4. Sensation is normal and deep tendon reflexes are reduced or absent.
5. Oral pharyngeal weakness leads to dysphagia and aspiration pneumonia.
6. Death is often due to respiratory failure related to diaphragmatic weakness.

Electrodiagnostic Features

1. Sensory nerve conduction studies (NCSs) are usually normal except in Kennedy disease in which the sensory nerve action potential (SNAP) amplitudes are reduced secondary to an associated sensory neuronopathy.

2. Motor NCS are normal or reveal diminished compound muscle action potential (CMAP) amplitudes.
3. Electromyography (EMG) reveals increased insertional and spontaneous activity in the form of fibrillation potentials, positive sharp waves, and fasciculation potentials as well as large, polyphasic fast-firing motor unit action potentials (MUAPs) (i.e., decreased recruitment).

Laboratory Features

1. Serum creatine kinase (CK) levels are normal or slightly increased.
2. DNA testing is available for the most common forms (SMA types. I–III, Kennedy disease).

TREATMENT

1. There is no proven medical therapy to improve strength and function in patients with different forms of SMA.
2. Major treatment is supportive therapies.
3. Physical and occupational therapy are key. Contractures develop in weak limbs and thus stretching exercises, particularly at the heal cords, iliotibial bands, and at the hips, must be started early.
4. Bracing:
   a. The appropriate use of bracing assist the child with SMA-2 and SMA-3 in ambulation or delay wheelchair dependence
   b. Long-leg braces (knee–foot orthosis) may stabilize the knees and prevent the knees from buckling.
   c. There may be some advantage to a lightweight, plastic knee-foot orthosis, but it is difficult to keep the foot straight with such a device, whereas the high-top boot worn with the double-upright brace provides excellent stability. The choice between plastic and metal often comes down to personal preference of the patient and physician.
   d. Night splints are used to maintain the feet at right angles to the leg to prevent ankle contractures, which will impair ambulation,
5. Surgery:
   a. Reconstructive surgery of the legs often accompanies bracing to keep the legs extended and prevent contractures of the iliotibial bands, hip and knee flexors, and ankle dorsiflexors.
   b. A simple way to maintain function in the legs with contractures in the iliotibial bands, hip flexors, and knee flexors is to perform percutaneous tenotomies of the Achilles tendons, knee flexors, hip flexors, and iliotibial bands. This procedure often allows a child who is becoming increasingly dependent on a wheelchair to resume walking.
   c. Scoliosis may develop, leading to pain, aesthetic damage, and perhaps respiratory compromise. Consider spinal fusion in children with 35-degree scoliosis or more and who are in significant discomfort. Ideally, forced vital capacity (FVC) should be greater than 35% to minimize the risk of surgery.
6. Respiratory failure:
   a. Respiratory muscle weakness may initially be managed by noninvasive methods (i.e., BiPAP). Consider bilevel positive airway pressure (BiPAP) in patients with dyspnea or evidence of nocturnal hypopnea (e.g., frequent nocturnal arousals, morning headaches, excessive daytime sleepiness), particularly if FVC is less than 50% of predicted.
   b. Tracheostomy and mechanical ventilation should be discussed with patient and families and offered if it is their wish.
7. Genetic Counseling:
   a. It is imperative to instruct parents of children with SMA-1, -2, and -3 that they have a 25% chance that any future children could have the disease.
   b. Kennedy disease is X-linked recessive, therefore their male children will not be affected but the female children will be obligate carriers.
   c. Prenatal diagnosis is available.

HEREDITARY SPASTIC PARAPLEGIA

BACKGROUND

1. The hereditary spastic paraplegias (SPGs) are a clinically and heterogeneous group of disorders characterized by progressive lower limb spasticity.
2. This group of disorders is subclassified by the pattern of inheritance, age of onset, and the presence of additional neurologic defects.
3. The prevalence of SPG ranges from 2.0 to 4.3/100,000.

PATHOPHYSIOLOGY

1. SPG may be inherited in an autosomal dominant, autosomal recessive, or X-linked nature.
2. Autosomal dominant inheritance accounts for approximately 70% of pure SPG. Most of these autosomal dominant families are linked to mutations in the spastin gene located on chromosome 2p22-p21.
3. Autosomal recessive SPG7 has been linked to mutations in the gene encoding for paraplegin.
4. X-linked SPG1 is caused by mutations in the gene encoding for the L1 cell adhesion molecule (L1CAM).
5. X-linked form of SGP2 is caused by mutations in the proteolipid protein gene.

PROGNOSIS

The disease is usually only slowly progressive and life expectancy is not affected in "pure" forms but may be reduced in "complicated" forms (see Clinical Features, below).

DIAGNOSIS

Clinical Features

1. Patients may be classified into "pure spastic paraplegia," if there is only spasticity and sensory involvement and "complicated spastic paraplegia," if there is associated optic atrophy, deafness, extrapyramidal disease, dementia, ataxia, peripheral neuropathy, or amyotrophy.
2. Onset is variable: childhood to adult life.
3. There is significant clinical and genetic heterogeneity between and within kinships with SPG.

Laboratory Features

1. Cerebrospinal fluid (CSF) is usually normal, although increased protein is noted in some patients.
2. Magnetic resonance imaging (MRI) scans may demonstrate atrophy of the spinal cords and occasionally the cerebra cortex.
3. Genetic testing is available for some forms of SPG.

TREATMENT

1. There are no specific medications to slow the progression of the disease.
2. Treatment is supportive with physical and occupational therapy.
3. Stretching exercises are important to prevent contractures.
4. Braces and or walkers may be necessary to stabilize the gait.
5. Spasticity:

     a. Baclofen 5 mg by mouth (p.o.) three times a day (t.i.d.) to start. May increase up to 80 mg daily [20 mg four times a day (q.i.d.)] as tolerated and as needed.

     b. Tizanidine 2 mg t.i.d. to start. May increase up to 12 mg t.i.d. as tolerated and as needed.

     c. Diazepam 2 mg twice a day (b.i.d.). May increase up to 10 mg q.i.d. as tolerated and as needed.

AMYOTROPHIC LATERAL SCLEROSIS

BACKGROUND

1. Motor neuron disease is often divided into four different clinical syndromes that may represent the spectrum of the same disease process:
   a. Primary muscular atrophy [anterior horn cell loss with no upper motor neuron (UMN) involvement]
   b. Adult-onset progressive bulbar palsy (preferential degeneration of bulbar nuclei not associated with significant spinal anterior horn cell dysfunction or upper motor neuron signs)
   c. Primary lateral sclerosis [corticospinal tract involvement sparing the lower motor neurons (LMNs)]
   d. Amyotrophic lateral sclerosis (ALS) (a variable combination of all of the preceding abnormalities; i.e., both UMN and LMN signs affecting both the bulbar and somatic musculature).
2. Progressive muscular atrophy (PMA) accounts for roughly 10% and primary lateral sclerosis (PLS) makes up at most only 1% to 3% of motor neuron disease cases. Progressive bulbar palsy accounts for approximating 1% to 2% of motor neuron disease.
3. ALS has an incidence of 0.4 to 3.0/100,000 and a prevalence of 4 to 6 cases/100,000.

PATHOPHYSIOLOGY

1. Most cases of ALS are sporadic, but as many as 10% of cases are inherited, so-called familial ALS (FALS). Approximately 25% of cases of FALS are caused by mutations in the gene encoding copper/zinc (Cu/Zn) superoxide dismutase (*SOD1*).
2. The pathogenic basis of sporadic ALS is unclear.

PROGNOSIS

1. The sporadic ALS and FALS forms of ALS are clinically and pathologically similar.
2. The course of ALS is relentless with a linear decline in strength with time. The median survival is approximately 3 years.

DIAGNOSIS

Clinical Features

1. Many patients exhibit only LMN signs or purely UMN signs early in the course of the disease.
2. In the limbs, muscle weakness and atrophy usually begin asymmetrically and distally and then spread within the neuroaxis to involve contiguous groups of motor neurons.
3. Bulbar involvement manifests initially as dysphagia or dysarthria.

4. El Escorial criteria for the diagnosis of ALS:

    a. A clinical diagnosis of "definite ALS" requires the presence of UMN and LMN signs in the bulbar region as well as at least two of the three other spinal regions (i.e., cervical, thoracic, and lumbosacral).

    b. "Probable ALS" is defined by the presence of UMN and LMN signs in at least two regions (some UMN signs must be rostral to the LMN deficits).

    c. "Possible ALS" requires UMN and LMN signs in only one region, UMN signs alone in two or more regions, or LMN signs are rostral to the UMN signs.

    d. Electrophysiologic criteria for definite LMN degeneration require: (a) the presence of fibrillation potentials; (b) large-amplitude, long-duration MUAPs; and (c) reduced recruitment. EMG evidence of LMN degeneration in two muscles supplied by two different nerve roots and nerves in an extremity can substitute for clinical evidence of LMN loss in the extremity. Fulfilling the El Escorial criteria for definite or even probable ALS can be difficult even for patients with advanced disease.

Electrodiagnostic Features

1. Sensory NCS results are normal.

2. Motor NCS results may be normal or demonstrate reduced amplitudes secondary to atrophy. Distal latencies and conduction velocities are normal or reveal only slight slowing proportional to the degree of axonal loss.

3. No evidence of conduction block or other features of primary demyelination.

4. EMG demonstrates evidence of active denervation in the form of fibrillation potentials and positive sharp waves as noted above. The earliest abnormality is fasciculation potentials due to motor unit hyperexcitability/instability that occur prior to motor unit degeneration.

TREATMENT

1. Riluzole:

    a. Two controlled trials have demonstrated that riluzole 50 mg p.o. b.i.d. extends tracheostomy-free survival by 2 to 3 months. Unfortunately, the studies did not find that riluzole improves strength or the quality of life.

    b. Riluzole is thought to act by inhibiting the release of glutamate at presynaptic terminals.

    c. Side effects include nausea, abdominal discomfort, and hepatotoxicity.

    d. Check hepatic function tests every month for 3 months and then every 3 months while on riluzole. Hepatotoxicity is reversible once riluzole is discontinued.

2. Supportive care:

    a. Despite that the lack of effective therapy to halt or reverse the progression of the disease, there are many therapeutic measures that improve the quality of life in patients with ALS.

    b. A multimodality approach in treating patients with ALS is essential.

    c. Patients are seen in clinic at least every 3 months in conjunction with physical, occupational, speech, and respiratory therapy.

    d. They are also evaluated by psychiatry, gastroenterology, pulmonary medicine, and social workers as necessary.

3. Physical therapy:

    a. Stretching exercises, passive and active, to prevent contractures.

    b. Assess gait and needs (i.e., cane, walker, wheelchair).

4. Occupational therapy:

    a. Patients should be evaluated for adaptive devices (e.g., ball-bearing feeders) that may improve function.

    b. The patient's home should be evaluated for equipment needs.

5. Dysarthria:

    a. Patients should be evaluated by a speech therapist.

    b. Techniques may be given to help patient with articulation.

    c. Patients may benefit from various speech augmentation devices and switch- or light-guided scanning computerized devices.
  6. Dysphagia:
    a. Because of the associated swallowing difficulties occurring with bulbar weakness, nutrition becomes impaired.
    b. High-calorie and protein-concentrated supplementation should be added to diet.
    c. When dysphagia is severe, a percutaneous endoscopy gastrostomy (PEG) is recommended. Some studies have demonstrated that nutrition by PEG or gastrojejunostomy improves quality of life and survival by a few months.
        1) Ideally, PEG placement should be done before FVC falls below 50% to reduce the risks of the surgical procedure.
        2) PEG placement does not prevent aspiration.
  7. Salivation:
    a. Drooling and hypersalivation can be a problem secondary to swallowing difficulties.
    b. TCAs [e.g., amitriptyline 10–100 mg p.o. at bed time (qhs)] have anticholinergic properties that can reduce secretions. In addition, patients not uncommonly have a reactive depression that may be helped by the addition of an antidepressant.
    c. Other medications that can be used include:
        1) Glycopyrrolate 1 to 2 mg p.o. b.i.d. to t.i.d.
        2) Benztropine 0.5 to 2.0 mg every day (qd)
        3) Trihexyphenidyl hydrochloride 1 mg qd to 5 mg t.i.d.
        4) Atropine 2.5 mg qd to 5 mg t.i.d.
  8. Thick mucus production:
    a. Some patients describe thick mucus, particularly when using the above medications to treat hypersalivation.
    b. Beta-blockers such as propranolol and metoprolol may help.
    c. Acetylcysteine 400 to 600 mg p.o. qd in one to three divided doses or as a nebulizer treatment (3–5 mL of 20% solution every 3–5 hours).
  9. Spasticity:
    a. Baclofen 5 mg p.o. t.i.d. to start. May increase up to 80 mg qd (20 mg q.i.d.) as tolerated and as needed.
    b. Tizanidine 2 mg t.i.d. to start. May increase up to 12 mg t.i.d. as tolerated and as needed.
    c. Diazepam 2 mg b.i.d. May increase up to 10 mg q.i.d. as tolerated and as needed.
 10. Pseudobulbar affect:
    a. An antidepressant medication can be used, particularly in patients with underlying depression.
    b. Amitryptiline 10 to 25 mg qhs increasing to 100 mg qhs as necessary.
 11. Constipation
    a. Constipation may result from weakness of the pelvic and abdominal muscles, diminished physical activity, anticholinergic and antispasticity medications, and opioids.
    b. Management includes increasing dietary fiber and fluid intake, adding bulk-forming laxatives, and using suppositories or enemas as needed.
 12. Ventilatory failure:
    a. Most patients with ALS die as a result of respiratory failure; therefore, it is important to assess for symptoms of signs of respiratory impairment during each clinic visit.
    b. Patients with forced vital capacities below 50% or those with symptomatic respiratory dysfunction are offered noninvasive ventilator support, usually BiPAP.
    c. Inspiratory and expiratory pressures are titrated to symptom relief and patient tolerability.
    d. In my experience, only a few patients desire tracheostomy and mechanical ventilation, because it prolongs expensive and often burdensome care for the

family. However, this is an individual decision that must be made by the patient. Tracheostomy needs to be offered to patients along with realistic counseling in regard to what this entails to the patient and the family.

   e. Intermittent dyspnea and the anxiety that accompanies it may be treated with lorazepam 0.5 to 2 mg sublingually, opiates (e.g., morphine 5 mg), or midazolam 5 to 10 mg intravenous (IV) (slowly) for severe dyspnea.

   f. Constant dyspnea can be managed with morphine starting at 2.5 mg q4h or continuous morphine infusion plus diazepam, lorazepam, or midazolam for associated anxiety.

   g. Thorazine 25 mg every 4 to 12 hours rectally or 12.5 mg every 4 to 12 hours IV should be considered for terminal restlessness.

13. Pain:

   a. Pain occurs in at least 50% of patients due to muscle cramps, spasticity, limited range of motion and contractures related to weakness, and skin pressure secondary to limited movement.

   b. Careful positioning and repositioning of the patient, physical therapy to help prevent contractures, antispasticity medications, antidepressants, nonsteroidal antiinflammatory medications, and opioids may be used to treat pain.

14. Psychosocial issues:

   a. Depression is not uncommon for patients and family members.

   b. Patients and family members may benefit from local support groups.

   c. Antidepressant medications.

ACUTE POLIOMYELITIS

BACKGROUND

1. Poliomyelitis is very uncommon in industrialized nations due to routine use of the polio vaccine.

2. However, not everyone is vaccinated, plus a poliomyelitis-like illness can be seen with other viruses (e.g., Coxsackie virus, West Nile virus).

PATHOPHYSIOLOGY

1. The virus gains access to the host usually through oral or respiratory route. The virus proliferates and viremia ensues.

2. The virus is taken up into the peripheral nervous system via binding to receptors and the distal motor nerve terminals.

3. Subsequent transport to the anterior horn cell in the spine occurs with degeneration of motor neurons.

PROGNOSIS

The degree of recovery is variable. Some patients develop weakness and achiness in muscles previously affected (postpolio syndrome, see below).

DIAGNOSIS

Clinical Features

1. Most people (98%), especially children, experience a minor nonspecific systemic illness for 1 to 4 days: sore throat, vomiting, abdominal pain, low-grade fever, easy fatigue, and minor headache.

2. A small percentage (2%) of individuals develop neck and back stiffness, fasciculations, and asymmetric weakness involving the extremities and/or bulbar musculature.
3. Following the initial illness and paralysis, recovery of function to varying degrees
   occurs over the ensuing 4 to 8 years.

Laboratory Features

1. CSF examination usually reveals increased protein and pleocytosis initially consisting of both polymorphonuclear leukocytes and lymphocytes and then later predominantly lymphocytes. The cell count is usually less than 100 cells/mm^3.
2. Diagnosis may be confirmed by culture of the offending virus, although
   the sensitivity is low. Also acute and convalescent antibody titers can be
   obtained.

Electrophysiologic Findings

1. Sensory NCSs are normal.
2. CMAP amplitudes may be reduced in patients with profound muscle atrophy.
3. The motor conduction velocities and distal latencies are normal or slightly abnormal in those individuals consistent with the degree of large fiber loss.
4. EMG demonstrates reduced recruitment of MUAP early with positive sharp
   waves and fibrillation potentials within 2 to 3 weeks following the onset of
   paralysis.

TREATMENT

1. There is no specific treatment other than supportive care.
2. Respiratory status needs to be monitored closely and patient mechanically venti-
   lated if necessary.
3. Nutritional support if patient is unable eat on his or her own.
4. Physical and occupation therapy are essential to improve function.
5. An antiepileptic medication (e.g., neurontin) or antidepressant medication
   can be used to treat associated pain that frequently accompanies the acute
   illness.

POSTPOLIOMYELITIS SYNDROME

BACKGROUND

As many as 25% to 60% of patients with a history of poliomyelitis infection develop subsequent neuromuscular symptoms 20 or 30 years after the initial acute
attack

PATHOPHYSIOLOGY

It is thought that motor neurons unaffected by the poliomyelitis sprout to reinnervate
previously denervated muscle fibers. These motor units that are increased in size
may be under increased stress compared with normal motor units, leading to gradual
degeneration over time in some.

PROGNOSIS

The course and the symptoms are highly variable but as a rule, actual muscle weakness is slowly progressive, if at all.

DIAGNOSIS

Clinical Features

1. Patients with postpolio syndrome complain of progressive fatigue (80%–90%), multiple joint pains (70%–87%), and muscle pain (70%–85%).
2. Fifty percent to 80% of patients also develop progressive loss of strength and muscle atrophy. This progressive weakness usually involves previously affected muscles but muscles thought to be clinically spared at the time of the acute infection may at times become affected.
3. Muscle cramps and fasciculations are also commonly noted.

Laboratory Features

1. Unlike acute poliomyelitis, the CSF does not demonstrate pleocytosis or viral particles.
2. Serum CK levels may be mildly elevated.

Electrophysiologic Findings

1. Sensory NCSs are normal.
2. CMAP amplitudes may be reduced in patients with profound muscle atrophy.
3. The motor conduction velocities and distal latencies are normal or only slightly abnormal proportionate to the degree of large fiber loss.
4. EMG demonstrates active denervation in the form of positive sharp waves and fibrillation potentials, fasciculation potentials, and reduced recruitment of long-duration, large-amplitude, polyphasic, unstable MUAPs.

TREATMENT

1. There are no specific therapies for postpolio syndrome.
2. Treatment is supportive similar to that for other motor neuron disorders.
3. Physical and occupational therapy can be beneficial.
4. A recent double-blind, placebo-controlled trial demonstrated no benefit with pyridostigmine.
5. Muscle pain may ease with TCA medications.
6. Severe dysphagia, dysarthria, and respiratory weakness are treated as discussed in the ALS section.

STIFF PERSON/STIFF LIMB SYNDROME

BACKGROUND

1. Moersh and Woltman were the first to describe 14 patients with the disorder, which they termed "stiff man syndrome."
2. Because the disorder is more common in women than in men, stiff person syndrome (SPS) has become the preferable name for the disorder.

3. Some authorities have clinically subdivided SPS into three subdivisions:
   a. Progressive encephalomyelitis with rigidity,
   b. Typical SPS, and
   c. Stiff limb syndrome.
4. There is an increased incidence of insulin-dependent diabetes mellitus (IDDM) and various autoimmune disorders.
5. There are reports of SPS associated with Hodgkin lymphoma, small cell carcinoma of the lung, and cancers of the colon and breast.
6. SPS also can occur in patients with myasthenia gravis or thymoma.

PATHOPHYSIOLOGY

SPS is an autoimmune disorder caused by antibodies directed against glutamic acid decarboxylase (GAD) and amphiphysin.

PROGNOSIS

Patients develop progressive stiffness and rigidity of the trunk and spine. Immunomodulating therapies may help somewhat, but most patients still have significant disability.

DIAGNOSIS

Clinical Features

1. Progressive encephalomyelitis with rigidity is a rapidly progressive disorder associated with generalized stiffness, encephalopathy, myoclonus, and respiratory distress that is usually fatal within 6 to 16 weeks.
2. Typical SPS:
   a. Characterized by muscular rigidity and episodic spasms involving truncal and limb muscles in the second to sixth decades of life.
   b. Superimposed "attacks" of intense muscle spasms or contractions.
   c. The stiffness and muscles spasms usually lead to gait impairment with occasional falls.
   d. Patients may complain of dyspnea secondary to chest restriction due to stiffness in the thoracic muscles.
   e. Paroxysmal autonomic dysfunction characterized by transient hyperpyrexia, diaphoresis, tachypnea, tachycardia, hypertension, pupillary dilation, and occasional sudden death may accompany the attacks of muscle spasm.
   f. Approximately 10% of patients also have generalized seizures or myoclonus.
   g. Physical examination is remarkable for exaggerated lumber lordosis and paraspinal muscle hypertrophy secondary to continuous paraspinal muscle contraction.
3. Stiff limb syndrome is characterized by asymmetric rigidity and spasms in the distal extremities or face.

Laboratory Features

1. Autoantibodies directed against the 64-kD GAD are evident in 60% of primary autoimmune cases of SPS.
2. Antibodies are directed against a 128-kD presynaptic protein, amphiphysin, are present in some patients with presumed paraneoplastic SPS.
3. The CSF is often abnormal in patients with SPS demonstrating increased immunoglobulin G (IgG) synthesis, oligoclonal bands, and anti-GAD antibodies.
4. Other autoantibodies and laboratory abnormalities associated with concomitant autoimmune disorders [e.g., Hashimoto thyroiditis, pernicious anemia,

hypoparathyroidism, adrenal failure, myasthenia gravis, systemic lupus erythematosus (SLE), rheumatoid arthritis].
5. Serum CK levels may be slightly elevated.

Electrophysiologic Findings

1. Sensory and motor conduction studies are normal.
2. EMG demonstrates normal-appearing MUAPs firing continuously.

TREATMENT

1. Symptomatic therapies:
   a. I usually initiate symptomatic treatment with diazepam 2 mg b.i.d. working up to a dosage of 5 to 20 mg three to four times a day.
   b. Next I start oral baclofen 5 mg t.i.d. which is increased up to 20 mg q.i.d.
   c. Intrathecal baclofen 300 to 800 μg/d may be tried if other agents are not tolerated or are unsuccessful.
   d. Other symptomatic agents with purported benefit include: clonazepam, dantrium, methocarbamol, valproate, vigabatrin, gabapentin, and botulinum toxin injection.
2. Various forms of immunotherapy may be tried to treat the underlying autoimmune basis and have been found to be beneficial in small trials.
   a. I usually give a treatment trial of intravenous immunoglobulin (IVIG) 2 g/kg monthly for 3 months and, if this is effective, subsequently spread out the dosing interval or reduce the dosage tailored to patient responsiveness.
   b. Plasma exchange can also be performed but needs to be repeated (as does IVIG) and thus is not curative.
   c. A trial of prednisone 0.75 to 1.5 mg/kg/d for 2 weeks, then 0.75 to 1.5 mg/kg ever other day for 2 to 4 months is tried if IVIG is ineffective. If prednisone is beneficial, I taper the prednisone to the lowest dose that controls the symptoms. I do not use prednisone in patients with diabetes mellitus (DM).
   d. Other immunosuppressive agents (e.g., azathioprine, mycophenolate mofetil; Table 8-1) may be tried singly or in combination with prednisone as a steroid-sparing agent.

TETANUS

BACKGROUND

1. Tetanus is a very serious and potentially life threatening medical condition arising from the *in vivo* production of a neurotoxin from the bacterium *Clostridium tetani*.
2. *C. tetani* produce tetanospasmin.
3. It is estimated that more than 1 million people per year demonstrate signs of clinical intoxication secondary to infections with *C. tetani*. About 150 cases of tetanus are noted each year in the United States by various governmental agencies.

PATHOPHYSIOLOGY

1. The bacteria or their spores gain access to the patient typically through a minor wound.
2. In the central nervous system (CNS), tetanus toxin lyses the SNARE proteins necessary for the release of inhibitory neurotransmitters [glycine and γ-aminobutyric acid (GABA)].

TABLE 8-1. IMMUNOSUPPRESSIVE / IMMUNOMODULATORY THERAPIES COMMONLY USED IN NEUROMUSCULAR DISORDERS

Therapy	Route	Dose	Side Effects	Monitor
Prednisone	p.o.	100 mg/d for 2–4 wk, then 100 mg every other day; single a.m. dose	Hypertension, fluid and weight gain, hyperglycemia, hypokalemia, cataracts, gastric irritation, osteoporosis, infection, aseptic femoral necrosis	Weight, blood pressure, serum glucose/potassium, cataract formation
Methylprednisolone	IV	1 g in 100 mL/normal saline over 1–2 h daily or every other day for 3–6 doses	Arrhythmia, flushing, dysgeusia, anxiety, insomnia, fluid and weight gain, hyperglycemia, hypokalemia, infection	Heart rate, blood pressure, serum glucose/potassium
Azathioprine	p.o.	2–3 mg/kg/d single a.m. dose	Flu-like illness, hepatotoxicity, pancreatitis, leukopenia, macrocytosis, neoplasia, infection, teratogenicity	Monthly CBC, liver enzymes
Methotrexate	p.o.	7.5–20 mg/wk; single or divided doses; 1 d/wk dosing	Hepatotoxicity, pulmonary fibrosis, infection, neoplasia, infertility, leukopenia, alopecia, gastric irritation, stomatitis, teratogenicity	Monthly liver enzymes, CBC; consider liver biopsy at 2 g accumulative dose
Cyclophosphamide	IV/IM	20–50 mg weekly; 1 d/wk dosing	Same as p.o.	Same as p.o.
	p.o.	1.5–2 mg/kg/d; single a.m. dose	Bone marrow suppression, infertility, hemorrhagic cystitis, alopecia, infections, neoplasia, teratogenicity	Monthly CBC, urinalysis
Chlorambucil	IV	1 g/m²	Same as p.o. (although more severe), and nausea/vomiting, alopecia	Daily to weekly CBC, urinalysis
	p.o.	4–6 mg/d single a.m. dose	Bone marrow suppression, hepatotoxicity, neoplasia, infertility, teratogenicity, infection	Monthly CBC, liver enzymes
Cyclosporine	p.o.	4–6 mg/kg/d split into two daily doses	Nephrotoxicity, hypertension, infection, hepatotoxicity, hirsutism, tremor, gum hyperplasia, teratogenicity	Blood pressure, monthly cyclosporine level, creatinine/BUN, liver enzymes
Mycophenolate mofetil	p.o.	Adults (1 g b.i.d. to 1.5 g b.i.d. Children (600 mg/m²/ dose b.i.d. (no more than 1 g/d in patients with renal failure)	Bone marrow suppression, hypertension, tremor, diarrhea, nausea, vomiting, headache, sinusitis, confusion, amblyopia, cough, teratogenicity, infection, neoplasia	CBCs are performed weekly for 1 mo, twice monthly for the second and third month, and then once a month for the first year
Intravenous Immunoglobulin	IV	2 g/kg over 2–5 d; then every 4–8 wk as needed	Hypotension, arrhythmia, diaphoresis, flushing, nephrotoxicity, headache, aseptic meningitis, anaphylaxis, stroke	Heart rate, blood pressure, creatinine/BUN

p.o., by mouth; IV, intravenous; IM, intramuscular; b.i.d., twice a day; CBC, complete blood count; BUN, blood urea nitrogen.
Modified from Amato AA, Barohn RJ. Idiopathic inflammatory myopathies. *Neurol Clin* 1997;15:615–648, with permission.

3. The result is hyperexcitability of motor neurons leading to continuous motor unit firing, opisthotonus, and hyperreflexia.

PROGNOSIS

1. The annual mortality rate due to this organism is variable depending upon the sophistication of emergent health care delivery and immunizations.
2. In Africa, the annual mortality rate is estimated at 28/100,000, while in Asia and Europe it is 15/100,000 and 0.5/100,00, respectively.
3. In the United States, the mortality due to tetanus intoxication is less than 0.1/100,000.
4. Worldwide, neonatal tetanus represents about 50% of the known cases with a mortality rate reaching 90%.

DIAGNOSIS

1. The clinical presentation of tetanus is subdivided into four major categories:
   a. Local,
   b. Generalized,
   c. Cephalic, and
   d. Neonatal.
2. Most patients complain of a feeling of increased "tightness" of the muscles about the wound in the affected extremity. Pain may also be noted.
3. Both the pain and muscle stiffness can persist for months and remain localized with an eventual spontaneous dissipation.
4. Some patients develop trismus (difficulty opening the mouth secondary to masseter muscle contraction).
5. Progression to generalized tetanus with tonic contraction of either entire limbs or the whole body secondary to relatively mild noxious stimuli. The generalized whole-body muscle contraction, opisthitonus, consists of extreme spine extension, flexion and adduction of the arms, fist clenching, facial grimacing, and extension of the lower extremities. This generalized contraction may impair breathing.
6. Neonatal tetanus is usually the result of an infected umbilical stump.
   a. Several hours to days of feeding difficulty (poor suck), general irritability, and possibly less than normal mouth opening or generalized "stiffness."
   b. Infants born to immunized mothers rarely have any difficulty with tetanus as the immunity is passively transferred from mother to infant. Once the massive whole-body contractions start, there is little doubt as to the diagnosis.

TREATMENT

1. Patients with suspected tetanus intoxication should be hospitalized immediately and evaluated for existent or impending airway compromise.
2. Human tetanus immunoglobulin should be administered as well as adsorbed tetanus toxoid at a different site.
3. The antibiotic of choice is metronidazole (500 mg IV every 6 hours for 7–10 days).
4. If airway compromise is noted, there is a good chance that this situation will persist for some time and a tracheotomy should be considered.
5. Benzodiazepines should be administered in rather large dosages to control muscle contractions. If this is ineffective, therapeutic neuromuscular blockade is warranted in addition to the benzodiazepines to maintain somnolence.
6. If autonomic symptoms or signs develop, these should be treated immediately with appropriate medications.
7. Physical and occupational therapy are usually needed during the recovery period to regain strength, endurance, and function.

GUILLAIN–BARRÉ SYNDROME AND RELATED NEUROPATHIES

BACKGROUND

1. There are three major subtypes of Guillain–Barré syndrome (GBS): acute inflammatory demyelinating polyradiculoneuropathy (AIDP), acute motor-sensory axonal neuropathy (AMSAN), and acute motor axonal neuropathy (AMAN).
2. The Miller–Fisher syndrome (ataxia, areflexia, and ophthalmoplegia) may share similar pathogenesis and can be considered a variant of GBS.
3. There is serologic evidence of recent infections with *Campylobacter jejuni* (32%), cytomegalovirus (CMV) (13%), Epstein–Barr virus (EBV) (10%), and *Mycoplasma pneumoniae* (5%).

PATHOPHYSIOLOGY

1. Molecular similarity between the myelin epitope(s) and glycolipids expressed on *Campylobacter, Mycoplasma,* and other infectious agents, which precede attacks of GBS, may be the underlying trigger for the immune attack.
2. Antibodies directed against these infectious agents may cross-react with specific antigens on Schwann cells or the axolemma.
3. Binding of these antibodies to target antigens on the peripheral nerve initially lead to conduction block.
4. In AIDP, demyelination ensues and in AMSAN and AMAN axonal degeneration occurs.

PROGNOSIS

1. The disease progression is usually over the course of 2 to 4 weeks. At least 50% of patients reach their nadir by 2 weeks, 80% by 3 weeks, and 90% by 4 weeks.
2. Progression of symptoms and signs for over 8 weeks excludes GBS and suggests the diagnosis of chronic inflammatory demyelinating polyneuropathy (CIDP) (see below). Subacute onset with progression of the disease over 4 to 8 weeks falls in a "gray zone" between typical AIDP and CIDP.
3. Respiratory failure develops in approximately 30% of patients. Neck flexion and extension and shoulder abduction correlate well with diaphragmatic strength and are thus important to closely follow.
4. Following the disease nadir, a plateau phase of several days to weeks usually occurs. Subsequently, most patients gradually recover satisfactory function over several months. However, only about 15% of patients are without any residual deficits 1 to 2 years after disease onset and 5 to 10% of patients have disabling motor or sensory symptoms.
5. The mortality rate is about 5% with patients dying as a result of respiratory distress syndrome, aspiration pneumonia, pulmonary embolism, cardiac arrhythmias, and sepsis related to secondarily acquired infections.
6. Risk factors for a poorer prognosis (slower and incomplete recovery) are age greater than 50 to 60 years, abrupt onset of profound weakness, the need for mechanical ventilation, and distal CMAP amplitudes less than 10% to 20% of normal.

DIAGNOSIS

Clinical Features

1. Most patients initially note weakness, numbness, and tingling in the distal aspects of the lower limbs that ascend to the proximal legs, trunk, arms, and face. Occasionally symptoms begin in the face or arms and descend to involve the legs.

2. Weakness is symmetric affecting proximal and distal muscles.
3. Large-fiber modalities (touch, vibration, and position sense) are more severely affected than small-fiber functions (pain and temperature perception).
4. Patients with AMAN have no sensory signs or symptoms.
5. Muscle stretch reflexes are reduced or absent.
6. Autonomic instability is common with hypotension or hypertension and occasionally cardiac arrhythmias.

Laboratory Features

1. Elevated CSF protein levels accompanied by no or only a few mononuclear cells is evident in over 80% of patients after 2 weeks. Within the first week of symptoms, CSF protein levels are normal in approximately one third of patients.
2. In patients with CSF pleocytosis of more than 10 lymphocytes/mm^3 (particularly with cell counts greater than 50/mm^3), GBS-like neuropathies related to Lyme disease, recent human immunodeficiency virus (HIV) infection, or sarcoidosis need to be considered.
3. Elevated liver function tests (LFTs) are evident in many patients. In such cases, it is important to evaluate the patient for viral hepatitis (A, B, and C), EBV, and CMV infection.
4. Antiganglioside antibodies, particularly anti-GM1 antibodies, are common. The presence of these antibodies correlates well with *C. jejuni* infection but are not specific or prognostic and there is no need to order this test in GBS.

Electrodiagnostic Features

1. In AIDP, the NCSs demonstrate evidence of a multifocal demyelination.
   a. Sensory conductions are often absent, but when present, the distal latencies are markedly prolonged, conduction velocities are very slow, and amplitudes may be reduced. Of note, sural SNAPs may be normal when median, ulnar, and radial SNAPs are abnormal as AIDP is not a length-dependent neuropathy.
   b. Motor conduction studies are most important for diagnosis: Distal latencies are very prolonged and conduction velocities are very slow. The distal amplitudes may be normal or reduced secondary to distal conduction block. Conduction block or temporal dispersion may be apparent on proximal stimulation.
   c. F-waves and H-reflexes are markedly delayed or absent.
   d. Prolonged distal motor latencies and prolonged or absent F-waves are the earliest abnormal features. Early abnormalities of the distal CMAP amplitude and latency and of the F-waves reflect the early predilection for involvement of the proximal spinal roots and distal motor never terminals in AIDP.
   e. Distal CMAP amplitudes less than 10% to 20% of normal are associated with a poorer prognosis.
2. In AMSAN, the NCSs demonstrate features of a primary axonopathy.
   a. Sensory NCSs are absent or show reduced amplitudes with normal distal latencies and conduction velocities.
   b. Motor NCSs likewise show absent or reduced amplitudes with normal distal latencies and conduction velocities.
3. In AMAN, the NCSs are similar to those in AMSAN except that sensory conductions are normal.

TREATMENT

1. There have been no treatment trials devoted to AMAN, AMSAN, or Miller–Fisher syndrome. Nevertheless, treatments used for AIDP are given to all patients with GBS-related neuropathies.
2. Plasma exchange (PE) and IVIG have been demonstrated in prospective controlled trials to be effective in the treatment of AIDP.

   a. The total amount of plasma exchanged is 200 to 250 mL/kg of patient body weight over 10 to 14 days. The removed plasma is generally replaced with albumin.
   b. Thus, a 70-kg patient would receive 14,000 to 17,500 mL (14–17.5 L) total exchange, which can be accomplished by four to six alternate-day exchanges of 2 to 4 L each.
3. IVIG has replaced PE in many centers as the treatment of choice because it is at least as effective as PE, more widely available, and easier to use than PE. The dosage of IVIG is 2.0 g/kg body weight infused over 5 days.
4. There is no added benefit of IVIG following PE.
5. Treatment with IVIG or PE should begin as soon as possible, preferably within the first 7 to 10 days of symptoms.
6. The mean time to improvement of one clinical grade in the various controlled, randomized PE and IVIG studies ranged from 6 days to as long as 27 days. Thus, one may not see dramatic improvement in strength in patients during the PE or IVIG treatments. There is no evidence that PE beyond 250 mL/kg or IVIG greater than 2 g/kg is of any added benefit.
7. As many as 10% of patients treated with either PE or IVIG develop a relapse following initial improvement. In patients who suffer such relapses, we give additional courses of PE or IVIG.
8. Respiratory care:
   a. Monitor FVC and negative inspiratory force (NIF) for signs of respiratory distress. FVC and NIF will decline prior to development of hypoxia and arterial blood gas.
   b. Consider elective intubation once the FVC declines to less than 15 mL/kg or NIF to less than −20 to −30.
9. Physical therapy:
   a. Careful positioning of patients is important to prevent bed sores and nerve compression.
   b. Range-of-motion exercises are started early to prevent contractures.
   c. As patient improves, exercises to improve strength, function, and gait.
10. Supportive care:
   a. Deep venous thrombosis prophylaxis with pneumonic devices and heparin 5,000 units subcutaneously b.i.d.
   b. Reactive depression is common in patients with severe weakness. Psychiatry consult can be beneficial.
11. Neuropathic pain control.

MILLER–FISHER SYNDROME

BACKGROUND

1. In 1956, C. Miller Fisher reported three patients with ataxia, areflexia, and ophthalmoplegia having a syndrome distinct from GBS.
2. There is a 2 to 1 male predominance with a mean age of onset in the early 40's.
3. An antecedent infection occurs over two thirds of the cases, usually *C. jejuni.*

PATHOPHYSIOLOGY

1. Perhaps through molecular mimicry, autoantibodies directed against these infectious agents cross-react with neuronal epitopes.
2. Anti-GQ1b antibodies can be detected in most patients with Miller–Fisher syndrome (MFS).
3. GQ1b is a ganglioside concentrated on oculomotor neurons, sensory ganglia, and cerebellar neurons.

PROGNOSIS

1. Clinical return of function usually begins within about 2 weeks.
2. Full recovery of function is typically seen within 3 to 5 months.

DIAGNOSIS

Clinical Features

1. Diplopia is the most common initial complaint (39%), while ataxia is evident in 21% of patients at the onset.
2. Ophthalmoparesis can develop asymmetrically but often progresses to complete ophthalmoplegia. Ptosis usually accompanies the ophthalmoparesis, but pupillary involvement is uncommon.
3. Other cranial nerves can also become involved. Facial weakness is evident in 57%, dysphagia in 40%, and dysarthria in 13% of patients.
4. Nearly half of the patients describe paresthesias of the face and distal limbs.
5. Areflexia is evident on examination in more than 82% of patients.
6. Mild proximal limb weakness can be demonstrated in the course of the illness in approximately one third of cases. Some patients progress to develop more severe generalized weakness similar to typical GBS.

Laboratory Features

1. Most of the patients with MFS have an elevated CSF protein without significant pleocytosis.
2. Serologic evidence of C. jejuni can also be demonstrated in some patients as well as antiganglioside antibodies, in particular anti-GQ1b.

Electrophysiologic Findings

1. The most prominent electrophysiologic abnormality in MFS is reduced amplitudes of SNAPs out of proportion to any prolongation of the distal latencies or slowing of sensory conduction velocities.
2. CMAPs in the arms and legs are usually normal.
3. In contrast to limb CMAPs, mild to moderate reduction of facial CMAPs can be demonstrated in over 50% of patients with MFS.
4. Blink reflex may be abnormal if there is facial nerve involvement. Reduced facial CMAPs coincide with the loss or mild delay of R1 and R2 responses on blink reflex testing.

TREATMENT

1. There are no controlled treatment trials of patients with MFS.
2. However, I treat patients with either IVIG 2 g/kg over 5 days or PE 250 mL/kg over 2 weeks similar to GBS.

CHRONIC INFLAMMATORY DEMYELINATING POLYRADICULONEUROPATHY

BACKGROUND

1. CIDP is an immune-mediated neuropathy characterized by a relapsing or progressive course.

2. CIDP most commonly presents in adults with a peak incidence at about 40 to 60 years of age, and there is a slightly increased prevalence in men.
3. The relapsing form has an earlier age of onset, usually in the 20's, compared to the more chronic progressive form of the disease.
4. Relapses have been associated with pregnancy.
5. The association of CIDP with infections has not been studied as extensively as in AIDP; however, an infection has been reported to precede 20% to 30% of CIDP relapses or exacerbations.

PATHOPHYSIOLOGY

The pathogenic basis of CIDP is autoimmune in nature.

PROGNOSIS

1. Approximately 90% of patients improve with therapy; however, at least 50% demonstrate a subsequent relapse within the next 4 years and less than 30% achieve remission off medication.
2. Patients treated early are more likely to respond, underscoring the need for early diagnosis and treatment.
3. Progressive course, CNS involvement, and particularly, axonal loss have been associated with a poorer long-term prognosis.

DIAGNOSIS

Clinical Features

1. Most patients present with relapsing or progressive, symmetric proximal and distal weakness of the arms and legs.
2. Although most patients (at least 80%) have both motor and sensory involvement, a few patients may have pure motor (10%) or pure sensory (5%–10%) symptoms and signs.
3. Most patients with CIDP have areflexia or hyporeflexia.
4. Cranial nerve involvement can occasionally occur but is usually mild and not the presenting feature in CIDP.

Laboratory Features

1. An elevated CSF protein (more than 45 mg/dL) is found in 80% to 95% of patients.
2. CSF cell count is usually normal, although up to 10% of patients have more than 5 lymphocytes/mm^3.
3. Elevated CSF cell counts should lead to the consideration of HIV infection, Lyme disease, and lymphomatous or leukemic infiltration of nerve roots.
4. As many as 25% of patients with CIDP or a CIDP-like neuropathy have an IgA, IgG, or IgM monoclonal gammopathy.
5. MRI with gadolinium may reveal hypertrophy and enhancement of the nerve roots and peripheral nerves.

Electrophysiologic Findings

1. Research criteria for demyelination include slow motor nerve conduction velocity to less than 70% to 80% of the lower limit of normal, prolonged distal motor latencies to 125% to 150% of the upper limit of normal, prolonged F-wave latencies to125% to 150%, conduction block, and temporal dispersion.
2. As many as 40% of patients with CIDP do not fulfill the strict research criteria for demyelination and yet are responsive to immunotherapy. Thus, do not withhold treatment in such patients if the diagnosis is considered likely on the basis of

clinical examination showing symmetric proximal and distal weakness in the arms and legs, diminished reflexes, and elevated CSF protein.

Histopathology

1. Nerve biopsies may reveal evidence of segmental demyelination and remyelination, endoneurial and perineurial edema, mononuclear inflammatory cell infiltrate in the epineurium, perineurium, or endoneurium that is often perivascular.
2. However, nerve biopsies can reveal mainly axonal degeneration or may be completely normal.
3. Nerve biopsies are not necessary if patients have characteristic clinical picture, increased CSF protein without pleocytosis, and demyelinating NCSs.

TREATMENT

Immunosuppressive and immunomodulatory therapies have been tried (see Table 8-1), albeit most have not been studied in a double-blind, placebo-controlled fashion. Randomized control trials have demonstrated efficacy of corticosteroids, PE, and IVIG in the treatment of CIDP. Patients may respond to one mode of treatment when other forms of treatment have failed or become refractory.

1. Corticosteroids:
   a. Initiate treatment with prednisone 1.5 mg/kg (up to 100 mg) daily for 2 to 4 weeks then switch to alternate-day treatment [e.g., 100 mg every other day (q.o.d.)].
   b. Patients with diabetes may not be able to be treated with alternate prednisone secondary to wide fluctuations in blood glucose. In such cases, treat with equivalent dose of daily prednisone (i.e., 50 mg/d).
   c. Patients are maintained on this dose of prednisone until their strength is normalized or there is a clear plateau in clinical improvement, which is usually occurs by 6 months.
   d. Subsequently, the dose of prednisone is slowly decreased by 5 mg every 2 to 3 weeks until they are on 20 mg q.o.d. At that point, we taper the prednisone no faster than 2.5 mg every 2 to 3 weeks.
   e. There are significant side effects related to long-term corticosteroid treatment including osteoporosis, glucose intolerance, hypertension, cataract formation, aseptic necrosis of the hip, weight gain, hypokalemia, and type 2 muscle fiber atrophy.
   f. Obtain baseline bone density studies and repeat the study every 6 months while patients are receiving prednisone.
   g. Start calcium (1,000–1,500 mg/d) and vitamin D (400–800 IU/d) for osteoporosis prophylaxis.
   h. Bisphosphonates are effective in the prevention and treatment of osteoporosis. If dual-energy x-ray absorptiometry (DEXA) scans demonstrate osteoporosis at baseline or during follow-up studies, I initiate alendronate 70 mg per week. In postmenopausal women, I start alendronate 35 mg orally once a week as prophylaxis for osteoporosis. The long-term side effects of bisphosphonates are not known especially in men and young premenopausal women. I start prophylactic treatment with alendronate 35 mg orally once a week if DEXA scans show bone loss at baseline (not as yet enough to diagnosis osteoporosis) or if there is significant loss on follow-up bone density scans. Alendronate can cause severe esophagitis and absorption is impaired if taken with meals. Therefore, patients must be instructed to remain upright and not to eat for at least 30 minutes after taking a dose of alendronate.
   i. Obtain baseline and periodic fasting blood glucose and serum electrolytes. Patients need to be instructed on a low-sodium, low-carbohydrate diet to avoid excessive weight gain, hypertension, and DM.
   j. I recommend physical therapy and an exercise program in order to reduce these side effects.

2. IVIG:

 a. A large double-blind, placebo-controlled, cross-over study demonstrated that IVIG was efficacious in CIDP.
 b. An observer-blinded, randomized trial of PE compared with IVIG found no clear difference in efficacy.
 c. For many authorities, IVIG has become the treatment of choice in CIDP. Similar to PE, patients require repeated courses of IVIG because the improvement is only transient. The timeframe and dose of IVIG treatments need to be individualized.
 d. Initially, I begin IVIG treatment with a dose of 2 g/kg over 5 days.
 e. Subsequently, I repeat IVIG 2 g/kg over 2 to 5 days every month for 2 months.
 f. Next, I try to adjust the total dose and dosing interval dependent on response. Some patients may get by with IVIG 1 g/kg every 2 to 3 months, whereas other patients may need infusions every couple of weeks.
 g. Serum IgA level should be assayed in patients prior to administering IVIG. Patients who are IgA-deficient may develop anaphylactic reactions to IVIG, which can contain some IgA.
 h. In addition, IVIG should be used cautiously in patients with diabetes and avoided in those with renal insufficiency because it has been associated with renal failure secondary to acute tubular necrosis in such cases.
 i. Many patients develop headaches (50%), diffuse myalgias, fever, blood pressure fluctuations, and flu-like symptoms. These side effects can be treated with prophylactic administration of hydrocortisone 100 mg IV, benadryl 25% to 50 mg IV, and Tylenol 650 mg p.o. 30 minutes prior to each IVIG infusion. Also lowering the rate of infusion should lessen side effects during the treatment.
 j. A few patients actually have aseptic meningitis. There are rare thrombotic complications (e.g., stroke, myocardial infarction), perhaps related to hyperviscosity.
 k. Neutropenia is common, but this is rarely clinically significant.

3. PE:

 a. Two prospective, randomized, double-blinded, placebo-controlled trials using sham PE demonstrated the efficacy of PE.
 b. Unfortunately, response to treatment is transient, usually lasting only a few weeks. Thus, chronic intermittent PE or the addition of immunosuppressive agents is required.
 c. I use PE, usually in combination with prednisone, in patients with severe generalized weakness because the response to PE may be quicker than that of using prednisone alone.
 d. I exchange approximately 200 to 250 mL/kg body weight over five to six exchanges over a 2-week period. Some patients will require more exchanges for maximum improvement to occur.
 e. Thereafter, exchanges can be scheduled every 1 to 2 weeks and the duration between exchanges gradually increased.
 f. I use PE alone in patients for whom we wish to avoid long-term prednisone (e.g., patients with poorly controlled DM or HIV infection) or in whom IVIG is contraindicated (e.g., patients with renal insufficiency).
 g. I also use a trial course of PE in patients who do not fulfill all the criteria for CIDP or those who have an underlying condition making the diagnosis difficult (e.g., patients with diabetes and superimposed CIDP-like neuropathy). Because the response to PE is generally faster than the response to prednisone, one can often determine earlier whether such patients could have an immune-responsive neuropathy.

4. Azathioprine:

 a. I usually do not treat CIDP with azathioprine alone, but it is an option in patients who cannot be given prednisone, PE, or IVIG.
 b. I use azathioprine in combination with prednisone in patients who have been resistant to prednisone taper.
 c. Begin azathioprine at a dose of 50 mg/d and gradual increase by 50 mg every week to a total dose of 2 to 3 mg/kg/d.

    d. Approximately 12% of patients receiving azathioprine develop fever, abdominal pain, nausea, and vomiting requiring discontinuation of the drug.

    e. Other side effects include bone marrow suppression, hepatotoxicity, and risk of infection and future malignancy.

    f. Monitor complete blood counts (CBCs) and LFTs every 2 weeks, while adjusting the dose of azathioprine and then every 3 months once the dose is stable.

5. Mycophenolate mofetil:

    a. Small anecdotal reports suggest that some patients may benefit from mycophenolate mofetil.

    b. I start at 1 g p.o. b.i.d. The dose can be increased by 500 mg per month up to 1.5 g p.o. b.i.d.

6. Cyclophosphamide:

    a. Both oral (50–150 mg/d) and monthly pulses of IV cyclophosphamide (1 g/m^2) have been reported to be beneficial in some patients either in combination with prednisone or in steroid refractory cases.

        1) Sodium 2-mercaptoethane sulfonate (Mesna) 20 mg/kg p.o. every 2 to 4 hours for 12 to 24 hours every month on day of IV infusions is given to reduce the incidence of bladder toxicity.

        2) Ondansetron 8 mg p.o. prior to cyclophosphamide infusion and 8 hours later is used to diminish nausea.

        3) Patients should be vigorously hydrated to minimize bladder toxicity.

    b. The major side effects of hemorrhagic cystitis, bone marrow suppression, increased risk of infection and future malignancy, teratogenicity, alopecia, nausea, and vomiting have limited its use.

    c. It is important to frequently monitor CBCs and urinalysis in patients treated with cyclophosphamide.

7. Cyclosporine:

    a. Several retrospective reports suggest that cyclosporine can be effective in some patients with CIDP, even in those refractory to other modes of therapy.

    b. I administer cyclosporine at a dose of 4 to 6 mg/kg orally per day, initially aiming for a trough level between 150 and 200 mg/dL.

    c. The major side effects of cyclosporine include nephrotoxicity, hypertension, tremor, gingival hyperplasia, hirsuitism, and increased risk of infection and future malignancies—mainly skin cancer and lymphoma.

    d. Electrolytes and renal function need to be monitored monthly while adjusting the dose and then every 3 months.

8. Supportive care:

    a. Physical and occupation therapy to improve strength, gait, and function and assess need for orthotic devices (e.g., ankle braces).

MULTIFOCAL MOTOR NEUROPATHY

BACKGROUND

1. Multifocal motor neuropathy (MMN) is commonly misdiagnosed as ALS, however, as noted above the muscle involvement is in the distribution of individual peripheral nerves, not spinal roots.

2. The incidence of MMN is much less than that of ALS with some large neuromuscular centers diagnosing one case of MMN for every 50 patients with ALS.

3. There is a male predominance with a male to female ratio of approximately 3 to 1.

4. The age of onset of symptoms is usually early in the fifth decade of life, ranging from the second to eighth decades of life.

PATHOPHYSIOLOGY

1. MMN is now generally regarded as a distinct entity because it represents a relatively uniform group of patients who differ significantly from patients with CIDP with respect to laboratory features, histopathology, and response to treatment.
2. The disparity between motor and sensory nerve involvement suggests that the autoimmune attack may be directed against an antigen specific for the motor nerve.
3. The pathogenic role for antiganglioside antibodies is not known.
4. An immune attack directed against an ion channel could account for conduction block of neural impulses and secondary inflammatory attack may result in demyelination.

PROGNOSIS

1. Approximately two thirds of patients improve with IVIG or cyclophosphamide.
2. Patients with long-standing disease with atrophy of muscles are less likely to respond.

DIAGNOSIS

Clinical Features

1. Characterized clinically by asymmetric weakness and atrophy, typically in the distribution of individual peripheral nerves, usually beginning in the arms.
2. Lack of atrophy in weak muscle groups early in the course of the illness; however, decreased muscle bulk can develop in time due to secondary axonal degeneration.
3. Fasciculations may be observed in affected limb muscles.
4. Sensory examination should be normal, as previously discussed.
5. Deep tendon reflexes are highly variable in that unaffected regions can be normal, whereas weak and atrophic muscles are usually associated with depressed or absent reflexes.

Laboratory Features

1. In contrast to CIDP and MADSAM, CSF protein is usually normal in patients with MMN.
2. Twenty-two percent to 84% of patients with MMN have detectable IgM antibodies directed against gangliosides, mainly GM1, but also asialo-GM1, and GM2, but the importance of these antibodies in terms of pathogenesis is unknown.
3. When present in high-titers the antibodies appear to be rather specific for MMN, but the sensitivity of the test is too low. The most sensitive and specific test is the nerve conduction study (see below) and the presence of absence of antiganglioside antibodies in a patient who has electrophysiologic abnormalities consistent with MMN adds little to the diagnosis.

Electrophysiologic Findings

1. In MMN, there is often evidence of conduction block in multiple upper and lower limb nerves. The locations of conduction block are not at the expected common nerve entrapment sites, but in the mid-forearm or leg, upper arm, across the brachial plexus, or nerve root region.
2. Other features of demyelination (i.e., prolonged distal latencies, temporal dispersion, slow conduction velocities, and prolonged or absent F-waves) are typically present on motor NCSs. In fact, conduction block need not be present for the diagnosis, if other features of demyelination are present.
3. The sensory NCSs are normal.
4. EMG reveals reduced recruitment in weak muscles. When secondary loss of axons has occurred, positive sharp waves and fibrillation potentials are commonly

detected in degrees commensurate with the amount of nerve injury and clinical wasting.

TREATMENT

1. IVIG is the treatment of choice in MMN.
   a. IVIG is initially given in a dose of 2 g/kg over 2 to 5 days with subsequent maintenance courses as necessary, similar to the management of CIDP.
   b. Unfortunately, not all patients with MMN respond to IVIG. Some series have noted that a later age of onset and patients who have significant muscle atrophy do not respond as well to treatment.
   c. I give three courses of monthly IVIG before concluding a patient has failed treatment.
2. IV cyclophosphamide was the first immunosuppressive agent demonstrated to be effective in MMN with over 70% of reported patients having clinically improved following treatment.
   a. I reserve cyclophosphamide for patients who failed to improve with IVIG or in whom IVIG is contraindicated (e.g., IgA deficiency, previous allergic reaction to IVIG, renal insufficiency, severe cardio- or cerebrovascular disease).
   b. My initial dosage of cyclophosphamide is 0.5 g/m^2 IV/mo.
   c. If no improvement is noted after 3 months, I increase the does to 0.75 g/m^2 IV/mo.
   d. If there is still no improvement after 3 months, I increase the dose to 1.0 g/m^2/mo.
   e. If there is no improvement after 3 months, I discontinue the cyclophosphamide. If improvement is noted, I continue monthly infusions for 12 months.
   f. Risks of cyclophosphamide include alopecia, nausea and vomiting, hemorrhagic cystitis, and significant bone marrow suppression. I have only rarely used cyclophosphamide given its short-term and long-term side effects since the reported efficacy of IVIG in MMN.
   g. Sodium 2-mercaptoethane sulfonate (Mesna) 20 mg/kg p.o. every 3 to 4 hours for 12 to 24 hours each month on day of IV infusions is given to reduce the incidence of bladder toxicity and ondansetron 8 mg p.o. prior to cyclophosphamide infusion and 8 hours later is used to diminish nausea.
   h. Patients should be vigorously hydrated to minimize bladder toxicity.
3. In contrast to CIDP and multifocal acquired demyelinating sensory and motor (MADSAM) neuropathy, few patients (less than 3% of reported cases) with MMN improve with high doses of corticosteroids or PE.

MULTIFOCAL ACQUIRED DEMYELINATING SENSORY AND MOTOR (MADSAM) NEUROPATHY

BACKGROUND

1. There have been several series of patients who resemble those with MMN but who have objective sensory abnormalities clinically, electrophysiologically, and histologically.
2. The terms "Lewis–Sumner syndrome" and "multifocal acquired demyelinating sensory and motor" (MADSAM) neuropathy have been used to describe this suspected variant of CIDP.

PATHOPHYSIOLOGY

1. The pathogenic basis for MADSAM neuropathy is not known.
2. MADSAM falls into the spectrum of CIDP and likely has a similar pathogenesis.

3. MADSAM neuropathy and CIDP are similar with respect to CSF and sensory nerve biopsy findings, as well as response to corticosteroids.

PROGNOSIS

Similar to CIDP, most patients improve with immunotherapy.

DIAGNOSIS

Clinical Features

1. Motor and sensory loss conforms to a discrete peripheral nerve distribution rather than a generalized stocking or glove pattern. Some patients describe pain and paresthesias.
2. Distal upper extremities are more commonly involved that the distal lower extremities. Cranial neuropathies can rarely occur.
3. There is a 2:1 male predominance. The average age of onset is in the early 50's (range, 14–77 years). Onset is usually insidious and slowly progressive.
4. Reflexes may be normal or decreased.

Laboratory Features

1. CSF protein is elevated in 60% to 82% of patients with MADSAM neuropathy.
2. Unlike MMN, GM1 antibodies are usually absent in MADSAM.
3. In patients with demyelination localized to the cervical roots or brachial plexus, MRI scans have revealed enlarged nerves that enhance in some, but not all, cases.

Histopathology

1. Sensory nerve biopsies demonstrate many thinly myelinated, large-diameter fibers and scattered demyelinated fibers.
2. Subperineurial and endoneurial edema and mild onion bulb formations may also be appreciated similar to CIDP.

Electrophysiologic Findings

1. As with CIDP and MMN, NCSs in MADSAM neuropathy demonstrate conduction blocks, temporal dispersion, prolonged distal latencies, prolonged F-waves, and slow conduction velocities in one or more motor nerves.
2. In contrast to MMN, the sensory studies are also abnormal. SNAPs are usually absent or small in amplitude, similar to those seen in patients with generalized CIDP.

TREATMENT

1. Most patients with MADSAM neuropathy improve with IVIG treatment.
2. I initiate treatment with IVIG 2 g/kg over 2 to 5 days and repeat every month for 3 months and then individualize subsequent doses and treatment intervals as described in the CIDP section.
3. If patients do not demonstrate a satisfactory response to IVIG, I start prednisone 1.5 mg/kg/d p.o. as discussed in the CIDP section.
4. In contrast to MMN but similar to CIDP, most patients with MADSAM neuropathy have also demonstrated improvement with steroid treatment.

5. This illustrates the importance of distinguishing MADSAM from MMN in which cyclophosphamide represents the only other medication reported to be beneficial besides IVIG.

ISAAC SYNDROME (SYNDROME OF CONTINUOUS MUSCLE FIBER ACTIVITY)

BACKGROUND

1. The disorder is caused by hyperexcitability of the motor nerves resulting in continuous activation of muscle fibers.
2. Most patients develop this disease sporadically; however, several families with apparent autosomal dominant inheritance have been reported. Isaac syndrome may occur in association with other autoimmune disorders (e.g., SLE, systemic sclerosis, celiac disease).
3. Paraneoplastic neuromyotonia has been reported with lung carcinoma, plasmacytoma, and Hodgkin lymphoma.
4. Isaac syndrome may occur in patients with myasthenia gravis or thymoma.
5. Generalized myokymia or neuromyotonia may complicate hereditary motor and sensory neuropathies [e.g., Charcot–Marie-Tooth disease(CMT)], acute or CIDPs, and autosomal dominant episodic ataxia.

PATHOPHYSIOLOGY

Isaac syndrome is an autoimmune disease caused by autoantibodies directed against voltage-gated potassium channels (VGKCs) located on peripheral nerves.

PROGNOSIS

Most patients respond well to treatment.

DIAGNOSIS

Clinical Features

1. Isaac syndrome usually occurs in adults but has been observed in a newborn.
2. Patients manifest with diffuse muscle stiffness, widespread muscle twitching (myokymia), cramps, increased sweating, and occasionally CNS symptoms (e.g., confusion, hallucinations, insomnia).
3. The myokymia is present continuously even during sleep.
4. The muscle stiffness worsens with voluntary activity of the affected body segment.
5. Patients may experience difficulty relaxing muscles following maximal contraction (i.e., pseudomyotonia).
6. Some patients experience numbness, paresthesiae, and weakness.

Laboratory Features

1. Antibodies directed against voltage-gated potassium channels (VGKC) are detectable in the serum and CSF.
2. Patients may have other laboratory features associated with concomitant autoimmune diseases.
3. CSF may demonstrate increased protein, increased immunoglobulins, and oligoclonal bands.

Electrophysiologic Findings

1. After-discharges are often evident following standard motor conduction studies.
2. EMG reveals continuous firing of MUAPs.
3. The most common abnormal discharges are combinations of fasciculation potentials, doublets, triplets, multiplets, complex repetitive discharges, and myokymic discharges.

TREATMENT

1. Various modes of immunomodulation appear to be beneficial in some patients, including plasmapheresis, IVIG, and corticosteroid treatment. I treat patients similar to those with CIDP, as discussed above.
2. Symptomatic treatment with antiepileptic medications (AEMs) (e.g., phenytoin, carbamazepine, and gabapentin) may also be useful as well perhaps by decreasing neuronal excitability by blocking sodium channels.

IDIOPATHIC AUTONOMIC NEUROPATHY

BACKGROUND

1. There is heterogeneity in the onset, the type of autonomic deficits, the presence or absence of somatic involvement, and the degree of recovery.
2. Approximately 20% of patients have selective cholinergic dysfunction, while 80% of patients have various degrees of widespread sympathetic and parasympathetic dysfunction.

PATHOPHYSIOLOGY

1. The disorder is suspected to be the result of an autoimmune attack directed against peripheral autonomic fibers or the ganglia.
2. A subset of patients may have antibodies directed against calcium channels, which are present on presynaptic autonomic nerve terminals.

PROGNOSIS

1. Most patients have a monopathic course with progression followed by a plateau and slow recovery or a stable deficit.
2. Although some patients exhibit a complete recovery, it tends to be incomplete in most.

DIAGNOSIS

Clinical Features

1. The most common symptom is orthostatic dizziness or lightheadedness occurring in about 80% of patients.
2. Gastrointestinal involvement as indicated by complaints of nausea, vomiting, diarrhea, constipation, ileus, or postprandial bloating is present in over 70% of patients.
3. Thermoregulatory impairment with heat intolerance and poor sweating is also present in most patients.
4. Blurred vision, dry eyes and mouth, urinary retention or incontinence, and impotence also are often present.
5. As many as 30% of patients also describe numbness, tingling, and dysesthesia of their hands and feet.
6. Muscle strength is normal.

Laboratory Features

1. The CSF often reveals slightly elevated protein without pleocytosis.
2. There are no serologic or immunologic abnormalities in the serum.
3. Supine plasma norepinephrine levels are not different, but standing levels are significantly reduced, when compared to normal controls.

AUTONOMIC TESTING

1. Cardiovascular studies reveal orthostatic hypotension and reduced variability of the heart rate to deep breathing in over 60% of patients.
2. An abnormal response to Valsalva maneuver can be demonstrated in over 40% of patients.
3. Summated quantitative sudomotor axon reflex test (QSART) scores are abnormal in 85% of patients. Most patients have abnormal thermoregulatory sweat tests with areas of anhidrosis in 12% to 97% of the body.
4. Gastrointestinal studies can demonstrate hypomotility anywhere from the esophagus to the rectum.

Electrophysiologic Findings

1. Routine motor and sensory NCSs and EMG are normal.
2. Quantitative sensory testing may reveal abnormalities in thermal thresholds.
3. Sympathetic skin response may be absent.

TREATMENT

1. Conclusions regarding the efficacy of immunotherapy are limited secondary to the retrospective and uncontrolled nature of most reports. Trials of PE, prednisone, IVIG, and other immunosuppressive agents have been tried with variable success.
2. I generally recommend a trial of IVIG 2 g/kg over 2 to 5 days.
3. The most important aspect of management is supportive therapy for orthostatic hypotension and bowel and bladder symptoms.
   a. Fluodrocortisone is effective at increasing plasma volume. Fluodrocortisone is administered only in the morning or in the morning and at lunch to avoid nocturnal hypertension. Initiate treatment at 0.1 mg/d and increase by 0.1 mg every 3 to 4 days until the blood pressure is controlled.
   b. Midodrine, a peripheral α_1-adrenergic agonist, is also effective and can be used in combination with fluodrocortisone. Midodrine is started at 2.5 mg/d and can be gradually increased to 40 mg/d in divided doses (every 2–4 hours) as necessary.
   c. Gastrointestinal hypomotility can be treated with metaclopramide, cisapride, or erythromycin.
   d. Bulking agents, laxatives, and enemas may be needed in patients with constipation. Urology should be consulted in patients with neurogenic bladders. Patient may require cholinergic agonists (e.g., bethanechol), intermittent self-catheterization, or other modes of therapy.

VASCULITIC NEUROPATHIES

BACKGROUND

1. Vasculitis is a histologic diagnosis requiring transmural inflammation and necrosis of the blood vessel walls.

2. Vasculitic disorders can be classified on the basis of caliber of vessel involved (i.e., small, medium, or large vessel), as to whether the vasculitis is primary [e.g., polyarteritis nodosa, Churg–Strauss syndrome (CSS), Wegener granulomatosis (WG)] or secondary to other systemic disorders (connective tissue diseases, infection, drug reactions, malignancy), or as to whether the vasculitis is systemic or isolated to the peripheral nervous system (PNS).

3. Polyarteritis nodosa (PAN) is the most common of the necrotizing vasculitides with an incidence ranging from 2 to 9/million.
   a. The onset is usually between 40 and 60 years of age.
   b. PAN is a systemic disorder involving small- and medium-caliber arteries in multiple organs.
   c. Vasculitis of the gastrointestinal tract can manifest as abdominal pain or bleeding.
   d. Ischemia of the kidneys can lead to renal failure.
   e. Orchitis is also a classic symptom of PAN.
   f. Weight loss, fever, and loss of appetite are also usually noted.

4. CSS manifests similar to PAN.
   a. The incidence is roughly one third that of PAN, but the frequency of PNS and CNS involvement in cases of CSS is similar to PAN.
   b. In contrast to PAN, patients with CSS usually present with respiratory involvement. Patients typically develop allergic rhinitis, nasal polyposis, and sinusitis followed by asthma.
   c. In CCS, asthma begins later in life, in contrast to common asthma, which usually develops before the age of 35 years.
   d. Pulmonary infiltrates are present in nearly half the patients, usually in association with asthma and hypereosinophilia.
   e. Symptoms and signs of systemic vasculitis occur an average of 3 years after the onset of asthma.
   f. Rather than an ischemic nephropathy as evident in PAN, 16% to 49% of patients with CSS develop a necrotizing glomerulonephritis.

5. WG is a rare disorder consisting of necrotizing granulomatous involvement of the upper and lower respiratory tract and glomerulonephritis
   a. The early symptoms of respiratory disease (nasal discharge, cough, hemoptysis, and dyspnea) and facial pain can help distinguish this from other vasculitic disorders.
   b. About 30% to 50% of patients may have some form of neurologic dysfunction, although only 15% to 20% of patients have peripheral neuropathy. Either a mononeuropathy multiplex or a generalized symmetric pattern of involvement can be found.
   c. Cranial neuropathies, particularly the second, sixth, and seventh nerves, are involved in approximately 10% of cases as a result of extension of the nasal or paranasal granulomas rather than vasculitis.

6. Microscopic polyangiitis (MPA):
   a. The clinical symptoms of MPA are similar to those of PAN, except that the lungs are often involved.
   b. MPA is about one third as common as PAN and has an average age of onset of 50 years.
   c. Polyneuropathy complicates MPA in 14% to 36% of cases.
   d. Impaired renal function as illustrated by increased blood urea nitrogen (BUN) and creatinine levels and hematuria is evident in most patients.

PATHOPHYSIOLOGY

The pathogenic basis is cytotoxic- or complement-mediated destruction of blood vessels (depending on the specific type of vasculitis) with ischemic damage to peripheral nerves

PROGNOSIS

1. Since the use of corticosteroids to treat systemic vasculitis began in the 1950's, the 5-year survival rate increased from 10% to 55% by the mid to late 1970's.
2. The addition of cyclophosphamide to corticosteroids further increased the 5-year survival rate to over 80%.
3. Nonsystemic vasculitis carries a better prognosis and often will respond to treatment with prednisone alone.

DIAGNOSIS

Clinical Features

1. Motor and sensory fibers are affected resulting in a numbness, pain, and weakness.
2. Three patterns of peripheral nerve involvement can be appreciated:
   a. Multiple mononeuropathies.
   b. Overlapping mononeuropathy multiplex.
   c. Generalized symmetric polyneuropathies. The mononeuropathy multiplex pattern (simple and overlap forms) are the most common, found in 60% to 70% of cases at the time of diagnosis, whereas a generalized polyneuropathy is evident in approximately 30% to 40% of patients.

Electrophysiologic Findings

1. Motor and sensory nerve conduction demonstrates unobtainable potentials or reduced amplitudes with relatively normal distal latencies and conduction velocities consistent with axonal degeneration.
2. EMG demonstrates evidence of active denervation in affected muscles.
3. There is asymmetric involvement of motor and sensory nerves and EMG abnormalities reflective of the multifocal pathophysiology.

Laboratory Features

1. Erythrocyte sedimentation rate (ESR), C-reactive protein, and rheumatoid factor are elevated in most patients.
2. PAN: As many as one third of cases are associated with hepatitis B antigenemia. In addition, hepatitis C and HIV infection have also been reported with PAN. Abdominal angiograms can reveal a vasculitic aneurysm. Abdominal angiograms can reveal a vasculitic aneurysm.
3. CCS: Evaluation is remarkable for eosinophilia and antineutrophil cytoplasmic antibodies (ANCAs), primarily myeloperoxidase or p-ANCA because of its perinuclear staining pattern. These p-ANCA antibodies are present in as many as two thirds of patients.
4. WG: Evaluation is remarkable for the presence of antineutrophil antibodies directed against proteinase-3 (c-ANCA). The specificity of c-ANCA for WG is 98% and the sensitivity is 95%. The vasculitis is similar to that of PAN, affecting medium and small blood vessels. Granulomatous infiltration of the respiratory tract and necrotizing glomerulonephritis are also seen.
5. The lack of peripheral eosinophilia and eosinophilic infiltrates on biopsy and absence of asthma help distinguish WG from CSS.
6. MPA: Laboratory evaluation usually demonstrates the presence of p-ANCA, although c-ANCAs can also occasionally be detected.

Histopathology

1. If involved, I prefer to biopsy the superficial peroneal nerve because the peroneus brevis muscle can also be biopsied at the same time. The diagnostic yield is increased when the nerve and muscle are both biopsied.

2. The definitive histologic diagnosis of vasculitis requires transmural inflammatory cell infiltration and necrosis of the vessel wall.

TREATMENT

1. Systemic vasculitis is treated initially with a combination of corticosteroids and cyclophosphamide.
2. Hypersensitivity vasculitis and isolated PNS vasculitis can be treated with prednisone alone.
3. Initiate corticosteroid treatment with pulsed methylprednisolone (1 g IV every day for 3 days) then switch to oral prednisone 1.5 mg/kg/d (up to 100 mg/d) as a single dose in the morning.
   a. After 2 to 4 weeks, I switch to alternate-day prednisone (i.e., 100 mg q.o.d.). After 4 to 6 months, I begin tapering prednisone by 5 mg every 2 weeks down to 20 mg q.o.d. and then by 2.5 mg every 2 weeks.
   b. Collateral treatment with calcium and vitamin D supplementation as well as bisphosphonates to prevent and treat steroid-induced osteoporosis are used as discussed in the section on CIDP.
4. Cyclophosphamide is started the same time as the corticosteroids and can be given orally or in IV pulses.
   a. Oral cyclophosphamide at a dose of 1.0 to 2.0 mg/kg is a more potent suppressor of the immune system, but is associated with more adverse side effects (e.g., hemorrhagic cystitis) than IV pulses.
   b. I prefer monthly IV pulses of cyclophosphamide at a dose of 500 to 1,000 mg/m^2 of body surface area.
   c. Sodium 2-mercaptoethane sulfonate (Mesna) 20 mg/kg p.o. every 3 to 4 hours for 12 to 24 hours each month on day of IV infusions is given to reduce the incidence of bladder toxicity and ondansetron 8 mg po prior to cyclophosphamide infusion and 8 hours later is used to diminish nausea.
   d. Patients should be vigorously hydrated to minimize bladder toxicity.
5. Following IV pulses of cyclophosphamide, the leukocyte count drops with a nadir between 7 to 18 days, during which time the risk of infection is greatest. Check CBCs and urinalysis prior to each treatment. Urinalysis is obtained every 3 to 6 months after treatment because of the risk of future bladder cancer.
6. Continue with the high-dose corticosteroids and cyclophosphamide treatment until the patient begins to improve or at least the deficit stabilizes, which is usually within 4 to 6 months. Subsequently, prednisone is gradually tapered by 5 mg every 2 to 3 weeks.
7. Pulsed cyclophosphamide is generally continued for at least 6 months after stabilization. Cyclophosphamide can then be discontinued and can be replaced by azathioprine or methotrexate (see Table 8-1). If patients do not respond to pulsed cyclophosphamide, oral dosing should be tried prior to concluding the patient failed cyclophosphamide treatment.
8. Patients with CSS often require continued low doses of prednisone secondary to their associated asthma. Relapses are uncommon in PAN, MPA, and isolated PNS vasculitis but occur in as many as 50% of cases of WG. Such patients may require life-long immunosuppressive therapy.
9. There is less experience with other immunosuppressive agents in the treatment of vasculitis. In an open-label study of low-dose methotrexate (0.15–0.3 mg/kg/wk) in combination with corticosteroids, marked improvement was noted in 76% of patients with WG and remission occurred in 69%.
10. Patients with hepatitis B– or C–related PAN require special treatment:
    a. Conventional treatment with high-dose corticosteroids and cyclophosphamide may allow the virus to persist and replicate, thus increasing the risk of liver failure.
    b. I use corticosteroids only during the first few weeks of treatment to manage life-threatening manifestations of systemic vasculitis. Afterward, the corticosteroids are abruptly discontinued.
    c. PE and antiviral agents such as vidarabine or α-interferon are used to control the course of the illness.

d. α-Interferon (3 million units three times a week) is efficacious in treating hepatitis C–related mixed cryoglobulinemia.

NEUROPATHY ASSOCIATED WITH SARCOIDOSIS

BACKGROUND

1. Sarcoidosis is a multisystem granulomatous disorder affecting the liver, spleen, mucous membranes, parotid gland, muscle tissue, CNS, and PNS.
2. Women are affected more commonly than men.
3. The PNS or CNS is involved in about 5% of patients with sarcoidosis.

PATHOPHYSIOLOGY

1. Sarcoidosis is an autoimmune disorder although the etiology and pathogenic mechanism of the disorder are unclear.
2. Peripheral neuropathy may result from direct compression, ischemia, a combination of these two insults, or other ill defined factors.

PROGNOSIS

1. Patients with neurosarcoidosis, particularly of the cranial nerves, may respond well to corticosteroid treatment.
2. If patients are resistant to corticosteroids, other immunosuppressive agents can be tried (e.g., cyclosporine).

DIAGNOSIS

Clinical Features

1. Nonspecific constitutional symptoms of fever, weight loss, and fatigue are usually the presenting complaints of most patients.
2. Palpable peripheral lymph nodes may be noted.
3. A common finding on presentation is acute granulomatous uveitis, which can progress to significant visual impairment or even blindness.
4. Patients may present with multiple cranial nerve involvement. The most common cranial nerve to be involved is the seventh nerve, which can be affected bilaterally. The second and eighth cranial nerves are also frequently affected.
5. Multiple peripheral mononeuropathies and polyradiculoneuropathy also occur. With a generalized root involvement, patients may present with signs and symptoms quite similar to AIDP or CIDP.
6. The most common involvement of the peripheral nervous system is a subclinical mononeuropathy multiplex, which can be demonstrated by electrodiagnostic medicine evaluation. Less commonly, some patients present with symptoms and signs suggestive of a slowly progressive primarily sensory, motor, or sensorimotor peripheral neuropathy.
7. Hilar adenopathy is noted on chest radiographs.

Histopathology

1. The major histopathologic finding is noncaseating granulomas in various tissues.
2. When the peripheral nerves are affected, nerve biopsy can reveal profuse infiltration of the nerve by multiple sarcoid tubercles affecting all regions of the supporting

neural structures (endoneurium, perineurium, and epineurium) associated with lymphocytic angiitis.

Electrophysiologic Findings

1. The most common finding is an absence or reduction in SNAP amplitudes and, much less frequently, CMAP amplitudes in a mononeuropathy multiplex pattern.
2. A few patients have more profound slowing indicating demyelinating as opposed to axonal component of nerve damage.

TREATMENT

1. I initiate treatment with prednisone 1.5 mg/kg/d p.o. and adjust the dose as described in the Treatment section on CIDP.
2. Second-line agents in patients unresponsive or refractory to steroids are azathioprine (2–3 mg/kg/d), methotrexate (7.5–20 mg/wk), cyclosporine (3–6 mg/kg/d), and cyclophosphamide (1–2 mg/kg/d) as described in the CIDP section (see Table 8-1).

NEUROPATHY ASSOCIATED WITH LEPROSY

BACKGROUND

1. The acid–fast bacteria *Mycobacterium leprae* causes leprosy.
2. It is most commonly found in Southeast Asia, Africa, South America, and Europe, but it is endemic in certain areas of the United States of America (i.e., Hawaii, Texas).
3. Three primary clinical manifestations of the disease are commonly recognized: tuberculoid, lepromatous, and borderline leprosy (Table 8-2).
4. It is the host's immunologic status that determines which form of the disease develops.

PATHOPHYSIOLOGY

1. The clinical and pathologic spectrum of the disease is dependent on the host's immune response to *M. leprae* and reflects the relative balance between T helper cell type 1 (T_H1; helper) and T_H2 (suppressor) cells.
2. Tuberculoid leprosy and lepromatous leprosy represent the two extremes of disease manifestation.
3. The tuberculoid form defines one end of the spectrum, in which the T_H1 cells predominate. The T_H1 cells produce interleukin-2 (IL-2) and γ-interferon, which in turn lead to activation of macrophages.
4. On the other extreme, the lepromatous form is dominated by T_H2 cells, which produce IL-4, -5, and -10, thereby down-regulating cell-mediated immunity and inhibiting macrophages.
5. The borderline subtypes exhibit immune responses spanning the spectrum between the tuberculoid and lepromatous forms.

PROGNOSIS

The neuropathy is very responsive to antibiotics.

TABLE 8-2. CLINICAL, LABORATORY, IMMUNOLOGIC, AND HISTOPATHOLOGIC FEATURES OF LEPROSY

	Tuberculous Leprosy (TT)	Mid-Borderline Leprosy (BB)	Lepromatous Leprosy (LL)
Lepromin Test	Positive (>5 mm induration)	+/− (2–5 mm induration)	Negative (0–2 mm induration)
Bacterial Index	0	2–4	5–6
Morphologic Index	Low (down to 0)	Moderate	High (up to 10)
Immunology	Cell-mediated immunity: intact; $T_H1 > T_H2$ lymphocytes; Cytokines expressed: IL-2, γ-IF	Cell-mediated immunity: unstable can range from intact to absent	Cell-mediated immunity: absent; $T_H2 > T_H1$ lymphocytes; cytokines expressed: IL-4, -5, -10
Skin Lesions	Few localized and well demarcated large skin lesions; erythematous macules and plaques with raised borders Centers of lesions may be hypopigmented	Size, number, and appearance of the skin lesions are intermediate between that seen in the TT and LL poles	Multiple, symmetric small macules and papules; older lesions form plaques and nodules
Histopathology	Localized granulomas and giant cells encompassed by dense lymphocytic infiltrate extending to epidermis Fite stain: negative for bacteria	Granulomas with epithelioid cells but no giant cells. Not localized by zones of lymphocytes. Lymphocytes, if present, are diffusely infiltrating Fite stain: slight positive	Scant lymphocytes, but if present are diffuse along with organismladen foamy macrophages Fite stain: marked positive
Neuropathies	Mononeuropathy of the superficial cutaneous nerves or large nerve trunks (i.e., ulnar, median, peroneal nerves), multiple mononeuropathies Pure neuritic leprosy may be seen	The neuropathies can range in the spectrum of that seen in TT to LL	Distal symmetric sensory and sensorimotor polyneuropathies are more common than mononeuropathy Pure neuritic leprosy is not seen
Treatment[a]	Dapsone 100 mg/d Rifampin 600 mg/d Duration 12 mo	As per LL	Dapsone 100 mg/d Rifampin 600 mg/d Clofazimine 50 mg/d Duration: 2 y or until skin smear (MI) is 0

T_H1, T helper type 1; TT, tuberculous leprosy; BB, mid-borderline leprosy; LL, lepromatous leprosy; IL, interleukin; IF, interferon; MI, morphologic index.
The features of the borderline tuberculoid (BT) form range between the TT and BB forms. The features of the borderline lepromatous (BL) form range between those seen in BB and LL forms of leprosy.
[a]Treatment is as recommended by the Hansen's Disease Center, Carville LA.
From Altman D, Amato AA. Lepromatous neuropathy. *J Clin Neuromusc Dis* 1999;1:68–73, with permission.

DIAGNOSIS

Clinical Features

1. In tuberculoid leprosy, the cell-mediated immune response is intact leading to focal, circumscribed inflammatory lesions involving the skin or nerves.
   a. The skin lesions appear as well-defined, scattered hypopigmented patches and plaques with central anesthesia and raised, erythematous borders.
   b. The organism has a predilection for the cooler regions of the body (e.g., face, limbs) rather than warmer regions such as the groin or axilla.
   c. The more superficial nerves in the vicinity of the skin lesions may also be affected.
   d. There is a predilection for involvement of specific nerve trunks: the ulnar nerve at the medial epicondyle, the median nerve at the distal forearm, the peroneal nerve at the fibular head, the sural nerve, the greater auricular nerve, and the superficial radial nerve at the wrist.
   e. The most common neurologic manifestation of tuberculoid leprosy is mononeuropathy or mononeuropathy multiplex.
2. In lepromatous leprosy, cell-mediated immunity is impaired resulting in an extensive infiltration of the bacilli process, anesthesia, and anhidrosis.
   a. Clinical manifestations tend to be more severe in the lepromatous subtype, but as in the tuberculoid form, cooler regions of the body are more susceptible.
   b. The organisms multiply virtually unchecked and hematogenously disseminate, producing confluent and symmetric areas of rash.
   c. A slowly progressive symmetric sensorimotor polyneuropathy develops over time.
   d. As with the tuberculoid subtype, nerve trunks can be affected with time leading to superimposed mononeuropathies.
3. Patients with borderline leprosy have the highest incidence of neurologic complications.
   a. These patients can show clinical and histologic features of both the lepromatous and tuberculoid forms of leprosy.
   b. Patients can develop generalized symmetric sensorimotor polyneuropathies, mononeuropathies, and mononeuropathy multiplex, including multiple mononeuropathies in atypical locations, such as the brachial plexus.
4. Rarely, patients with leprosy present with isolated peripheral neuropathy without skin lesions.
   a. Lepromatous neuropathy should be suspected in individuals without skin lesions who live in endemic areas.
   b. Virtually all the cases of pure neuritic leprosy have the tuberculoid or borderline tuberculoid subtypes of the disease.

Electrophysiologic Studies

EMG and NCS findings are consistent with multiple axonal mononeuropathies.

Histopathology

Diagnosis of leprosy can be confirmed with a skin or nerve biopsy (see Table 8-2).

TREATMENT

1. Multidrug therapy with dapsone, rifampin and clofazimine is presently the mainstay of treatment, although a number of other agents have recently demonstrated efficacy, including thalidomide, pefloxacin, ofloxacin, sparfloxacin, minocycline, and clarithromycin (see Table 8-2).
2. Treatment typically requires 2 years of therapy in order to achieve full eradication of the organism.
3. A potential complication of therapy, particularly in the borderline leprosy, is

the reversal reaction, which can occur at any time during treatment of the disease.

   a. The reversal reaction occurs as a result of a shift to the tuberculoid end of the spectrum with an increase in cellular immunity.

   b. Up-regulation of the cellular response is characterized by excessive release of tumor necrosis factor-α, γ-interferon, and IL-2 with new granuloma formation.

   c. Prednisone 50 mg/d appears to blunt this adverse reaction and may even be used prophylactically in high-risk patients at treatment onset.

4. A second type of reaction to treatment is erythema nodosum leprosum (ENL), which occurs in patients at the lepromatous pole of the disease.

   a. ENL is associated with the appearance of multiple erythematous, sometimes painful, subcutaneous nodules; exacerbation of the neuropathy can also occur.

   b. ENL is due to the slow degradation of antigens (bacterial debris) resulting in antigen–antibody complex and complement deposition in affected tissue.

   c. ENL can be treated with prednisone 50 mg/d or thalidomide.

5. Prevention of leprosy is the ultimate goal and involves multiple strategies, starting with the prompt diagnosis and treatment of suspected cases, often with brief hospitalizations to ensure understanding and compliance with multidrug regimens.

6. Chemoprophylaxis of childhood contacts with daily rifampin for 6 months is currently recommended.

7. Various vaccinations are available in endemic areas, including BCG, killed leprae, and chemically modified organism.

NEUROPATHY ASSOCIATED WITH LYME DISEASE

BACKGROUND

1. *Borrelia burgdorferi,* a spirochete transmitted by ticks:

2. Is transmitted by the deer tick, *Ixodes dammini.*

3. A spirochete acquired by a tick by feeding on an infected host animal, who then transmits the spirochete to its next host when feeding.

4. Approximately 12 to 24 hours of tick attachment are required to accomplish this secondary host infection.

PATHOPHYSIOLOGY

1. The pathogenic mechanism for the Lyme neuropathy is unknown.

2. The neuropathy may be the result of an indirect immunologic response and/or some form of vasculopathy.

PROGNOSIS

Patients improve with appropriate antibiotic treatment.

DIAGNOSIS

Clinical Features

1. Three stages of the disease are recognized:

   a. Early infection (erythema migrans: localized)

   b. Disseminated infection

   c. Late-stage infection

2. Within 1 month following a bite from an infected tick, an expanding erythematous circular region surrounding the original tick bite is noted. However, erythema migrans is not noticed by all patients.
3. With respect to the PNS manifestations, the findings can vary depending upon the stage of the disease.
4. In stage 2 disease, cranial mononeuropathies can be documented. Facial nerve palsy is the most common and is bilateral in about 50% of cases.
5. Asymmetric polyradiculoneuropathies, plexopathies, or multiple mononeuropathies can also occur.
6. Rarely, the patients may be mistaken to have AIDP.
7. In stage 3, a distal symmetric sensorimotor polyneuropathy can occur.

Laboratory Features

1. Antibodies directed against the spirochete can be measured using immunofluorescent or enzyme-linked immunosorbent assay (ELISA). False-positive reactions are not uncommon.
2. Western blot analysis is useful to confirm a positive ELISA.

Electrophysiologic Findings

Nerve conduction studies reveal reduced CMAP and SNAP amplitudes and denervation changes on EMG in the distribution of affected nerves.

TREATMENT

1. Adults with facial nerve palsies secondary to Lyme disease should be treated with amoxicillin 500 mg p.o. q.i.d. plus probenecid 500 mg q.i.d. for 2 to 4 weeks. If they are allergic to penicillin, doxycycline 100 mg p.o. b.i.d. for 2 to 4 weeks should be given.
2. Children younger than 4 years with facial palsies can be treated with amoxicillin 20 to 40 mg/kg/d in four divided doses for 2 to 4 weeks. If allergic to penicillin, children can be treated with erythromycin 30 mg/kg/d in four divided doses for 2 to 4 weeks.
3. Adult patients with other types of peripheral neuropathy are treated with IV penicillin 20 to 24 million U/d for 10 to 14 days or ceftriaxone 2 g IV daily for 2 to 4 weeks. Adults who are allergic to penicillin should receive doxicycline 100 mg p.o. b.i.d. for 30 days.
4. Children with Lyme neuropathy (other than facial nerve palsy) can receive IV penicillin G 250,000 U/kg/d in divided doses for 10 to 14 days or ceftriaxone 50 to 80 mg/kg/d IV for 2 to 4 weeks.

HUMAN IMMUNODEFICIENCY VIRUS–ASSOCIATED DISTAL SYMMETRIC POLYNEUROPATHY

BACKGROUND

Distal symmetric polyneuropathy (DSP) is usually seen in patients with acquired immunodeficiency syndrome (AIDS).

PATHOPHYSIOLOGY

1. Vitamin B_{12} deficiency has been noted in some series, but other studies have suggested that vitamin B_{12} metabolism does not play a significant role in the neurologic complications of HIV infection.

2. Nerve biopsies may demonstrate perivascular inflammation (mainly macrophages and T cells) suggesting a possible immune-mediated basis.

PROGNOSIS

The neuropathy is unfortunately poorly responsive to treatment.

DIAGNOSIS

Clinical Features

1. Patients often complain of numbness and painful paresthesias of the hands and feet.
2. Some patients are asymptomatic but are found to have diminished sensation to all modalities on examination.

Electrophysiologic Findings

The electrodiagnostic medicine examination reveals evidence of a symmetric, axonal, sensory polyneuropathy greater than motor polyneuropathy.

TREATMENT

1. Antiretroviral agents have no demonstrable affect on the course of DSP.
2. Treatment is largely symptomatic pain relief (Table 8-3).

HUMAN IMMUNODEFICIENCY VIRUS–ASSOCIATED POLYRADICULONEUROPATHY

BACKGROUND

Patients with advanced AIDS can develop acute, progressive polyradiculopathy, plexopathy, or multiple mononeuropathies secondary to CMV infection.

PATHOPHYSIOLOGY

The basis is believed to be secondary to infection and secondary inflammation of neurons by CMV.

PROGNOSIS

The prognosis in most patients is poor, with most reported patients with this complication dying within several weeks or months.

DIAGNOSIS

Clinical Features

1. Patients have severe numbness, pain, and weakness in the legs, which is usually asymmetric.
2. They also note a reduction in perineal sensation with painful paresthesias. Incontinence of urine and stool are common.
3. Occasionally, the upper limbs and cranial nerves become involved.

TABLE 8-3. TREATMENT OF PAINFUL SENSORY NEUROPATHIES

Therapy	Route	Dose	Side Effects
First-line			
Tricyclic antidepressants (e.g., amitryptiline, nortriptyline)	p.o.	10–100 mg qhs	Cognitive changes, sedation, dry eyes and mouth, urinary retention, constipation
Gabapentin	p.o.	300–1,200 mg t.i.d.	Cognitive changes, sedation
Second-line			
Carbamezepine	p.o.	200–400 mg q6–8h	Cognitive changes, dizziness, leukopenia, liver dysfunction
Phenytoin	p.o.	200–400 mg qhs	Cognitive changes, dizziness, liver dysfunction
Tramadol	p.o.	50 mg q.i.d.	Cognitive changes, gastrointestinal upset
Third-line			
Mexiletine	p.o.	200–300 mg t.i.d.	Arrhythmias
Other Agents			
Lidocaine 2.5%/pylocaine 2.5% cream	Apply cutaneously	q.i.d.	Local erythema
Lidoderm 5% patch	Apply to painful area	Up to three patches daily	Local erythema
Capsaicin 0.025%–0.075% cream	Apply cutaneously	q.i.d.	Painful burning skin

p.o., by mouth; t.i.d., three times a day; q.i.d, four times a day; qhs, at bedtime.

4. Patients may have evidence of CMV infection in other parts of the body (i.e., CMV retinitis).

Laboratory Features

1. CSF reveals an increased protein, neutrophilic pleocytosis, and decreased glucose.
2. CMV can be cultured from the CSF, blood, and urine.

Electrophysiologic Findings

EMG/NCS demonstrate evidence of an axonal, multifocal polyradiculoneuropathy.

TREATMENT

1. A trial of gancyclovir or foscarnet is warranted, although prognosis is very poor.
2. Pain should be managed similar to other painful neuropathies (see Table 8-3).

HERPES VARICELLA ZOSTER–RELATED NEUROPATHY

BACKGROUND

1. Herpes varicella-zoster (HVZ) infection can result from reactivation of latent virus, or from a primary infection.
2. Primary acquired HVZ infection is frequently associated with severe disseminated zoster in the immunocompromised patients.
3. The incidence of HVZ infection is approximately 480 persons per 100,000.
4. The peak age of developing the disease is between 55 and 75 years of age.

PATHOPHYSIOLOGY

1. Following initial infection, the HZV migrates to the sensory ganglia.
2. With reactivation, the virus replicates and travels down the sensory nerves and results in the typical skin lesions.
3. Motor paresis is postulated to develop by the virus causing local neuritis in the spinal nerve and subsequently gaining access to the motor axons.

PROGNOSIS

Roughly 25% of affected patients have a significant residual of pain referred to as postherpetic pain, which can be quite disabling.

DIAGNOSIS

1. Two thirds of infections are manifested by dermal zoster.
2. Pain and paresthesias in the dermatome region may precede the vesicular rash by a week or more.
3. Five percent to 30% of patients with typical cutaneous herpes zoster can develop some form of motor weakness affecting the myotomal muscles corresponding to the dermatomal distribution of skin lesions.

TREATMENT

1. IV acyclovir can be lifesaving in immunocompromised patients with severe infections.

2. The treatment of postherpetic neuralgia is symptomatic (see Table 8-3).
3. Neurontin and carbamezapine have been noted to be affective in postherpetic neuralgia.
4. Placebo-controlled studies have demonstrated that tricyclic antidepressants reduce the pain in many postherpetic neuralgia patients.
5. Lidoderm 5% patches can be applied over the painful sites. Up to three patches can be used per day.

DIABETIC DISTAL SYMMETRIC SENSORY AND SENSORIMOTOR POLYNEUROPATHY

BACKGROUND

1. The most common form of diabetic neuropathy is distal symmetric sensory polyneuropathy (DSPN).
2. The risk of developing peripheral neuropathy correlates with the duration of DM, the control of hyperglycemia, and the presence of retinopathy and nephropathy.

PATHOPHYSIOLOGY

1. The pathogenic basis for DSPN in unknown and controversial.
2. The major theories involve a metabolic process, ischemic damage, or an immunologic disorder.

PROGNOSIS

The neuropathy is slowly progressive but can be stabilized or improved with good control of the diabetes.

DIAGNOSIS

Clinical Features

1. This is a length-dependent neuropathy, which manifests clinically with sensory loss beginning in the toes and gradual progression over time to involve the legs.
2. The sensory neuropathy can progress to affect the hands, again beginning with the fingers and progressing proximally to result in the commonly referred to "glove and stocking" distribution.
3. When severe, a patient may exhibit sensory loss over the abdominal region progressing from the midline laterally toward, but not typically affecting the back.
4. Patients often complain of tingling, lancinating pains, burning, and a deep aching.
5. While there may be mild atrophy and weakness of foot intrinsics and ankle dorsiflexors, significant weakness is uncommon.
6. Patients with DSPN can also develop symptoms and signs of an autonomic neuropathy.

Electrophysiologic Findings

EMG/NCS demonstrate evidence of a length-dependent, generalized, symmetric, and sensory greater than motor polyneuropathy that is primarily axonal in nature.

TREATMENT

1. Several studies have demonstrated that tight control of glucose can reduce the risk of developing neuropathy or improve the underlying neuropathy.
2. Pancreatic transplantation also results in stabilization or slight improvement.
3. A variety of medications have been used to treat painful symptoms associated with DSPN, including AEMs, antidepressants, sodium channel blockers, and other analgesics with variable success. My approach to treating diabetic neuropathic pain is similar to that of any form of painful sensory neuropathies (see Table 8-3).
4. I usually initiate treatment with gabapentin, generally starting at a dosage of 300 to 400 mg t.i.d. and gradually increasing as tolerated and necessary up to 1,200 mg t.i.d. Other AEMs can be tried in lieu of neurontin including dilantin, carbamezepine, topirmimate, and so forth. There has not been a study clearly demonstrating one agent to be superior to another in neuropathic pain relief.
5. At the same time I give a trial of Lidoderm 5% patches, which can be applied to the feet. Up to 1 ½ patches can be applied to each foot per day.
6. If gabapentin and Lidoderm patches are insufficient to control the pain, I add a tricyclic antidepressant (TCA) (e.g., nortriptyline, amitryptiline) at a dosage of 10 to 25 mg qhs. I increase the dose by 25 mg/mo up to 100 mg qhs or as tolerated.
7. Tramadol 50 mg q.i.d. is given in patients refractory to an AEM in combination with a TCA and Lidoderm patches.
8. Unfortunately, we have not found capsaicin cream to be particularly useful.
9. Treatment of autonomic neuropathy is largely symptomatic.
   a. Orthostatic hypotension can be treated with fluodrocortisone (starting at 0.1 mg b.i.d.) or midodrine (10 mg t.i.d.).
   b. Nonsteroidal antiinflammatory agents may also be of benefit.
   c. Metaclopramide is used to treat diabetic gastroparesis.
   d. Clonidine may help with persistent diarrhea.
   e. Sildenafil has gained popularity in treatment of impotence.

DIABETIC RADICULOPLEXUS NEUROPATHY

BACKGROUND

1. Also known as diabetic amyotrophy, Burns–Garland syndrome, diabetic lumbosacral radiculoplexopathy, and proximal diabetic neuropathy.
2. The polyradiculoneuropathy more commonly affects older patients with DM type II, but it can affect type I diabetics. In approximately one third of patients, the polyradiculoneuropathy is the presenting manifestation of DM.

PATHOPHYSIOLOGY

An immune-mediated microangiopathy has been speculated but not proven.

PROGNOSIS

1. Although the onset is typically unilateral, it is not uncommon for the contralateral leg to become affected several weeks or months later. Rarely, diabetic amyotrophy begins in both legs at the same time.
2. The neuropathy progresses gradually or in a stepwise fashion, usually over several weeks or months, but documented cases of worsening over 18 months have been described.

DIAGNOSIS

Clinical Features

1. The neuropathy usually begins unilaterally with severe pain in the low back, hip, and thigh.
2. Within a few days or weeks, atrophy and weakness of proximal and distal muscles in the affected leg are apparent. About half of the patients complain of numbness and paresthesia.
3. The polyradiculoneuropathy is often heralded by severe weight loss.
4. Thoracic mono- or polyradiculopathies and cervical polyradiculoneuropathy may also occur.

Laboratory Features

1. CSF protein concentration is usually elevated, while cell count is normal.
2. ESRs may be increased.
3. MRI scans of the lumbosacral roots and plexus can reveal inflammatory changes.

Electrophysiologic Findings

1. In patients with underlying DSPN, electrophysiologic features of a generalized axonal sensorimotor polyneuropathy as described above are evident.
2. The NCSs and EMG of diabetic amyotrophy reflect multifocal axonal damage to the roots and plexus.
3. Needle EMG demonstrates positive sharp waves and fibrillation potentials in proximal and distal muscles in the affected limbs and in paraspinal muscles. Recruitment of MUAPs is reduced in weak muscle groups. As reinnervation occurs over time, large-amplitude, long-duration, polyphasic MUAPs can be appreciated.

TREATMENT

1. Small retrospective studies have reported that IVIG, prednisone, and other forms of immunosuppressive therapy are effective in treating patients with diabetic amyotrophy.
2. I generally avoid treating with IVIG given the increased risk of renal failure due to acute tubular necrosis in diabetics.
3. I have been impressed that short courses of corticosteroids can help ease the pain associated with the severe polyradiculoneuropathy. This may allow the patients to undergo physical therapy.
   a. I start prednisone 50 mg/d for 1 week, then taper by 10 mg/wk.
   b. This should be done in conjunction with the patients primary care provider as the glucose needs to be monitored closely and insulin/oral hypoglycemic agents adjusted during this short course of prednisone.

CRITICAL ILLNESS POLYNEUROPATHY

BACKGROUND

1. As opposed to AIDP and myasthenia gravis, which are the most common neuromuscular causes for admission to intensive care units (ICUs), weakness that develops in critically ill patients in the ICU setting usually is secondary to critical illness polyneuropathy, critical illness myopathy, or much less commonly, prolonged neuromuscular blockade.

2. In my experience, critical illness myopathy is much more common than critical illness neuropathy.

PATHOPHYSIOLOGY

The pathogenic basis of critical illness polyneuropathy is not clear.

PROGNOSIS

In patients who survive the underlying sepsis and multiorgan failure, muscle strength recovers slowly over several months.

DIAGNOSIS

Clinical Features

1. The peripheral neuropathy is often first suspected when the patient is unable to be weaned from a ventilator.
2. It is often difficult to ascertain the degree of sensory loss and modalities if the patient's mental status is altered. Nevertheless, generalized weakness of the limb muscles can be appreciated.
3. Deep tendon reflexes are absent or reduced.

Laboratory Features

1. CSF is usually normal or only mildly elevated, unlike AIDP and CIDP in which there is usually significantly increased CSF protein.
2. Serum CK levels are normal.

Electrophysiologic Features

1. Motor and sensory nerve NCS are remarkable for reduced or absent potentials.
2. EMG reveals profuse positive sharp waves and fibrillation potentials and decreased recruitment of MUAPS. It is not unusual in patients with severe weakness to be unable to recruit MUAPs.

TREATMENT

1. There is no specific therapy for critical illness neuropathy other than supportive care and treatment of the underlying sepsis and organ failure.
2. Physical and occupational therapy are essential to prevent contractures and build strength and endurance as the patient recovers.

PARANEOPLASTIC SENSORY NEUROPATHY/GANGLIONOPATHY

BACKGROUND

1. Small cell lung carcinoma is the most common associated malignancy, but cases of carcinoma of the esophagus, breast, ovaries, and kidney and lymphoma have also been reported.
2. The disorder is rare and most commonly effects females in late middle life with a mean age of onset of 59 years.

PATHOPHYSIOLOGY

Antigenic similarity between proteins in the tumor cells and the neuron cells may lead to an immune response directed against both tumor and neuronal cells.

PROGNOSIS

Unfortunately the neuropathy generally does not improve with treatment of the tumor or with immunosuppressive/immunomodulatory therapy.

DIAGNOSIS

Clinical Features

1. The predominant symptoms are the subacute onset of numbness, dysesthesia and paresthesia, beginning distally then spreading proximally.
2. These symptoms begin in the arms in over 60% and is asymmetric in approximately 40% of cases.
3. The onset can be quite acute or insidiously progressive.
4. Alterations in mental status, autonomic dysfunction, and cranial nerve abnormalities occur in about two thirds of patients as a result of a superimposed paraneoplastic encephalomyelitis.
5. While most cases of sensory neuronopathy have only sensory abnormalities, mild weakness may occasionally be evident.
6. The symptoms of the neuropathy may precede those of the cancer by several months or years. Discovery of a sensory neuronopathy should lead to an aggressive evaluation for an underlying malignancy. I obtain a chest CT scan, mammogram, pelvic CT or ultrasound, and antineuronal nuclear antibodies (anti-Hu).

Laboratory Features

1. CSF may be normal or may demonstrate mild lymphocytic pleocytosis and elevated protein.
2. Type 1 antineuronal nuclear antibody (ANNA-1), also known as "anti-Hu," can be demonstrated in serum and CSF in patients with small cell carcinoma of the lung complicated by paraneoplastic sensory or sensorimotor polyneuropathy, encephalitis and cerebellar degeneration.
3. I advise obtaining a chest radiograph every 3 months and chest CT or MRI every 6 months in patients who initially have no identifiable cancer but have a sensory neuronopathy with a positive ANNA-1.

Electrophysiologic Findings

1. NCS reveal low-amplitude or absent SNAPs with normal CMAPs.
2. Further, one can see abnormal SNAPs in the hands when SNAPs are normal in the legs. This feature is suggestive of a ganglionopathy as opposed to the much more common length-dependent axonopathies in which the sural SNAPs are affected earlier and more severely than the upper limb SNAPs.

TREATMENT

1. Treatment of the underlying cancer may prolong survival but generally does not affect the course of the underlying neuronopathy. However, there are rare cases of remission following treatment of the tumor.
2. Immunosuppressive and immunomodulatory therapy with prednisone, plasma exchange, and IVIG are typically not effective.
3. Supportive care with treatment of associated neuropathic pain (see Table 8-3).
4. Physical and occupational therapy are helpful.

NEUROPATHY ASSOCIATED WITH POEMS SYNDROME

BACKGROUND

1. Crow–Fukase or POEMS syndrome (P = polyneuropathy, O = organomegaly, E = endocrinopathy, M = monoclonal gammopathy, S = skin changes).
2. Patients may display all or none of these features.
3. Most patients have osteosclerotic myeloma, but POEMS can also be seen with Castleman disease, extramedullary plasmacytomas, or a solitary lytic plasmacytomas.

PATHOPHYSIOLOGY

The pathogenesis of POEMS syndrome is not clear, but likely autoimmune in nature.

PROGNOSIS

1. The neuropathy improves in almost 50% of cases treated with radiation, prednisone with or without some other form of chemotherapy.
2. However, the neuropathy and plasmacytoma can recur even in patients with an initial positive response to treatment.

DIAGNOSIS

Clinical Features

1. The neuropathy manifests as tingling, numbness, and weakness of the distal lower limbs that gradually progresses proximally in the lower limbs into the upper limbs similar to CIDP.
2. The peripheral neuropathy is usually present for several years prior to establishing the correct diagnosis.

Laboratory Features

1. Most patients have a IgG or IgA lambda chain monoclonal gammopathy.
2. In up to 20% of patients, the monoclonal protein is demonstrated in the urine but not in serum.
3. CSF protein levels are often elevated similar to CIDP.

Radiographic Studies

1. Skeletal survey reveals characteristic sclerotic (two thirds of cases) or mixed sclerotic and lytic bony lesions (one third of cases) usually in the vertebral bodies, pelvis, or ribs.
2. In 50% of cases, these skeletal lesions, which represent focal plasmacytomas, are multiple.

Electrophysiologic Findings

1. NCSs are suggestive of a demyelinating or mixed axonal and demyelinative sensorimotor peripheral neuropathy similar to CIDP.
2. Needle electromyographic examination can demonstrate fibrillation potentials and positive sharp waves with reduced recruitment of MUAPs of long duration and increased amplitude.

TREATMENT

1. The neuropathy may respond to radiation or a surgical excision of the isolated plasmacytoma or to chemotherapy.
2. The neuropathy can also improve with usual treatment given to patients with idiopathic CIDP (e.g., corticosteroids) (see Table 8-1).

NEUROPATHY ASSOCIATED WITH PRIMARY AMYLOIDOSIS

BACKGROUND

1. Amyloidosis is a relatively nonspecific name coined to designate a heterogeneous collection of various disorders all sharing the unified theme of amyloid deposition in different organs.
2. Classification of amyloidosis is based on the hereditary or acquired nature of the disease and the identification of the major protein constituent of the accumulating amyloid.
3. Familial amyloidosis is caused by mutations in the genes for transthyretin, apolipoprotein A-1, or gelsolin. Familial amyloidosis is discussed in the section on Hereditary Neuropathies.
4. Secondary amyloidosis (AA) is seen in patients with rheumatoid arthritis and other chronic inflammatory diseases and is associated with the accumulation of protein A. Peripheral neuropathy is uncommon.
5. Primary amyloidosis (AL amyloidosis) is the designation given when the amyloid is composed of light chains, thus the term "AL amyloidosis." Primary amyloidosis can occur in the setting of multiple myeloma, Waldenström macroglobulinemia, lymphoma, other plasmacytomas or lymphoproliferative disorders, or without any other identifiable disease.

PATHOPHYSIOLOGY

Light chains deposit in peripheral nerves.

PROGNOSIS

The prognosis of patients with primary amyloidosis is poor with a median survival of 2 years. Death is generally secondary to progressive congestive heart failure or renal failure.

DIAGNOSIS

Clinical Features

1. Primary (AL) amyloidosis is a systemic disorder that typically affects men past the sixth decade of life.
2. Peripheral neuropathy occurs in 1% to 30% of patients with AL amyloidosis and may be the presenting manifestation in one sixth of cases.
3. Initially small-fiber modalities are affected, resulting in painful dysesthesias along with diminished pain and temperature sensation.
4. The neuropathy is slowly progressive and eventually symmetric weakness develops, beginning in the distal lower limbs along with large fiber, discriminatory sensory loss.
5. Most patients develop autonomic involvement with postural hypertension, syncope, impotence, gastrointestinal disturbance, impaired sweating, loss of bladder control.

6. Carpal tunnel syndrome (CTS) occurs in 25% of patients and may be the presenting manifestation.

Laboratory Features

1. The amyloid is composed of the complete or variable portion of the monoclonal light chain.
2. Lambda (λ) is more common than kappa (κ) light chains (2:1) in AL amyloidosis.

Histopathology

1. Nerve biopsies may reveal amyloid deposition in either the globular or diffuse pattern infiltrating the epineurial and endoneurial connected tissue and in blood vessel walls.
2. Congo red or metachromatic staining confirms amyloidosis.
3. Immunohistochemistry is used to demonstrate that the amyloid deposits are secondary to light chain accumulation as opposed to transthyretin [familial amyloid polyneuropathy (FAP)].

Electrophysiologic Findings

1. NCSs may be normal early on secondary to a propensity to damage small fibers initially.
2. Median neuropathy at the wrist (CTS) is also a common finding.
3. With time, an axonal or mixed-axonal demyelinating sensory greater than motor neuropathy picture develops.

TREATMENT

1. Chemotherapy with melphalan, prednisone, colchicine that reduce the concentration of monoclonal proteins have generally been unsatisfactory.
2. Treatment is directed at supportive care (e.g., physical and occupational therapy).
3. Treat autonomic dysfunction as per section on Idiopathic Autonomic Neuropathy.
4. Neuropathic pain can be treated with a variety of medications (see Table 8-3).

NEUROPATHY ASSOCIATED WITH MONOCLONAL GAMMOPATHY OF UNCERTAIN SIGNFICANCE (MGUS)

BACKGROUND

1. MGUS is a term referring to monoclonal gammopathies occurring in the absence of a defined myeloma, plasmacytoma, lymphoma and so forth.
2. Cancer subsequently develops in some patients over time.
3. MGUS neuropathy is heterogeneic in regards to clinical, laboratory, and electrophysiologic features.
4. The neuropathies can be either demyelinating or axonal. Neuropathies associated with an IgM monoclonal protein are typically demyelinating, while IgG and IgA monoclonal gammopathies can be axonal or demyelinating in nature.

PATHOPHYSIOLOGY

1. The demyelinating neuropathies are likely immunologic in nature.

2. The relationship of the axonal neuropathies and the monoclonal gammopathies are less clear. The monoclonal proteins in such cases are not necessarily pathogenic, thus explaining the lack of efficacy in treatments dedicated to lowering the concentration of the monoclonal protein.

PROGNOSIS

1. Demyelinating proteins associated with IgM monoclonal gammopathy (often antibodies directed against myelin-associated glycoprotein) are usually associated with distal sensory loss and minimal weakness. This so-called distal acquired demyelinating neuropathy is generally refractory to immunosuppressive and immunomodulating therapies.
2. Demyelinating neuropathies associated with IgG or IgA monoclonal gammopathies are indistinguishable from CIDP and are similarly responsive to immunosuppressive and immunomodulatory therapies.
3. Axonal neuropathies and IgM, IgG, or IgA monoclonal gammopathies are typically not responsive to immunotherapy.

DIAGNOSIS

Clinical Features

1. Patients can present with symmetric proximal and distal weakness typical of idiopathic CIDP.
2. Patients with an axonal neuropathy present with distal sensory loss in a length-dependent fashion.

Laboratory Features

1. At least 50% of the patients with IgM-MGUS neuropathy have antibodies directed against myelin-associated glycoprotein (MAG).
2. Elevated CSF levels are common in patients with a demyelinating neuropathy.

Electrophysiologic Findings

1. IgG and IgA MGUS neuropathies can be either axonal or demyelinating in nature.

TREATMENT

1. Patients with MGUS-neuropathy who fulfill clinical and electrophysiologic criteria for CIDP should be treated with immunotherapy as recommended in the CIDP section (see Table 8-1).
2. Patients with IgM-MGUS demyelinating neuropathy and predominantly sensory symptoms are refractory to treatment and I generally to not treat these patients with immunosuppressive agents, IVIG or PE. There have been a number of anecdotal reports and small retrospective studies suggesting benefit but subsequent double-blind, controlled studies have all failed to demonstrate efficacy.

NEUROPATHY ASSOCIATED WITH LEAD INTOXICATION

BACKGROUND

1. Lead neuropathy is increasingly rare.

2. Seen in children who consume lead-based paints in older buildings and in industrial workers dealing with metals, batteries, or paints containing lead products.

PATHOPHYSIOLOGY

It is unclear whether the primary target of the toxic insult is the anterior horn cell or more distally in the peripheral or motor nerve.

PROGNOSIS

Progressive disorder if untreated.

DIAGNOSIS

Clinical Features

1. Patients may note the insidious and progressive onset of upper limb weakness. Classically, there is noticeably motor involvement of the radial nerve with a wrist/finger extensor weakness. When the lower limbs are involved, an asymmetric foot drop is likely to noted.
2. There are few or no sensory complaints and sensory examination to all modalities is usually found to be well-preserved.

Laboratory Features

1. Elevated serum coproporphyrin level, basophilic stippling of erythrocytes, and reduced hemoglobin content suggesting a microcytic/hypochromic anemia.
2. A 24-hour urine collection reveals elevated levels of lead excretion.

Electrophysiologic Findings

Motor and sensory NCSs and EMG findings are consistent with an axonal, motor greater than sensory neuropathy.

TREATMENT

1. The most important treatment is removing the source of the exposure and chelation therapy with calcium disodium ethylenediamine tetraacetate (EDTA) 25 mg/kg/d (up to 1 g/d) IV for 3 days.
2. British anti-Lewisite (BAL) and pencillamine also demonstrate variable efficacy.

NEUROPATHY ASSOCIATED WITH THALLIUM INTOXICATION

BACKGROUND

Thallium is available as a rodenticide and occasionally may be recognized in persons who are the victim of homicide attempts.

PATHOGENESIS

It is not known whether the primary insult is on the neuronal cell body or the axons. Neither is the pathogenic basis for the toxicity known.

PROGNOSIS

A lethal dose of thallium in humans is rather variable, but averages about 1 g or 8 to 15 mg/kg and death can result in less than 48 hours following a particularly large dose.

DIAGNOSIS

Clinical Features

1. Patients usually present with burning pain and paresthesias in the feet bilaterally, abdominal pain, and vomiting.
2. With severe intoxication, proximal weakness and involvement of the cranial nerves can occur. Some patients require mechanical ventilation due to respiratory muscle involvement.
3. The hallmark of thallium poisoning is alopecia, however, this may not be evident until the third or fourth week after exposure and can be rather mild in some patients.

Laboratory Features

1. Serum and urine levels of thallium are increased.
2. Routine laboratory testing can reveal anemia, azotemia, and liver function abnormalities.
3. CSF protein levels are elevated.

Electrophysiologic Findings

EMG and NCSs are consistent with a severe axonal sensorimotor polyneuropathy.

TREATMENT

1. In acute intoxication, potassium ferric ferrocyanide II may be effective in preventing absorption of thallium from the gut. However, it is not clear if the medication is effective once thallium has been absorbed.
2. Unfortunately, chelating agents have not been found to be particularly useful.
3. Maintaining adequate diuresis will help in eliminating thallium from the body without increasing tissue availability from the serum.

NEUROPATHY ASSOCIATED WITH ARSENIC INTOXICATION

BACKGROUND

Arsenic is another heavy metal that can cause a toxic sensorimotor polyneuropathy. The neuropathy begins 5 to 10 days after ingestion of arsenic and progress for several weeks.

PATHOPHYSIOLOGY

The pathogenic basis of arsenic toxicity is not known.

PROGNOSIS

If the dosage ingested is large enough, rapid progression to death secondary to vascular collapse may ensue.

DIAGNOSIS

Clinical Features

1. Abrupt onset of abdominal discomfort, nausea, vomiting, pain, and diarrhea followed within several days by the development of a burning sensation in the feet and hands.
2. Soon thereafter, progressive loss of muscle strength distally develops.
3. With severe intoxication, weakness progresses to proximal muscles and the cranial nerves. Some patients may require mechanical ventilation.
4. These symptoms and signs can be suggestive of GBS.
5. Mees lines, which are transverse line at the base of the fingernails and toenails, may become evident by 1 or 2 months.

Laboratory Features

1. Clearance from blood is rapid, therefore serum concentration of arsenic is not diagnostically helpful.
2. Arsenic levels are increased in the urine, hair, or fingernails of affected patients.
3. Similar to lead intoxication, basophilic stippling of erythrocytes can occasionally be observed as well as an aplastic anemia with pancytopenia. Increased CSF protein levels without pleocytosis as seen in AIDP can be demonstrated as well.

Electrophysiologic Findings

EMG and NCSs are consistent with a severe axonal sensorimotor polyneuropathy.

TREATMENT

1. Chelation therapy with British anti-Lewisite (BAL) has yielded inconsistent results in small retrospective studies.
2. The beneficial effect, if any, from BAL is not dramatic and therefore is not recommended.
3. Treatment is supportive.

NEUROPATHY ASSOCIATED WITH VITAMIN B$_{12}$ DEFICIENCY

BACKGROUND

1. Vitamin B$_{12}$–deficient states can thus occur as a result of dietary deficiency (vegetarian diet), lack of intrinsic factor (pernicious anemia with autoimmune destruction of parietal cells, or gastrectomy), malabsorption syndromes (sprue or lower ileum resection), genetic defects in methionine synthetase, and bacteria (blind-loop syndrome) or parasites (tapeworm).
2. Cobalamin is necessary for demethylation of methyltetrahydrofolate.
3. Tetrahydrofolate, in turn, is important in the production of folate coenzymes, which are required for DNA synthesis.

PATHOPHYSIOLOGY

1. The pathogenic mechanism for the neuropathy associated with cobalamin deficiency is not known.
2. The neuropathy may result from the above-noted impairment in DNA synthesis or secondary to some other biochemical defect.

PROGNOSIS

Although the neuropathy may not improve, further deterioration may be prevented by treatment with vitamin B_{12}.

DIAGNOSIS

Clinical Features

1. Patients present with numbness in the distal lower extremities.
2. Numbness may begin in the hands and mimic CTS but this is secondary to the myelopathy associated with B_{12} deficiency and not the neuropathy.
3. The combination of hyporeflexia and extensor plantar responses in a patient with numb extremities and gait instability should make one suspicious for B_{12} deficiency.

Laboratory Features

1. Serum B_{12} levels are decreased or in the low range of normal.
2. In patients with B_{12} levels in the low normal range but with symptoms and signs suggestive of cobalamine deficiency, it is important to assess for serum or urine levels of methylmalonic acid and homocysteine. These metabolites are increased in patients with cobalamine deficiency and can precede abnormalities in serum B_{12} concentrations.
3. A CBC and smear can reveal megaloblastic anemia. Importantly, the neurologic complications of cobalamine deficiency can be evident before the hematologic abnormalities are appreciated.
4. Patients with an autoimmune basis for their B_{12} deficiency may demonstrate autoantibodies directed against gastric parietal cells.

Electrophysiologic Findings

1. EMG and NCS reveal features of an axonal sensory greater than motor polyneuropathy.
2. Somatosensory evoked potentials and magnetic stimulation demonstrate slowing of central conduction.

TREATMENT

Cobalamin deficiency is treated with intramuscular injections of vitamin B_{12} 1 g every day for 5 days then 1 g IM every month.

NEUROPATHY ASSOCIATED WITH VITAMIN E DEFICIENCY

BACKGROUND

Three major conditions are associated with vitamin E deficiency:
1. Deficient fat absorption (e.g., cystic fibrosis, chronic cholestasis, short-bowel syndrome, and intestinal lymphangiectasia)
2. Deficient fat transport (abetalipoproteinemia, hypobetalipoproteinemia, normotriglyeridemic abetalipoproteinemia, and chylomicron retention disease)
3. A genetically based abnormality of vitamin E metabolism

PATHOPHYSIOLOGY

1. The pathogenic basis for the neuropathy is unknown.
2. Vitamin E has antioxidant properties and may serve to modulate glutamate excitotoxicity.
3. The dorsal root ganglia and posterior column nuclei have the lowest concentrations of vitamin E in the nervous system.
4. Low concentrations of vitamin E may leave these neurons particularly vulnerable to deficiency of the vitamin and its possible neuroprotective effects.

PROGNOSIS

Early recognition is imperative since treatment can arrest and sometimes reverse the neurologic symptoms.

DIAGNOSIS

Clinical Features

1. Patients present with numbness, incoordination, and gait instability.
2. Physical examination reveals loss of vibratory perception, proprioception, a positive Romberg test, and ataxia. Ocular examination reveals ophthalmoplegia and retinopathy in patients with significant disease. Muscle stretch reflexes are reduced.

Laboratory Features

Serum vitamin E level is reduced.

Electrophysiologic Findings

1. Sensory NCSs reveal reduced amplitudes or are absent.
2. Somatosensory evoked potentials demonstrate normal peripheral nerve potentials with marked slowing and attenuation of central responses documenting slowing of central conduction with loss of posterior column fibers.
3. Motor conduction studies are normal.

TREATMENT

1. Treatment is initiated with vitamin E 400 mg b.i.d. and is gradually increased up to 100 mg/kg/d until vitamin E levels normalize.
2. Patients with malabsorption syndromes require water-miscible vitamin E preparations or IM injections of vitamin E in doses of 100 mg/wk.

CHRONIC IDIOPATHIC SENSORY OR SENSORIMOTOR POLYNEUROPATHY

BACKGROUND

1. Chronic acquired chronic sensory or sensory motor polyneuropathies occur in approximately 3% of middle-aged to older adults.
2. Despite extensive evaluation, as many as 50% of all polyneuropathies cannot be determined and thus are categorized as chronic idiopathic polyneuropathy.

PATHOPHYSIOLOGY

The pathogenic basis is not known.

PROGNOSIS

1. Sensory symptoms begin in the toes, slowly progress up the legs, and eventually reach the distal upper limbs.
2. In about 50% of patients, sensory symptoms are confined to the lower limbs.
3. The average time to involvement of the upper limbs is about 5 years.
4. Mild distal weakness and atrophy involving foot intrinsic muscles may develop over time.

DIAGNOSIS

Clinical Features

1. Most patients present with sensory symptoms between the ages of 45 and 70 years.
2. Patients often complain of numbness, tingling, or pain (e.g., sharp stabbing paresthesias, burning, or deep aching sensation) in the feet.

Laboratory Features

1. The diagnosis of chronic idiopathic polyneuropathy is one of exclusion.
2. Laboratory testing for DM, ANA, erythrocyte sedimentation rate (ESR), serum and urine protein electropheresis (SPEP, UPEP), B_{12} level, and thyroid, liver, and renal functions should all be normal.

Electrophysiologic Findings

1. Sensory NCSs demonstrate either absent or reduced amplitudes, particularly of the sural SNAPs.
2. Motor conduction tests demonstrate reduced amplitudes of peroneal and posterior tibial nerves in about 60%.
3. EMG reveals positive sharp waves, fibrillation potentials, and reduced recruitment in distal lower limb muscles.
4. Within the category of idiopathic sensory or sensorimotor polyneuropathies are patients that appear to have pure small-fiber sensory neuropathies.
   a. By definition, these patients have normal nerve conduction.
   b. Skin biopsies can be performed to measure the density of intraepidermal nerve fibers.

TREATMENT

1. There is no treatment for slowing the progression or reversing the "numbness" or lack of sensation.
2. My approach to treating the painful paresthesias and burning sensation associated with chronic idiopathic sensory neuropathy is similar to the treatment of neuropathic pain regardless of etiology (e.g., painful sensory neuropathies related to DM, HIV infection, herpes zoster infection) (see Table 8-3).

ENTRAPMENT/COMPRESSION NEUROPATHIES

BACKGROUND

1. The most common entrapment neuropathies in the arms involve the median nerve at the wrist (CTS) and ulnar neuropathies at the elbow and lesser extent at the wrist.
2. In the legs, peroneal neuropathy across the fibular head is the most common.

PATHOPHYSIOLOGY

Compression of these nerves initially leads to focal demyelination and block of conduction. If compression is severe and prolonged, secondary axonal loss ensues.

PROGNOSIS

Most patients improve with surgery if conservative treatment fails.

DIAGNOSIS

1. Patients describe numbness, paresthesias, and weakness in the distribution of affected nerves.
2. NCSs are used to demonstrate focal slowing across area of compression.

TREATMENT

1. CTS:
   a. Conservative therapy with neutral angle wrist splints, a nonsteroidal medication (e.g., ibuprofen 200–800 mg t.i.d. to q.i.d.) are initiated in patients with suspected CTS.
   b. If no relief with conservative management, I refer patients to a hand surgeon.
2. Ulnar neuropathy at elbow:
   a. Instruct patients on not leaning on elbow.
   b. Elbow pad to buffer the ulnar nerve against compression.
   c. If no improvement with conservative management, I refer for surgery.
3. Ulnar neuropathy at the wrist:
   a. It is important to image the hand with MRI to look for structural abnormalities (e.g., ganglion cysts) that might be compressing the nerve).
   b. If such abnormalities are evident, surgery is recommended, otherwise management is supportive with physical and occupational therapy.
4. Peroneal neuropathy at the fibular head:
   a. Cause is external compression (e.g., crossing legs), rather than entrapment.
   b. Treatment is conservative: avoid crossing legs, physical therapy, ankle–foot orthosis for foot drop.

CHARCOT–MARIE–TOOTH DISEASE

BACKGROUND

The various categories of CMT are subclassified according to the nature of the pathology (e.g., demyelinating or axonal), mode of inheritance (autosomal dominant, autosomal recessive, or X-linked), age of onset (e.g., infancy or childhood/adulthood) and the specific mutated gene (Table 8-4).

PATHOPHYSIOLOGY

Mutations have been identified in various genes in the different forms of CMT. New mutations responsible for different forms of CMT are found at a fast pace. Recent information can be found on the internet: http://molgen-www.uia.ac.be/CMTMutations/.

TABLE 8-4. CLASSIFICATION OF CHARCOT-MARIE–TOOTH DISEASE AND RELATED NEUROPATHIES

Name	Pathology	Inheritance	Gene Location	Gene Product
CMT1	Demyelination and onion bulbs			
CMT1A		AD	17p11.2	PMP-22
CMT1B		AD	1q21-23	P_0
CMT1C		AD	?	?
CMT1D		AD	10q21.1-22.1	ERG2
CMT2	Axonal atrophy and degeneration			
CMT2A		AD	1p35-p36	KIF1B β
CMT2B		AD	3q13-q22	?
CMT2C with vocal cord and diaphragm paralysis		AD	?	?
CMT2D		AD	7p14	?
CMT2E (allelic to SMA5)		AD	8p21	Neurofilament light chain
CMT2X		X-linked	Xq24	?
CMT3 (Dejerine–Sottas disease, congenital hypomyelinating neuropathy)	Severe hypomyelination, classic onion bulbs, or basal lamina onion bulbs			
		AD	17p11.2	PMP-22
		AD	1q21-23	P_0
		AD	10q21.1-22.1	ERG2
		There may be AR and sporadic forms as well		
CMT4	All forms have hypomyelination			
CMT4A	Basal lamina onion bulbs	AR	8q13-21.1	GDAP1
CMT4B	Focally folded myelin sheaths	AR	11q23	MTMR2
CMT4C	Classic onion bulbs	AR	5q23-33	?
CMT4E (HMSN-Lom)	Demyelination	AR	8q24	NDRG1
CMT4F	Severe hypomyelination, onion bulbs	AR	19q13.1-13.3	Periaxin
CMTX	Mixed axonal and demyelinating features	X-linked dominant	Xq13	Connexin-32
HNPP	Demyelination, axonal atrophy, and tomacula	AD	17p11.2	PMP-22
		AD	1q21-23	P_0
HNA	Axonal degeneration	AD	17q24	?
HMSN-P	Neuronopathy	AD	3q13-q14	?
Giant axonal neuropathy	Giant axonal swellings	AR	16q24	Gigaxonin

CMT, Charcot-Marie–Tooth; HNPP, hereditary neuropathy with liability to pressure palsies; HNA, hereditary neuralgic amyotrophy; SMA, spinal muscular atrophy; HMSN-P, hereditary motor and sensory neuropathy—proximal; AD, autosomal dominant; AR, autosomal recessive; PMP-22, peripheral myelin protein-22; P_0, myelin protein zero protein; ERG2, early growth response-2 protein; MTMR2, myotubularin-related protein-2; NDRG1, N-myc-downstream-regulated gene; KIF1B β, kinesin; GDAP1, ganglioside-induced differentiation-associated protein-1

PROGNOSIS

There is a broad spectrum of severity even within the specific subtypes of CMT.

DIAGNOSIS

1. CMT1:
   a. Usually manifests in the first to third decades, with atrophy and weakness of the peroneal muscle groups resulting in progressive foot drop. Atrophy and weakness of the hand intrinsics follows.
   b. Most patients have pes cavus or equinovarus and hammertoes.
   c. Electrophysiologic findings:
      1) The sensory NCS in both the upper and lower limbs are usually markedly abnormal in most patients with CMT1.
      2) Motor NCS reveal markedly prolonged distal latencies and slow conduction velocities, usually in the range of 20 to 25 m/s. Unlike acquired demyelinating neuropathies (AIDP/GBS and CIDP), conduction block and temporal dispersion are not seen.
   d. Genetic testing is available to look for mutations involving *PMP22* (CMT1A), P_0 (CMT1B), and *ERG2* (CMT1D).
2. CMT2:
   a. The peak age of symptom onset in CMT2 is usually in the second decade, with some patients becoming symptomatic only in their seventh decade.
   b. Clinical features are very similar to those of CMT1. CMT2C is associated with vocal cord pararesis and diaphragmatic weakness and may present in infancy or early childhood.
   c. Electrophysiologic findings:
      1) The electrodiagnostic medicine findings in the various subtypes of CMT2 are quite distinct from those in CMT1.
      2) Sensory and motor NCS reveal reduced or absent SNAP amplitudes in both the upper and lower limbs.
      3) Distal latencies are either normal or only mildly prolonged and conduction velocities are also normal or only mildly slow.
   d. Genetic testing is available for only some types of CMT2 (e.g., *NFL* gene mutations in CMT2E).
3. CMT3 (Dejérine–Sottas disease, congenital hypomyelinating neuropathy):
   a. Manifests as generalized weakness and hypotonia at birth.
   b. Respiratory distress and swallowing difficulties are not uncommon, and unfortunately, the course is usually terminal in days to a few months.
   c. In less severe cases, infants appear normal at birth, but motor milestones are delayed. Some children achieve independent ambulation, although it may take several years.
   d. Electrophysiologic findings:
      1) The characteristic nerve conduction findings in CMT3 are the profound demyelinating features.
      2) SNAPs are usually unobtainable.
      3) Motor nerve conduction velocities are markedly slow (typically 5–10 m/s or less), distal latencies very prolonged with only moderately reduced amplitudes.
   e. Genetic testing is available to document mutations in *PMP22,* P_0, and the *ERG2* genes. As evident from the gene mutations, CMT3 is just a more severe form of CMT1.
4. CMT4:
   a. Resembles CMT1/CMT3 clinically and electrophysiologically.
   b. Onset can be in infancy or early adulthood.
   c. Nerve biopsies reveal severe hypomyelination with basal lamina onion bulbs in CMT4A, excessively fold myelin sheaths in CMT4B, classic onion bulbs in CMT4C.
   d. Electrophysiologic findings:

      1) SNAPs are generally unobtainable.

      2) CMAPs are usually reduced in amplitude.

      3) Motor NCSs are slow, ranging from less than 10 m/s to 30 m/s.

   e. Genetic testing is available for some types of CMT4

5. X-Linked Charcot–Marie–Tooth Disease (CMTX):

   a. CMTX is an X-linked dominant disorder, which has clinical features similar to CMT1, except that the neuropathy is much more severe in men than in women.

   b. CMTX comprises approximately 12% of the overall CMT cases.

   c. Onset in men usually occurs in the first two decades of life. In contrast to men, obligate women carriers are frequently asymptomatic.

   d. Electrophysiologic findings:

      1) NCS abnormalities consistent with demyelination and axonal degeneration and are much more prominent in men compared to women.

      2) SNAPs are reduced in amplitude or absent in most patients. When obtainable, the distal latencies and conduction velocities of the SNAPs are slow.

      3) Motor nerve conductions reveal normal or moderately reduced amplitudes.

      4) Distal motor latencies are prolonged in men more than women.

      5) In men, motor conduction velocities are in the range of 30 m/s, whereas in women they are slightly faster, in the range of 35 to 45 m/s.

   e. Genetic testing is available to screen for mutations in the connexin 32 gene.

TREATMENT

1. There are no specific medical therapies available to reverse or slow the progression of the various forms of CMT.

2. Primary treatment is supportive.

3. When cramping pain is severe, quinine sulfate 325 mg qhs is given.

4. Physical and occupational therapy are essential to prevent contractures and optimize the patient's functional capabilities.

5. Some patients with foot drop will benefit from bracing (e.g., ankle foot orthotics for foot drop). Bracing of the hands and fingers at night, although cumbersome, may help prevent claw deformities of the fingers.

6. Other orthotic devices may be useful to help with distal hand intrinsic weakness.

7. Genetic counseling is imperative for the patient and other family members.

HEREDITARY SENSORY AND AUTONOMIC NEUROPATHIES

BACKGROUND

There are a group of rare disorders described as hereditary sensory and autonomic neuropathies (HSANs), which have traditionally been classified into five different types.

PATHOPHYSIOLOGY

Mutations have been identified in various genes for the different subtypes of HSAN.

PROGNOSIS

These disorders are progressive but the morbidity and mortality are variable in the different subtypes.

DIAGNOSIS

See Table 8-5.

TREATMENT

1. There are no specific medical therapies available.
2. Treatment is primarily supportive.
3. Prevention of mutilating skin lesions with instruction to patients and families regarding the risk of trauma due to insensitivity of pain.
4. Appropriate antibiotics to treat skin ulcerations and osteomyelitis bone lesions.
5. Physical and occupational therapy.

FAMILIAL AMYLOID POLYNEUROPATHIES

BACKGROUND

There are several forms of FAP.

PATHOPHYSIOLOGY

Mutations in the genes for transthyretin (*TTR*), apolipoprotein A1, or gelsolin are responsible for the various forms of FAP. Mutations in *TTR* are the most common cause.

PROGNOSIS

Most patients die by the age of 50 years from systemic complications, although some patients do not manifest symptoms until late in life.

DIAGNOSIS

1. TTR-associated FAP.
   a. Characterized by the development of a generalized or multifocal sensorimotor polyneuropathy.
   b. Superimposed CTS is common and may be presenting feature.
   c. Patients usually develop numbness in the distal lower limbs in the third decade of life. Pain and temperature sensation are the most common modalities affected. Patients often describe stabbing, lancinating pains in the feet.
   d. Autonomic dysfunction can be quite severe resulting in impotence, postural hypotension, constipation, or persistent diarrhea.
   e. Later in the course of the illness, distal limb atrophy and weakness can be appreciated.
   f. Occasionally, cranial neuropathies develop.
   g. Vitreous opacities may also be apparent.
2. Apolipoprotein A1-associated FAP:
   a. Patients develop numbness and painful dysesthesias in the lower limbs in the fourth decade of life. Muscle weakness and atrophy is also seen.
   b. Symptoms progress to the distal upper limbs and more proximally.
   c. Autonomic neuropathy is not severe, but some patients develop diarrhea, constipation, and gastroparesis.
3. Gelsolin-associated FAP:

TABLE 8-5. HEREDITARY SENSORY AND AUTONOMIC NEUROPATHIES

Type	Inheritance	Chromosome	Gene	Onset	Clinical Features	Neurophysiology	Pathology
HSAN1	AD; rare AR and X-linked cases also reported	9q22	SPTLC1	Second to fourth decades	Loss of pain and temperature sensation; autonomic functions relatively spared (except for reduced sweating); atrophaties and foot ulcers are common; distal weakness may develop	Normal or only mildly reduced CMAPs and SNAPs amplitudes; near nerve recordings: reduced amplitudes of Aδ and C-fibers; abnormal QST (particularly temperature perception); SSR, absent	Distal greater than proximal loss of small myelinated and unmyelinated fibers more than large myelinated fibers
HSAN2	AR	?	?	Infancy–early childhood	Severe loss of sensation to all modalities (particularly touch-pressure/vibration); mutilation of hands and feet; impaired sweating, impotence, and bladder function	Absent SNAPs; normal or only mildly reduced CMAPs amplitudes; abnormal QST (particularly vibratory perception)	Virtual absence of large myelinated fibers; mild loss of small myelinated and unmyelinated fibers
HSAN3	AR	9q21	IKAP	Infancy	Severe autonomic dysfunction (labile BP, sweating, and temperature); decreased pain-temperature sensation more than touch/vibration; absence of fungiform papillae and taste; increased mortality	Decreased SNAP amplitudes; mild slowing of CMAP velocities; abnormal QST; normal SSR	Marked reduction of small myelinated and unmyelinated fibers and to a lesser extent large myelinated fibers; loss of neurons in sympathetic ganglia

HSAN4	AR	3q	trkA/NGF receptor	Infancy	Absence of pain and temperature sensation; episodic fevers, postural hypotension, anhidrosis; self-mutilation; mental retardation	Mildly reduced amplitudes and slow CVs of SNAPs and to a lesser extent of CMAPs; abnormal QST (particulary temperature perception); SSR, intact	Virtual absence of small myelinated and unmyelinated fibers and a moderate loss of large myelinated fibers
HSAN5	AD or AR	?	?	Infancy	Congenital indifference to painful stimuli despite intact sensation to all modalities and normal deep tendon reflexes	Normal SNAPs, CMAPs, QST, and SSR	Normal nerve biopsies or only mild loss of small myelinated and unmyelinated fibers

HSAN, hereditary sensory and autonomic neuropathy; AD, autosomal dominant; AR, autosomal recessive; TrkA/NGF, tyrosine kinase A/nerve growth factor; SPTLC1, serine palmitoyltransferase long chain base 1; IKAP, I$_\kappa$B kinase complex–associated protein; SNAP, sensory nerve action potential; CMAP, compound muscle action potential; QST, quantitative sensory testing; SSR, sympathetic skin response; BP, blood pressure.

a. Characterized by the combination of lattice corneal dystrophy and multiple cranial neuropathies (e.g., facial palsies and bulbar weakness).
b. Onset of symptoms is usually in the third decade of life.
c. Over time, a mild generalized sensorimotor polyneuropathy develops.
4. Electrophysiologic studies reveal abnormalities consistent with a generalized or multifocal, axonal sensorimotor polyneuropathy.
5. Diagnosis of FAP can be made on genetic testing or by detection of amyloid deposition in abdominal fat pad, rectal, or nerve biopsies.

TREATMENT

1. Because the liver produces 90% of the body's TTR, liver transplantation has been used to treat FAP related to *TTR* mutations. Serum TTR levels decrease after transplantation and improvement in clinical and neurophysiologic features has been reported. However, abnormal TTR can continue to be synthesized in the CNS (by the choriod plexus) and within the eyes and potentially result in progressive deficits form local accumulation in these areas.
2. There are no other specific medical or surgical therapies for the different FAPs.
3. Treatment is largely supportive.
4. Neuropathic pain can be treated with a variety of medications (see Table 8-3).
5. Autonomic symptoms also may be partially responsive to therapy (see section on Idiopathic Autonomic Neuropathy).

FABRY DISEASE

BACKGROUND

Fabry disease (angiokeratoma corporis diffusum) is an X-linked disorder, which manifests in males in childhood or adolescence.

PATHOPHYSIOLOGY

The disorder is caused by mutations in the α-galactosidase gene located on chromosome Xq21-22.

PROGNOSIS

The course of the disease is slowly progressive. The major manifestation of the disorder is premature atherosclerosis leading to hypertension, renal failure, cardiac disease, stroke, and death by the fifth decade of life.

DIAGNOSIS

Clinical Features

1. Patients present with burning or stabbing pain in the hands and feet.
2. Characteristic skin lesions (angiokeratomas), which appear as a reddish purple maculopapular rash around the umbilicus, scrotum, inguinal, and perineum can be seen. In addition, punctate red angiectasias are present in the nailbeds, oral mucosa, and conjunctiva.
3. Occasionally, female carriers develop a mild painful sensory neuropathy but only rarely do they have significant atherosclerotic disease.

Laboratory Features

A decrease in α-galactosidase activity can be demonstrated in leukocytes and cultured fibroblasts.

Electrophysiologic Findings

As this disorder affects mainly small myelinated and unmyelinated nerve fibers, NCSs and needle EMG are typically normal.

TREATMENT

1. Treatment of systemic manifestations (e.g, hypertension, cardiac disease, renal insufficiency, and stroke).
2. Treat neuropathic pain (see Table 8-3).
3. Recombinant α-galactosidase is not as yet FDA-approved or available, but trials are ongoing.

REFSUM DISEASE

BACKGROUND

1. Refsum diseases is a peroxisomal disorder of lipid metabolism in which phytanic acid fails to undergo α-oxidation.
2. The disease can manifest in infancy to early adulthood.
3. A tetrad of symptoms form the cardinal clinical features of the disorder:
   a. Peripheral neuropathy,
   b. Retinitis pigmentosa (often the earliest symptom which manifests as night blindness),
   c. Evidence of cerebellar dysfunction, and
   d. Elevated protein content in the CSF.

PATHOPHYSIOLOGY

1. This disease is inherited in an autosomal recessive manner and appears to be genetically heterogeneic.
2. Classic Refsum disease with childhood or early adulthood onset has been linked to mutations in the phytanoyl-CoA α-hydroxylase gene. Phytanic acid accumulates in various organs including the central and peripheral nervous systems leading to neuronal degeneration.
3. Mutations in various genes encoding for peroxins (proteins involved in the peroxisomal transport/import, biogenesis, and proliferation) are suspected to be alternative causes of Refsum disease, especially in the infantile type.

PROGNOSIS

It is important to diagnose Refsum syndrome early because it is a treatable disorder.

DIAGNOSIS

Clinical Features

1. Infantile Refsum disease falls within the clinical spectrum of Zellweger syndrome and neonatal ALD, albeit much milder in severity.

2. Classic Refsum disease is associated with sensorineural hearing loss, cardiac conduction abnormalities, neuropathy, and dermal alterations (ichthyosis) that usually manifest in most patients by the end of the second decade.
3. Distal lower limb muscle wasting and weakness (e.g., bilateral foot drop) are evident early. The relentless nature of the disease results in muscle weakness progressing proximally to involve both the lower and upper limbs.
4. Some patients may complain of paresthesias and spontaneous pain sensations in the limbs.
5. The neuropathy can have a fluctuating course.

Laboratory Features

Serum phytanic acid levels are increased.

Electrophysiologic Findings

1. Motor and sensory NCS may demonstrate features suggestive of a primary demyelinating or axonal, generalized sensorimotor polyneuropathy.

TREATMENT

Elimination of phytanic precursors (phytols: fish oils, dairy products, and ruminant fats) from the diet may help patients with respect to reducing the clinical complications of the disease.

PORPHYRIC NEUROPATHIES

BACKGROUND

1. The porphyrias are a group of inherited disorders caused by defects in heme biosynthesis. There are three major forms of porphyria that are associated with neuropathy: acute intermittent porphyria (AIP), hereditary coprophyria (HCP), and variegate porphyria (VP).
2. Regardless of the type of porphyria inherited, the acute neurologic manifestations are quite similar and can affect the CNS and PNS.
3. Patients with HCP and VP can exhibit photosensitive skin lesions, which are not seen in AIP.
4. Attacks of porphria can be precipitated by certain drugs, hormonal changes (e.g., pregnancy, luteal phase of the menstrual cycle), and dietary restrictions.
5. Any drug that is metabolized by the P450 system in the liver can induce an attack of porphyria.

PATHOPHYSIOLOGY

The porphyrias are inherited in an autosomal dominant fashion. AIP is associated with porphobilinogen deaminase deficiency, HCP is caused by defects in coproporhyrin oxidase, and VP is associated with protoporphyrinogen oxidase deficiency.

PROGNOSIS

The neuropathy improves with treatment.

DIAGNOSIS

Clinical Features

1. Patients experiencing an attack of porphyria often complain of acute abdominal pain that can mimic a surgical abdomen.
2. Soon thereafter is the development of agitation, and restlessness that can progress to overt hallucinations and seizures.
3. Within 48 to 72 hours, the onset of lower limb and back pain followed by motor weakness resembling GBS occurs.
4. Patients may complain of numbness and paresthesias, although sensory loss can be hard to determine given the patient mental state.
5. The deep tendon reflexes are variably diminished.
6. Autonomic dysfunction manifested by signs of sympathetic overactivity (e.g., pupillary dilatation, tachycardia, and hypertension) is common.

Laboratory Features

1. The CSF protein can be normal or mildly elevated.
2. The urine may be brown secondary to the high concentration of porphyrin metabolites.
3. The diagnosis is made by evaluating the urine or stool for the accumulating intermediary precursors of heme (i.e., δ-aminolevulinic acid, porphobilinogen, uroporphobilinogen, coproporphyrinogen, and protoporphyrinogen). The specific lowered enzyme activities can also be measured in erythrocytes and leukocytes.
4. Genetic screening for AIP is routinely available

Electrophysiologic Findings

1. Motor NCS reveal decreased amplitudes with normal or only mildly reduced nerve conduction velocities, and normal and occasional mild prolongation of the distal motor latencies.
2. Sensory NCS usually demonstrates preservation of SNAP conduction velocities and distal sensory latencies. A reduction in SNAP amplitudes can be seen in some patients, but this is not as common as the finding of reduced CMAP amplitudes.
3. EMG during the acute stage of weakness demonstrates primarily a reduced recruitment. Over the course of the next 4 to 6 weeks, in those patients with significant clinical weakness, fibrillation potentials and positive sharp waves can be observed in the affected muscles.

TREATMENT

1. The primary treatment is prevention by awareness of drugs that can precipitate the acute porphyric attack in patients with known porphyria.
2. Once an attack occurs, hematin and glucose should be administered to prevent the accumulation of heme precursors.
3. IV glucose is started at a rate of 10 to 20 g/hr.
4. If there is no improvement within 24 hours, IV hematin 1 to 5 mg/kg/d for 3 to 14 days should be given. This hematin dose can be infused over a 30- to 60-minute period.
5. Autonomic symptoms are treated as discussed in Idiopathic Autonomic Neuropathy section.
6. Supportive therapy as discussed in the Guillain–Barré Syndrome section.

BIBLIOGRAPHY

Motor Neuron Diseases

Amato AA, Cornman EW, Kissel JT. Treatment of stiff-man syndrome with intravenous immunoglobulin. *Neurology* 1994;44:1652–1654.

Barker RA, Revesz T, Thom M, et al. Review of 23 patients affected by the stiff man syndrome: clinical subdivision into stiff trunk (man) syndrome, stiff limb syndrome, and progressive encephalomyelitis with rigidity. *J Neurol Neurosurg Psychiatry* 1998;65;633–640.

Brooks BR. Natural history of ALS: symptoms, strength, pulmonary function, and disability. *Neurology* 1996;47[Suppl 2]:S71–S82.

Brown P, Marsden CD. The stiffman and stiffman-plus syndromes. *J Neurol* 1999;246:648–652.

Caress JB, Abend WK, Preston DC, et al. A case of Hodgkin's lymphoma producing neuromyotonia. *Neurology* 1997;49:258–259.

Dalakas M, Illa I. Post-polio syndrome: concepts in clinical diagnosis, pathogenesis, and etiology. *Adv Neurol* 1991;56:495–511.

Dalakas MC, Fujii M, Li M, et al. The clinical spectrum of anti-GAD antibody postive patients with stiff-person syndrome. *Neurology* 2000;55:1531–1535.

Dalakas MC, Fujii M, Li M, et al. High-dose intravenous immune globulin for stiff-person syndrome. *N Engl J Med* 2001;345:1870–1876.

Desport JC, Preux PM, Truong CT, et al. Nutritional assessment and survival in ALS patients. *Amyotroph Lateral Scler Other Motor Neuron Disord* 2000;1:91–96.

Dumitru D, Amato AA. Disorders of motor neurons. In: Dumitru D, Amato AA, Swartz MJ, eds. *Electrodiagnostic medicine,* 2nd ed. Philadelphia: Hanley & Belfus, 2002:581–651.

Harding AE, Thompson PD, Kocen RS, et al. Plasma exchange and immunosuppression in the stiff man syndrome. *Lancet* 1989;1:915.

Iannaccone ST, Russman BS, Brown RH, et al. Prospective analysis of strength in spinal muscular atrophy. *J Child Neurol* 2000;15:97–101.

Isaacs H, Heffron JJA. The syndrome of continuous muscle fiber activity cured: further studies. *J Neurol Neurosurg Psychiatry* 1974;37:1231–1235.

Lacomblez L, Bensimon G, Leigh P, et al. Dose-ranging study of riluzole in amyotrophic lateral sclerosis. *Lancet* 1996;347:1425–1431.

MacGowan DJL, Scelsa SN, Waldron M. An ALS-like syndrome with new HIV infection and complete response to antiretroviral therapy. *Neurology* 2001;57:1094–1097.

Miller F, Korsvik H: Baclofen in the treatment of stiff-man syndrome. *Ann Neurol* 1981;9:511–512.

Miller RG, Rosenberg JA, Gelinas DF, et al. Practice parameter: the care of the patient with amyotrophic lateral sclerosis (an evidence-based review)—report of the Quality Standards Subcommittee of the American Academy of Neurology. *Neurology* 1999;52:1311–1321.

Moulingnier A, Moulonguet A, Pialoux G, et al. Reversible ALS-like disorder with HIV infection. *Neurology* 2001;57:995–1001.

Munsat TL, Andres PL, Finison L, et al. The natural history of motor neuron loss in ALS. *Neurology* 1988;38:452–458.

Rowland LP, Shneider NA. Amyotrophic lateral sclerosis. *N Engl J Med* 2001;344:1688–1699.

Sharoqi IA. Improvement of stiff man syndrome with vigabatrin [letter]. *Neurology* 1998;50:833–834.

Silbert PL, Matsumoto JY, McManis PG, et al. Intrathecal baclofen therapy in stiff-man syndrome: a double-blind, placebo-controlled trial. *Neurology* 1995;45:1893–1897.

Souza-Lima CF, Ferraz HB, Braz CA, et al. Marked improvement in a stiff-limb patient treated with intravenous immunoglobulin. *Move Disord* 2000;15:358–359.

Spehlmann R, Norcross K, Rasmus SC, et al. Improvement of stiff-man syndrome with sodium valproate. *Neurology* 1981;31:1162–1163.

Stayer C, Tronnier V, Dressnandt J, et al. Intrathecal baclofen therapy for stiff-man syndrome and progressive encephalomyelopathy with rigidity and myoclonus. *Neurology* 1997;49:1591–1597.

Tan E, Lynn J, Amato AA, et al. Immunosuppressive treatment of motor neuron syndromes. *Arch Neurol* 1994;51:194–200.

Thorsteinsson G: Management of postpolio syndrome. *Mayo Clin Proc* 1997;72:627–638.

World Federation of Neurology Research Group in Neuromuscular Disease. El Escorial Criteria for the diagnosis of amyotrophic lateral sclerosis. *J Neurol Sci* 124[Suppl]:96–107.

Zerres K, Rudnik-Schoneborn S, Forrest E, et al. A collaborative study in the natural history of childhood and juvenile onset spinal muscular atrophy (type II and III SMA): 569 patients. *J Neurol Sci* 1997;146:67–72.

Zeres K, Wirth B, Rudnik-Schoneborn S. Spinal muscular atrophy: clinical and genetic correlations. *Neuromusc Dis* 1997;202–207.

Acquired Neuropathies

Altman D, Amato AA. Lepromatous neuropathy. *J Clin Neuromusc Dis* 1999;1:68–73.

Amato AA, Collins MP. Neuropathies associated with malignancy. *Semin Neurol* 1998;18:125–144.

Amato AA, Barohn RJ. Diabetic lumbosacral radiculoneuropathyies. *Curr Treat Op Neurol* 2001;3:139–146.

Amato AA, Anderson MP. A 51-year-old woman with lung cancer and neuropsychiatric abnormalities. *N Engl J Med* 2001;345:1758–1765.

Amato AA, Dumitru D. Acquired neuropathies. In: Dumitru D, Amato AA, Swartz MJ, eds. *Electrodiagnostic medicine,* 2nd ed. Philadelphia: Hanley & Belfus, 2002:937–1041.

Azulay JP, Rihet P, Pouget J, et al. Long term follow up of multifocal motor neuropathy with conduction block under treatment. *J Neurol Neurosurg Psychiatry* 1997;62:391–394.

Backonja M, Beydoun A, Edwards KR, et al. Gabapentin for the symptomatic treatment of painful neuropathy in patients with diabetes mellitus: a randomized control trial. *JAMA* 1998;280:1831–1836.

Balart LA, Perillo R, Roddenberry J, et al. Hepatitis C RNA in liver of chronic hepatitis C patients before and after interferon alpha treatment. *Gastroenterology* 1993;104:1472–1477.

Barohn RJ. Approach to peripheral neuropathy and neuronopathy. *Semin Neurol* 1998;18:7–18.

Bolton CF, Young GG. Critical illness polyneuropathy. *Curr Treat Op Neurol* 2000;2:489–498.

Bonomo L, Casato M, Afeltra A, et al. Treatment of idiopathic mixed cryoglobulinemia with alpha interferon. *Am J Med* 1987;83:7266–730.

Callabrese LH. Therapy of systemic vasculitis. *Neurol Clin* 1997;15:973–991.

Dalakas MC, Quarles RH, Farrer RG, et al. A controlled study of intravenous immunoglobulin in demyelinating neuropathy with IgM gammopathy. *Ann Neurol* 1996;40:792–795.

Diabetes Control and Complications Trial Research Group. The effect of diabetes on the development and progression of long-term complications in insulin-dependent diabetes mellitus. *N Engl J Med* 1993;329:977–986.

Diabetes Control and Complications Trial. Effect of intensive diabetes treatment on nerve conduction in the Diabetes Control and Complications Trial. *Ann Neurol* 1995;38:869–880.

Dutch Guillain-Barré Study Group. Treatment of Guillain–Barré syndrome with high-dose immune globulins combined with methylprednisolone: a pilot study. *Ann Neurol* 1994;35:749–752.

Dyck PJ, O'Brien PC, Oviatt KF, et al. Prednisone improves chronic inflammatory demyelinating polyradiculoneuropathy more than no treatment. *Ann Neurol* 1982;11:136–141.

Dyck PJ, Daube J, O'Brien PC, et al. Plasma exchange in chronic inflammatory demyelinating polyradiculoneuropathy. *N Engl J Med* 1986;314:461–465.

Dyck PJ, Benstead TJ, Conn DL, et al. Nonsystemic vasculitic neuropathy. *Brain* 1987;110:843–854.

Dyck PJ, Low PA, Windebank AJ, et al. Plasma exchange in polyneuropathy associated with monoclonal gammopathy of undetermined significance. *N Engl J Med* 1991;325:1482–1486.

Dyck PJ, Litchey WJ, Kratz KM, et al. A plasma exchange versus immune globulin infusion trial in chronic inflammatory demyelinating polyradiculoneuropathy. *Ann Neurol* 1994;36:838–845.

Enevoldson TP, Wiles CM. Severe vasculitic neuropathy in systemic lupus erythematosis and response to cyclophosphamide. *J Neurol Neurosurg Psychiatry* 1991;54:468–469.

Feldman EL, Bromberg MB, Albers JW, et al. Immunosuppressive treatment in multifocal motor neuropathy. *Ann Neurol* 1991;30:397–401.

Galer BS. Painful polyneuropathy. *Neurol Clin* 1998;791–811.

Ghini M, Mascia MT, Gentilini M, et al. Treatment of cryoglobulinemic neuropathy with α-interferon [letter]. *Neurology* 1996;46:588–589.

Graus F, Keimer-Guibert F, Rene R, et al. Anti-Hu associated paraneoplastic encephalomyelitis: analysis of 200 patients. *Brain* 2001;124:1138–1148.

Hahn AF, Bolton CF, Pillay N, et al. Plasma-exchange therapy in chronic inflammatory demyelinating polyneuropathy: a double-blind, sham-controlled, cross-over study. *Brain* 1996;119:1055–1066.

Hahn AF, Bolton CF, Zochodne D, et al. Intravenous immunoglobulin treatment in chronic inflammatory demyelinating polyneuropathy: a double-blind, placebo-controlled, cross-over study. *Brain* 1996;119;1067–1077.

Halperin JJ, Little BW, Coyle PK, et al. Lyme disease: cause of a treatable peripheral neuropathy. *Neurology* 1987;37:1700–1706.

Harati Y, Gooch C, Swenson M, et al. Double-blind randomized trial of tramadol for the treatment of the pain of diabetic neuropathy. *Neurology* 1998;50:1842–1846.

Heafield MTE, Gammage MD, Nightingale S, et al. Idiopathic dysautonomia treated with intravenous immunoglobulin. *Lancet* 1996;347:28–29.

Hodgkinson SJ, Pollard JD, McLeod JG. Cyclosporine A in the treatment of chronic demyelinating polyradiculopathy. *J Neurol Neurosurg Psychiatry* 1990;53:327–330.

Hughes R, Bensa S, Willison H, et al. Randomized controlled trial of intravenous immunoglobulin versus oral prednisolone in chronic inflammatory demyelinating polyradiculoneuropathy. *Ann Neurol* 2001;50:195–201.

Jankovic J, Gilden JL, Hiner BC, et al. Neurogenic orthostatic hypotension: a double-blind, placebo-controlled study with midodrine. *Am J Med* 1993;95:34–48.

Janssens J, Peeters TL, Vantrappen G, et al. Improvement of gastric emptying in diabetic gastroparesis by erythromycin: preliminary studies. *N Engl J Med* 1998;338:1397–1404.

Jaradeh SS, Prieto TE, Lobeck LJ. Progressive polyradiculoneuropathy in diabetes: correlation with variables and clinical outcome after immunotherapy. *J Neurol Neurosurg Psychiatry* 1999;67:607–612.

Kieburtz K, Simpson D, Yiannoutsos C, et al. A randomized trial of amitriptyline and mexiletine for painful neuropathy in HIV infection. *Neurology* 1998;51:1682–1688.

Lacomis D, Petrella JT, Giuliani MJ. Causes of neuromuscular weakness in the intensive care unit: a study of ninety-two patients. *Muscle Nerve* 1998;21:610–617.

Léger J-M, Chassande B, Musset L, et al. Intravenous immunoglobulin therapy in multifocal motor neuropathy: a double-blind, placebo-controlled study. *Brain* 2001;124:124–153.

Low PA, Gilden JL, Freeman R, et al. Efficacy of midodrine vs. placebo in neurogenic orthostatic hypotension: a randomized, double-blind multicenter study. *JAMA* 1997;227:1046–1051.

Mahttanakul W, Crawford TO, Griffin JW, et al. Treatment of chronic demyelinating polyneuropathy with cyclosporine-A. *J Neurol Neurosurg Psychiatry* 1996;60:185–187.

Max MB, Lynch SA, Muir J, et al. Effects of desipramine, amitriptyline, and fluoxetine on pain in diabetic neuropathy. *N Engl J Med* 1992;326:1250–1256.

Max MB. Treatment of post-herpetic neuralgia: antidepressants. *Ann Neurol* 1994;35:S50–S53.

Mendell JR, Barohn RJ, Freimer ML, et al. Randomized controlled trial of IVIG in untreated chronic inflammatory demyelinating polyradiculoneuropathy. *Neurology* 2001;56:445–449.

Plasma Exchange/Sandoglobulin Guillain–Barré Syndrome Trial Group. Randomized trial of plasma exchange, intravenous immunoglobulin, and combined treatments in Guillain–Barré syndrome. *Lancet* 1997;349:225–230.

Quan D, Rich MM, Bird SJ. Acute idiopathic dysautonomia: electrophysiology and response to intravenous immunoglobulin. *Neurology* 2000;54:770–771.

Saperstein DS, Katz JS, Amato AA, et al. Clinical spectrum of chronic acquired demyelinating polyneuropathies. *Muscle Nerve* 2001;24:311–324.

van der Meche FGA, Schmidtz PIM, and the Dutch Guillain–Barré Study Group. A randomized trial comparing intravenous immunoglobulin and plasma exchange in Guillain–Barré syndrome. *N Engl J Med* 1992;326:1123–1129.

van Doorn PA, Brand A, Strengers PFW, et al. High dose intravenous immunoglobulin treatment in chronic inflammatory demyelinating polyneuropathy: a double-blind placebo controlled cross-over study. *Neurology* 1990;40:209–212.

van Doorn PA, Vermeulen M, Brand A, et al. Intravenous immunoglobulin treatment in patients with chronic inflammatory demyelinating polyneuropathy. *Arch Neurol* 1991;48:217–220.

Vermeulen M, van Doorn PA, Brand A, et al. Intravenous immunoglobulin treatment in patients with chronic inflammatory demyelinating polyneuropathy: a double blind, placebo controlled study. *J Neurol Neurosurg Psychiatry* 1993;56:36–39.

Wolfe GI, Baker NS, Amato AA, et al. Chronic cryptogenic sensory polyneuropathy: clinical and laboratory characteristics. *Arch Neurol* 1999;56:540–547.

Hereditary Neuropathies

Amato AA, Dumitru D. Hereditary neuropathies. In: Dumitru D, Amato AA, Swartz MJ, eds. *Electrodiagnostic medicine,* 2nd ed. Philadelphia: Hanley & Belfus, 2002:889–936.

Barohn RJ. Approach to peripheral neuropathy and neuronopathy. *Semin Neurol* 1998;18:7–18.

Bergethon PR, Sabin TD, Lewis D, et al. Improvement in the polyneuropathy associated with familial amyloid polyneuropathy after liver transplantation. *Neurology* 1996;47:944–951.

Bosch EP, Pierach CA, Bossenmaier I, et al. Effect of hematin in porphyric neuropathy. *Neurology* 1977;27:1053–1056.

Coehlo T. Familial amyloid polyneuropathy: new developments in genetics and treatment. *Curr Opin Neurol* 1996;9:355–359.

Mendell JR. Charcot-Marie-Tooth neuropathies and related disorders. *Sem Neurol* 1998;18:41–47.

Steinberg D, MIze CE, Herndon JH, et al. Phytanic acid in patients with Refsum's syndrome and response to dietary treatment. *Arch Intern Med* 1970;125:75–87.

9. NEUROMUSCULAR JUNCTION DISORDERS AND MYOPATHIES

Anthony A. Amato

MYASTHENIA GRAVIS

BACKGROUND

1. Myasthenia gravis is an autoimmune disease caused by an immunologic attack directed against the postsynaptic neuromuscular junction (NMJ).
2. The incidence of myasthenia gravis ranges between 1 and 9/million, whereas the prevalence ranges between 25 and 142/million. The incidence of myasthenia gravis is slightly greater in women than in men. The age of onset is bimodal for both men and women. Women demonstrate annual peak incidences at ages 20 to 24 years and 70 to 75 years, while men have peak rates between 30 and 34 years and 70 and 74 years.
3. Patients with myasthenia gravis can be classified according to the Osserman criteria:
   a. Group 1: ocular, 15% to 20%
   b. Group 2A: mild generalized, 30%
   c. Group 2B: moderately severe generalized, 20%
   d. Group 3: acute fulminating, 11%
   e. Group 4: late severe, 9%
4. As many as 70% of patients with myasthenia gravis have thymic hyperplasia while approximately 10% have a thymoma. Thymomas are much more common in patients between the ages of 50 and 70 years. Importantly, the thymomas can be malignant and invasive. The role of the thymus in myasthenia gravis is unclear.

PATHOPHYSIOLOGY

Myasthenia gravis is an acquired autoimmune disorder of neuromuscular transmission resulting from antibodies directed against the acetylcholine receptor (AChR) or against the muscle-specific receptor tyrosine kinase (MuSK).

PROGNOSIS

1. At least 50% of patients initially presenting with purely ocular symptoms eventually develop a more generalized form of the disease.
2. Most patients evolve to their weakest within the first 3 years.
3. Patients may develop severe generalized weakness with respiratory failure or inability to swallow. Severe respiratory and bulbar weakness can develop in absence of ocular or extremity weakness.
4. Patients with only mild weakness may respond to anticholinesterase medications. However, patients with moderate or severe weakness require immunosuppressive or immunomodulating agents.

DIAGNOSIS

Clinical Features

1. The clinical hallmarks of myasthenia gravis are fluctuating weakness characterized by abnormal fatigability that improves with rest.

2. Patients often complaining of drooping eyelids, blurred vision, or frank diplopia, particularly after prolonged reading or at the end of the day. Ptosis is the presenting symptom in 50% to 90% of patients, whereas 15% complain of blurred vision or frank diplopia. At some point, about 90% to 95% of patients complain of diplopia.
3. Dysphagia and dysarthria occur in as many as one third of patients.
4. Proximal limb and neck weakness is a presenting symptom in approximately 20% to 30% of individuals. Importantly, approximately 3% of patients manifest with predominantly distal weakness. Head drop secondary to neck extensor weakness is not uncommon and can be the presenting feature. There may be a gradual but definite onset of fatigue after repetitive activities.
5. Occasionally, patients can present in respiratory failure due to weakness of the diaphragm and accessory muscles of respiration.
6. Patients with MuSK antibodies often manifest with balbar or respiratory weakness without ocular involvement.

PHARMACOLOGIC TESTING

1. The edrophonium (i.e., Tensilon) test can be helpful in diagnosing myasthenia gravis. Edrophonium is an anticholinesterase and will result in transient increase in AChR in the NMJ.
   a. Anticholinergic side effects of edrophonium include fasciculations, bradycardia, nausea, vomiting, increased tearing, and lacrimation.
   b. Monitor the pulse and blood pressure of patients and be prepared to administer atropine to counteract the anticholinergic effects of edrophonium.
   c. Place a butterfly needle in the antecubital vein and give a 2-mg test dose of edrophonium. If there is not response after 30 seconds, the remaining 8 mg is administered in increments (2 mg every 15 seconds).
   d. It is most important to assess an objective sign of weakness not the patient's subjective response. In this regard, evaluating improvement of measured ptosis or ophthalmoparesis are most useful.
   e. A test is not considered positive if the patients states that they feel stronger.

Laboratory Features

1. AChR antibodies are detected in about 80% to 90% of patients with generalized myasthenia gravis with a slightly lower value in the ocular form (70%).
2. Antibodies directed against the muscle-specific receptor tyrosine kinase, MuSK, are seen in approximately one-third of patients without AChR antibodies.
3. Antistriatal muscle antibodies (also know as antititin antibodies) are evident in approximately 30% of adult patients with myasthenia gravis and 80% of patients who have thymomas.
4. Antinuclear antibodies (ANAs) and thyroid function tests may be abnormal in patients with other associated autoimmune conditions.

Electrophysiologic Findings

1. Repetitive stimulation is typically performed on an intrinsic hand muscle such as the abductor digiti minimi first, however, in patients with only proximal weakness, the trapezius can be assessed. In patients with only ocular or bulbar weakness, a facial muscle (orbicularis oculi or nasalis, or orbicularis oris) should be studied.
   a. First, perform a 2- to 3-Hz repetitive stimulation with the patient at rest. Normally, there should be less than a 10% decrement.
   b. If an abnormal decrement is demonstrated, the patient is instructed to exercise the muscle for 10 seconds in order to assess for postexercise facilitation and the resulting improvement in the decrement on 2- to 3-Hz stimulation immediately postexercise.
   c. If no decrement is appreciated at rest, the muscle is exercised for 1 minute in order to see if postexercise exhaustion will bring out an abnormal decrement. Repetitive stimulation at 2- to 3-Hz stimulation is performed immediately

TABLE 9-1. ANTICHOLINESTERASE DRUGS COMMONLY USED FOR MYASTHENIA GRAVIS

Drug	Route	Adult Dose	Children's Dose	Infant Dose	Frequency
Neostigmine bromide (Prostigmin)	p.o.	15 mg	10 mg	1–2 mg	q2–3 h
Neostigmine methyl sulfate (Prostigmin injectable)	IM, IV	0.5 mg	0.1 mg	0.05 mg	q2–3 h
Pyridostigmine bromide (Mestinon)	p.o., IM, IV	60 mg 2 mg	30 mg 0.5–1.5 mg/kg	4–10 mg 0.1–0.5 mg	q3–6 h q3–6 h
Mestinon Timespan	p.o.	180 mg			qHS

p.o., by mouth; IM, intramuscular; IV, intravenous; q, every; HS, at bed time.

postexercise and once per minute for the next 5 to 6 minutes following 1 minute of exercise.
2. If repetitive nerve stimulation is normal, a single-fiber electromyogram (EMG) should be performed. Single-fiber EMG documents increased jitter in 77% to 100% of patients depending upon disease severity.

TREATMENT

1. There are various treatment strategies commonly used for treatment of myasthenia gravis:
   a. Acetylcholinesterase inhibitors (Table 9-1)
   b. Immunosuppressive/Immunomodulating agents
   c. Plasma exchange (PE)
   d. Thymectomy
2. The regimen used in patients with myasthenia gravis is individualized and dependent upon the severity of the myasthenia, age of the patient, the presence of absence of an enlarged thymus, and concurrent medical problems.
3. I try to treat patients with ocular myasthenia only with Mestinon. If patients are still symptomatic on Mestinon, I will treat with a short course (2–3 months) of prednisone in a slowly incrementing fashion (see "start-low, go-slow approach" to prednisone treatment below).
4. Patients in myasthenic crisis (severe respiratory distress or bulbar weakness) represent the opposite end of the spectrum.
   a. Patients should be admitted to an intensive care unit (ICU) and followed closely, particularly concerning pulmonary function.
   b. When the forced vital capacity declines to less than 15 ml/kg or the negative inspiratory pressure is less than 30 cm H_2O, consider elective intubation of the patient to protect the airway and begin mechanical ventilation. Alternative, bilevel positive airway pressure (BiPAP) may be initiated and may alleviate the need for intubation in patients who are not hypercapnic (i.e., $Paco_2$ above 50 mm Hg).
   c. Initiate PE until the patients has had significant return of strength and can be weaned off the ventilator. Intravenous immunoglobulin (IVIG) may be an alternative treatment.
   d. In addition to starting PE, I usually begin corticosteroids at or around the same time
5. Specific therapies:
   a. Acetylcholinesterase inhibitors:

1) The acetylcholinesterase inhibitor, pyridostigmine bromide (Mestinon), usually improves weakness in patients with myasthenia gravis.
2) Start pyridostigmine in adults at a dose of 30 to 60 mg every 6 hours. In children, I start pyridostigmine at a dose of 1.0 mg/kg. The dosage is gradually titrated as necessary to control myasthenic symptoms and reduce side effects. Most adults require between 60 and 120 mg of pyridostigmine every 4 to 6 hours.
3) There is a timed-released form of pyridostigmine (Mestinon Timespan, 180 mg). A Mestinon Timespan tablet can be given at night for patients who have severe generalized weakness upon awakening. Alternately, in patients with only mild or moderate weakness, it is equally efficacious to have the patient set their alarm 30 minutes before they need to arise from bed and take a regular pyridostigmine dose at that time.
4) Patients can develop cholinergic side effects secondary to the build up of AChR at muscarinic and nicotinic receptors. Muscarinic side effects include nausea, vomiting, abdominal cramping, diarrhea, increased oral and bronchial secretions, bradycardia, and rarely, confusion or psychosis. In patients with significant side effects, I pretreat with anticholinergic medications [e.g., anaspaz one tablet four times a day (q.i.d.)] 30 minutes prior to their pyridostigmine doses.

b. Corticosteroids:
1) Most of our patients with moderate to severe generalized myasthenia gravis receive prednisone. There are two treatment strategies generally used when using prednisone in patients with myasthenia gravis:
    a) Aggressive high-dose daily steroids at the onset of treatment approach.
    b) "A start low and go slow approach." The high-dose daily regimen leads to a much quicker improvement of weakness.
2) I initiate treatment with prednisone 1.5 mg/kg/d (up to 100 mg) for 2 weeks and then switch to alternate-day prednisone (e.g., 100 mg every other day). I maintain the patients on this high dose of prednisone until their strength has normalized or there is a clear plateau in improvement. Subsequently, I slowly taper the prednisone by 5 mg every 2 to 3 weeks down to 20 mg every other day. At this point, I taper even slower by 2 mg every 4 weeks. It is usually at these low doses that patients may have a relapse.
3) Most patients will require some amount of immunosuppressive medication but I try to find the lowest doses necessary to maintain their strength.
4) The addition of other immunosuppressive agents (e.g., azathioprine or mycophenolate) may also have a prednisone-sparing effect and allow for lower doses of the corticosteroid. Many authorities initiate treatment with one of these agents at the same time as prednisone is started in hope that the prednisone may be tapered quicker and to a lower dose than could be achieved by prednisone monotherapy. However, in general I try to see if patients can be treated on low dosages of prednisone alone because of the possible long-term side effects of other immunosuppressive agents.
5) About 5% to 15% of patients experience a varying degree of initial worsening after they are started on high doses of steroids. Therefore, I usually hospitalize patients for the first week after initiating treatment with high-dose corticosteroids.
6) Because of the risk of exacerbation with high-dose corticosteroids, some have advocated the start-low and go-slow approach. Patients are started at a dose of 15 to 20 mg/d and the dose is slowly increased by 5 mg every 2 to 4 days or so until definite improvement is noted. Unfortunately, improvement takes much longer with this approach and is thus not very useful in patients with severe weakness. I reserve this approach for patients with mild generalized disease not controlled with Mestinon or the patients with ocular myasthenia who I treat with immunosuppression.
7) There are multitude of potentially serious side effects to the chronic administration of corticosteroids (e.g., risk of infection, diabetes mellitus, hypertension, glaucoma, osteoporosis, and aseptic necrosis of the joints).

8) Obtain a chest radiograph and a purified protein derivative (PPD) skin test with controls on all patients prior to initiating immunosuppressive medications. Patients with a history of tuberculosis or those with a positive PPD result may need to be treated prophylactically with isoniazid.

9) Measure bone density with dual-energy x-ray absorptiometry (DEXA) at baseline and every 6 to 12 months while patients are receiving corticosteroids.

10) Calcium supplementation (1 g/d) and vitamin D (400–800 IU/d) are started for prophylaxis against steroid-induced osteoporosis. I usually recommend Tums for calcium as it can also help with the dyspepsia associated with steroid use.

11) Bisphosphonates are effective in the prevention and treatment of osteoporosis. If DEXA scans demonstrate osteoporosis at baseline or during follow-up studies, I initiate alendronate 70 mg/wk. In postmenopausal women, I start alendronate 35 mg orally once a week as prophylaxis for osteoporosis. The long-term side effects of bisphosphonates are not known, especially for men and young premenopausal women. For these patients, I start prophylactic treatment with alendronate 35 mg orally once a week if DEXA scans show bone loss at baseline (not as yet enough to diagnosis osteoporosis) or if there is significant loss on follow-up bone density scans. Alendronate can cause severe esophagitis and absorption is impaired if taken with meals. Therefore, patients must be instructed to remain upright and not to eat for at least 30 minutes after taking a dose of alendronate.

12) I do not prophylactically treat with histamine-H_2 receptor blockers, unless the patient develops gastrointestinal discomfort or has a history of peptic ulcer disease. Tums can help prevent any discomfort and also serve as a source of calcium.

13) Patients are instructed to start a low-sodium, low-carbohydrate, high-protein diet to prevent excessive weight gain.

14) Patients are also given physical therapy and encouraged to slowly begin an aerobic exercise program.

15) Blood pressure is measured with each visit along with periodic eye examinations for cataracts and glaucoma. Fasting blood glucose and serum potassium levels are periodically checked. Potassium supplementation may be required if the patient becomes hypokalemic.

16) Steroid myopathy versus relapse of myasthenia gravis: High-dose, long-term steroids and lack of physical activity can cause type 2 muscle fiber atrophy with proximal muscle weakness. This needs to be distinguished from weakness due to relapse of the myasthenia. Patients who become weaker during prednisone taper and have worsening of their decrement repetitive stimulation or increasing jitter and blocking on single-fiber EMG are more likely experiencing a flare of the myasthenia. In contrast, patients with continued high doses of corticosteroids, normal repetitive stimulation and single-fiber EMG results, and other evidence of steroid toxicity (i.e., cushingoid appearance) may have type 2 muscle fiber atrophy and could benefit from physical therapy and reducing the dose of steroids.

c. Azathioprine:

1) I prescribe azathioprine for patients with moderate to severe generalized myasthenia gravis whose disease is not well controlled on prednisone and Mestinon. I start azathioprine at a dose of 50 mg/d in adults and gradually increase by 50 mg/wk to a total dose of 2 to 3 mg/kg/d.

2) A systemic reaction characterized by fever, abdominal pain, nausea, vomiting, and anorexia occurs in 12% of patients requiring discontinuation of the drug. This reaction generally occurs within the first few weeks of therapy and resolves within a few days of discontinuing the azathioprine.

3) A major drawback of azathioprine is that it often takes 6 months or longer to be effective.

4) Monitor complete blood counts (CBC) and liver function tests (LFTs)—aspartate aminotransferase (AST), alanine aminotransferase (ALT), bilirubins, and γ-glutamyl transpeptidase (GGT)—every week until the patient is on a stable dose of azathioprine, then every 3 months. If the white blood cell (WBC) count falls below 4,000/mm^3, decrease the dose.

5) Azathioprine is held if the WBC declines to 2,500/mm^3 or the absolute neutrophil count falls to 1,000 per mm^3. Leukopenia can develop as early as 1 week or as late as 2 years after initiating azathioprine. The leukopenia usually reverses within 1 month, and it is possible to then rechallenge the patient with azathioprine without recurrence of the severe leukopenia.

6) Discontinue azathioprine if the LFTs increase more than twice the baseline values. Liver toxicity generally develops within the first several months of treatment and can take several months to resolve. Patients can occasionally be successfully rechallenged with azathioprine after LFTs return to baseline without recurrence of hepatic dysfunction.

d. Cyclosporine:

1) Cyclosporine inhibits primarily T-cell–dependent immune responses. I tend to use cyclosporine mainly in patients who are refractory to prednisone and azathioprine.

2) Most patients notice improvement within 2 to 3 months of initiating treatment, thus it works much faster than azathioprine.

3) I start cyclosporine at a dose of 3.0 to 4.0 mg/kg/d in two divided doses and gradually increase to 6.0 mg/kg/d as necessary.

4) The cyclosporine dose is initially be titrated to maintain trough serum cyclosporine levels of 50 to 150 ng/mL. Adjust the dose to keep the trough less than 150 ng/mL and the creatinine level less than 150% of baseline.

5) Blood pressure, electrolytes, renal function, and trough cyclosporine levels need to be monitored.

e. Mycophenolate mofetil:

1) Mycophenolate mofetil is a newer immunosuppressive agent that inhibits the proliferation of T- and B-lymphocytes by blocking purine synthesis in only lymphocytes.

2) Improvement has been noted as early as 2 weeks (most within the first 3 months) after starting the medication, but benefit can be delayed up to 12 months.

3) The starting dose is 1 g twice daily. I increase the dose by 500 mg/mo up to 1.5 g twice a day (b.i.d.).

4) Mycophenolate is renally excreted, therefore the dose should be no more than 1 g/d (i.e., 500 mg b.i.d.) in patients with renal insufficiency.

5) A benefit of mycophenolate compared to other immunosuppressive agents is the lack of renal or liver toxicity with the drug.

6) The major side effect is diarrhea. Less common side effects include abdominal discomfort, nausea, peripheral edema, fever, and leukopenia.

f. IVIG:

1) Some studies have found that IVIG is equivalent to PE in the treatment of myasthenic crisis, whereas other studies have suggested that PE is more efficacious. I have successfully used IVIG in patients in myasthenic crisis and believe it is an equal alternative to PE until proven otherwise.

2) IVIG has not been compared to the above-mentioned immunosuppressive agents.

3) I usually use IVIG for patients in crisis or to increase their strength before thymectomy. I also use IVIG in patients who are refractory to other forms of immunotherapy or in combination with prednisone for a steroid-sparing effect.

4) I initiate IVIG (2 g/kg) slowly over 2 to 5 days and repeat infusions at monthly intervals for at least 3 months. Thereafter treatment is individualized. Some patient may need treatment (0.4–2 g/kg) every week, while others may go several months between IVIG courses.

      5) All patients should have an IgA level checked prior to treatment, because those with low IgA levels may be at risk for anaphylaxis. Patients should also have renal functions checked, especially those with diabetes mellitus, because of a risk of IVIG-induced renal failure.

      6) Flu-like symptoms—headaches, myalgias, fever, chills, nausea, and vomiting—are common and occur in as many as half the patients receiving IVIG. Theses symptoms can be reduced by premedication with a corticosteroid and lowering the rate of infusion.

      7) Rash, aseptic meningitis, myocardial infarction, and stroke may also complicate IVIG infusions. IVIG should be avoided in patients with hypercoagulable states and significant atherosclerotic cardiovascular disease.

  g. PE:

      1) PE is used in patients with myasthenic crisis or those with moderate weakness prior to thymectomy in order to maximize their preoperative strength.

      2) The typical course involves exchange of 2 to 3 L of plasma three times a week until strength is significantly improved (at least five to six total exchanges). Improvement is noticeable after two to four exchanges.

      3) PE lowers the serum concentration of anti-AChR antibodies, but it must be repeated at relatively regular intervals due to its limited duration of effect.

      4) Within a week following PE, the autoantibodies begin to rebound. Therefore, patients will also need to be also started on an immunosuppressive agent.

  h. Thymectomy:

      1) Thymectomy is clearly indicated in patients with a thymoma.

      2) The role of thymectomy in patients with myasthenia gravis without thymoma is unclear and was the subject of a *Practice Guideline* in 2000 by the American Academy of Neurology. The recommendation of the panel was that thymectomy is an option to increase the probability of improvement or remission in patients with nonthymomatous myasthenia gravis.

TRANSIENT NEONATAL AUTOIMMUNE MYASTHENIA GRAVIS

BACKGROUND

Transient neonatal autoimmune myasthenia gravis develops in approximately 10% of infants born to mothers with myasthenia gravis.

PATHOPHYSIOLOGY

Weakness results from the passive transfer through the placenta of the mother's antibodies against AChRs.

PROGNOSIS

1. Onset is usually within the first 3 days of life and manifests with a weak cry, difficulty feeding due to a poor suck, generalized weakness and decreased tone, respiratory difficulty, ptosis, and diminished facial expression (facial muscle weakness).

2. Weakness is temporary with a mean duration of about 18 to 20 days.

DIAGNOSIS

1. The diagnosis should be suspected in any infant born to a mother with myasthenia gravis.

2. Mothers of floppy infants should be examined for signs of myasthenia gravis because not all mothers are symptomatic.
3. Diagnosis can be confirmed by demonstrating AChR antibodies in the infant's serum or decrementing response to repetitive nerve stimulation.

TREATMENT

1. Infants with neonatal myasthenia and weakness may be treated with anticholinesterase medications for 3 to 6 weeks until such time that the antibody levels have diminished to the point where sufficient safety factors are reestablished at significant number of NMJs.
2. Those infants with severe weakness may require mechanical ventilation and treatment with PE.

LAMBERT–EATON MYASTHENIC SYNDROME

BACKGROUND

1. Lambert–Eaton Myasthenic syndrome (LEMS) is the second most common NMJ disorder following myasthenia gravis.
2. LEMS is an immunologic disorder caused by antibodies directed against voltage-gated calcium channels (VGCCs).
3. Approximately 84% of patients with LEMS are older than 40 years, with a mean age at presentation of 54 years.
4. In approximately two thirds of cases, LEMS arises as a paraneoplastic disorder, usually secondary to small cell carcinoma of the lung. Small cell carcinoma of the lung is the culprit of approximately 90% of the paraneoplastic cases of LEMS. Other malignancies associated with LEMS include lymphoproliferative disorders, pancreatic cancer, and breast and ovarian carcinoma. The LEMS symptoms usually precede tumor diagnosis by about 10 months (5 months to 3.8 years).
5. In the other third of patients, LEMS occurs as an autoimmune disorder without an underlying cancer. Such cases are more common in females and younger patients and are associated with other autoimmune disorders
6. The paraneoplastic and nonparaneoplastic forms of LEMS are otherwise clinically and electrophysiologically indistinguishable.

PATHOPHYSIOLOGY

1. LEMS is caused by antibodies directed against VGCCs on the presynaptic motor nerve terminals.
2. The antibodies bind to the VGCCs and subsequently inhibit the entry of calcium into the nerve terminal, which is required for the release of AChR. Additionally, the antibodies may cross-link neighboring calcium channels thus precipitating the process of internalization and degradation of the calcium channels.

PROGNOSIS

1. Patients generally improve with treatment.
2. Patients with primary autoimmune LEMS without underlying malignancy tend to do well. However, the prognosis in patients with an underlying cancer is more related to that of the malignancy, which generally is poor.

DIAGNOSIS

Clinical Features

1. Patients with the LEMS usually complain of proximal weakness and easy fatigability.
2. Ptosis and diplopia are often transient and mild. Some patients develop dysarthria or dysphagia but theses are more commonly secondary to dryness of the mouth.
3. Autonomic dysfunction as reduced saliva, dry eyes, blurred vision, constipation, decreased sweating, and impotence are commonly seen in patients with LEMS.
4. Although, most patients do not have respiratory problems related to the NMJ defect (they may have dyspnea related to their lung cancer), rare cases of LEMS presenting with respiratory failure have been described.
5. Neurologic examination demonstrates symmetric, proximal greater than distal, weakness affecting the legs more than the arms. Mild ptosis, ophthalmoparesis, and bulbar weakness may be apparent but these signs are not as common or as severe as typically seen in myasthenia gravis. Deep tendon reflexes may be diminished or absent, but then become significantly more easy to obtain once a slight contraction of the muscle has been performed.

Laboratory Features

1. Antibodies directed against the P/Q-type VGCCs of the motor nerve terminals are detected in the serum in more than 90% of patients with LEMS (both paraneoplastic and non–cancer-related cases).
2. Antibodies directed against the N-type calcium channels, which are located on autonomic and peripheral nerves as well as cerebellar, cortical, and spinal neurons are present in 74% of patients with LEMS and lung cancer and 40% of patients without cancer.
3. Some patients with paraneoplastic LEMS also have anti-Hu antibodies and the associated sensory ganglionopathy, cerebellar degeneration, and encephalopathy.
4. As many as 13% of patients with LEMS also have AChR binding antibodies. The anti-AChR antibodies are not necessarily pathogenic in patients with LEMS and may just represent an epiphenomenona.

Electrophysiologic Findings

1. Motor nerve conduction studies reveal a marked reduction in the compound muscle action potential (CMAP) amplitude.
2. With 10 seconds of exercise, repeated stimulation of the nerve elicits an increment in the CMAP amplitude due to postexercise facilitation.
3. If patients are unable to cooperate, high rates of repetitive stimulation at 20 to 50 Hz for up to 10 seconds will produce the same incrementing response. I do not routinely use high rates of repetitive stimulation, unless necessary, as it can be quite painful.
4. Repetitive stimulation at 2 to 3 Hz demonstrates an abnormal decrement.
5. Single-fiber EMG demonstrates increased jitter.

TREATMENT

1. Patients with LEMS should undergo an immediate and thorough investigation for underlying carcinoma, particularly involving the thoracic cavity (i.e., small cell lung cancer). In patients with paraneoplastic LEMS, muscle strength may improve with surgical removal of the tumor, radiation therapy, and chemotherapy.
2. In patients with and without tumor, a number of therapeutic medications can be given to assist with the symptoms of weakness and fatigue.
   a. Acetylcholinesterase inhibitors:
      1) I generally treat patients with Mestinon 60 mg four to five times a day as in patients with myasthenia gravis.

    2) The response is variable and often modest in comparison to that of myasthenia gravis.
  b. 3,4-diaminopyridine (3,4-DAP)
    1) The aminopyridines block voltage-dependent potassium conductance thereby prolonging nerve terminal depolarization and facilitate AChR release.
    2) The 3,4-DAP is not yet approved by the Food and Drug Administration (FDA). However, the medication can be obtained on a compassionate-use basis for patients with LEMS from Jacobus Pharmaceutical Co. (Princeton, NJ) pending approval from the FDA. Information regarding the application process to receive 3,4 DAP can be obtained by faxing the drug company at (609) 799-1176.
    3) The starting dose is 20 mg three times daily (t.i.d.) and is gradually increased up to 80 mg/d to achieve a maximal benefit.
    4) The medication appears to be well tolerated with a few patients experiencing perioral and acral paresthesias. It is recommended that doses not exceed 80 mg/d as higher doses may result in seizures.
  c. Immunosuppressive agents and immunomodulating therapies (see Table 8-1 in Chapter 8)
    1) Corticosteroids, azathioprine, cyclosporine, and mycophenolate are helpful.
    2) Dosing is similar to that described in the Myasthenia Gravis section.
    3) Unlike, myasthenia gravis, there is no role for thymectomy in the treatment of LEMS.
    4) Plasmapheresis may be helpful in patients with LEMS but the effect wears off after a few weeks and must be repeated.
    5) IVIG has been noted to be beneficial in small, uncontrolled series of patients with LEMS. Dosing is similar to that outlined for myasthenia gravis.

BOTULISM

BACKGROUND

1. Botulism is a serious and potentially fatal disease caused by one of several protein neuroexotoxins produced by the bacterium *Clostridium botulinum*.
2. There are eight immunologically distinct types of botulinus neurotoxin (BTX) designated alphabetically in their order of discovery: A, B, C1, C2, D, E, F, and G.
3. Types A, B, and E, account for most reported food poisoning cases; however, D, F, and G have been responsible for a few deaths. Toxin type C affects animals and not humans.
4. Five clinical forms of botulism have been described: (a) classic or food-borne botulism, (b) infant botulism, (c) hidden botulism, (d) wound botulism, and (e) inadvertent botulism.
  a. Classic or Food-borne Botulism
    1) The method of transmitting the botulinus toxin is usually through poorly prepared home-canned vegetables.
    2) The number of fatalities resulting from food-borne botulism has declined from about 50% prior to 1950, to approximately 7.5% from 1976 to 1984.
    3) Those persons over 60 years of age are particularly prone to more serious complication, possibly less complete recovery, and certainly a higher mortality rate.
  b. Infant Botulism
    1) This is the most common form of botulism in the United States with an incidence of 1/100,000 live births.

     2) The mortality rate among recognized infants infected with botulinus spores is under 4%.

     3) Spores of the *C. botulinum* inadvertently enter the infants intestinal tract, germinate and colonize this region, and then produce the toxin which is then absorbed through the intestinal tract's lumen.

     4) Epidemiologic studies reveal risk for botulism in infants consuming honey. As many as 25% of tested honey products contain clostridia spores. As a result, honey should be avoided in infants.

  c. Hidden botulism:

     1) Hidden botulism is believed to be a form of "infantile" botulism occurring in individuals older than 1 year.

     2) Patients have a typical clinical presentation suggestive of botulinus intoxication with supportive laboratory findings but do not have an obvious food or wound source for the disease.

     3) The disorder usually manifests in individuals who usually have an intestinal abnormalities (e.g., such as Crohn disease or following gastrointestinal surgery) that allows the colonization by the *C. botulinum* leading to the *in vivo* production of the toxin.

  d. Wound botulism:

     1) A wound is infected by *C. botulinum* with the subsequent production of toxin *in vivo*. The typical insult is some type of focal trauma to a limb with or without a compound fracture.

     2) There have been increasing reports of wound botulism occurring in intravenous (IV) drug abusers. BTX A is more often the offending agent, however, type B has also been implicated.

  e. Inadvertent botulism:

     1) This is the most recent form of botulism and refers to iatrogenic cases. BTX is now commonly used to treat focal dystonias and other movement disorders.

     2) Rarely, patients may develop distant or generalized weakness after focal injections of BTX. The mechanism is likely hematogenous spread of the toxin.

PATHOPHYSIOLOGY

The net affect of BTX intoxication is the inhibition of release of AChR vesicles.

PROGNOSIS

1. In the adult, the clinical presentation of botulinus intoxication is similar regardless of whether the disease is acquired through the food-borne, wound, or hidden (i.e., suspected gastrointestinal route).

  a. Patients develop dysphagia, dry mouth, diplopia, and dysarthria beginning rather acutely and progressing over the course of 12 to 36 hours. The time course is dependent in part on the amount of toxin consumed.

  b. Gastrointestinal symptoms of nausea, occasional vomiting, and initial diarrhea followed by constipation may occur just before or coincident with the above-noted neurologic symptoms. Associated complaints of abdominal cramps, undue fatigue, and dizziness may also be described during the disease's evolution.

  c. Then patients develop progressive weakness affecting first the upper and then the lower extremities. The patient may begin to notice shortness of breath prior to extremity involvement.

2. In wound botulism, gastrointestinal complaints of nausea, vomiting, and usually abdominal cramps are less common than food-borne botulism. The period of symptom development is longer in wound botulism as 4 to 14 days are required for an incubation period compared to hours for toxin or spore ingestion.

3. In infants, botulinus intoxication can manifest with an entire spectrum of disease from mild symptoms to sudden death.

  a. A relatively early sign is constipation.

b. The infant may later appear listless with a diminution in spontaneous movements. Parents may note that the child has a poor ability to take in nutrition secondary to a diminished suck.

c. Respiratory function should be closely monitored as approximately 50% of infants require assisted mechanical ventilation. This necessity of respiratory assistance may be because of not only respiratory muscle weakness, but also airway obstruction secondary to pharyngeal muscle weakness and loss of tonus.

d. Several weeks may be required before the patient shows any signs of recovery. The duration of required mechanical ventilation is dependent on the severity of the illness and serotype of the infecting organism with a mean of 58 days for type A and 26 days for type B botulism.

e. Recovery is usually satisfactory in all patients provided they are cared for in a hospital setting from the first manifestations of the disease. In the elderly, associated complications can lead to unavoidable death. There are long-term sequelae of fatigue and some mild reduction in respiratory capacity in selected patients.

DIAGNOSIS

Clinical Features

1. Cranial nerve evaluation reveals ptosis, diminished gag reflex, dysphagia, dysarthria, and weakness of the face, jaw opening and closing, and tongue.
2. Depending on the length of time between presentation and examination, the upper and lower limbs may be involved to varying degrees. The upper limbs are typically more affected than the lower limbs with an occasional asymmetry noted.
3. Deep tendon reflexes may be normal or diminished initially, with progression to complete loss in severely affected individuals.
4. Careful patient examination can reveal disturbances of autonomic function affecting both the sympathetic and parasympathetic systems. Pupils are often poorly reactive to light. In addition, there can be loss of vagal cardiac control, ileus, hypothermia, and urinary retention possibly requiring catheterization. In addition, hypotension without tachycardia may be present and a lack of vasomotor responses to postural change may be observed.
5. In cases of suspected wound botulism, the integument should be carefully searched for not only gross disruption and wound contamination, but also for apparently minor appearing bruises with or without signs of infection.

Laboratory Features

1. Stool and serum samples can be sent for toxin identification; however, this is a time-consuming process.
2. Less commonly, the organism can be cultured from the stool or a wound site.

Electrophysiologic Findings

1. CMAP amplitudes become reduced; however, it is not uncommon for patients examined relatively early after symptom onset to demonstrate normal amplitudes.
2. At low rates of repetitive stimulation (2–3 Hz), over 50% demonstrate a decremental response. Approximately 25% do not reveal a decrement at low stimulation rates whereas 20% have an increment.
3. About 90% of infants with botulism demonstrate an increment on 20- to 50-Hz repetitive stimulation.
4. The needle EMG examination can be somewhat variable depending on the time of examination.
   a. Early in the course of the disease, there is usually normal needle insertional activity and a lack of abnormal spontaneous activity.

   b. Fibrillation potentials and positive sharp waves may be found in severely affected muscles.
   c. The motor unit action potentials (MUAPs) have a myopathic appearance.
   d. Abnormal increases in jitter can be observed very early in the disease in 40% to 50% of single-fiber EMG studies.

TREATMENT

1. Antitoxin should be administered within 24 hours of symptom onset, before the toxin binding and entry into the nerve terminals. Once nerve terminal entry has been accomplished, the antitoxin is no longer capable of neutralizing the toxin.
2. The mainstay of care is supportive from the perspective of maintaining adequate ventilation and being prepared for prompt mechanical ventilation intervention.
3. Secretions must be handled as well as adequate nutrition provided.
4. Constipation must be kept under control.

TICK PARALYSIS

BACKGROUND

1. There are three major families of ticks, Ixodidae (hard body ticks), Argasidae (soft body ticks), and Nuttalliellidae. Ticks belonging to the first two families are responsible for causing human paralysis. These creatures are found worldwide primarily inhabiting rural and wilderness areas.
2. In North America, the tick, *Dermacentor andersoni* (common wood tick) usually causes the disease, but *Dermacentor variabilis* (dog tick) can also cause the disorder. Occasionally, ticks such as *Amblyomma americanum*, *Amblyomma maculatum*, as well as others have been implicated in human paralysis.
3. In Australian, *Ixodes holocyclus* (Australian marsupial tick) causes especially severe disease in humans.
4. Peak occurrences of paralysis caused by ticks are in the spring and summer months. Children are three times as likely to be involved as adults.

PATHOPHYSIOLOGY

1. Gravid female ticks are more commonly implicated because they feed for considerably longer times (days) and inject more toxin into their hosts compared to nongravid females and males.
2. In North American cases of tick paralysis, the toxin may block the sodium channel at the nodes of Ranvier and the distal motor nerve terminals.
3. Ixovotoxin released by the Australian *Ixodes holocyclus* tick most likely interferes with the release of ACh at the NMJ, perhaps similar to the effect of botulinus toxin.

PROGNOSIS

1. Patients develop acute or subacute progressive weakness that may require ventilatory support.
2. Removal of the tick results in prompt improvement in strength except for the Australian variety in which weakness may continue to progress to respiratory failure even after the tick is removed.

DIAGNOSIS

Clinical Features

1. Patients typically present with ascending weakness developing over the course of a few hours or days to flaccid paralysis that can mimic Guillain–Barré syndrome (GBS), myasthenia gravis, and botulism.
2. Early cranial nerve involvement including internal and external ophthalmoplegia, facial weakness, dysarthria, dysphagia, and respiratory muscle weakness is a salient feature.
3. Patients may complain of pain, itching, burning, or numbness in the extremities.
4. Deep tendon reflexes are diminished or absent.
5. If there is a recent history of camping or other types of leisure activity involving wooded or high grassy areas, the suspicion of tick paralysis should be raised.

Laboratory Features

1. Cerebrospinal fluid (CSF) protein concentration is usually normal in tick paralysis.
2. AChR antibodies are absent.

Electrophysiologic Findings

1. The sensory nerve conduction studies usually reveal normal amplitudes, latencies, and velocities.
2. Motor conduction velocity is usually slow or borderline in weak extremities. The CMAP amplitudes are borderline or decreased in size.
3. Removal of the tick within several days of clinical presentation results in the prompt resolution of amplitude and conduction velocity abnormalities.
4. Repetitive nerve stimulation at low and high rates usually fails to reveal either a significant decrement or increment.

TREATMENT

1. The treatment of tick paralysis is prompt removal of the tick with hospitalization for observation of potential impending respiratory failure.
2. Begin supportive and respiratory therapies as outlined in the GBS section.
3. A meticulous and comprehensive search for a tick is required. Common places for a tick to be present include the inferior hairline in the neck, periauricular area and the ear itself, the hair about the parietal scalp, the axilla, and the inguinal region.
4. Use a pair of tweezers or forceps and firmly grasp the tick as close to the patient's skin as possible (i.e., near the tick's mouth parts). A firm steady pull should then be applied. The body of the tick should never be pierced as more toxin may be released.
5. Within 24 to 48 hours of tick removal, most patients are well enough to be discharged from the hospital provided the tick is removed prior to profound functional loss.
6. An exception is the Australian variety of the tick, which produces such a virulent toxin that weakness may continue to progress to respiratory failure even after the tick is removed.
   a. An antitoxin in the form of polyclonal dog antiserum is available for the Australian form of the disease.
   b. The antiserum treatment is expensive and only effective if given in the early stages of paralysis and it may be associated with serum sickness,
   c. Continued ventilator support is required for several additional hours or until the patient can once again sustain voluntary ventilation.

CONGENITAL MYASTHENIC SYNDROMES

BACKGROUND

An increasing number of distinct congenital myasthenic syndromes (CMSs) are becoming better characterized. Within the category of CMSs, the individual types of CMS are subdivided according to the previously used scheme of presynaptic, synaptic space, and postsynaptic locations of the presumed site for the abnormality. Unlike autoimmune myasthenia gravis, these disorders may manifest with the first year of life.

PATHOPHYSIOLOGY

1. Presynaptic disorders
   a. Familial infantile myasthenia (defective AChR resynthesis or packaging)
   b. Congenital paucity of synaptic vesicles and reduced quantal release
2. Postsynaptic disorders:
   a. End-plate acetylcholinesterase deficiency
   b. Slow-channel syndrome
   c. Low-affinity, fast-channel syndrome
   d. Primary AChR deficiency
   e. Congenital myasthenia with mode-switching kinetics

PROGNOSIS

1. Weakness is stable or only slowly progressive.
2. Patients may develop respiratory failure at times of intercurrent illness.
3. Although patients may improve with various forms of treatment (see below), the improvement is not as dramatic as that seen in myasthenia gravis or LEMS.

DIAGNOSIS

Clinical Features

1. Onset may be congenital or in early adulthood.
2. Ptosis and ophthalmoparesis are common.
3. Fatigable weakness of the extremities as well as ocular and bulbar muscles.
4. Response to Tensilon is variable and dependent on the specific subtype of CMS. Patients with acetylcholinesterase deficiency and slow-channel syndromes may actually do worse with Tensilon.

Laboratory Features

1. Serum creatine kinase (CK) levels are normal.
2. AChR antibodies are absent.

Electrophysiologic Studies

1. Motor nerve conduction studies demonstrate repetitive after-discharges in patients with acetylcholinesterase deficiency and slow-channel syndromes.
2. Repetitive nerve conduction studies at 2 to 3 Hz reveal abnormal decrement.
3. EMG shows small myopathic MUAPs without abnormal insertional or spontaneous activity.
4. Single-fiber EMG demonstrates increased jitter.
5. Sophisticated electrophysiologic studies in intercostal muscles are used to define the different subtypes but are not readily available.

6. Genetic testing for mutations of genes encoding various proteins comprising the AChR and collagen Q are available only at research laboratories.

TREATMENT

1. These are not autoimmune in etiology, and thus, antibodies to AChR are not present. Therefore, treatments aimed at modulating the immune system (e.g., PE, IVIG, thymectomy, corticosteroids, and other immunosuppressive agents) are not effective in the CMS.
2. Mestinon 60 mg q.i.d. may improve strength in patients with presynaptic defects, primary AChR deficiency, and fast-channel syndrome.
3. 3,4 DAP 1 mg/kg/d is helpful in patients with the fast-channel syndrome. In some studies, only a few of the patients with primary AChR deficiency responded, while the other patients with CMS failed to improve.
4. Mestinon and 3,4 DAP may lead to worsening in patients with the slow-channel syndrome and end-plate acetylcholinesterase deficiency.
5. Quinidine may be helpful in slow-channel syndromes by shortening and even normalizing the duration of mutant channel openings. Administration of quinidine with serum levels of 0.7 to 2.5 μg/mL improved the clinical and electrophysiologic features in patients with slow-channel syndrome.
6. Patients with respiratory weakness may benefit from BiPAP treatment.

INFLAMMATORY MYOPATHIES

BACKGROUND

1. Inflammatory myopathies are a heterogeneous group of disorders characterized by muscle weakness, elevated serum CK levels, and inflammation on muscle biopsy.
2. The inflammatory myopathies can be divided into the more common idiopathic group, in which the etiology is unknown; myositis associated with connective tissue disease and of inflammatory disorders; and myositis due to various infections.
3. There are three major categories of idiopathic inflammatory myopathies:
   a. Dermatomyositis (DM)
   b. Polymyositis (PM)
   c. Inclusion body myositis (IBM)
4. Overlap syndromes refer to DM and PM occurring in association with another autoimmune connective tissue disorder (CTD): systemic lupus erythematosus, mixed connective tissue disease, scleroderma, rheumatoid arthritis, Sjögren syndrome.
5. The annual incidence of the idiopathic inflammatory myopathies is approximately 1/100,000.
   a. DM and IBM are the most common myositides.
   b. DM can occur in childhood through adulthood.
   c. IBM is the most common myopathy in patients older than 50 years.
   d. PM is rare and is overdiagnosed. Many cases of "PM" turn out to be IBM, DM with minimal rash, or muscular dystrophy with inflammation.

PATHOPHYSIOLOGY

1. DM is a humerally mediated microangiopathy leading to destruction of capillaries and arterioles supplying skin and muscle. Weakness is related to ischemia/infarction of muscle.
2. PM is caused by an HLA-restricted, antigen-specific, cell-mediated autoimmune response directed against muscle fibers.

3. IBM has an unclear pathogenesis.
   a. The inflammatory changes on muscle biopsy are similar to PM and suggest a cell-mediated autoimmune attack.
   b. The lack of improvement with various immunosuppressive and immunomodulatory therapies suggest that IBM could be a primary degenerative myopathy (i.e., a dystrophy) with secondary inflammation.

PROGNOSIS

1. DM and PM are responsive to immunotherapies.
2. IBM is refractory to immunotherapy.

DIAGNOSIS

Clinical Features

1. DM:
   a. May present with acute or insidious onset of proximal greater than distal weakness.
   b. Characteristic skin rash (e.g., heliotrope, forehead and malar regions, chest and neck, extensor surface of extremities/joints, Gottron sign and papules, periungual telangiectasias) usually accompany or precede muscle weakness.
   c. Other organ systems may be involved: interstitial lung disease (ILD) in 10% to 20%, myocarditis, gastrointestinal bleed secondary to vasculopathy of gut, arthritis.
   d. Increased risk of malignancy.
2. PM:
   a. May present with acute or insidious onset of proximal greater than distal weakness.
   b. No rash.
   c. Other organ systems may be involved: ILD in 10% to 20%, myocarditis, arthritis.
   d. May have increased risk of malignancy.
3. IBM:
   a. Presents with an insidious onset of proximal and distal weakness.
   b. Early involvement of wrist and finger flexors in arms with relative sparing of the deltoids and of the quadriceps and ankle dorsiflexors in the legs helps distinguish from other myopathies.
   c. Weakness is often asymmetric. Severe dysphagia can develop.
   d. Other organs are not involved.
   e. No increased risk of malignancy.

Laboratory Features

1. DM/PM:
   a. Serum CK level can be normal in DM, particularly early in the course or with insidious onset but more commonly is moderately elevated more than ten times normal.
   b. Serum CK level is not a good indicator of disease activity.
   c. ANAs may be detected in patients with overlap syndrome (e.g., myositis associated with and underlying CTD).
   d. Anti–Jo-1 antibodies should be ordered as they are associated with ILD, which can influence therapy (see below).
2. PM:
   a. Serum CK levels are elevated, often more than ten times normal.
   b. Serum CK level is not a good indicator of disease activity.
   c. ANAs may be detected in patients with overlap syndrome (e.g., myositis associated with and underlying CTD).
   d. Anti–Jo-1 antibodies should be ordered, as they are associated with ILD, which can influence therapy (see below).

3. IBM:
   a. Serum CK level is normal or only mildly elevated (less than ten times normal).
   b. Autoantibodies are uncommon (present in fewer than 20% of patients) and are of uncertain significance in this elderly population.

Electrodiagnostic Features

1. EMG demonstrates increased insertional and spontaneous activity (fibrillation potentials and positive sharp waves).
2. MUAPs are usually small in amplitude, short in duration, polyphasic, and recruit early.
3. Long duration units, which are often seen in neurogenic disorders, also may be seen, particularly in IBM. This abnormality reflects chronicity of the myopathic process as opposed to a superimposed neurogenic disorder.

Histologic Features

1. DM:
   a. The characteristic histopathologic abnormality is perifascicular atrophy but this is seen in less than 30% of cases and is seen for the most part in patients with long-standing weakness.
   b. Inflammatory cell infiltrate, when evident, is seen in the perimysium and around blood vessels (perivascular).
   c. Unlike PM and IBM, there is no endomysial inflammation and invasion of nonnecrotic muscle fibers.
   d. Earliest histologic abnormalities are deposition of immune complex of small blood vessels and tubuloreticular inclusions in endothelial walls.
2. PM:
   a. Muscle biopsy demonstrates endomysial mononuclear inflammatory cell infiltrate surrounding and invading nonnecrotic muscle fibers.
   b. Immune complex deposition on small blood vessels is not seen.
3. IBM:
   a. Muscle biopsy demonstrates endomysial mononuclear inflammatory cell infiltrate surrounding and invading nonnecrotic muscle fibers similar to PM.
   b. Muscle fibers with one or more rimmed vacuoles are often but not invariably seen.
   c. Increased number of ragged red and cytochrome oxidase–negative fibers are seen, indicative of mitochondrial abnormalities.
   d. Amyloid deposition in vacuolated muscle fibers may be seen.
   e. Electron microscopy may demonstrate 15- to 21-nm tubulofilaments in the cytoplasm of vacuolated muscle fibers and less commonly in myonuclei.
   f. Because of sampling error, as many as 20% to 30% of muscle biopsies will not demonstrate all these histologic abnormalities leading to erroneous diagnosis of PM unless the clinical pattern of weakness that is specific for IBM is not recognized by the clinician.

TREATMENT

Immunotherapy is recommended for DM, PM, and overlap myositis. I do not recommend such treatment for IBM as this myopathy is refractory to such therapies.
1. Corticosteroids:
   a. In patients with severe weakness (unable to ambulate) or with severe systemic involvement (myocarditis, dyspnea related to ILD), I initiate treatment with Solumedrol 1 g IV daily for 3 days and then start oral prednisone.
   b. In patients with mild or moderate weakness, I begin treatment with single-dose prednisone (1.5 mg/kg up to 100 mg) by mouth (p.o.) every morning.
   c. After 2 to 4 weeks of daily prednisone, I switch directly to alternate day dosing [i.e., 100 mg every other day (q.o.d.)].

   d. Patients with more severe disease are more slowly tapered to alternate-day dosing over 2 to 3 months. Decrease the dose by 10 mg a week (e.g., 100 mg alternating with 90 mg daily for 1 week then 100 mg alternating with 80 mg daily for 1 week until they are on 100 mg q.o.d.).

   e. Patients are initially seen every 2 to 4 weeks and I maintain the high-dose prednisone until the patients are back to normal strength or until improvement in strength has reached a plateau (usually 4 to 6 months).

   f. Subsequently, the prednisone dose is tapered by 5 mg every 2 to 3 weeks.

   g. Once the dose is reduced to 20 mg q.o.d., prednisone is tapered no faster than 2.5 mg every 2 weeks.

   h. If a patient does not significantly improve after 4 to 6 months of prednisone, or if there is an exacerbation during the taper, I add a second-line agent (e.g., methotrexate, azathioprine, mycophenolate mofetil, or IVIG).

      1) At the same time, the prednisone dose is doubled and given daily (no more than 100 mg/d) for at least 2 weeks before switching back to q.o.d. dosing.

      2) Once a patient has regained his or her strength, I resume the prednisone taper at a slower rate.

   i. Although serum CK levels are monitored, adjustments of prednisone and other immunosuppressive agents should be based on the objective clinical examination and not the CK levels or the patient's subjective response.

      1) An increasing serum CK level can herald a relapse but without objective clinical deterioration, I would not increase the dose of the immunosuppressive agent.

      2) However, I may hold the dose or the slow the taper.

   j. A maintenance dose of prednisone is often required to sustain the clinical response.

   k. High-dose, long-term steroids and lack of physical activity can cause type 2 muscle fiber atrophy with proximal muscle weakness that needs to be distinguished from weakness due to relapse of the myositis.

      1) Patients who become weaker during prednisone taper, have increasing serum CK levels, and abnormal spontaneous activity on EMG are more likely experiencing a flare of the myositis.

      2) In contrast, patients with normal serum CK levels and EMG findings and other evidence of steroid toxicity (i.e., cushingoid appearance) may have type 2 muscle fiber atrophy and could benefit from physical therapy and reducing the dose of steroids.

2. Concurrent management with steroids:

   a. Obtain a chest radiograph and a PPD skin test with controls on all patients before initiating immunosuppressive medications. Patients with prior history of tuberculosis or those with a positive PPD may need to be treated prophylactically with isoniazid.

   b. Measure bone density with DEXA at baseline and every 6 months while patients are receiving corticosteroids.

      1) A bone density less than 2.5 standard deviations below normal is considered positive for osteoporosis.

      2) Calcium supplementation (1 g/d) and vitamin D (400 IU/d) are started for prophylaxis against steroid-induced osteoporosis.

      3) Bisphosphonates are effective in the prevention and treatment of osteoporosis. If DEXA scans demonstrate osteoporosis at baseline or during follow-up studies, I initiate alendronate 70 mg per week. In postmenopausal women, I start alendronate 35 mg orally once a week as prophylaxis for osteoporosis. The long-term side effects of bisphosphonates are not known especially in men and young premenopausal women. In those patients, I start prophylactic treatment with alendronate 35 mg orally once a week if DEXA scans show bone loss at baseline (not as yet enough to diagnosis osteoporosis) or if there is significant loss on follow-up bone density scans.

      4) Alendronate can cause severe esophagitis and absorption is impaired if taken with meals. Therefore, patients must be instructed to remain upright and not to eat for at least 30 minutes after taking a dose of alendronate.

   c. I do not prophylactically treat with histamine-H_2 receptor blockers unless the patient develops gastrointestinal discomfort or has a history of peptic ulcer disease. Tums can be used for calcium supplementation and dyspepsia.

   d. Patients are instructed to start a low sodium, low-carbohydrate, high-protein diet to prevent excessive weight gain.

   e. Physical therapy is initiated and patients are encouraged to slowly begin an aerobic exercise program.

   f. Blood pressure is measured with each visit along with periodic eye examinations for cataracts and glaucoma.

   g. Fasting blood glucose and serum potassium levels are periodically checked.

      1) Potassium supplementation may be required if the patient becomes hypokalemic.

      2) Oral hypoglycemic agents or insulin may be required in patients who become hyperglycemic.

3. Second-line therapies:

   a. These agents have been used primarily in patients poorly responsive to prednisone or who relapse during prednisone taper as well as for their potential steroid-sparing effect.

   b. Methotrexate is my second-line agent of choice unless the patient has ILD, as methotrexate can cause pulmonary fibrosis.

   c. Azathioprine is my choice in patients with ILD.

   d. IVIG is effective in DM. I have not found it to be helpful in PM.

   e. Mycophenolate mofetil may prove useful as a second line agent but there is limited published experience with this medication in myositis. See Treatment of Myasthenia Gravis for details.

4. Methotrexate:

   a. I usually begin methotrexate orally at 7.5 mg/wk given in three divided doses 12 hours apart.

   b. The dose is gradually increased by 2.5 mg/wk up to 20 mg/wk.

   c. If there is no improvement after 1 month of 20 mg/wk of oral methotrexate, switch to weekly parenteral [intramuscular (IM) or IV] methotrexate and increase the dose by 5 mg/wk up to 60 mg/wk.

   d. In patients with severe muscle weakness and/or myocarditis, I initiate methotrexate parenterally in doses of 20 to 25 mg/wk in combination with corticosteroids.

   e. The major side effects of methotrexate are alopecia, stomatitis, ILD, teratogenicity, oncogenicity, risk of infection, and bone marrow, renal, and liver toxicities.

   f. Folate is started at the same time. Doses over 50 mg/wk require leukovorin rescue.

   g. Because methotrexate can cause ILD, I do not recommend its use in patients with myositis who already have the associated ILD. I also always check for an anti–Jo-1 antibody titer in the serum because of the risk of ILD in patients with these antibodies.

   h. Baseline and periodic pulmonary function tests need to be checked on patients treated with methotrexate.

   i. CBCs and LFTs (AST, ALT, and GGT) need to be followed closely. It is important to check the GGT, as elevations are specific for hepatic dysfunction, whereas the AST and ALT may be elevated from myositis.

5. Azathioprine:

   a. I start azathioprine at a dose of 50 mg/d in adults and gradually increase by 50 mg/wk to a total dose of 2 to 3 mg/kg/d.

   b. The major drawback is that it can take 9 months or more to see an effect from azathioprine.

   c. A systemic reaction characterized by fever, abdominal pain, nausea, vomiting, and anorexia occurs in 12% of patients requiring discontinuation of the drug. This systemic reaction generally occurs within the first few weeks of therapy and resolves within a few days of discontinuing the azathioprine. Rechallenge with azathioprine usually results in the recurrence of the systemic reaction.

d. Other major complications of azathioprine are bone marrow suppression, hepatic toxicity, pancreatitis, teratogenicity, oncogenicity, and risk of infection.
e. Allopurinol should be avoided, because combination with azathioprine increases the risk of bone marrow and liver toxicity. A major drawback of azathioprine is that it often takes 6 months or longer to be effective.
f. Monitor CBC and LFTs every 2 weeks until the patient is on a stable dose of azathioprine, then monitor once a month.
g. If the WBC count falls below 4,000 per mm^3, I decrease the dose. Azathioprine is held if the WBC declines to 2,500 per mm^3 or the absolute neutrophil count falls to 1,000 per mm^3. Leukopenia can develop as early as 1 week or as late as 2 years after initiating azathioprine. The leukopenia usually reverses within 1 month, and it is possible to then rechallenge the patient with azathioprine without recurrence of the severe leukopenia.
h. Discontinue azathioprine if the LFTs increase more than twice the baseline values. Liver toxicity generally develops within the first several months of treatment and can take several months to resolve. Patients can occasionally be successfully rechallenged with azathioprine after LFTs return to baseline without recurrence of hepatic dysfunction. Again it is important to check the GGT, which is specific for the liver, as opposed to just AST and ALT, which could be elevated secondary to hepatotoxicity or exacerbation of the myositis.

6. IVIG:
a. A prospective, double-blind, placebo-control study of 15 patients with DM demonstrated significant clinical improvement with IVIG.
b. All patients should have an IgA level checked before treatment. Patients with low IgA levels may be at risk for anaphylaxis.
c. I start IVIG (2 g/kg) slowly over 2 to 5 days and repeat infusions at monthly intervals for at least 3 months.
d. Patients should have renal functions checked, especially those with diabetes mellitus because of a risk of IVIG-induced renal failure. IVIG is avoided in patients with renal insufficiency.
e. There is a low risk of thrombosis with subsequent myocardial infarction or stroke. For this reason, I avoid IVIG in patients with significant atherosclerotic cardiovascular disease
f. Flu-like symptoms—headaches, myalgias, fever, chills, nausea, and vomiting—are common and occur in as many as half the patients. Rash and aseptic meningitis may occur.
g. I premedicate patients 30 minutes prior to IVIG infusions with hydrocortisone 100 mg IV, Benadryl 25 mg IV, and Tylenol 650 mg p.o. This reduces the incidence of headaches and myalgias.

7. Third-line agents when the above treatments fail include cyclophosphamide and cyclosporine.

8. Cyclophosphamide:
a. The efficacy of cyclophosphamide is controversial, and it has usually been reserved for patients refractory to prednisone, azathioprine, methotrexate, and IVIG.
b. Cyclophosphamide has also been advocated in patients with severe ILD as improvement generally begins faster than that seen in treatment with azathioprine.
c. Cyclophosphamide can be given orally at a dose of 1.0 to 2.0 mg/kg/d or by IV at a dose of 1 g/m^2/mo for patients with severe myositis and ILD.
d. The major side effects are gastrointestinal upset, bone marrow toxicity, alopecia, hemorrhagic cystitis, teratogenicity, sterilization, and increased risk of infections and secondary malignancies.
e. It is important to maintain a high fluid intake to avoid hemorrhagic cystitis. Urinalysis and CBCs need to be followed closely (every 1 to 2 weeks at the onset of therapy and then at least monthly).
f. Cyclophosphamide should be decreased if the WBC count decreases below 4,000/mm^3. Cyclophosphamide is held if the WBC declines below 3,000/mm^3, the absolute neutrophil count falls below 1,000/mm^3, or if there is evidence

of hematuria. Cyclophosphamide can be restarted at a lower dose once the leukopenia has resolved, but I do restart the medication in patients with hematuria.

9. Cyclosporine:
   a. I start cyclosporine at a dose of 3.0 to 4.0 mg/kg/d in two divided doses and gradually increase to 6.0 mg/kg/d as necessary.
   b. The cyclosporine dose should initially be titrated to maintain trough serum cyclosporine levels of 50 to 200 ng/mL.
   c. Blood pressure, electrolytes and renal function, and trough cyclosporine levels need to be monitored periodically.
   d. Side effects of cyclosporine and tacrolimus are renal toxicity, hypertension, electrolyte imbalance, gastrointestinal upset, hypertrichosis, gingival hyperplasia, oncogenicity, tremor, and risk of infection.
10. Supportive therapy:
    a. Physical therapy:
       1) Range-of-motion exercises are started early to prevent contractures.
       2) As patient improves, exercises to improve strength, function, and gait.
    b. Speech therapy:
       1) Patients with dysphagia should undergo a swallowing study.
       2) If severe dysphagia or recurrent aspiration is documented, a percutaneous gastrostomy tube or cricopharyngectomy (in IBM) may be warranted.
11. Malignancy workup:
    a. There is an increased risk of cancer in patients with DM and perhaps PM.
    b. The malignancies generally occur within 3 years of the presentation of the myositis.
    c. Patients should have a complete history and physical examination, including rectal, breast, and pelvic examinations.
    d. Chest radiography should be performed on every patient and pelvic ultrasound or computed tomography (CT) scans and mammograms on women.
    e. Colonoscopy should be performed on everyone older than 50 years, those patients with heme-positive stool, and those with gastrointestinal symptoms (e.g., abdominal pain, persistent constipation, blood in stool).

TRICHINOSIS

BACKGROUND

Trichinosis is the most common parasitic disease of skeletal muscle.

PATHOPHYSIOLOGY

1. Following ingestion of meat infected with encysted larvae, gastric juices liberate the larvae that infect the gut.
2. Maturation of the parasite occurs in the gut. Next, second generation larvae migrate into the bloodstream and lymphatics to invade the muscle and provoke the inflammatory response.
3. The organism matures and remains within single muscle fibers until consumed by another organism, thereby completing the life cycle.

PROGNOSIS

1. Myalgias and weakness peak in the third week of the infection but can last for several months.

2. Severe disease can be complicated by myocarditis and central nervous system (CNS) infection.
3. In nonimmunocompromised patients, there is usually complete recovery within several months.

DIAGNOSIS

Clinical Features

1. Two to 12 days following ingestion of inadequately cooked meat (usually pork), the larval form of the nematode disseminates through the blood stream and invades the musculature.
2. The most frequent muscles invaded, in order of frequency, are the diaphragm, extraocular, tongue, laryngeal, jaw, intercostal, trunk, and limbs.
3. Patients develop fever, abdominal pain, diarrhea, generalized myalgias, and weakness.
4. Periorbital edema, ptosis, subconjunctival hemorrhage, and an erythematous urticaria or petechial rash are often present.

Laboratory Features

1. Most patients have eosinophilic leukocytosis and elevated serum CK level.
2. Serum antibodies against *Trichinella spiralis* can be demonstrated in 3 to 4 weeks after infection.

Histopathology

1. Infiltration of the muscle by inflammatory cells is more common.
2. Larvae, cysts, focal calcification of the cysts, fibrosis, and granulomas may be observed.

TREATMENT

1. Thiobendazole 25 mg/kg b.i.d. for 10 days is the treatment of choice for larvae and the mature nematode, but efficacy has not been established against the encysted larvae.
2. Mebendazole may be effective against both circulating and encysted larvae.
3. Because a Herxheimer-like reaction can develop following degeneration of the larvae, concurrent corticosteroid administration is beneficial. Prednisone is started at a dose of 60 mg p.o. daily for the first 2 days of treatment followed by a reduction by 10 mg every 2 days

---

CRITICAL ILLNESS MYOPATHY (ACUTE QUADRIPLEGIC MYOPATHY)

BACKGROUND

1. Weakness developing in a patient in the ICU may be secondary to critical illness polyneuropathy, prolonged neuromuscular blockage, or myopathic process.
2. This myopathic disorder has been termed "critical illness myopathy" (CIM), acute quadriplegic myopathy, acute illness myopathy, and myopathy associated with thick filaments (myosin).
3. CIM is at least three times more common than critical illness polyneuropathy.

PATHOPHYSIOLOGY

1. The mechanism of muscle fiber necrosis is not known.
2. Myosin is selectively lost in some patients.
3. Decreased muscle membrane inexcitability that occurs with this myopathy.

PROGNOSIS

1. The mortality is high, approximately 30% in one large series, secondary to multiple organ failure and sepsis rather than the myopathy.
2. The morbidity and mortality in CIM appears to be similar to that of critical illness neuropathy.
3. In patients who survive, muscle strength recovers slowly over several months.

DIAGNOSIS

Clinical Features

1. CIM usually developing in patients who received high-dose IV corticosteroids and/or nondepolarizing neuromuscular blockers.
2. The disorder has also been reported in critically ill patients with sepsis or multi-organ failure who have not received other corticosteroids or nondepolarizing neuromuscular blocking agents.
3. There may be a predilection for development of CIM in transplant recipients who receive high doses of IV corticosteroids during the perioperative period.
4. Patients with CIM exhibit severe generalized muscle weakness that develops over a period of several days. Occasionally the weakness can be quite asymmetric and mimic a stroke.
5. The myopathy may be first recognized by the inability to wean the patient from the ventilator.
6. Sensory examination is usually normal, albeit sometimes difficult to interpret in an intubated patient with concurrent altered mental status. Deep tendon reflexes are decreased or absent.

Laboratory Features

Serum CK levels can be normal, but is moderately elevated in about 50% of patients.

Histopathology

1. Muscle biopsies often demonstrates type 2 muscle fiber atrophy with or without type 1 fiber atrophy, muscle fiber necrosis, and focal or diffuse loss of reactivity for myosin adenosine triphosphatase (ATPase).
2. A loss of thick filaments (myosin) is often apparent on immunohistochemistry and electron microscopy (EM).

Electrophysiologic Findings

1. Nerve conduction studies demonstrate significantly diminished amplitudes of CMAPs with normal distal latencies and conduction velocities.
2. In contrast, SNAP amplitudes are normal or mildly reduced (greater than 80% of the lower limit of normal).
3. EMG frequently demonstrates prominent fibrillation potentials and positive sharp waves. Short-duration, small-amplitude, polyphasic MUAPs that recruit early are evident. In severe cases, it may be difficult to recruit any MUAP.

TREATMENT

1. There is no medical therapy other than supportive care and treating underlying systemic abnormalities (e.g., antibiotics in sepsis, dialysis in renal failure).

2. If patients are still receiving high doses of corticosteroids or nondepolarizing neuromuscular blockers, the medications should be stopped.
3. Patients will require extensive physical therapy to prevent contractures and help regain muscle strength and functional abilities.

DUCHENNE AND BECKER MUSCULAR DYSTROPHY

BACKGROUND

1. The best known of the muscular dystrophies is the X-linked recessive Duchenne muscular dystrophy (DMD). The incidence is roughly 1/3,500 male births with a prevalence approaching 1/18,000 males. Approximately one third of cases of DMD are a result of spontaneous mutations in the dystrophin gene located on chromosome Xp21.
2. Becker muscular dystrophy (BMD) represents a form of dystrophinopathy that is milder than the more severe DMD phenotype with which it is allelic. BMD can be distinguished from DMD primarily by its rate of progression combined with dystrophin analysis. The incidence of this disorder is approximately 5/100,000 with a prevalence of 2.4/100,000. Approximately 10% of cases are the result of spontaneous mutations.

PATHOPHYSIOLOGY

1. Dystrophin is a structural protein that is intimately bound to the sarcolemma and provides structural integrity to the muscle membrane.
2. The large size of the gene accounts for the high mutation rate and the one third of cases caused by new spontaneous mutations. Large deletions, ranging from several kilobase to more than 1 million base pair, can be demonstrated in approximately two thirds of patients with dystrophinopathy. Approximately 5% to 10% of DMD cases are caused by point mutation resulting in premature stop codons. Duplications are evident in another 5% of cases. Smaller mutations, which are not readily detectable, account for the remainder.
3. Mutations disrupting the translational reading frame of the gene result in near total loss of dystrophin and usually lead to DMD, while in-frame mutations result in the translation of semifunctional dystrophin of abnormal size and/or amount typically resulting in outlier or BMD clinical phenotypes. Although there are exceptions to the "reading-frame rule," 92% of phenotypic differences are explained by in-frame and out-of-frame mutations.

PROGNOSIS

1. Children with DMD are confined to a wheelchair by the age of age 12 and most die from respiratory complications in their late teenaged year or early 20's.
2. The severity of BMD is quite variable. Patients with BMD are ambulatory past the age of 15 years. The life expectancy is reduced with an age of death ranging from 23 to 89 years (mean, 42 years).

DIAGNOSIS

Clinical Features

1. Most male children with DMD appear normal at birth and achieve the anticipated milestones of sitting and standing either normally or with only slight delay.
2. A "clumsy" walk and frequent falls is noted by about 2 to 6 years of age.

3. Weakness is characteristically worse proximally than distally and more so in the lower compared to upper limbs.
4. Children are confined to a wheelchair by the age of 12 years.
5. Cardiac dysrhythmias and congestive heart failure can occur late in the disease.
6. Smooth muscle is also affected and patients can develop gastroparesis and intestinal pseudoobstruction.
7. The CNS is also involved in DMD and the average IQ of the affected children is one standard deviation below the normal mean.
8. BMD has a milder course, with patients remaining ambulatory past the age of 15 years. The mean age of losing the ability to ambulate independently is in the fourth decade.
9. Some patients with BMD manifest with only myalgias, myoglobinuria, cardiomyopathy, and asymptomatic hyper–CK-emia.

Laboratory Features

1. The serum CK levels are markedly elevated (as much as 50–100 times normal or greater).
2. Patients with BMD with only exertional myalgias may have only slightly elevated serum CK levels (three times normal).

Histopathology

1. Muscle biopsy reveals evidence of muscle fiber degeneration and regeneration. There is considerable fiber size variation with scattered hypertrophic and hypercontracted fibers in addition to small, rounded, regenerating fibers. There is increased endomysial and perimysial connective tissue.
2. Immunohistochemistry demonstrates absent dystrophin staining on the muscle membrane in most cases of DMD and diminished dystrophin staining.
3. Western blot analysis of muscle tissue assesses both the quantity and size of the dystrophin present. In DMD, there is a marked reduction in dystrophy (typically less than 3% of normal). In BMD, Western blot analysis reveals an abnormal quantity and/or size of the dystrophin to a lesser degree than seen in DMD.

TREATMENT

1. Steroids:
   a. Prednisone (0.75 mg/kg/d) is effective in increasing strength and function (peaking at 3 months) and the subsequent slowing of the rate of deterioration in children with DMD. The beneficial effects are noted as early as 10 days and are sustained for at least 3 years. Lower doses of prednisone (less than 0.75 mg/kg/d) are not as effective.
   b. Unfortunately high-dose prednisone is associated with significant side effects including weight gain, stunted growth, cushingoid appearance, excessive hair growth, irritability, and hyperactivity. In addition, prednisone is associated with an increased risk of infections, cataract formation, hypertension, glucose intolerance, osteoporosis, and osteonecrosis.
   c. Because of the severe side effects associated with high-dose steroids, I try to hold off using it until patients are having significant ambulatory difficulty in an attempt to stave off wheelchair dependence for a period. Once the child is confined to the wheelchair, I taper him or her off the prednisone.
   d. An analog of prednisone, deflazacort (not as yet FDA-approved in the United States), has been studied in a few clinical trials. Deflazacort at doses of 0.9 mg/kg/d and 1.2 mg/kg/d may be as effective as prednisone 0.75 mg/kg/d and associated with fewer side effects.
   e. Creatine monohydrate (5–10 g/d) is often prescribed for patients with DMD or BMD. Creatine supplementation may increase the muscle supply of phosphocreatine and increase the ATP resynthesis; however, large clinical trials demonstrating efficacy are lacking.

2. Supportive therapy:
   a. The best management should involve neurologists, physiatrists, physical therapists, occupational therapists, speech therapists, respiratory therapists, dietitians, psychologists, and genetic counselors to assess all the needs of individual patients.
   b. Physical therapy is a key component in the treatment of patients with muscular dystrophy. Contractures develop early in the disease, particularly at the heal cords, iliotibial bands, and hips; therefore, stretching exercises must also be started early (i.e., at 3–4 years of age).
3. Bracing:
   a. The appropriate use of bracing may delay the child's progression to a wheelchair by approximately 2 years.
   b. A major factor responsible for the children's inability to stand or walk is weakness of the quadriceps. The addition of a long-leg brace (knee–foot orthosis) may stabilize the knee and prevents the knee from flexing. The children walk stiff-legged, but they do not have the same problem with falling that they had previously. Generally, children are ready for bracing when they have ceased to climb stairs, are having great difficulty arising from the floor, and are having frequent daily falls.
   c. There may be some advantage to a lightweight, plastic knee—foot orthosis, but it is difficult to keep the foot straight with such a device, whereas the high-top boot worn with the double-upright brace provides excellent stability. The choice between plastic and metal often comes down to the personal preference of the patient and physician.
   d. A night splint to maintain the feet at right angles to the leg is important at an early age. Ankle contractures are almost never seen in patients who use these splints conscientiously.
4. Surgery:
   a. Reconstructive surgery of the leg often accompanies bracing to keep the leg extended and prevent contractures of the iliotibial bands, hip and knee flexors, and ankle dorsiflexors.
   b. A simple way to maintain function in the legs with contractures beginning in the iliotibial bands, hip flexors and knee flexors is to perform percutaneous tenotomies of the Achilles tendons, knee flexors, hip flexors, and iliotibial bands. This procedure often allows a child who is becoming increasingly dependent on a wheelchair to resume walking.
   c. Scoliosis is a universal complication of DMD and results in patient pain, aesthetic damage, and perhaps respiratory compromise. I consider spinal fusion in children with 35-degree scoliosis or more and who are in significant discomfort. Ideally, forced vital capacity (FVC) should be greater than 35% to minimize the risk of surgery. Quality of life seems to be improved following spinal stabilization, however, scoliosis surgery does not appear to increase respiratory function.
5. Ventilatory failure:
   a. Most patients with DMD die as a result of respiratory failure; therefore, it is important to assess for symptoms or signs of respiratory impairment during each clinic visit.
   b. Patients with FVCs below 50% or those with symptomatic respiratory dysfunction are offered noninvasive ventilator support, usually BiPAP.
   c. Inspiratory and expiratory pressures are titrated to symptom relief and patient tolerability.
   d. In my experience, only a few patients desire tracheostomy and mechanical ventilation. However, this is an individual decision that must be made by the patient. Tracheostomy needs to be offered to patients along with realistic counseling in regard to what this entails to the patient and the family.
6. Genetic counseling:
   a. The daughters of males with BMD (males with DMD are usually infertile) and the mothers of affected children who also have a family history of DMD or BMD are obligate carriers of the mutated dystrophin gene.

b. Mothers and sisters of isolated DMD or BMD patients are at risk for being carriers.

c. It is always essential to determine the carrier status of "at-risk" females for genetic counseling (see below). There is a 50% chance that males born to carrier females will inherit the disease, whereas 50% of the daughters born will become carriers themselves.

d. Carrier females are usually asymptomatic, but rarely, dystrophinopathies clinically manifest in females. Approximately 8% of DMD carriers have mild muscle weakness.

e. Serum CK levels may be elevated in female carriers early in life. However, a normal serum CK level does not exclude a carrier status. Elevated serum CK levels are identified in less than 50% of obligate carriers and there is a false-positive rate of 2.5%.

f. The most reliable method of detecting carrier status is with DNA analysis.

  1) First, affected male relatives should be evaluated for mutations in the dystrophin gene. The detection of a mutation in such patients with DMD makes carrier detection of at-risk female relatives much easier and allows subsequent prenatal detection in at-risk fetuses. If a mutation is demonstrated in an affected male relative, at-risk females can be screened for the same mutation.

  2) Carrier status of a mother of a sporadic DMD case must be interpreted cautiously because of the potential for germ-line mosaicism. In a germ-line mosaic, the mutation involves only a percentage of the germ cells (i.e., oocytes), but is not present in the leukocytes in which DNA analysis is performed. An affected child may have an identifiable mutation on DNA analysis, whereas the mother could have no demonstrable mutation in the leukocytes, but she might still be a carrier. The recurrence rate in germ-line carriers is unknown and dependent on the number of mutated oocytes but has been estimated to be as high as 14%.

g. Prenatal diagnosis can be made with DNA analysis of chorionic villi or amniotic fluid cells when there is an identifiable mutation in the family.

h. When mutations are not evident in affected DMD cases, carrier detection depends on the less reliable linkage analysis of many family members using restriction fragment length polymorphisms.

LIMB–GIRDLE MUSCULAR DYSTROPHY

BACKGROUND

1. The limb–girdle muscular dystrophies (LGMDs) are a heterogeneous group that clinically resembles the dystrophinopathies except for the equal occurrence in males and females (Table 9-2).

2. The reported incidence and prevalence of LGMD is approximately 6.5/100,000 live births and 2/100,000 population, respectively.

3. These disorders are inherited in an autosomal recessive, or less commonly, autosomal dominant fashion. Autosomal dominant LGMDs are classified as type 1 (e.g., LGMD-1), while recessive forms are classified as type 2 (e.g., LGMD-2). Further alphabetic subclassification has been applied to these disorders as they have become genotypically distinct (e.g., LGMD-2A, LGMD-2B, etc.).

PATHOPHYSIOLOGY

Mutations have been described in various genes encoding for sarcolemmal and sarcomeric structural proteins as well as cytosolic enzymes.

TABLE 9-2. MOLECULAR CLASSIFICATION OF THE MUSCULAR DYSTROPHIES

Disease	Chromosome	Protein
X-linked recessive dystrophies		
DMD/BMD	Xp21	Dystrophin
EDMD	Xq28	Emerin
Autosomal dominant dystrophies		
LGMD 1A	5q22-31	Myotilin
LGMD 1B	1q11-12	Nuclear lamin A/C
LGMD 1C	3p25	Caveolin-3
LGMD 1D	6q23	?
LGMD 1E	7q	?
Myotonic dystrophy type 1	19q13.2	Myotonin protein kinase
Myotonic dystrophy type 2	3q	DM2
FSHD	4q35	?
Oculopharyngeal dystrophy	14q	Polyalanine binding protein 2 (*PABP2*)
Bethlem myopathy 1	21q22.3	Collagen type VI (α_1 or α_2 subunits)
Bethlem myopathy 2	2q37	Collagen type VI (α_6 subunit)
Autosomal recessive dystrophies		
LGMD 2A	15q15	Calpain-3
LGMD 2B / Miyoshi myopathy	2p13	Dysferlin
LGMD 2C	13q13	γ-Sarcoglycan
LGMD 2D	17q21	α-Sarcoglycan
LGMD 2E	4q12	β-Sarcoglycan
LGMD 2F	5q33	δ-Sarcoglycan
LGMD 2G	17q11-12	Telethonin
LGMD 2H	9q31-q33	TRIM 32
LGMD 2I	19q13.3	Fukutin-related protein, *FKRP1*
Congenital muscular dystrophy		
Classic CMD Type 1	6q21-22	Merosin (α_2 subunit)
Classic CMD Type 2	12q13	α_7 integrin
Classic CMD Type 2	19q13.3	Fukutin-related protein, *FKRP1*
Fukuyama type	9q31-33	Fukutin
Walker–Warburg type	9q31-33	?
MEB	1p32-p34	POMGnT1
CMD with rigid spine syndrome	1p35-36	Selenoprotein N1

DMD, Duchenne muscular dystrophy; LGMD, limb–gridle muscular dystrophy; BMD, Becker muscular dystrophy; FSHD, facioscapulohumeral muscular dystrophy; EDMD, Emery–Dreifuss muscular dystrophy; MEB, muscle–eye–brain disease; POMGnT1, *O*-mannose-β-1,2-*N*-acetylglucosaminlyl transferase; CHD, congenital muscular dystrophy.

PROGNOSIS

Similar to that for DMD and BMD.

DIAGNOSIS

1. Patients can manifest with severe early childhood-onset weakness similar to DMD or with a more benign phenotype similar to BMD.
2. For the most part, the clinical, laboratory, and histopathologic features of the LGMDs are nonspecific.
3. Serum CK levels are elevated
4. Muscle biopsies demonstrate dystrophic features similar to those described with DMD and BMD.

5. Immunohistochemistry and immunoblotting demonstrate normal dystrophin. Immunostaining for sarcoglycans, merosin, and dysferlin can be used for diagnosis in some subtypes of LGMD

TREATMENT

1. Treatment is largely supportive, similar to DMD and BMD.
2. Physical and occupational therapy are important to prevent contractures and improve function.
3. Whether corticosteroids can improve strength and delay progression similar to that observed in DMD is not known, although some patients with LGMD reported benefit from such treatment.
4. Modest improvement in strength has been reported in a small number of patients with LGMD treated with short courses of creatine monohydrate (5–10 g/d).

CONGENITAL MUSCULAR DYSTROPHY

BACKGROUND

The congenital muscular dystrophies (CMDs) are a heterogeneous group of autosomal recessive inherited disorders characterized by perinatal onset of hypotonia with proximal weakness, joint contractures affecting the elbows, hips, knees, and ankles (arthrogryposis).

PATHOPHYSIOLOGY

Mutations in various genes have been identified (Table 9-2). These mutations seem to affect the ability of sarcolemmal proteins to bind to the extracellular matrix.

PROGNOSIS

The prognoses for merosin-negative classical CMD, Fukuyama-type, Walker–Warburg, and the Santivouri-type are quite poor, with death in early childhood. Some patients with only partial merosin deficiency and those classic CMDs with normal merosin can live to adulthood and manifest mild phenotypes similar to BMD.

DIAGNOSIS

1. The CMDs are classified according to clinical, ophthalmologic, radiologic, and pathologic features.
2. The major categories of CMDs are as follows:
   a. The classic or occidental/Western type
   b. Fukuyama-type characterized by defects in neuronal migration (i.e., polymicrogyria) with severe mental retardation, seizures, and a progressively deteriorating course
   c. Walker–Warburg or the cerebral–ocular–dysplasia syndrome
   d. Santivouri-type or muscle–eye–brain disease
3. Serum CK levels are elevated.
4. EMG and nerve conduction studies are myopathic. In merosinopathies, mild slowing of motor and sensory nerve conductions may be apparent.
5. Magnetic resonance imaging (MRI) of the brain demonstrates migrational disturbances in Fukuyama type, Walker–Warburg, and the Santivouri types and evidence of cerebral hypomyelination in merosin-deficient CMD.

6. Muscle biopsies appear dystrophic. Immunostaining for merosin is negative in merosin-deficient CMD.

TREATMENT

1. Treatment of the CMD is supportive.
2. Physical therapy is important to prevent contractures.
3. Antiepileptic medications are used for control of seizures.

FACIOSCAPULOHUMERAL MUSCULAR DYSTROPHY

BACKGROUND

1. The incidence of facioscapulohumeral muscular dystrophy (FSHD) approximates 4/million with a prevalence of roughly 50/million population.
2. The disease is inherited in an autosomal dominant fashion. However, there is a variable degree of penetrance of clinical findings within families.

PATHOPHYSIOLOGY

1. FSHD is an autosomal dominant disorder linked to the telomeric region of chromosome 4q35.
2. The gene has not yet been isolated, but an *Eco*RI polymorphism in this region is present on chromosome 4q35 in most patients with FSHD as noted above.
3. This *Eco*RI polymorphism is variable in size but is reduced compared to normal [FSHD, 10–30 kilobase (kb); normal, 50–300 kb].
4. The mutation results in the FSHD gene lying closer to the telomere, a process that may cause altered transcription of the nearby gene(s).

PROGNOSIS

1. Some patients with FSHD experience a late exacerbation of muscle weakness. They may only have mild weakness for years, then there is a marked increase of weakness in the typical distribution over the course of several years.
2. Approximately 20% of patients with FSHD eventually will require wheelchairs.
3. FDHD is usually associated with a normal life span.

DIAGNOSIS

Clinical Features

1. The age of onset is usually between 3 and 44 years, although onset has been described as late as 75 years.
2. The muscles of facial expression are typically affected early. Patients are unable to fully close their eyes against resistance and sleep with incomplete eyelid closure.
3. Weakness of the scapula stabilizer muscles leads to upward and lateral rotation of the shoulder blades with scapular winging. There is also significant weakness and atrophy of the biceps brachii and triceps with relatively normal bulk of the forearm muscles producing the so-called Popeye arms. Wrist extensors are weaker than wrist flexors. The characteristic facial and upper torso appearance led to the designation of FSHD.
4. Some patients with FSHD manifest only with scapular winging.

5. The tibialis anterior muscles are the earliest lower limb muscle to manifest weakness and occasionally patients present with foot drop.
6. The muscle involvement may progress to the pelvic musculature producing a hyperlordotic posture and a waddling gait. As in the face, weakness in the arms and legs is often asymmetric.
7. Weakness can be strikingly asymmetric in the face and limbs.
8. Rare patients can manifest similar to a LGMD with sparing of facial muscles.

Laboratory Feature

1. Serum CK levels may be only mildly to moderately elevated or may be normal in some persons.
2. Genetic testing is available to confirm the diagnosis.

TREATMENT

1. Modest improvement in strength has been reported in a small number of patients with FSHD treated with short courses of creatine monohydrate (5–10 g/d).
2. Treatment is largely supportive with physical therapy to decrease contractures.
3. If the patient is unable to raise the arms above the head because of the lack of scapular fixation, surgical stabilization of the scapula to the thorax may be beneficial and increase range of motion and function of the arm. I reserve this for ambulatory patients.
4. Patients with severe biceps, triceps, and forearm weakness may benefit from a forearm orthosis or ball-bearing feeder device.
5. Ankle–foot orthotics are useful in patients with foot drop secondary to tibialis anterior and peroneal muscle weakness.
6. Surgical transposition of the posterior tibial tendon to the dorsum of the foot is particularly useful in patients who have a marked intorsion of the foot when walking.

EMERY–DREIFUSS MUSCULAR DYSTROPHY

BACKGROUND

1. Emery–Dreifuss muscular dystrophy (EDMD) is characterized by the triad of the following:
   a. Early contractures of the Achilles tendons, elbows, and posterior cervical muscles
   b. Slowly progressive muscle atrophy and weakness with a predominantly humeroperoneal distribution in early stages
   c. Cardiomyopathy with conduction defects
2. Prominent contractures are evident prior to the development of significant weakness.

PATHOPHYSIOLOGY

1. EDMD is caused by mutations in a gene (STA) located on chromosome Xq28, which encodes for the protein emerin.
2. Emerin is localizes to the inner nuclear membranes of skeletal, cardiac and smooth muscle fibers as well as skin cells.
3. Mutations in emerin result in the disorganization of the nuclear lamina and heterochromatin.

PROGNOSIS

1. The disorder is slowly progressive and even severely affected patients are usually able to ambulate into the third decade.
2. Potentially lethal cardiac abnormalities by the end of the second or beginning of the third decade. Conduction defects range from first-degree atrioventricular (AV) block to complete heart block.
3. Although female carriers do not manifest muscle weakness or contractures, they may develop cardiopathy.

DIAGNOSIS

Clinical Features

As noted in Background.

Laboratory Features

1. The serum CK levels are either normal or only mildly to moderately elevated.
2. Electrocardiograms (ECGs) frequently reveal sinus bradycardia, prolongation of the PR interval, or more severe degrees of conduction block.

Histopathology

Muscle biopsy and skin biopsies reveal absence of emerin on the nuclear membrane.

TREATMENT

1. It is important to monitor cardiac function because of the risk of arrhythmias and sudden death.
2. I obtain yearly ECGs on all patients (as well as on possible female carriers) and cardiology consultations on patients with significant abnormalities.
3. Patients may require pacemakers and some authorities have even recommended prophylactic pacemakers.
4. Stretching exercises are indicated to minimize contractures.
5. Otherwise, there is no specific medical therapy.

OCULOPHARYNGEAL MUSCULAR DYSTROPHY

BACKGROUND

1. Oculopharyngeal muscular dystrophy (OPMD) is inherited in an autosomal dominant fashion and usually manifests in the fourth to sixth decades of life.
2. There is an increased incidence in French Canadians.

PATHOPHYSIOLOGY

1. OPMD is caused by mutations involving expansions of a short GCG repeat within the poly(A) binding protein 2 gene (PABP2) on chromosome 14q11.
2. Normally, there are six GCG repeats encoding for a polyalanine tract at the N-terminus of the protein. Approximately 2% of the population has polymorphism with seven GCG repeats.
3. In OPMD, there is an expansion to eight to 13 repeats.

4. The function of *PABP2* and how the mutation in the gene leads to muscle degeneration are unknown.

PROGNOSIS

The late onset of the disease in most patients combined with slow progression usually does not alter the patient's life span provided adequate medical attention is sought with regard to the nutritional aspect of this disease.

DIAGNOSIS

Clinical Features

1. Most patients present with bilateral ptosis. As many as 25% present initially with difficulty swallowing.
2. The extraocular muscles are affected in approximately 50% of patients, but diplopia is not a common symptom.
3. Mild weakness of the neck and proximal limbs can be detected in some patients.

Laboratory Features

1. Serum CK levels are normal or only mildly elevated.
2. Diagnosis can be confirmed by genetic testing.

TREATMENT

1. Eyelid crutches on glasses or even taping the eyelids open can be used to treat the ptosis.
2. Ptosis surgery can also be performed if patients have sufficient orbicularis oculi strength to allow complete closure of the eyelids postoperatively.
3. Swallowing studies should be obtained to delineate the degree of pharyngeal and esophageal dysmotility.
4. Patients with severe dysphagia may benefit from cricopharyngeal myotomy.
5. Some patients will require percutaneous endoscopic gastrostomy (PEG) tube placement secondary to severe dysphagia.

MYOTONIC DYSTROPHY TYPE 1 (DM1)

BACKGROUND

1. Myotonic dystrophy type 1 (DM1) is inherited in an autosomal dominant manner.
2. The incidence of this disorder is 13.5/100,000 live births and the prevalence is 3 to 5/100,000.
3. DM1 can present at any age; onset in infancy is known as congenital myotonic dystrophy.

PATHOPHYSIOLOGY

1. DM1 is caused by an expansion of unstable polymorphic cytosine-thymine-guanine (CTG) trinucleotide repeat in the 3′ untranslated region of the myotonin protein kinase gene on chromosome 19q13.2.
2. Nuclear retention of mutant messenger RNA (mRNA) containing expanded CTG repeats sequesters RNA-binding proteins, which impairs normal transcription and splicing of other mRNAs leading to abnormal translation of many different proteins.

PROGNOSIS

1. The severity of myotonic dystrophy directly correlates with the size of the CTG repeat.
2. The size of the repeat is unstable and typically expands from one generation to the next, which accounts for the anticipation phenomena (i.e., the earlier presentation and/or more severe disease in each generation).
3. Life expectancy is reduced. The higher mortality is reflective of death from the associated respiratory weakness and cardiomyopathy.

DIAGNOSIS

Clinical Features

1. Frontal balding, posterior subscapular cataracts, ptosis, and wasting of the facial and masseter/temporalis muscles are characteristic.
2. Limb weakness begins distally and progresses rather slowly to affect proximal muscles.
3. The myotonia is most prominent in the hands.
4. The smooth muscles of the gastrointestinal tract are also involved leading to dysphagia and chronic pseudoobstructions.
5. Involvement of the diaphragm and intercostal muscles are common, leading to alveolar hypoventilation.
6. Decreased central drive contributes to hypoventilation leading to symptoms suggestive of sleep apnea: frequent nocturnal arousals, excessive daytime hypersomnolence, and morning headaches.
7. Cardiac abnormalities are common with approximately 90% of patients having conduction defects on ECG.
8. Sudden cardiac death secondary to arrhythmia is well documented; however, the severity of the cardiomyopathy does not necessarily correlate with the severity of skeletal muscle weakness.
9. Cognitive impairment, particularly in memory and spatial orientation, may be evident, although these abnormalities are not as severe in adult-onset cases as they are in the congenital form of the disorder.

Laboratory Features

1. Serum CK level may be normal or mildly increased.
2. Genetic testing can confirm the disorder.
3. EMG demonstrates myotonic discharges.

TREATMENT

1. There is no treatment available clearly shown to improve muscle strength.
2. Myotonia rarely warrants treatment. In fact, some drugs that improve myotonia (i.e., quinine, procainamide, and tocainide) can potentiate cardiac arrhythmias and should be avoided.
3. If myotonia is severe enough to require treatment, phenytoin 100 to 300 mg daily or mexiletine150 mg daily to 300 mg t.i.d. may be tried.
4. Obtain yearly ECGs to monitor for evidence of conduction defects/arrhythmias and right-sided heart failure due to pulmonary hypertension.
5. Cardiology consultation, 24-hour Holter monitoring and echocardiograms are ordered in patients with significant ECG abnormalities.
6. Some patients will ultimately require antiarrhythmic medication or pacemaker insertion.
7. Patients with myotonic dystrophy are at risk for pulmonary and cardiac complications from general anesthesia and neuromuscular blocking medications. These agents should be avoided if possible.
8. Pulmonary function tests are routinely performed.

9. Obtain overnight polysomnography in patients with symptoms and signs of cor pulmonale or sleep apnea.
10. Patients with significant hypoventilation or sleep apnea may benefit from noninvasive ventilatory assistance with BiPAP.
11. Modafinil 200 to 400 mg/d has been demonstrated to improve hypersomnolence.
12. Some patients require excision of their cataracts.
13. Ankle braces are indicated in patients with foot drop to assist their gait.
14. Genetic counseling:
    a. Patients need to know that the risk of passing the disease on to their children is 50% with each pregnancy.
    b. The disease severity is generally worse from one generation to the next especially in children born to mothers with myotonic dystrophy.
    c. Prenatal diagnosis is possible via amniocentesis or chorionic villous sampling.

MYOTONIC DYSTROPHY TYPE 2 OR PROXIMAL MYOTONIC MYOPATHY

BACKGROUND

1. Myotonic dystrophy type 2 (DM2) or proximal myotonic myopathy (PROMM) is a multisystem, autosomal dominant disorder characterized by proximal muscle weakness, myotonia, myalgias, and cataracts.
2. Some patients have features almost identical to DM2.

PATHOPHYSIOLOGY

1. DM2 is caused by mutations in the gene that encodes for zinc finger 9 (*ZNF9*) on chromosome 3q21.
2. The mutations are expanded CCTG repeats in intron 1.
3. As with DM1, this expanded repeat likely leads to the expression of a toxic pre-mRNA that sequesters RNA-binding proteins, which impairs the splicing of other mRNA species, including those of ion channels.

PROGNOSIS

Slowly progressive proximal weakness develops in most patients.

DIAGNOSIS

1. Clinical features are similar to DM1 except that weakness is much less severe and predominantly affects proximal muscles and patients with PROMM more often complain of muscle stiffness and aching.
2. Cardiac involvement is also much less common.
3. Onset is in middle or late adulthood.
4. Serum CK level is mildly elevated.
5. EMG demonstrates myotonic discharges.
6. Genetic testing is available to confirm the diagnosis.

TREATMENT

1. Treatment is similar to that described in the section on Myotonic Dystrophy Type 1 section, although cardiac and pulmonary complications are less frequent.
2. Genetic counseling.

MYOTONIA CONGENITA

BACKGROUND

There are autosomal dominant (Thomsen disease) and autosomal recessive (Becker disease) forms of myotonia congenita.

PATHOPHYSIOLOGY

Both the autosomal dominant and recessive forms of myotonia congenita are caused by mutations in the muscle chloride channel gene (*CLCN1*) on chromosome 7q35.

PROGNOSIS

The life span is not adversely affected.

DIAGNOSIS

1. Autosomal dominant myotonia congenital:
   a. Muscle stiffness that usually manifests in early childhood.
   b. Patients have generalized muscle hypertrophy leading to Herculean physique.
   c. Action and percussion myotonia are evident.
   d. Patients are generally not weak.
   e. Serum CK level is normal or only slightly elevated.
   f. EMG demonstrates myotonic discharges.
2. Autosomal recessive myotonia congenita:
   a. The severity of the myotonia is worse in the recessive form and gradually increases during the first two decades of life.
   b. Patients develop proximal muscle weakness.
   c. Action and percussion myotonia are evident.
   d. Patients are generally not weak.
   e. Serum CK level is usually increased two to four times normal.
   f. EMG demonstrates myotonic discharges.

TREATMENT

1. Most patients with myotonia congenita do not require medical treatment.
2. When the myotonia is severe and limits function, antiarrhythmic and antiepileptic medications, which interfere with the muscle sodium channel, can be beneficial.
3. I initiate treatment with mexiletine 150 mg daily and gradually increase as tolerated and as necessary to control the symptoms to a maximum of 300 mg t.i.d. The major side effects of mexiletine are lightheadedness, diarrhea, and dyspepsia.
4. If mexiletine is ineffective, dilantin 100 to 300 mg daily is the next step.

POTASSIUM-SENSITIVE PERIODIC PARALYSIS

BACKGROUND

1. Primary hyperkalemic periodic paralysis is transmitted in an autosomal dominant fashion, and there is a high degree of penetrance in both females and males.
2. "Potassium-sensitive periodic paralysis" is the preferred term, because attacks of weakness are not necessarily associated with hyperkalemia in all patients.

However, all patients are sensitive to potassium as they can become weak when given potassium.

PATHOPHYSIOLOGY

Potassium-sensitive periodic paralysis is caused by mutations in the α-subunit of the voltage-dependent sodium channel (*SCN4A*).

PROGNOSIS

The frequency of attacks tends to diminish with time, although fixed proximal weakness may also develop.

DIAGNOSIS

Clinical Features

1. In most patients, symptoms manifest within the first decade of life.
2. Attacks of weakness usually develop in the morning but can occur at any time and are precipitated by rest following exercise or fasting.
3. Unlike hypokalemic periodic paralysis (discussed later), there is rarely generalized flaccid paralysis.
4. The duration of weakness is usually less than 2 hours, although mild weakness can persist for a few days.
5. The frequency of attacks is highly variable with some persons afflicted several times a day, whereas others experience difficulty once a year.
6. Some patients have clinical myotonia.
7. Secondary hyperkalemia can cause generalized weakness mimicking primary hyperkalemic periodic paralysis and must be excluded, particularly in patients with no family history. Patients with secondary causes of hyperkalemia do not exhibit clinical or electrical myotonia.

Laboratory Features

1. Between attacks of weakness, serum potassium levels are normal.
2. The attacks of weakness are usually associated with an increase in serum potassium levels (up to 5–6 mmol/L). Secondary causes of hyperkalemia need to be excluded.
3. Serum CK levels can be normal or mildly elevated in patients even between attacks of weakness.
4. Genetic testing is available to confirm the diagnosis.

Electrophysiologic Findings

1. Both motor and sensory nerve conduction studies are normal between and during attacks of weakness. During an attack, the CMAP amplitudes may be reduced or absent in patients with severe weakness. CMAP amplitudes may also decrease in response to brief excercise.
2. The needle EMG may reveal myotonic discharges that may also be seen in patients without apparent clinical myotonia.

Histopathology

Muscle biopsy frequently reveals vacuoles.

TREATMENT

1. Preventive therapy with a low-potassium, high-carbohydrate diet and avoidance of fasting, strenuous activity, and cold is recommended.
2. The acute attacks of weakness are often mild in severity, short lasting, and do not require treatment.

3. Ingestion of simple carbohydrates (e.g., fruit juices, glucose-containing candies) results in insulin excretion, which diminishes serum potassium levels, and can improve strength.
4. Beta-adrenergic agonists (e.g., metaproterenol, albuterol, salbutamol) can be affective in improving strength and used safely provided there are no associated cardiac arrhythmias.
5. Only rarely with severe attacks is treatment with IV glucose, insulin, or calcium carbonate indicated.
6. Prophylactic treatment with acetazolamide (125–1,000 mg/d), chlorothiazide (250–1,000 mg/d), and dichlorphenamide (50–150 mg/d) may be beneficial in reducing the frequency of attacks and may help with myotonia as well

---

PARAMYOTONIA CONGENITA

BACKGROUND

1. Paramyotonia congenita is an autosomal dominant disorder with high penetrance, which as noted above is allelic to hyperkalemic periodic paralysis.
2. Some kinships have clinical features of both hyperkalemic periodic paralysis and paramyotonia congenita.
3. The name derives from the "para"-doxic reaction to exercise. In contrast to the warm-up phenomena observed in the other myotonic syndromes, repeated exercise worsens the muscle stiffness in patients with paramyotonia congenita.

PATHOPHYSIOLOGY

Paramyotonia congenita with and without episodes of periodic paralysis are caused by mutations in the α subunit of the voltage-gated sodium channel ($SCN4A$).

PROGNOSIS

Some patients develop attacks of weakness and mild fixed proximal weakness over time.

DIAGNOSIS

Clinical Features

1. Muscle stiffness with or without attacks of periodic paralysis is evident within the first decade of life.
2. Cold temperature also precipitates myotonia and weakness.
3. Percussion myotonia can be demonstrated, although usually is not prominent.
4. Paramyotonia particularly of the eyelids is typically evident in most patients. Myalgias are not a common complaint.
5. Muscle strength is normal in patients between attacks of paralysis.

Laboratory Features

1. Serum CK levels can be mildly to moderately elevated.
2. Serum potassium levels may be elevated in some patients during an attack of paralysis.
3. Genetic testing is available to confirm the diagnosis.

Electrophysiologic Findings

1. Both motor and sensory nerve conduction studies are normal between and during attacks of weakness. During an attack, the CMAP amplitudes may be reduced or

absent in patients with severe weakness. CMAP amplitudes also diminish if the limb is cooled with cold water.

2. The needle EMG may reveal myotonic discharges that can also be seen in patients without apparent clinical myotonia.

TREATMENT

1. Mexiletine 150 mg daily to 300 mg t.i.d. has been used to prevent weakness and myotonia induced by cold in patients with associated paramyotonia congenita.
2. Chlorothiazide 50 to 100 mg daily is also sometimes effective in relieving the myotonia.

ACETAZOLAMIDE-RESPONSIVE MYOTONIA

BACKGROUND

This disorder was previously known as acetazolamide-responsive myotonia congenital.

PATHOPHYSIOLOGY

The disorder is now known also to be caused by mutations in the α-subunit of the voltage-gated sodium channel and not the chloride channel as in myotonia congenita.

PROGNOSIS

Usually responsive to acetazolamide.

DIAGNOSIS

Clinical Features

1. Patients develop painful muscle stiffness/myotonia in childhood that is most severe in the face and hands. Severity and frequency increase with age at least into early adulthood.
2. Myotonia is provoked by fasting, potassium, and to a lesser extent by exercise. Myotonia is eased by ingestion of high carbohydrate meals.
3. Examination reveals normal muscle strength.

Laboratory Features

Serum CK level can be normal or mildly elevated.

Electrophysiologic Findings

1. Routine motor and sensory studies are normal.
2. Needle EMG examination demonstrates significant runs of myotonic potentials, but MUAP morphology and recruitment are normal.

TREATMENT

1. Acetazolamide is affective in reducing myotonia and associated muscle pain.
2. Acetazolamide is started at 125 mg/d and titrated as tolerated to 250 mg t.i.d.
3. Mexiletine 150 mg daily to 300 mg t.i.d. is also effective in some patients.

FAMILIAL HYPOKALEMIC PERIODIC PARALYSIS

BACKGROUND

1. Hypokalemic periodic paralysis type 1 is the most frequent form of periodic paralysis with an estimated prevalence of 1/100,000.
2. It is an autosomal dominant disorder, with reduced penetrance in women (a male-to-female ratio of 3 or 4 to 1).
3. It is genetically heterogeneic.

PATHOPHYSIOLOGY

1. Most cases of familial hypokalemic periodic paralysis (hypoKPP type 1) are caused by mutations in the skeletal muscle voltage-gated calcium channel α-1 subunit (*CACL1A3*) gene (see below in the section on hypoKPP).
2. However, several kinships have been identified with mutations in *SCN4A*, so-called hypoKPP type 2.
3. Still other kinships, hypoKPP type 3, have been linked to mutations in the potassium channel.

PROGNOSIS

The frequency of attacks generally decreases after the age of 30 years and some patients become free of attacks in their 40's or 50's.

DIAGNOSIS

Clinical Features

1. Symptom onset is usually in the first two decades when patients note the development of episodic weakness.
2. Most patients note that some form of atypical strenuous exercise or exertion followed by rest or sleep usually precipitates an attack.
3. Other aggravating factors include heavy meals rich in carbohydrates and sodium, alcohol consumption, exposure to cold, and emotional stress. The bouts of weakness can occur at any time of day, although early morning hours appears to have a slightly higher propensity for being associated with weakness.
4. Severity of an attack can range from mild weakness of an isolated muscle group to severe generalized paralysis.
5. The frequency of these attacks of weakness is also highly variable and can occur several times a week or once a year.

Laboratory Features

1. Attacks of weakness are associated with decreased serum potassium levels usually below 3.0 mEq/L. Secondary causes of hypokalemia periodic paralysis need to be excluded.
2. Between bouts of weakness, the serum potassium is normal.
3. During severe attacks of weakness, there is oliguria with urinary retention of sodium, potassium, chloride, and water.
4. Genetic testing is available to confirm the diagnosis.
5. The ECG may demonstrate bradycardia, flattened T waves, prolonged PR and QT intervals, and notably U waves secondary to the hypokalemia.
6. Serum CK levels are normal or only mildly elevated between attacks and increased during an attack of weakness.

Histopathology

1. The muscle biopsy may demonstrate multiple or single intracellular vacuoles, tubular aggregates, and dilatation of the sarcoplasmic reticulum
2. Patients with the typical *CACNL1A* mutations are more likely to have vacuoles, while tubular aggregates are more commonly seen in patients with *SCNA4* mutations.

Electrophysiologic Findings

1. Sensory and motor nerve conduction studies are normal between attacks of weakness.
2. During the paralytic attack, the CMAP amplitude declines precipitously secondary to muscle membrane inexcitability. CMAP amplitudes may also decrease following brief exercise.
3. The needle EMG examination between attacks of muscle paralysis usually reveals no abnormalities.
4. Early in an attack of weakness, a slight increase in spontaneous potentials (fibrillation potentials and positive sharp waves) and insertional activity may be noted. As the paralytic attack progresses, one observes a decrease in the amplitude and duration of voluntary MUAPs as well as an overall decrease in the number of MUAPs contributing to the interference pattern.

TREATMENT

1. Preventive measures include avoidance of provocative factors (e.g., ingestion of high-carbohydrate meals, strenuous exercise).
2. Acetazolamide (125–1,500 mg/d) and potassium salts (0.25–0.5 mEq/kg) can also be prophylactically administered to prevent hypokalemia and attacks of weakness. However, acetazolamide may exacerbate attacks of weakness in patients with hypokalemic periodic paralysis type 2 caused by *SCNA4* mutations.
3. Dichlorphenamide (50–150 mg/d) appears to be at least as effective in reducing attack frequency and severity as acetazolamide.
4. Triamterene (25–100 mg/d) and spironolactone (25–100 mg/d) may be used to prevent attacks and improve interattack weakness, when acetazolamide and dichlorphenamide are not effective.
5. Acute attacks of weakness are treated with oral potassium salts (0.25 mEq/kg) every 30 minutes until strength improves.
6. If the patient's condition precludes oral potassium, IV potassium (KCL bolus 0.05–0.1 mEq/kg or 20–40 mEq/L of KCL in 5% mannitol) may be administered.
7. Cardiac monitoring is essential during treatment.

KLEIN–LISAK–ANDERSEN OR ANDERSEN–TAWIL SYNDROME

BACKGROUND

Klein–Lisak–Andersen, also known as Andersen–Tawil, syndrome is a distinct autosomal dominant disorder characterized by the triad of periodic paralysis, ventricular dysrhythmias, and dysmorphic features.

PATHOPHYSIOLOGY

Mutations in potassium channel gene (*KCNJ2*) located on chromosome 17q23 are the same families.

PROGNOSIS

Some patients develop mild fixed proximal weakness. Life-threatening cardiac dysrhythmias can also occur.

DIAGNOSIS

Clinical Features

1. This form of periodic paralysis could be associated with hypokalemia, normal kalemia, or hyperkalemia.
2. The cardiopathy ranges from an asymptomatic long QT interval to potentially fatal ventricular tachyarrhythmias.
3. The major dysmorphic features described include short stature, scaphocephaly, hypertelorism, low-set ears, broad nose, micrognathia, high arched palate, clindactyly and short fingers, syndactyly, and scoliosis.
4. The episodes of periodic weakness and cardiac arrhythmia can manifest in early childhood.
5. There is no evidence of myotonia or paramyotonia.

Laboratory Features

1. Serum CK level is normal or only mildly elevated (less than five times normal).
2. Serum potassium levels can be normal, elevated, or decreased during attacks of weakness.
3. A prolonged QT interval is present in 80% of patients, while some have even more ominous ventricular tachyarrhythmias.

Histopathology

Muscle biopsies frequently reveal tubular aggregates similar to those observed in other forms of periodic paralysis.

Electrophysiologic Findings

1. Motor and sensory nerve conduction studies are normal.
2. Likewise electromyography is normal interictally. Importantly, there are no myotonic discharges.

TREATMENT

1. Early recognition of the potential cardiac conduction abnormalities is important, because they may be treated with antiarrhythmic agents or pacemaker insertion.
2. Acetazolamide (125–1,500 mg/d) may prevent paralytic attacks in some patients.

MALIGNANT HYPERTHERMIA

BACKGROUND

1. The incidence of malignant hyperthermia (MH) in patients exposed to general anesthesia ranges from 0.5% to 0.0005%.
2. At least 50% of patients with MH have had previous anesthesia without clinically manifesting the disorder.

PATHOPHYSIOLOGY

1. MH is thought to arise secondary to excessive calcium release by the sarcoplasmic reticulum calcium channel, the ryanodine receptor.
2. Increased intracytoplasmic calcium leads to excessive muscle contraction, increased utilization of oxygen and ATP, and overproduction of heat.
3. MH susceptibility is genetically very heterogeneic with at least six different genes identified.

PROGNOSIS

Patients and family members should be warned of increased risk of subsequent episodes of MH with anesthesia.

DIAGNOSIS

Clinical Features

1. MH is an autosomal dominant disorder characterized by severe muscle rigidity, myoglobinuria, fever, tachycardia, cyanosis, and cardiac arrhythmias precipitated by depolarizing muscle relaxants (e.g., succinylcholine) and inhalational anesthetic agents (e.g., halothane).
2. MH usually occurs during surgery, but it can manifest in the postoperative period. Rarely, attacks of MH have developed following exercise, ingestion of caffeine, or stress.

Laboratory Features

1. Serum CK level can be normal or mildly elevated interictally in patients susceptible to MH.
2. During attacks of MH, serum CK levels are markedly elevated and myoglobinuria can develop.
3. Hyperkalemia and metabolic and respiratory acidosis are evident.

TREATMENT

1. Patients at risk for MH should not be given known triggering anesthetic agents.
2. MH is a medical emergency requiring several therapeutic steps.
   a. The anesthetic agent must be discontinued while 100% oxygen is delivered.
   b. Dantrolene 2 to 3 mg/kg every 5 minutes for a total of 10 mg/kg should be administered.
   c. The stomach, bladder, and lower gastrointestinal tract are lavaged with iced saline solution and cooling blankets are applied.
   d. Acidosis and hyperkalemia are treated with sodium bicarbonate, hyperventilation, dextrose, insulin, and occasionally calcium chloride.
   e. Urinary output must be maintained with hydration, furosemide, or mannitol.
   f. The patient must be monitored and treated for cardiac arrhythmias.

CONGENITAL MYOPATHIES

BACKGROUND

The term "congenital myopathy" refers to myopathic disorders presenting preferentially, but not exclusively, at birth (Table 9-3).

TABLE 9-3. CONGENITAL MYOPATHIES

Disease	Inheritance	Gene/Chromosome	Clinical Features
Central core myopathy	AD	Ryanodine receptor (RYR1)/19q13.1	Onset: Infancy or childhood, occasionally adulthood; proximal limbs and mild facial weakness; skeletal anomalies; risk for MH
Multicore/minicore myopathy	AD, AR, sporadic	Some caused by mutations in Selenoprotein N1	Onset: Infancy or childhood; proximal and facial muscles; rare EOM weak; cardiomyopathy and respiratory weakness; skeletal anomalies; risk for MH
Nemaline myopathy			
Severe infantile form	AR AR/AD	Nebulin/2q21.2-q22; α-actin/1q42	Infantile onset: severe generalized hypotonia/weakness; respiratory weakness; skeletal anomalies; usually fatal in first year of life
Mild early onset form	AD	Rare: α-tropomyosin (TMP3)/1q21-q23 NOTE: Most AD kinships do not map to this locus	Most common subtype Onset: Infancy or childhood; mild generalized hypotonia and weakness; facial muscles; rare ptosis, EOM weak; dysmorphic facies and skeletal anomalies
Adult onset form	Sporadic	Unknown	Onset in adult life; mild proximal and occasionally distal weakness; no facial or skeletal anomalies
Centronuclear/myotubular myopathy			
Severe neonatal type	X-linked	Myotubularin/Xp28	Severe neonatal hypotonia and weakness; respiratory weakness; ptosis and EOM weak; poor prognosis in most
Late infantile type	AR, perhaps AD	Unknown	Most common subtype Onset: Late infancy or early childhood; generalized weakness and hypotonia; facial and EOM weakness, ptosis; facial anomalies
Late childhood/adult type	AD	Unknown	Onset in late childhood or adulthood; mild proximal and/or distal predominance; facial and EOM muscles variable involved: no skeletal or facial anomalies

Congenital fiber type disproportion	Sporadic	Unknown	Onset in infancy; generalized nonprogressive weakness; occasional respiratory weakness; skeletal and facial anomalies
Reducing body myopathy	Most appear sporadic; ? AR in some	Unknown	Onset in infancy to adulthood; generalized or proximal weakness; May have facial, respiratory or asymmetric weakness; skeletal anomalies
Fingerprint body myopathy	Most sporadic	Unknown	Infantile onset; Slowly or nonprogressive proximal weakness
Sarcotubular myopathy	Unknown; Single report in two brothers	Unknown	Onset: Infancy; slow progressive proximal with or without distal weakness
Trilaminar myopathy	Unknown; single case	Unknown	Infantile onset; generalized weakness; skeletal anomalies
Hyaline body myopathy	Sporadic or AR	Unknown	Onset in infancy or early childhood; proximal or scapuloperoneal weakness
Cap myopathy	Unknown	Unknown	Onset in infancy; generalized weakness; skeletal anomalies
Zebra body myopathy	Unknown	Unknown	Onset in infancy or childhood; generalized weakness that may be asymmetric and worse in arms
Myofibrillar myopathy (desmin myopathy, cytoplasmic or spheroid body myopathy)	AD AR Sporadic	Desmin/2q35 αB-crystallin/11q21 ?/ chromosome 12 Desmin/2q35 unknown	Onset in infancy or late adulthood; distal, scapuloperoneal, or generalized weakness; cardiomyopathy
Tubular aggregate myopathy			
Type 1	AD	Unknown	Onset: Childhood or early adulthood; limb-girdle weakness
Type 2	AR	Unknown	Onset: Infancy; congenital myasthenia; fatigable weakness
Type 3	Sporadic	Unknown	Adult onset: myalgia

AD, autosomal dominant; AR, autosomal recessive; EOM weakness, ophthalmoparesis; BSAPPs, brief duration, small amplitude, polyphasic potentials.

PATHOPHYSIOLOGY

A variety of mutations has been identified for the specific forms of congenital myopathy.

PROGNOSIS

The congenital myopathies were initially considered as nonprogressive, although it is now clear that progressive weakness can occur. Some forms are particularly associated with a poor prognosis and death in infancy or early childhood (e.g., X-linked myotubular myopathy, infantile-onset nemaline rod myopathy).

DIAGNOSIS

1. Congenital myopathies can be inherited in an autosomal dominant, autosomal recessive, or X-linked pattern.
2. The serum CK level is either normal or only mildly elevated.
3. Nerve conduction studies are normal. EMG demonstrates increased muscle membrane instability and myopathic motor units in myotubular/centronuclear, myofibrillar, and occasionally nemaline and central core myopathies.
4. Definitive diagnosis of a congenital myopathies requires muscle biopsy.
5. Genetic testing is not commercially available.

TREATMENT

1. There are no medical treatments available to improve strength or slow deterioration.
2. Treatment is largely supportive as discussed with the muscular dystrophies.
3. Physical and occupational therapies are important to reduce contractures and improve mobility and function.
4. Patients may benefit from bracing and other orthotic devices.
5. It is important to advise patients and families of the risk of MH in central core and multicore myopathies.

ACID MALTASE DEFICIENCY

BACKGROUND

1. Acid maltase deficiency is an autosomal recessive disorder caused by defects in the lysosomal acid maltase (α-glucosidase) pathway.
2. There are three recognized clinical subtypes of acid maltase deficiency:
   a. A severe infantile form (also known as Pompe disease)
   b. A juvenile-onset type
   c. An adult-onset variant
3. The incidence is the less than 1/100,000 newborns.

PATHOPHYSIOLOGY

The disorder is caused by mutations encoding for acid maltase (α-glucosidase) on chromosome 17q21-23.

PROGNOSIS

Infantile acid maltase deficiency is progressive and invariably fatal by 2 years of age secondary to cardiorespiratory failure. Respiratory failure usually leads to death in the second or third decade of life in the juvenile form of the disease.

DIAGNOSIS

Clinical Features

1. Infantile acid maltase deficiency:
   a. The cardinal features of the disease include profound cardiomegaly, macroglossia, and mild to moderate hepatomegaly.
   b. Infants demonstrate progressive weakness and hypotonia within the first 3 months of life. Feeding difficulties and respiratory muscle weakness are common.
2. The juvenile form of the disease usually presents in the first decade of life with proximal greater than distal weakness and respiratory muscle weakness.
3. The adult-onset form of acid maltase deficiency usually begins in the third or fourth decade with generalized proximal greater than distal muscle weakness and the respiratory muscles weakness.

Laboratory Features

1. Deficiency of α-glucosidase activity can be demonstrated in muscle fibers, fibroblasts, leukocytes, lymphocytes, and urine.
2. Serum CK levels are elevated to variable degrees in all forms of the disease.
3. ECGs can demonstrate left axis deviation, a short PR interval, large QRS complexes, inverted T waves, ST depression, or persistent sinus tachycardia.
4. Echocardiograms can show progressive hypertrophic cardiomyopathy.
5. Pulmonary function tests show a restrictive defect with decreased FVC, reduced maximal inspiratory and expiratory pressures, and early fatigue of the diaphragm.

Electrophysiologic Findings

1. Sensory and motor nerve conduction are typically normal.
2. Needle EMG reveals abundant fibrillation potentials, positive sharp waves, and myotonic or pseudomyotonic potentials. Voluntary MUAPs demonstrate the typical alterations noted in chronic myopathic disorders.

Histopathology

1. The characteristic light microscopy feature is the formation of vacuoles within type 1 and 2 fibers.
2. The vacuoles react strongly to periodic acid–Schiff (PAS) and are sensitive to diastase. These vacuoles also stain intensely to acid phosphatase confirming that the vacuoles filled with glycogen are secondary lysosomes.

TREATMENT

1. There is no specific treatment for acid maltase deficiency other than supportive therapy for associated cardiorespiratory complications.
2. Respiratory muscles can be affected preferentially and therefore one must follow the pulmonary functions closely.
3. Early respiratory insufficiency may be managed by noninvasive mechanical ventilatory support (e.g., BiBAP).
4. Prenatal diagnosis is possible with amniocentesis or chorionic villous sampling.

DEBRANCHER ENZYME DEFICIENCY

BACKGROUND

Debrancher enzyme deficiency, also known as Cori–Forbes disease, accounts for approximately 25% of glycogen storage disease.

PATHOPHYSIOLOGY

Caused by mutations in the debrancher enzyme gene located on chromosome 1p21.

PROGNOSIS

The course is slowly progressive but mild, and life span is not affected.

DIAGNOSIS

Clinical Features

1. Onset of muscle weakness is usually in the third to fourth decade of life and is slowly progressive.
2. Approximately, one third of the cases begin in infancy or early childhood, and motor milestones can be delayed.
3. There is prominent atrophy and weakness of distal limb muscles in about 50% of patients.
4. Cardiomyopathy can also complicate debrancher deficiency.

LABORATORY FEATURES

1. Debrancher enzyme deficiency can be demonstrated with biochemical assay of muscle, fibroblasts, or lymphocytes.
2. Serum CK levels are elevated two to 20 times normal.
3. ECGs can reveal conduction defects and arrhythmias.
4. Echocardiogram may reveal findings suggestive of hypertrophic obstructive cardiomyopathy.

Electrophysiologic Findings

1. Sensory and motor nerve conduction are typically normal.
2. Needle EMG reveals abundant fibrillation potentials, positive sharp waves, and myotonic or pseudomyotonic potentials. Voluntary MUAPs demonstrate the typical alterations noted in chronic myopathic disorders.

Histopathology

1. Muscle biopsies demonstrate a vacuolar myopathy with abnormal accumulation of glycogen in the subsarcolemmal and intermyofibrillar regions of muscle fibers.
2. These vacuoles stain intensely with PAS but are partially diastase-resistant. Furthermore, in contrast to acid maltase deficiency, these vacuoles do not stain with acid phosphatase, suggesting that the glycogen does not primarily accumulate in lysosomes.

TREATMENT

1. There is no specific medical therapy for the muscle weakness.

2. Patients are best managed by preventing fasting hypoglycemia through frequent low-carbohydrate feedings and maintaining a high-protein intake.
3. Supportive therapy is required for patients with clinical manifestations of congestive heart failure.

BRANCHING ENZYME DEFICIENCY

BACKGROUND

Branching enzyme deficiency, also known as Andersen disease and polyglucosan body disease, is caused by the deficiency of the enzyme capable of creating the branched glycogen molecule, which results in an accumulation of polysaccharide in the liver, CNS, and skeletal and cardiac muscles.

PATHOPHYSIOLOGY

Caused by mutations within the gene for glycogen branching enzyme located on chromosome 3.

PROGNOSIS

Course is variable.

DIAGNOSIS

Clinical Features

1. There is a neuromuscular form of the disease with which patients manifest primarily with muscle weakness and cardiomyopathy.
2. Weakness and atrophy can be predominantly proximal or distal.
3. There is also a form of branching enzyme deficiency, often referred to as polyglucosan body disease, which manifests mainly in adults as progressive upper and lower motor neuron loss, sensory nerve involvement, cerebellar ataxia, neurogenic bladder, and dementia.

Laboratory Features

1. Deficiency of branching enzyme may be demonstrated in muscle.
2. The serum CK level may be normal or slightly elevated.
3. ECG can demonstrate progressive conduction defects leading to complete AV block.
4. Echocardiogram may reveal a dilated cardiomyopathy.

Electrophysiologic Findings

1. Sensory and motor nerve conduction findings are typically normal.
2. Needle EMG reveals abundant fibrillation potentials, positive sharp waves, and myotonic or pseudomyotonic potentials. Voluntary MUAPs demonstrate the typical alterations noted in chronic myopathic disorders.

Histopathology

1. Routine light and electron microscopy reveal deposition of varying amounts of finely granular and filamentous polysaccharide (polyglucosan bodies) in the CNS, peripheral nerves (axons and Schwann cells), skin, liver, and cardiac and skeletal muscles.
2. These polyglucosan bodies are PAS-positive and diastase-resistant.

TREATMENT

1. Liver transplantation has been performed in some children.
2. Long-term follow-up (mean, 42 months) has shown that most of the patients became free of liver, neuromuscular, and cardiac dysfunction.
3. No other medical therapies have been demonstrated to be effective.
4. Treatment is otherwise supportive.

DYNAMIC GLYCOGEN STORAGE DISORDERS

BACKGROUND

1. These include myophosphorylase (McArdle disease), phosphofructokinase, phosphorylase b kinase, phosphoglycerate kinase, phosphoglycerate mutase, lactate dehydrogenase, and β-enolase deficiencies and are very similar and are associated with exertional cramps and occasionally myoglobinuria with mild exercise.
2. Thus, these are considered the dynamic glycogen storage disorders as opposed to the above-described acid maltase, debrancher, and branching enzyme deficiencies that are associated with nondynamic, fixed weakness.

PATHOPHYSIOLOGY

These disorders are caused by mutations in the respective genes.

PROGNOSIS

1. Approximately 50% of patients experience myoglobinuria related to exercise, while a third of these individuals have various degrees of renal failure.
2. As many as one third of patients develop mild, fixed proximal weakness as a result of recurrent bouts of rhabdomyolysis.

DIAGNOSIS

Clinical Features

1. The major symptom is exercise intolerance, which usually starts in childhood. Exertional muscle pain, cramps, and myoglobinuria develop later and the diagnosis is usually made by the second or third decade of life.
2. Some patients note a second-wind phenomena in which after the onset of mild exertional myalgias or cramps, the individual may continue with the exercise at the previous or a slightly reduced level following a brief period of rest.
3. Overt myoglobinuria is rarely noted in children and primarily manifests in the second or third decades.
4. Most patients essentially have normal physical examinations between attacks of muscle cramping.

Laboratory Features

1. Serum CK levels are invariably elevated at baseline.
2. The exercise forearm test can be used to diagnosis various disorders of glycolysis.
   a. The forearm muscles are exercised by having the patient rapidly and strenuously open and close the hand for 1 minute. Immediately after exercise and then 1, 2, 4, 6, and 10 minutes after exercise, blood samples are again taken and analyzed for lactate and ammonia.

b. The normal response is for lactate and ammonia levels to rise three to four times the baseline levels.
c. If neither the lactate nor the ammonia levels increase, the test is inconclusive and implies that the muscles were not sufficiently exercised.
d. A rise in lactate levels but not ammonia is seen in myoadenylate deaminase deficiency (probably nonpathogenic deficiency).
e. In myophosphorylase, phosphofructokinase, phosphoglycerate mutase, phosphoglycerate kinase, phosphorylase B kinase, β-enolase, and lactate dehydrogenase deficiencies, the ammonia levels rise appropriately, but the lactic acid does not.

Electrodiagnostic Findings

EMG and nerve conduction studies are usually normal.

Histopathology

1. Excessive accumulation of glycogen in the subsarcolemmal and intermyofibrillar areas are usually observed on light microscopy and EMG.
2. Staining for myophosphorylase and phosphofructokinase can be performed and absence of staining is evident in these disorders.
3. Enzyme activities can be assayed for definitive diagnosis of the specific subtypes of glycogen storage disease.

TREATMENT

1. Intense isometric exercises such as weight lifting and maximum-aerobic exercises such as sprinting should be avoided.
2. Patients may benefit from a mild to moderate aerobic conditioning. A mild to moderate exercise program improves exercise capacity by increasing cardiovascular fitness and the supply of necessary metabolic substrates to muscle.
3. Patients with McArdle disease should be instructed on moderating their physical activity and in obtaining a "second wind" response. Any bout of moderate exercise should be preceded by 5 to 15 minutes of low-level warm-up activity to promote the transition to the second wind.
4. Oral glucose or fructose loading before activities may be effective in McArdle disease but may be deleterious in phosphofructokinase deficiency.
5. Patients with myoglobinuria should be admitted to the hospital and hydrated to prevent acute tubular necrosis.

CARNITINE DEFICIENCY

BACKGROUND

1. Carnitine deficiency is the most common disorder of lipid metabolism.
2. Carnitine deficiency systemic or only evident in muscle. Muscle carnitine deficiency may be primary or secondary to some other myopathic disorder.

PATHOPHYSIOLOGY

Primary carnitine deficiency has been linked to mutations in the sodium-dependent carnitine transporter protein gene (*OCTN2*) located on chromosome 5q33.1.

PROGNOSIS

Course and response to replacement therapy with carnitine are variable.

DIAGNOSIS

Clinical Features

1. Primary muscle carnitine deficiency usually manifests in childhood or early adult life, but infantile onset has also been described.
2. Progressive proximal muscle weakness and atrophy develop.
3. Cardiac involvement with ventricular hypertrophy, congestive heart failure, and arrhythmias occurs in some patients.
4. A secondary deficiency of carnitine may result from a variety of disorders, including respiratory chain defects, organic aciduria, endocrinopathies, dystrophies, renal and liver failure, and malnutrition or as a toxic effect of certain medications. It is not clear whether patients with secondary carnitine deficiency truly develop myopathic symptoms.

Laboratory Features

1. Plasma and tissue carnitine levels are severely decreased in the primary systemic carnitine deficiency, whereas the deficiency is much less (25%–50% normal) in secondary forms of carnitine deficiency.
2. Only muscle carnitine levels are decreased in primary muscle carnitine deficiency.
3. Serum CK levels are normal in approximately 50% of patients with the myopathic form of the disease but can be elevated to as much as 15 times normal.

Electrophysiologic Findings

1. Motor and sensory nerve conduction studies are normal.
2. Needle EMG is often normal but some patients with profound weakness have increased insertional activity. Short-duration, small-amplitude, polyphasic MUAPs that recruit early can be observed.

Histopathology

1. Muscle fibers contain numerous vacuoles and abnormal accumulation of lipid.
2. Muscle carnitine level is dramatically decreased (less than 2 to 4% of normal).

TREATMENT

1. Oral L-carnitine (2–6 g/d) has benefited some, but not all patients, with carnitine deficiency.
2. Treatment is otherwise supportive.

CARNITINE PALMITYLTRANSFERASE (CPT) DEFICIENCY

BACKGROUND

Carnitine palmitoyltransferase (CPT) deficiency is the most common cause of myoglobinuria.

PATHOPHYSIOLOGY

1. Caused by mutations in the *CPT2* gene located on chromosome 1p32.
2. Deficiency of CPT impairs the transport of acylcarnitine across the inner mitochondrial membrane.
3. Thus, the generation of ATP from fatty-acid metabolism is impaired.

PROGNOSIS

Persistent weakness after attacks of myoglobinuria is uncommon but may occur.

DIAGNOSIS

Clinical Features

1. The typical clinical presentation is muscular pain and cramping following intense or prolonged exertion. Symptoms may also be triggered by fasting or recent infection.
2. Myoglobinuria is a common feature of this disease and renal failure can occur.
3. Most patients become symptomatic by the second decade.
4. Between attacks, the physical examination is usually normal.

Laboratory Features

Serum CK levels are usually normal, except when the patient performs intense physical activities or fasts for prolonged periods.

Electrophysiologic Findings

EMG and NCS findings are typically normal between attacks of myoglobinuria.

Histopathology

1. There is usually no gross abnormality noted on light microscopic examination of muscle tissue. An increase in the lipid content of muscle is detectable in muscle tissue examined by EMG.
2. Enzyme analysis on muscle tissue can confirm the deficiency.

TREATMENT

1. Patients with CPT deficiency should be cautioned to avoid any situation that provokes muscle pain and puts them at risk for myoglobinuria.
2. The physiologic effect of fasting should be explained, and the patient should be warned not to attempt exercise under such conditions.
3. The use of glucose tablets or candy bars during exercise may raise exercise tolerance slightly.
4. If myoglobinuria is noted, the patient should be admitted to the hospital, and renal function should be monitored.

MITOCHONDRIAL MYOPATHIES

BACKGROUND

1. Refers to disorders with identifiable mitochondrial DNA mutations, enzyme deficiencies, and structural abnormalities.

2. Mitochondrial DNA (mtDNA) encodes for 22 transfer RNA (tRNAs), two ribosomal RNAs (rRNAs), and 13 mRNAs.
3. The 13 mRNAs are translated into 13 polypeptide subunits of the respiratory chain complexes.
4. Most mitochondrial proteins are encoded by nuclear DNA and these proteins are translated in the cytoplasm and subsequently are transported into the mitochondria.
5. There appears to be some nuclear control of replication of the mitochondrial genome.

PATHOPHYSIOLOGY

1. Mutations have been identified in several of the mtDNA genes encoding for tRNA. Disorders with these mutations [e.g., myoclonic epilepsy and ragged red fibers (MERRFs) and mitochondrial myopathy lactic acidosis and stroke (MELAS)] have a typical mitochondrial inheritance pattern (e.g., only from mother to both male and female children).
2. Some disorders are caused by mutations in nuclear genes responsible for replication of mtDNA [e.g., mitochondrial DNA-depletion syndromes, mitochondrial neurogastrointestinal encephalomyopathy (MNGIE), and progressive external ophthalmoplegia (PEO)]. These disorders may be inherited in an autosomal recessive or dominant manner.
3. Other disorders are associated with single large deletions of mtDNA but occur sporadically [e.g., Kearn–Sayre syndrome (KSS)].

PROGNOSIS

Dependent of the specific subtype. A reduced life expectancy is associated with most of the disorders.

DIAGNOSIS

Clinical Features

1. The clinical presentations of the different forms of mitochondrial myopathies are quite heterogeneous.
2. Findings include short stature, scoliosis, ptosis, ophthalmoparesis, proximal weakness, cardiomyopathy, neuropathy, hearing loss, optic neuropathy, pigmentary retinopathy, endocrinopathy, myoclonic seizures, ataxia, headaches, stroke-like symptoms (including cortical blindness), gastroparesis, and intestinal pseudoobstruction.

Laboratory Features

1. Serum CK may be normal or elevated.
2. ECG may show conduction abnormalities in some disorders (e.g., KSS).
3. Serum and CSF lactate levels may be normal or elevated.

Histopathology

1. The histopathologic abnormalities on muscle biopsies of the various mitochondrial myopathies are nonspecific.
2. Mitochondrial abnormalities are reflected on the modified Gomori trichrome stain in which subsarcolemmal accumulation of abnormal mitochondria stains red and gives the abnormal muscle fibers their characteristic appearance (ragged red fibers).
3. Oxidative enzyme stains (NADH, SDH, and COX) are also routinely used to diagnose mitochondrial myopathies.

4. Ultrastructural alterations in mitochondria are apparent on EMG. These abnormalities include an increased number of normal-appearing mitochondria, enlarged mitochondria with abnormal cristae, and mitochondria with paracrystalline inclusions.
5. Specific mitochondrial enzymes (components of the respiratory chain) may show reduced activity.
6. Genetic testing:
   a. Mutations in mitochondrial DNA may be demonstrated in leukocytes but specificity is increased looking for the mutations in muscle tissue.

TREATMENT

1. There are no proven medical therapies for most mitochondrial myopathies.
2. I recommend patients take coenzyme Q (children's dose is 30 mg daily; adults are given 150–1,200 mg daily).
3. Likewise, I tell patients to take creatine monohydrate (5–10 g/d).
4. Patients with MERRF and an associated myoclonic seizure disorder should be treated with antiepileptic medication (e.g., valproic acid).
5. Patients and their physicians need to be aware that patients with mitochondrial myopathies can be very sensitive to sedating medications and anesthetic agents leading to alveolar hypoventilation and respiratory failure.
6. Hormone replacement is given for associated specific endocrinopathies.
7. Pacemaker insertion may be required because of the associated cardiac conduction defects.
8. Eyelid surgery to correct ptosis can be performed provided there is sufficient facial strength to allow full eye closure.
9. Patients with severe gastrointestinal dysmotility may require PEG tube placement or parenteral feedings for nutritional support.
10. Ankle foot orthoses may be beneficial in patients with distal lower limb weakness.

BIBLIOGRAPHY

Neuromuscular Junction Disorders

Achiron A, Barak Y, Miron S, et al. Immunoglobulin treatment in refractory myasthenia gravis. *Muscle Nerve* 2000;23:551–555.
Agius MA. Treatment of ocular myasthenia gravis with corticosteroids: yes. *Arch Neurol* 2000;57:750–751.
Chaudhry V, Cornblath DR, Griffin JW, et al. Mycophenolate mofetil: a safe and promising immunosuppressant in neuromuscular diseases. *Neurology* 2001;56:94–96.
Cherington M. Clinical spectrum of botulism. *Muscle Nerve* 1998:21:701–710.
Ciafaloni E, Nikhar NK, Massey JM, et al. Retrospective analysis of the use of cyclosporine in myasthenia gravis. *Neurology* 2000;55:448–450.
Ciafaloni E, Massey JM, Tucker-Lipscomb B, et al. Mycophenolate mofetil for myasthenia gravis: an open-label pilot study. *Neurology* 2001;56:97–99.
Dumitru D, Amato AA. Disorders of the neuromuscular junction. In: Dumitru D, Amato AA, Swartz MJ, eds. *Electrodiagnostic medicine,* 2nd ed. Philadelphia: Hanley & Belfus, 2002:1127–1227.
Drachman DB. Myasthenia gravis. *N Engl J Med* 1994;330:1797–1810.
Engel AG, Ohno K, Sine SM. Congenital myasthenic syndrome: recent advances. *Arch Neurol* 1999;56:163–167.
Evoli A, Batocchi AP, Minisci C, et al. Therapeutic options in ocular myasthenia gravis. *Neuromusc Dis* 2001;11:208–216.
Gajdos P, Chevret S, Clair B, et al. Clinical trial of plasma exchange and high-dose intravenous immunoglobulin in myasthenia gravis. *Ann Neurol* 1997;41:789–796.
Gronseth GS, Barohn RJ. Practice parameter: thymectomy of autoimmune myasthenia gravis (an evidence-based review): report of the Quality Standards Subcommittee of the American Academy of Neurology. *Neurology* 2000;55:7–15.

Harper CM, Engel AG. Quinidine sulfate therapy for the slow-channel myasthenic syndrome. *Ann Neurol* 1998;43:480–484.

Hauser RA, Malek AR, Rosen R. Successful treatment of a patient with severe refractory myasthenia gravis using mycophenylate mofetil. *Neurology* 1998;51:912–913.

Hoch W, McConville J, Helms S, et al. Autoantibodies to the receptor tyrosine kinase MuSK in patients with myasthenia gravis without acetylcholine receptor antibodies. *Nat Med* 2001;7:365–368.

Howard JF. Intravenous immunoglobulin for the treatment of acquired myasthenia gravis. *Neurology* 1998;51[Suppl 5]:S30–S36.

Kaminski HJ, Daroff RB. Treatment of ocular myasthenia: steroids only when compelled. *Arch Neurol* 2000:57:752–753.

Kincaid JC. Tick bite paralysis. *Sem Neurol* 1990;10:32–34.

Newsom-Davis J. Lambert-Eaton myasthenic syndrome. *Curr Treat Op Neurol* 2001;3:127–131.

Palace J, Newsom-Davis J, Lecky B. A randomized double-blind trial of prednisolone alone or with azathioprine in myasthenia gravis. *Neurology* 1998;50:1778–1783.

Palace J, Wiles CM, Newsom-Davis J. 3,4-diaminopyridine in the treatment of congenital (hereditary) myasthenia. *J Neurol Neurosurg Psychiatry* 1991;54:1069–1072.

Rabinstein A, Wijdicks EFM. BiPAP in acute respiratory failure due to myasthenic crisos may prevent intubation. *Neurology* 2002;59:1647–1649.

Sanders DB, Massey JM, Sanders LL, et al. A randomized trial of 3,4-diaminopyridine in Lambert-Eaton myasthenic syndrome. *Neurology* 2000;54:603–607.

Tindall RSA, Phillips JT, Rollins JA, et al. A clinical therapeutic trial of cyclosporine in myasthenia gravis. *Ann N Y Acad Sci* 1993;681:539–551.

Acquired Myopathies

Amato AA, Barohn RJ. Idiopathic inflammatory myopathies. *Neurol Clinics* 1997;15:615–648.

Amato AA, Dumitru D. Acquired myopathies. In: Dumitru D, Amato AA, Swartz MJ, eds. *Electrodiagnostic medicine,* 2nd ed. Philadelphia: Hanley & Belfus, 2002:1265–1432.

Amato AA, Gronseth GS, Jackson CE, et al. Inclusion body myositis: clinical and pathological boundaries. *Ann Neurol* 1996;40:581–586.

Badsrising UA, Maat-Schieman MLC, Ferrari MD, et al. Comparison of weakness progression in inclusion body myositis during treatment with methotrexate or placebo. *Ann Neurol* 2002;51:369–372.

Campellone JV, Lacomis D, Kramer DJ, et al. Acute myopathy after liver transplantation. *Neurology* 1998;50:46–53.

Dalakas MC. Polymyositis, dermatomyositis, and inclusion body myositis. *N Engl J Med* 1991;325:1487–1498.

Dalakas, Illa I, Dambrosia JM, et al. A controlled trial of high dose intravenous immunoglobulin infusions as treatment for dermatomyositis. *N Engl J Med* 1993;329:1993–2000.

Dalakas MC, Saries B, Dambrosia, et al. Treatment of inclusion body myositis with IVIG: a double-blind, placebo-controlled study. *Neurology* 1997;48:712–716.

Dalakas MC, Koffman B, Fujii M, et al. A controlled study of intravenous immunoglobulin combined with prednisone in the treatment of IBM. *Neurology* 2001;56:323–327.

Darrow DH, Hoffman HT, Barnes GJ, et al. Management of dysphagia in inclusion body myositis. *Arch Otolaryngol Head Neck Surg* 1992;118:313–317.

Gherardi R, Baidrimont M, Lionnet F, et al. Skeletal muscle toxoplasmosis in patients with acquired immunodeficiency syndrome: a clinical and pathological study. *Ann Neurol* 1992;32:535–542.

Greenberg SA, Amato AA. Inflammatory myopathy associated with mixed connective tissue disease and scleroderma renal crisis. *Muscle Nerve* 2001;24:1562–1566.

Joffe MM, Love LA, Leff RL. Drug therapy of idiopathic inflammatory myopathies: predictors of response to prednisone, azathioprine, and methotrexate and a comparison of their efficacy. *Am J Med* 1993;94:379–387.

Lacomis D, Zochodne DW, Bird SJ. Critical illness myopathy. *Muscle Nerve* 2000;23:1785–1788.

Levin MI, Mozaffar T, Al-Lozi MT, et al. Paraneoplastic necrotizing myopathy: clinical and pathologic features. *Neurology* 1998;50:764–767.

Hereditary Myopathies

Amato AA, Dumitru D. Hereditary myopathies. In: Dumitru D, Amato AA, Swartz MJ, eds. *Electrodiagnostic medicine,* 2nd ed. Philadelphia: Hanley & Belfus, 2002:1265–1370.

Andrews CT, Taylor TC, Patterson VH. Scapulothoracic arthrodesis for patients with facioscapulohumeral muscular dystrophy. *Neuromusc Dis* 1998;8:580–584.

Angelini C, Pegoraro E, Turella E, et al. Deflazacort in Duchenne dystrophy: study of long-term effect. *Muscle Nerve* 1994;17:386–391.

Askanas V, Engel WK, Kwan HH, et al. Autosomal dominant syndrome of lipid neuromyopathy with normal carnitine: successful treatment with long-chain fatty acid free diet. *Neurology* 1985;35:66–72.

Backman E, Henriksson KG. Low-dose prednisone treatment in Duchenne and Becker muscular dystrophy. *Neuromusc Disord* 1995;5:233–241.

Bonifati MD, Ruzza G, Bonometto P, et al. A multicenter, double-blind, randomized trial of deflazacort versus prednisone in Duchenne muscular dystrophy. *Muscle Nerve* 2000;23:1344–1347.

DiMauro S, Lamperti C. Muscle glycogenoses. *Muscle Nerve* 2001;24:984–999.

Fenichel GM, Florence JM, Pestronk A, et al. Long-term benefit from prednisone therapy in Duchenne muscular dystrophy. *Neurology* 1991;41:1874–1877.

Fenichel G, Pestronk A, Florence J, et al. A beneficial effect of oxandrolone in the treatment of Duchenne muscular dystrophy: a pilot study. *Neurology* 1997;48:1225–1226.

Fenichel GM, Griggs RC, Kissel J, et al. A randomized efficacy and safety trial of oxandrolone in the treatment of Duchenne dystrophy. *Neurology* 2001;56:1075–1079.

FSH Study Group. A prospective, quantitative study of the natural history of facioscapulohumeral muscular dystrophy (FSHD): implications for therapeutic trials. *Neurology* 1997;48:38–46.

Griggs RC, Moxley RT, Mendell JR, et al. Duchenne Dystrophy: randomized, controlled trial of prednisone (18 months) and azathioprine (12 months). *Neurology* 1993;43:520–527.

Griggs RC, Mendell JR, Miller RG. Periodic paralysis and myotonia. In: *Evaluation and treatment of myopathies.* Philadelphia: FA Davis Co, 1995:318–354.

Haller RG. Treatment of McArdle's disease. *Arch Neurol* 2000;57:923–924.

Iannaccone ST, Nanjiani Z. Duchenne muscular dystrophy. *Curr Treat Op Neurol* 2001;3:101–117.

Jackson CE, Barohn RJ, Ptacek LJ. Paramyotonia congenita: abnormal short exercise test, and improvement after mexiletine therapy. *Muscle Nerve* 1994;17:763–768.

Ketenjian AY. Scapulocostal stabilization for scapular winging in facioscapulohumeral muscular dystrophy. *J Bone Joint Surg Am* 1978;60:476–484.

Moxley RT III. Myotonic disorders in childhood: diagnosis and treatment. *J Child Neurol* 1997;12:116–129.

Selby R, Starzl TE, Yunis E, et al. Liver transplantation for type IV glycogen storage disease. *N Engl J Med* 1991;324:39–42.

Shapira Y, Glick B, Harel S, et al. Infantile idiopathic myopathic carnitine deficiency: treatment with L-carnitine. *Pediatr Neurol* 1993;9:35–38.

Snyder TM, Little BW, Roman-Campos G, et al. Successful treatment of familial idiopathic lipid storage myopathy with L-carnitine and modified lipid diet. *Neurology* 982;32:1106–1115.

Tarnopolsky M, Roy BD, MacDonald JR. A randomized, controlled trial of creatine monohydrate in patients with mitochondrial cytopathies. *Muscle Nerve* 1997; 20:1502–1509.

Tarnopolsky M, Martin J. Creatine monohydrate increases strength in patients with neuromuscular disase. *Neurology* 1999;52:854–857.

Tawil R, McDermott MP, Brown R Jr, et al. Randomized trials of dichlorphenamide in the periodic paralyses. *Ann Neurol* 2000;47:46–53.

10. CHRONIC PAIN

Robert D. Helme and Ian Yi-Onn Leong

BACKGROUND

Definitions

1. *Pain* is an unpleasant sensory and emotional experience associated with actual or potential tissue damage or described in terms of such damage.
2. *Chronic pain* is described as pain continuing after the time of normal healing or pain present for more than 6 months.
3. Other useful terms, especially in cancer pain:
   a. *Breakthrough pain* is pain that occurs unexpectedly in the presence of stable background analgesia.
   b. *End-of-dose failure* is pain that occurs between regular doses of analgesic due to decreasing effective tissue levels between doses.
   c. *Incident pain* is pain on movement and implies a musculoskeletal origin or bony involvement by cancer.

Epidemiology

1. Depending on the definition used, approximately 20% of patients seen by primary care physicians have chronic pain.
2. Chronic pain increases with age from 20 to 60. It probably reaches a plateau and declines from age 80.
3. About 50% of patients with cancer will experience pain at some stage of their disease, with 60% to 80% of patients experiencing pain in the advanced stages of their disease.
4. Annual costs of pain treatment both direct and indirect is estimated to be $125 billion in the United States.

The Biopsychosocial Model of Chronic Nonmalignant Pain

1. The relationship between the amount of nociceptive stimulus and the pain reported or the pain behaviors exhibited are dependent on social, psychological, and biomedical factors.
2. The level of pain experienced (suffering) and the affective and behavioral expression of the pain are mediated by the cognitive appraisal of the nociceptive stimulus and its environmental variables.
3. Changes in the pain experienced, the mood of the patient, and the behaviors exhibited by the patient is often not synchronous. An improvement in pain is not always followed by a similar improvement in mood and function.
4. Management of the chronic pain syndrome frequently requires the treating physician to be aware of the multidimensional nature of the pain experience and to adjust treatments accordingly.

Classification

Pain can be classified by its pathogenetic mechanism.
1. Nociceptive pain: Caused by direct tissue injury with resultant stimulation of nociceptors on afferent Aδ and C fibers.
   a. Examples of deep somatic nociceptive pain include arthropathy and back pain.
   b. Superficial somatic nociceptive pain includes painful skin and mucous ulcers.
   c. Visceral nociceptive pain can result from lesions in solid organs or may result from distention of a hollow viscus.
2. Neuropathic pain: Caused by damage to the nervous system.
   a. Peripheral neuropathic pain is derived from activation of afferent nerves

especially those associated with nociceptors; for example post surgical injury, post herpetic neuralgia, diabetic neuropathy, neuroma, nerve root irritation, phantom limb pain, neuralgias and causalgia, complex regional pain syndrome type 2 (CRPS2).

   b. Central neuropathic pain occurs when there is involvement of the central neuraxis involved in the transmission of nociceptive stimuli; for example, stroke, syringomyelia, and multiple sclerosis.
3. Psychological: Examples are found in *Diagnostic and Statistical Manual of Mental Disorders, Fourth Edition (DSM-IV)*. The most common is pain disorder.
4. Mixed: Examples include cancer and vertebral canal stenosis.
5. Uncertain: examples include fibromyalgia and CRPS-1.

PATHOPHYSIOLOGY

Physiologic Mechanisms

1. Pain pathways:
   a. Nociceptors (e.g., ion gated–vannilloid, ligand gated–opioid, 5-hydroxy tryptamine [5HT]) attached to small-diameter primary afferents (mechanical, thermal, chemical) enter the dorsal horn of the spinal cord terminating in laminae 1, 2, 4, and 5.
   b. Modified afferent information is transmitted to relay nuclei in the brainstem and the thalamus predominantly via the spinothalamic pathways.
   c. Thalamic input is transmitted to primary somatic cortex ([sensorimotor cortex] SM1, SM2), limbic cortex (cingulate and insula), and prefrontal cortex.
   d. Descending modulation occurs via the periaqueductal gray matter and reticulospinal pathways (dorsolateral fasiculus).
2. Sensitization:
   a. Peripheral sensitization occurs in nociceptors to noxious and nonnoxious stimulation. Mechanisms include
      1) Inflammatory mediators, prostaglandins, neuromediators, and trophic factors
      2) Ephaptic transmission
      3) Sympathetic modulation
   b. Central sensitization occurs through
      1) Up-regulation of excitatory systems [e.g., glutamate via N-methyl D-aspartate (NMDA) receptors]
      2) Inhibition of inhibitory systems (e.g., GABA, glycine)
      3) Altered nervous system tissue (e.g., glial proliferation, neuronal dropout, axonal sprouting, sodium channel overexpression)

Neuropathic Pain Mechanisms

1. Increased ectopic activity in damaged afferent mechanosensitive neurons and in the spared neighboring fibers.
2. Increased ectopic activity in spared C fibers; this is responsible for maintenance of central sensitization in many instances of neuropathic pain.
3. Central sensitization

Visceral Pain Mechanisms

1. High-threshold receptors that are normally active when there is acute injury become sensitized with prolonged stimulation. They respond to physiologic stimuli until the peripheral sensitization settles.
2. "Silent" receptors which are quiescent normally become active during visceral inflammation.
3. The dorsal column transmits some visceral nociceptive information, together with other traditional nociceptive pathways.
4. Visceral pain causes activation of a different part of the anterior cingulate cortex compared to somatic pain.

5. With a lower density of innervation, there is less temporal and spatial resolution of visceral pain.
6. Autonomic responses are often more obvious with visceral pain.

PROGNOSIS

1. Outcomes in chronic pain should not be narrowly defined in terms of pain intensity only, but should be defined in the broader context of physical function, mood, and social function.
2. Psychosocial factors predict outcome (physical and psychosocial functioning) better than the physical characteristics of the pain in chronic nonmalignant pain. When maladaptive, these are known as "yellow flags" and comprise negative factors.
3. Factors that predict a poor response in cancer pain include: neuropathic pain, incident pain, a patient with multiple pains from differing mechanisms, pain that has been persistent, adverse effects that are difficult to control, and a history of drug or alcohol abuse.

Attitudes and Beliefs

1. Belief that pain implies ongoing damage or is potentially severely disabling.
2. Belief that pain must be abolished before improvement in physical function is possible.
3. Catastrophic misinterpretation of events.
4. Belief that pain is uncontrollable.
5. Belief that passive treatment (e.g., medications) is more helpful than active (participatory) treatment (e.g., rehabilitation).

Behaviors

1. Use of extended rest
2. Reduced activity levels such as activities of daily living (ADLs)
3. Active avoidance of normal activity
4. Excessive reliance on aids
5. High intake of alcohol and other substances since the onset of pain
6. Irregular participation in physical exercise

Diagnostic and Treatment Experiences

1. Health care professional sanctioning disability and not providing interventions that will improve function
2. Experience of conflicting diagnoses or function
3. Healthcare professional functioning from a wholly biomedical perspective

Emotions

Emotions include depression, anger, anxiety (including heightened sensitivity to benign bodily sensations), and fear of movement.

Family and Spousal Relationships

1. Presence of an overprotective spouse
2. Solicitous behavior from spouse
3. Poor familial relationship
4. Lack of social support

Work Conditions

1. Unsupportive management at the workplace
2. Unhappy work environment
3. Limited possibilities for a graduated return to work

Response to Pharmacologic Therapy

1. Chronic pain responds poorly to pharmacologic therapy.
2. About 30% of patients will have a satisfactory long-term response to opioid therapy alone and these patients will show good response early in the course of treatment. Half of them, however, discontinue opioids because of toxicity or for other reasons.
3. About 50% of patients with neuropathic pain will have moderate pain reduction with adjuvants. However, only 10% to 20% of patients will have complete pain relief. The analgesic effect of adjuvants is likely to decrease with time.
4. About 85% of patients with cancer pain will show satisfactory response to conventional management.

DIAGNOSIS

Diagnostic Formulation

1. Should include a medical diagnosis (where possible), the psychologic (both affective and cognitive) and social factors that are modulating the pain experience, and the behaviors exhibited by the patient and the family.

General Assessment

1. Should also include an assessment of the goals and targets of the patient.

Medical Assessment

1. Should include a thorough description of the pain complaint:
2. The site of pain and its radiation.
3. The severity of the worst pain, least pain, and average pain should be scaled using a rating scale:
   a. Numeric rating scale (0–10, 0–20, or 0–100)
   b. Verbal rating scale (for example, mild, moderate, severe, horrible, excruciating)
   c. Visual analog scale (VAS) (marking on a 10-cm line how severe the pain is with anchors of "no pain" and "most severe pain" on the ends)
4. The temporal profile: continuous, intermittent, paroxysmal, or persistent pain.
5. Factors modulating the intensity of pain, in particular precipitating, aggravating, and relieving factors.
6. Quality descriptors. Examples could be taken from the McGill Pain Questionnaire: aching, sharp, burning, stabbing, throbbing.
7. Accompanying autonomic features including dystrophic skin, nail and hair changes, and localized changes in temperature and color should be noted.
8. Other neurologic symptoms (like paraesthesia, analgesia, weakness) and muscular symptoms (like stiffness and joint restriction) should be noted.
9. At all times, correctable pathologies should be identified if possible.
10. Certain features suggest serious disease in pain conditions and warrant further evaluation: pains that wake the patient in the night; pains that are persistent and are not at all modified by any analgesia; systemic features like unexplained weight loss, fever, or the patient complaining that they feel unwell; symptoms that suggest other organ disease; and progressive neurologic deficit.
11. Beyond a reasonable workup, the relentless pursuit of a "definitive" diagnosis is discouraged.

Affective Presentation

1. Should be defined and quantified, either by the means of standardized psychometric questionnaires or by the means of self-monitoring methods (numeric measures, diaries).
2. Anxiety can range from a mild irritation to a psychiatric disorder with concurrent panic attacks (e.g., posttraumatic stress disorder). Frequently there is increased

somatic awareness of benign symptoms and there is often misinterpretation (often exaggeration) of these symptoms. The Beck Anxiety Inventory is one good measure for quantifying anxiety symptoms.

3. Depression can vary from a mild dysphoria to severe depression. Importantly, somatic symptoms of depression (insomnia, lack of energy, weight change) are also frequently found in chronic pain and should not be automatically attributed to depression. Suicidal ideation should be assessed in all patients with chronic pain. The Beck Depression Inventory, the Zung Depression Scale and the Center for Epidemiological Studies-Depression Scale have been used in the context of pain assessment. The Geriatric Depression Scale is more suitable for older people.

4. Fear of movement has been identified as a strong affective factor predicting disability. The Tampa Kinesophobia Scale is one measure to quantify this factor.

5. Anger and hostility toward health professionals, relatives, and workplace management should be identified. Patients are also often frustrated by the lack of improvement in their condition.

Psychiatric Disorders as an Explanation

1. Should be diagnosed with care. The prevalence of true psychogenic pain is low. Preferably, this should only be diagnosed by a psychiatrist or psychologist in the setting of a multidisciplinary clinic. Examples would include somatoform disorders, conversion disorders, hypochondriasis, and pain disorder (see *DSM-IV* for diagnostic details).

Behavior Assessment

1. Verbal behaviors.
2. Health-seeking behaviors, for example the number of times the patient visited his or her local doctor in the previous week, the number of specialists that the patient has consulted or intends to consult, and the number of medications taken.
3. Pain-specific behaviors such as wincing, guarding, and moaning.
4. Activity-related behaviors such as avoidance of certain activities and extended rest periods should be evaluated. The ADLs, instrumental activities of daily living, and social activities the patient still participates in should be quantified.
5. Target behaviors. During assessment, the patient should be asked to identify realistic goals that he or she can work toward in the course of treatment.

Cognitive Processes

1. Cognitive processes are important modifying factors in the pain experience. These attitudes, beliefs, or perceptions should be identified and corrected in the course of treatment. Examples of psychometrics relevant to this area include the Survey of Pain Attitudes and the Coping Strategies Questionnaire.
2. Beliefs about pain include the following:
   a. Beliefs about the nature of their pain, for example that it implies a serious or potentially terminal illness.
   b. Beliefs about control. Patients who believe that they can control their pain have better moods, whereas patients who believe that their pain is not controllable, or controllable by medication or their health care providers have poorer moods.
   c. Self-efficacy beliefs. Patients who believe that they can achieve their goals despite their pain function better and have a more positive affect.
   d. Beliefs about hurt, harming, and further injury frequently result in avoidance behaviors.
3. Coping styles and strategies. Patients who are avoiders tend to fare worse than those who confront their problems. Passive coping strategies and emotion-focused strategies tend to lead to a worse prognosis.

Psychosocial Variables

1. May be important in the management of chronic pain, including the following:
   a. Relationships with significant others, in particular the degree of solicitousness in the relationship
   b. Work environment
   c. Social supports
   d. Home environment and immediate environs

Other Issues

1. Include litigation and spiritual attitudes. The latter is particularly relevant in cancer pain management.

Signs Relevant in the Examination of the Patient with Chronic Pain

1. A thorough musculoskeletal and neurologic examination must be performed.
2. Apart from a rheumatologic examination, examination for myofascial trigger points should be elicited. Features of trigger points include the following:
   a. Taut bands of muscle.
   b. Palpation of these taut bands can reproduce the usual pain and the pattern of radiation of pain.
   c. Local twitch response during palpation.
   d. Associated muscular and autonomic dysfunction.
3. Neurologic signs include:
   a. Hyperalgesia: Increased pain report to a stimulus that is normally painful (mechanical, thermal or chemical), including a lowered threshold response.
   b. Hyperpathia: Increased reaction to a painful stimulus, especially a repetitive stimulus, and often accompanied by an increased threshold to a noxious stimulus.
   c. Allodynia: Pain due to a stimulus that does not normally provoke pain (examples include brushing and cold).

Other Measurement Methods in Chronic Pain

1. Psychophysical: threshold, tolerance, suprathreshold scaling to electrical, thermal, and chemical stimuli.
2. Physiologic:
   a. Microneurography: small afferent fibers and sympathetics
   b. Nerve conduction studies: large fiber (nonnoxious fibers)
   c. Autonomic: lacks specificity
   d. Imaging: anatomic proximity of tissue pathology to nervous system elements

Features of Some Conditions

Nociceptive Pain

1. This is generally pain arising from primary afferent nerves in bones, muscles, and joints, as well as superficially from skin-associated elements.
2. It is frequently described as dull or aching, although other descriptors may also be used. The pain is well localized to the site of pathology and there is frequently tenderness (mechanical hyperalgesia).
3. There may be referral of pain, which can sometimes seem to mimic neuropathic type pain. For example, internal disc disruption can often produce a sciatic nerve–like pattern of pain radiation.
4. Movement tends to exacerbate the pain.

Neuropathic Pain

1. Peripheral neuropathic pain can arise from peripheral (small fiber) neuropathies, entrapment neuropathies, localized neuropathies, and phantom limb pain.

2. Central neuropathic pain includes central poststroke pain and pain from myelopathies, such as multiple sclerosis and human immunodeficiency virus (HIV)–related myelopathy.
3. Neuropathic pain is frequently described as lancinating, burning, and shooting. There may be pain in the numb area, tingling, or a sensation of pins-and-needles. Pain arising from an area of anesthesia is called "anesthesia dolorosa."
4. The pain has a dermatomal pattern and follows a nerve distribution or pattern suggestive of a spinal cord or cortical lesion.
5. Certain movements may produce nerve traction and exacerbate the pain; for example, straight leg raising.
6. There is stimulus-evoked pain on examination.

Complex Regional Pain Syndrome

1. This occurs days to weeks after an injury, which may have been trivial, and there is a distal predominance of abnormal findings, which exceeds that which would be expected from the injury (CRPS-1).
2. There is spontaneous and evoked pain (allodynia and hyperalgesia) in a nondermatomal pattern.
3. There are accompanying autonomic signs (edema, changes in temperature and color, and changes in sweating levels), and occasional motor signs (wasting, weakness, tremor and dystonia) and dystrophic signs (skin and hair changes, nail changes and osteoporosis).
4. In CRPS-2 (causalgia), there is nerve injury. This is absent in CRPS-1. The pain usually occurs at the time of injury. The signs are greatest in the anatomic distribution of the nerve, but may spread beyond it. Limb protection is often evident and tremor or dystonia may develop.

Fibromyalgia Syndrome

1. This describes a syndrome of chronic widespread pain.
2. Eleven of 18 specific tender points should be identified.
3. Fatigue and insomnia are usually prominent.
4. It is associated with restless legs syndrome, irritable bowel syndrome, irritable bladder syndrome, cold intolerance, cognitive dysfunction, and neurally mediated hypotension.
5. Depression is often present.

TREATMENT

Overview

Management of chronic nonmalignant pain should be directed to all aspects of the pain experience.
1. The pain sensation may be modified with the use of pharmacologic agents, anesthetic procedures, physical treatments, and, less commonly, neurosurgical interventions.
2. Where possible, disease-modifying medication or procedures should be offered in the context of an overall pain management program.
3. Emotional difficulties in the context of chronic pain can be dealt with using cognitive behavioral therapy (CBT), or emotional expression techniques. Concomitant use of anxiolytics or antidepressants is indicated when the problem is resistant to conservative measures.
   a. Fear and avoidance can also be managed using CBT and specific behavioral therapy methods such as *in vivo* exposure. Reassurance alone is almost always unhelpful.
4. Physical functioning should be improved with the use of graded physical activity.
5. Dysfunctional attitudes, perceptions, or beliefs should be managed using education and CBT.

6. Efforts should be taken to counsel the spouse or care giver. Workplace and home environmental interventions should be done to improve the independent functioning of the patient. Socialization and assertiveness skills are also sometimes required.
7. Other aspects requiring management may be insomnia and sexual dysfunction.
8. Relapse prevention also forms a vital part of the overall management strategy.
9. Pain intensity reduction is not the only goal in the management of the patient. Physical and psychosocial functioning are just as important. Improving the self-efficacy of the individual is important for achieving these goals.

Evaluation

Patients should be evaluated and treated in a multidisciplinary pain clinic if they do not respond adequately in a reasonable time to individual therapies.

Principles of Pharmacologic Management

1. Pharmacologic management should be targeted toward the suspected mechanism of the pain.
2. Principles of analgesic administration.
   a. The goal is for medication to be used in a time-contingent manner.
   b. Additional analgesia can be taken prophylactically if a pain-provoking activity is planned.
   c. Pain-contingent administration of medications should only be considered in the presence of an unpredicted exacerbation of pain (breakthrough pain) that cannot be controlled by other methods.

Simple Analgesics

1. Acetaminophen (paracetamol):
   a. This is used in mild nociceptive pain. It does not attenuate neuropathic pain, but may be helpful in patients for whom neuropathic pain is exacerbated by a nociceptive component.
   b. The dosage is 500 to 1,000 mg by mouth (p.o.) every 6 hours.
   c. It should be abandoned if a dose of 4 g/d for a week produces no significant analgesia.
   d. Side effects are minimal. Overdose results in hepatic failure. Prolongation of prothrombin times has been reported and care must be taken with patients taking anticoagulants.
2. Nonsteroidal antiinflammatory drugs (NSAIDs):
   a. These drugs are best used in the context of moderate inflammatory pain. Long-term use of NSAIDs is best avoided where possible.
   b. The efficacy of one NSAID over another has never been clearly established. However, a patient may respond better to one class than another. A trial may be attempted in the presence of an inflammatory pain.
   c. They have the potential for allergic reactions and gastrointestinal side effects, renal failure, hypertension, and cardiac failure.
   d. Risk factors for gastrointestinal toxicity include:
      1) Concomitant use of two NSAIDs
      2) Concomitant use of anticoagulants or steroids
      3) Age more than 65
      4) History of peptic ulceration
      5) History of gastrointestinal bleeding
      6) High doses of NSAID use
      7) Presence of serious comorbidity, such as hypertension, diabetes mellitus, or renal, hepatic, or cardiovascular disease
   e. Strategies to reduce gastrointestinal toxicity:
      1) Avoiding NSAIDs with higher toxicity (e.g., Piroxicam and Ketoprofen) and using agents with lower toxicity (e.g., Ibuprofen and Diclofenac).

TABLE 10-1. TYPICAL DOSING SCHEDULES

	Dose Range (mg)	Dosing Intervals (h)
Indomethacin	50–100	6–12
Diclofenac	25–150	8–12
Ibuprofen	200–1,600	6–8
Ketoprofen	100–200	12–24
Naproxen	250–1,000	12
Meloxicam	7.5–15	24
Celecoxib	100–200	12–24
Rofecoxib	12.5–25	24

2) Using a proton pump inhibitor (e.g., Omeprazole 20 mg/d) or a prostaglandin analog [e.g., Misoprostol 200 μg four times a day (q.i.d.)].

3) Use of a COX-II inhibitor

  f. COX-II–specific inhibitors
  1) COX-II inhibitors have less gastroduodenal toxicity compared with conventional NSAIDs. However, celecoxib loses its protective effect when aspirin is coadministered.
  2) Rofecoxib has been demonstrated to have higher cardiovascular risk than naproxen.
  3) COX-II inhibitors should be used when clearly indicated in patients with rheumatoid arthritis or osteoarthritis at high risk of gastrointestinal toxicity.
  4) Typical dosing schedules are shown in Table 10-1.

Tramadol

1. Tramadol acts at μ-opioid receptors and also increases serotonergic and noradrenergic inhibition of nociceptive transmission.
2. It is used for moderate to severe pain.
3. Tramadol may induce seizures and should be used with caution in patients with epilepsy or concurrently with selective serotonin reuptake inhibitors (SSRIs) or tricyclic antidepressants. Other common side effects include nausea, sedation and sweating.
4. The immediate-release formulation can be administered every 4 to 8 hours and the slow-release formulation can be given every 12 hours.
5. The maximum daily dose is 400 mg/d.

Opioids

Overview

1. Weak opioids such as codeine or dextropropoxyphene are used for moderate pain and stronger opioids are used for severe malignant and nonmalignant pain when other analgesics provide insufficient pain relief. There should be clear objective evidence of underlying pathology that is known to be opioid-responsive.
2. Side effects include constipation, nausea, vomiting, respiratory failure, confusion, sedation, hypotension, and rash.
3. Principles of prescribing opioids:
  a. Long-acting opioids should be given in a time-contingent manner after titration using a short-acting formulation.
  b. Combinations of opioids should be avoided.
  c. Meperidine/pethidine should be avoided in chronic pain as there is a high risk of neurotoxicity from accumulation of metabolites.
  d. Interindividual variation to different opioids: Individuals may have to try different opioids to decide on the one with the best efficacy and with the least side effects.

    e. In malignant pain, if tolerance develops, opioid rotation may be attempted or other strategies to increase the therapeutic window could be used. In nonmalignant pain, the patient should undergo a multidisciplinary assessment before opioid rotation is considered.

    f. Driving, operating heavy machinery, and tasks requiring delicate psychomotor skills should be avoided during dose titration, but are not contraindicated when stable doses are reached.

Examples of Opioids

1. Codeine:
    a. Usually used alone or as part of a compound analgesic.
    b. Metabolized to morphine in the body, which is the active compound. Ten percent of white individuals are unable to metabolize codeine and will not experience analgesia.
    c. Orally, 10 mg of codeine is approximately equivalent to 1 mg of morphine.
    d. At higher doses, it does not have any advantages over morphine and may be more constipating.

2. Morphine:
    a. Metabolized to morphine-3-glucuronide and morphine-6-glucuronide (which is a potent analgesic).
    b. Can be given orally as an immediate-release formulation or a slow-release formulation. Slow-release formulations differ slightly in pharmacokinetics and patients should not be switched from one to another.
    c. Other routes of administration are subcutaneous (s.c.), intramuscular (IM), intravenous (IV), intrathecal, and epidural.
    d. A usual oral starting dosage would be 5 to 10 mg every 4 hours. Half this dose should be used in older patients.
    e. Long-acting compounds should be used when a satisfactory dose is reached.

3. Oxycodone:
    a. This is one and a half times to two times as potent as morphine.
    b. A controlled-release formulation is available with onset of analgesia at 30 minutes to 1 hour and lasting for up to 12 hours.

4. Hydromorphone:
    a. Hydromorphone is approximately five times as potent as morphine.
    b. It can be given orally, parenterally, or intraspinally.
    c. It is highly soluble and high doses can be given in small volumes via the parenteral route. This is also advantageous when using the s.c. route (e.g., in palliative care). It is the preferred opioid in acute renal failure.

5. Fentanyl:
    a. This is available as transdermal, parenteral, and transmucosal formulations.
    b. The transdermal patches are available in 25, 50, 75, and 100 μg/h patches.
    c. Patches are effective for 3 days and the half-life of fentanyl is 15 to 20 hours after removal of the patch.
    d. It is to be avoided in opioid naive patients. A stable dose of opioids should be arrived at before conversion to fentanyl patches.
    e. The 25 μg/h patch is equivalent to 60 to 100 mg of oral morphine. Increasing strengths of patches correspond to multiples of that equivalence value.
    f. Transmucosal fentanyl is used for breakthrough pain in cancer. It is most useful in incident pain.

6. Methadone:
    a. It is also an NMDA receptor antagonist and may be useful in chronic pain.
    b. It has a variable half-life, which increases with prolonged use.
    c. Its use in detoxification programs has limited its application in pain control.
    d. It should only be used by physicians who have experience in its use.

Opioid Rotation

1. Opioid rotation is a strategy that uses the fact that there is incomplete cross-tolerance among opioids.

TABLE 10-2. EXAMPLES OF EQUIVALENCE VALUES

Opioid	Approximate Oral Morphine Equivalent (mg)
Codeine 30 mg p.o.	3
Buprenorphine 0.2 mg SL	7.5
Pethidine 50 mg IM	20
Hydromorphone 1 mg p.o.	5
Oxycodone 10 mg p.o.	15–20

p.o., by mouth; SL, sublingual; IM, intramuscular.

2. It should be considered in cases of tolerance or dose-related side effects.
3. The total 24-hour dose of the present opioid is calculated and converted to the equivalent dose in oral morphine. This is then converted to the 24-hour dose of the desired opioid in its desired route.
4. If switching to an opioid other than methadone or fentanyl, reduce the dose by 25% to 50%.
5. If switching to transdermal fentanyl, do not reduce the dose.
6. Switches to methadone should be performed by physicians who have expertise in its use or who are supervised by such.
7. Examples of equivalence values are given in Table 10-2.

Opioids for Nonmalignant Pain
1. The patient should be informed that this is a trial because clear efficacy of opioids in this situation is not fully proven.
2. Preferably a psychologic assessment should be performed. In particular, the risk for drug-related harm and addiction should be identified.
3. The patient should be informed of risk and benefits of opioid treatment and informed consent should be obtained.
4. A contract between patient and prescriber should be drawn up that includes information on dose, side effects, outcome measures and limits to prescriber numbers.
5. The prescriber should assess the patient at regular intervals to assess aberrant behaviors and benefits of treatment.
6. Clear documentation should be maintained.
7. Physicians must be vigilant of their own intentions when prescribing opioids to a patient and must be ready to curtail its use if necessary.
8. While physicians should not treat patients who require opioids as potential drug addicts, they should be aware of aberrant behavior that may suggest potential for drug-related harm.
9. Major aberrant behaviors include the following:
   a. Selling prescription drugs.
   b. Forging prescriptions.
   c. Stealing or borrowing drugs.
   d. Injecting oral formulations of drugs.
   e. Obtaining prescription drugs from nonmedical sources.
   f. Concurrently abusing illicit drugs or alcohol.
   g. Repeatedly increasing dose without approval.
   h. Repeatedly losing prescription.
   i. Repeatedly seeking prescription from other physicians or from the emergency department without informing the prescriber or after being warned to desist.
   j. Deteriorating function that appears to be drug related.
   k. Repeatedly avoiding changes to treatment despite physical or psychological side effects.
10. Minor aberrant behaviors include the following:
    a. Aggressively complaining about the need for more drug.

   b. Drug hoarding during periods of reduced symptoms.
   c. Requesting specific drugs.
   d. Openly acquiring similar drugs from other sources.
   e. Increasing the dose without approval.
   f. Using drugs to treat other symptoms without approval.
11. Management of aberrant behavior:
   a. Major aberrant behavior should be managed by weaning and ceasing opioids, joint management with an addiction medicine specialist, or giving very frequent supplies (e.g., daily or weekly).
   b. Minor aberrant behavior requires reassessment of the patient (expectations, medication suitability, pathology) with a consideration of changing the drug, urine testing, or reducing the time interval for supplying the medication. Previous discussions about the conditions for prescription should be reinforced.

Adjuvants

Antidepressants

1. These are best used in the context of neuropathic pain. They have been shown to have some effect in musculoskeletal conditions, such as chronic low back pain and osteoarthritis. Analgesic effects are independent of mood-modifying effects. Tricyclic antidepressants have the best efficacy. The SSRIs and other new classes of antidepressants have a less certain role.
2. Tricyclic antidepressants:
   a. The best studied is amitriptyline. Other commonly used tricyclics are nortriptyline and desipramine.
   b. The starting dosage for amitriptyline is 10 to 25 mg at night. Dosages can be increased by 10 to 25 mg at night every 3 to 7 days. The ideal dose will be the best efficacy with the least side effects. If there is no benefit at 75 mg at night, this strategy should be abandoned. The dose range for desipramine is 25 to 300 mg daily, for nortriptyline it is 50 to 150 mg daily, and for dothiepin it is 100 to 200 mg/d.
   c. The side effects are sedation, nausea, constipation, postural hypotension, visual blurring, dry mouth, precipitation of narrow angle glaucoma, and urinary retention especially in the elderly. Arrhythmias may occur in those who are predisposed.
3. Other antidepressants:
   a. SSRI. Paroxetine (20–40 mg daily) and citalopram (20–40 mg daily) have been used.
   b. Venlafaxine has been used at doses of 37.5 mg to 300 mg daily for chronic pain. There is only anecdotal evidence of efficacy.
   c. These drugs are best reserved for patients for whom depression is prominent and requires pharmacologic treatment or when other adjuvants have not been shown to be effective.

Antiepileptic Drugs

1. Antiepileptics are used as adjuvant analgesics in neuropathic pain. Carbamazepine and gabapentin are used more often than phenytoin, sodium valproate, and lamotrigine.
2. Carbamazepine:
   a. This has been shown to be most useful in trigeminal neuralgia. Its role in postherpetic neuralgia, diabetic peripheral neuropathy, and other conditions is less clear.
   b. The starting dose is 50 mg/d and this dose is titrated upward every 3 days by 50 mg/d until the appearance of side effects or clinical response. Lack of effect in an antiepileptic dose range suggests a lack of efficacy.
   c. Common side effects include central nervous system toxicity (nausea, dizziness, ataxia and diplopia), rash, sedation, hyponatremia, and hepatic or bone marrow toxicity.

3. Gabapentin:
   a. Gabapentin has been shown to work via calcium channel blockade in neuropathic pain. The main conditions for which gabapentin has been shown to be effective include diabetic peripheral neuropathy and postherpetic neuralgia.
   b. The starting dose is 300 mg/d and this dose can be increased by 300 mg/d every day for 3 days and then every week until the appearance of clinical response or toxicity. Maximum dose is 2,400 mg/d given in three divided doses.
   c. Side effects include dizziness, ataxia and somnolence. Its side effect profile is superior to that of the older antiepileptic medications.
4. Lamotrigine
   a. There has been some anecdotal evidence to suggest that lamotrigine is useful in refractory trigeminal neuralgia, pain from spinal cord injury, and other neuralgias. One trial has shown benefit in pain after stroke. Effective doses have been shown to be around 400 mg/d.
5. Sodium valproate
   a. There is also limited evidence for this antiepileptic drug in a wide range of presumed neuropathic pain conditions. Dosages are generally kept low [e.g., 200 mg twice a day (b.i.d.)] increasing to 400 mg b.i.d. thus reducing the side effects commonly encountered at higher doses such as nausea, weight gain, and tremor.

Other Agents for Neuropathic Pain

1. Mexiletine has been used in diabetic neuropathy at doses of up to 750 mg/d. The starting dose is 50 mg/d and the dose is increased by 50 mg/d every 3 days until there is clinically relevant benefit or until intolerable side effects. Side effects include cardiac arrhythmias, gastrointestinal disturbances, and tremors. A cardiac evaluation, including an electrocardiogram (ECG), prior to use is required.
2. IV/s.c. lignocaine can be helpful in some instances of intractable neuropathic pain.

Topical Agents

1. Numerous prescription and over-the-counter topical medications are available.
2. Topical lignocaine has been shown to be efficacious in neuropathic pain, in particular postherpetic neuralgia.
3. Topical capsaicin preparations have been used in musculoskeletal pain and neuropathic pain with varying effects. Topical NSAIDs have been used for musculoskeletal pain, again with variable effects.
4. Overall, topical agents are reasonably safe and worth a trial. Topical NSAIDs, however, may be systemically absorbed and care should be taken in patients with renal failure. Topical capsaicin is associated with a burning sensation.

Other Classes of Medications

1. Ketamine has NMDA receptor antagonist activity and has been used in chronic malignant and nonmalignant pain. Its efficacy remains debatable.
2. One regimen is a continuous s.c. infusion of ketamine starting at a dose of 100 mg over 24 hours and increasing by 200 mg/24 hours every day up to a maximum dose of 500 mg/24 hours. The clinically effective dose is maintained for 72 hours.
3. Low-dosage levodopa (e.g., 100 mg at night) has been used for pain and dysesthesias accompanying restless legs syndrome (also long-acting dopamine agonists) and in neuropathic pain (acute herpes zoster pain and diabetic neuropathy).

Physical Therapies

1. Physical exercise is an intrinsic part of most pain management programs. It is best delivered along with concepts from cognitive behavioral therapy. *In vivo* exposure concepts should also be incorporated.

2. Other modalities are used more in the setting of acute pain or may be used as adjuncts in chronic pain. Care must be taken that the patient does not develop an overreliance on these passive measures.
3. Manipulation and mobilization have been found to be better than rest for acute back pain.
4. Methods of stimulation induced analgesia include transcutaneous electrical nerve stimulation and acupuncture.
5. Other physical modalities include massage and other forms of "bodywork," heat, cold, and ultrasound.

Cognitive Behavioral Therapy and Other Psychological Therapies

Overview

1. The cognitive-behavioral conception of chronic pain views that the cognitions (appraisals, beliefs, and expectancies) can modify the relationship between a nociceptive stimulus and the resultant pain-associated behaviors and mood changes and their social consequences. The patient is encouraged to take an active role in the treatment process.
2. A person's cognitions can also be affected by his or her mood, environment, behavior, and physiology.
3. CBT attempts to help the patient identify maladaptive cognitions and behaviors and develop more adaptive strategies.
4. Methods include behavioral techniques (goal setting, graded activity, goal-contingent activity) and cognitive strategies (cognitive reconceptualization, medication reduction). The patient is also taught other coping strategies such as attentional control, relaxation, and problem solving. Maladaptive strategies are discouraged. Finally relapse prevention is also taught.

Goal Setting, Pacing of Activities and Goal Contingent Activity

1. The patient is taught to set realistic physical and social goals. These are then broken down to manageable steps and the patient is taught to pace up gradually toward these goals. Graded physical exercise serves as a platform to introduce these skills and as a means to combat deconditioning.
2. Activity charts and charts of short- and long-term goals are used as motivating tools and as a demonstration and reminder of success.
3. Using these strategies, the patient is taught to develop goal-contingent activity strategies rather than pain-contingent strategies.
4. This reinforces the patients' sense of control and they learn to attribute success to their own efforts.

Cognitive Reconceptualization

1. The patient is led away from a solely biomedical conception of his or her problems to one incorporating biopsychosocial components.
2. The patient is taught that how the pain sensation is interpreted can change some of the consequences of pain.
3. The Gate Control Theory is often used as a model to illustrate that cognitive factors are capable of modifying the incoming nociceptive stimulus.
4. The patient is also taught the Antecedent–Belief (or automatic thought)–Consequence (both emotional and behavioral) model and is taught to dispute maladaptive beliefs or thoughts and to arrive at more adaptive cognitions.
5. Some typical beliefs would be "I cannot control the pain" or "I'd better not move because I am harming myself" and this may result in consequences such as depression and avoidance of activity. These can be disputed and replaced with more healthy beliefs such as "I have many strategies to control my pain such as ... " or "Increased pain can happen at any time and does not mean I am harming myself." These thoughts can help to lessen depression and improve activity.

Medication Reduction

1. Some patients are overmedicated and reduction in medication may be beneficial. It is also a means of improving self-efficacy, in that the patients come to realize that they have other strategies that can be used to manage pain and they do not have to rely on medications.
2. This is done using a graded reduction schedule with the patient fully involved in the decision-making process.

Attentional Control Strategies

The patient is taught distraction techniques and the use of imagery to help in the management of pain.

Relaxation

Methods used include progressive muscular relaxation and deep breathing as a means of reducing muscular tension.

Problem Solving

1. The patient is presented with a variety of situations and is asked to generate alternatives, to weigh the advantages and disadvantages of these alternatives, and then to implement them.
2. This is operationalized into real problems that the patient may be encountering now. The other strategies are used as means to achieve these goals.

Relapse Prevention

The patient is taught to expect setbacks and is helped to develop strategies to cope with these setbacks.

In Vivo Exposure

1. *In vivo* exposure is a behavioral technique that specifically helps to deal with fear related to movement and activity.
2. The patient, with the aid of the therapist, develops a hierarchy of feared activities. The patient is then asked to perform the least-feared activities until there is a significant reduction in fear. This must be repeated by the patient on a daily basis until it no longer evokes fear. The next task that is least feared is then addressed in the same manner until all such activities are dealt with.
3. Frequently, the patient is capable of exposing him- or herself to the feared activity once he or she has experienced some degree of success and the rationale of the therapy is well understood.

Emotional Expression

Patients are asked to write about their most distressing thoughts or fears. Such outpouring of emotion has been shown to decrease pain and inflammatory activity in patients with rheumatoid arthritis.

Management of Cancer Pain

1. Cancer pain frequently occurs in the setting of role changes, spiritual and emotional distress, other physical symptoms, physically and emotionally demanding therapies, and impending death.
2. These should preferably be addressed by a multidisciplinary team.
3. Frequently, there may be more than one pain and these should each be assessed and treated.
4. Tumor reduction therapy should be considered as part of the overall pain control strategy.
5. Time-contingent medication is nearly always mandatory and breakthrough doses should always be ordered.

6. The pharmacologic treatment should be directed to the suspected mechanism of pain.
7. An immediate-release formulation of opioid is the best means of starting therapy. Converting to a long-acting formulation is advisable.
8. The breakthrough dose is usually calculated as one sixth of the 24-hour dose and should be an immediate-release formulation. Incident pain can be effectively treated with transmucosal fentanyl. End-of-dose failure implies that the background dose of analgesia should be increased.
9. Side effects should be treated aggressively. Opioid rotation may be attempted when the pain is opioid-responsive but side effects are limiting the use of the current opioid.
10. Multimodal pharmacologic therapy can be used to decrease opioid requirement.
11. Pain from bone metastases should be treated either with an NSAID, a bisphosphonate (if it is due to breast cancer or multiple myeloma), radiotherapy, or radioisotope therapy.
12. Opioid myths (e.g., "I will become an addict," "Increasing opioid doses means I will die earlier," "If I increase doses now, I will have nothing to fall back on when I get more advanced disease") must be addressed in all patients.

Management of Pain in the Elderly

1. Older people are a heterogenous group.
2. On one hand, some elderly are more prone to side effects and usually require lower doses of medications than the younger person due to altered pharmacokinetics and pharmacodynamics. Others are able to tolerate the same medication doses as their younger counterparts.
3. Doses should be halved. Dose escalations should occur more cautiously.
4. Drug–drug and drug–disease interactions must be considered when new medications are added. Polypharmacy increases the risk of iatrogenic complications.
5. Drugs with sedating side effects should be used cautiously as this may increase falls. Tricyclic antidepressants can cause incontinence or retention of urine.
6. Nonpharmacologic methods should be encouraged as a means to decrease the risk of polypharmacy.
7. Other factors such as relational losses, loss of life roles, decrease socialization, increase in medical comorbidity, presence of other geriatric syndromes and changes in physical function need to be considered in the overall management of the patient.
8. Patients with dementia who report that they are in pain usually are.
9. The usual methods of assessment of pain severity would be applicable in patients with mild dementia.
10. Those who have severe dementia will need observation by caregivers for evidence of pain behaviors. Agitation and behavioral changes may be a sign of ongoing pain and an analgesic trial should be attempted.

Invasive Therapies

1. Invasive therapies may be required for poorly controlled cancer pain. In nonmalignant pain, the patient should be chosen with care; this should only take place in a multidisciplinary pain center.
2. Surgical procedures include spinal anterolateral tractomy, dorsal rhizotomy, and exploration of neuromas and nerve decompression as well as stimulation procedures such as in the periaqueductal gray matter.
3. Nerve lesioning is never indicated in nonmalignant pain.
4. Dorsal column stimulation is helpful in selected cases where other therapies have been tried and found to be inadequate. A full psychosocial assessment is mandatory before implementation in chronic nonmalignant pain.
5. Chemical sympathectomy is indicated in carefully chosen cases of CRPS-1 where other therapies have been unsuccessful. It should always be used with an active

physical rehabilitation program. Surgical sympathectomy is no longer indicated as a pain management strategy.

BIBLIOGRAPHY

Diagnostic and statistical manual of mental disorders, 4th ed. Washington, DC: American Psychiatric Association, 1994.

Loeser JD, Butler SH, Chapman CR, and Turk D, eds. *Bonica's management of pain.* Philadelphia: Lippincott Williams & Wilkins, 2001.

Main CJ, Spanswick CC. *Pain management: an interdisciplinary approach.* Edinburgh: Churchill Livingstone, 2000.

Mersky H, Bogduk N, eds. *Classification of chronic pain: task force on taxonomy—International Association for the Study of Pain.* Seattle, WA: IASP Press, 1994.

Passik SD, Portenoy RK. Substance abuse issues in palliative care. In: Berger A, Portenoy RK, Weissman D, eds. *Principles and practice of supportive oncology,* 2nd ed. Philadelphia: Lippincott–Raven Publishers, 1998:513–529.

Turk DC, Melzack R, eds. *Handbook of pain assessment.* New York: The Guilford Press, 2001.

11. HEADACHE AND FACIAL PAIN

Egilius L. H. Spierings

TENSION HEADACHE

BACKGROUND

1. Also known as muscle-contraction or tension-type headache.
2. In its episodic form (fewer than 15 d/mo), almost ubiquitously experienced with a lifetime prevalence of 69% in men and 88% in women.
3. Unless frequent, if not daily, unlikely to come to medical attention because the headaches are relieved abortively by nonprescription analgesics.
4. In susceptible individuals, may trigger migraine headache.

PATHOPHYSIOLOGY

Sustained contraction of the craniocervical muscles, caused by such trivial issues as stress, fatigue, and lack of sleep.

PROGNOSIS

Over time, due to a gradual increase in frequency and progressive earlier occurrence during the day, may develop into chronic tension headache. From there, due to the secondary development of migraine or migraine-like headaches, may develop into tension-vascular headache. The progression from intermittent to daily headaches takes, on average, a decade.

DIAGNOSIS

1. Mild or moderate headaches, intermittently occurring, usually coming on in the late afternoon, lasting for up to several hours.
2. Headaches generally bilateral and diffuse in location, located across the forehead or on top or in the back of the head.
3. Pain described as tightness or pressure and not associated with other symptoms, except sometimes for mild photophobia and/or phonophobia.
4. Headaches generally not associated with significant tightness of the neck and/or shoulder muscles, which is more common in migraine, especially when the headaches occur frequently.

TREATMENT

1. Although generally taken, use of analgesics abortively should be discouraged and use of muscle relaxants encouraged.
2. Use fast- and short-acting muscle relaxants abortively, such as
   a. Carisoprodol, 350 mg;
   b. Chlorzoxazone, 500 mg;
   c. Metaxalone, 800 mg; and
   d. Methocarbamol, 500 mg.
3. Encourage rest and relaxation along with medication for abortive therapy.
4. When preventive therapy is required, using a heating pad daily on the neck and shoulder muscles can be helpful. Otherwise, physical therapy of the neck, shoulder,

and upper-back muscles, with modalities such as heat, ultrasound, massage, stretching, myofascial release, and so forth.

5. Effective preventive medications are tricyclics, such as:
   a. Amitriptyline;
   b. Doxepin; and
   c. Imipramine.
6. Amitriptyline and doxepin are particularly helpful when there is also insomnia because the medications are sedating. Imipramine is less sedating and otherwise better tolerated. It causes less weight gain and has less anticholinergic side effects, including dry mouth and constipation.
7. A good starting dose is 25 mg at bedtime, after which the dose is gradually increased until some dryness of the mouth develops. The dose of a tricyclic usually required to achieve a beneficial effect in tension headache lies between 25 and 75 mg/d.

SINUS HEADACHE

BACKGROUND

1. Also known as sinus-vacuum headache or barosinusitis, not to be confused with acute bacterial sinusitis, characterized by yellow–green postnasal drip, bad smell or taste, and sometimes fever.
2. Prevalence unknown but probably the most common cause of facial pain and the second most common headache condition after tension headache.
3. Unless frequent, if not daily, unlikely to come to medical attention because the headaches are relieved abortively by nonprescription antihistamines and/or decongestants.
4. In susceptible individuals, may trigger migraine headache.

PATHOPHYSIOLOGY

1. Headache caused by underpressure in the sinuses due to obstruction of the orifices, in particular the ostiomeatal complexes (maxillary sinuses) and nasofrontal ducts (frontal sinuses).
2. Obstruction generally caused by swelling of the nasal mucosa, often on the basis of anatomically relatively narrow orifices, and involving all sinuses.
3. Sometimes, obstruction caused by a mucus plug and involving a single sinus, particularly the maxillary sinus, resulting in severe pain through the ipsilateral eye.

PROGNOSIS

Good if recognized and treated correctly; treatment sometimes requires surgery to relieve anatomic cause of orifice narrowing, for example, concha bullosa or Haller cell.

DIAGNOSIS

1. Headache located in the center of the forehead, bridge of the nose, and/or cheeks, generally described as pressure.
2. Associated with nasal congestion and/or postnasal drip.
3. Brought on by exposure to allergen or irritant, such as perfume or cigarette smoke, and also typically by a decrease in barometric pressure (oncoming rain or snow).

4. Sinus computed tomography (CT) scan with coronal cuts recommended when chronic bacterial sinusitis is suspected.

TREATMENT

1. Corticosteroid nasal spray used daily or as needed.
2. When allergy based, an antihistamine orally (cetirizine, fexofenadine, loratadine) or intranasally (azelastine), if necessary in combination with a mucolytic (guaifenesin) or leukotriene antagonist (montelukast, zafirlukast).

MIGRAINE HEADACHE

BACKGROUND

1. Most common cause of severe headache:
   a. One-year population prevalence of self-defined severe headache: 21%; incidence of severe/disabling headache: 1.3%/yr;
   b. One-year population prevalence of migraine as defined by the International Headache Society criteria: 12.6%; male-to-female ratio, 1 to 3.
2. When preceded by transient focal neurologic symptoms, known as classic migraine or migraine with aura; otherwise known as common migraine or migraine without aura.

PATHOPHYSIOLOGY

1. Headache is caused by arterial vasodilation in combination with neurogenic inflammation, probably in the extracranial circulation, preferentially involving the frontal branch of the superficial temporal artery, giving rise to the characteristically throbbing pain in the temple.
2. Associated autonomic and sensory symptoms are probably caused by activation of the sympathetic nervous system and ascending reticular arousal system, respectively, secondary to the pain of the headache.

PROGNOSIS

1. Often does not abate until age 50 or 60; in women, usually related to the cessation of menstruation, provided estrogen replacement therapy is *not* initiated.
2. May progress over time with a gradual increase in frequency of the migraine headaches and a progressive interposition of these headaches with tension headaches, ultimately resulting in tension-vascular headache (chronic/transformed migraine).

DIAGNOSIS

1. Recurring moderate or severe headaches, typically lasting for one half to several days, on average occurring once or twice a month.
2. The headaches often start between age 5 and 15, commonly with similar headaches occurring in first-degree relatives.
3. The headaches are generally of such intensity that they interfere with the ability to function physically and sometimes require bed rest. They are generally also of such intensity that they interfere with the functioning of other systems in the body, resulting in a plethora of associated symptoms.
4. Common associated symptoms of the migraine headache are:

a. Pallor of the face;
b. Coldness of the hands and feet;
c. Increased sensitivity to light, noise, and smell; and
d. Anorexia, nausea, vomiting, and diarrhea.
5. When brought on by stress, the headache typically comes afterwards; in women, migraine headaches usually occur in relation to the menstrual cycle:
   a. One or 2 days premenstrually;
   b. Mid-cycle at ovulation; and/or
   c. At the end of menstruation.
6. Other common triggers of migraine headache are:
   a. Vasodilators:
      1) Alcohol;
      2) Histamine (red wine); and
      3) Sodium nitrate (cured-meat products).
   b. Vasoconstrictors:
      1) Caffeine; and
      2) Sympathomimetic amines:
         a) Tyramine (red wine, aged cheese); and
         b) Phenylethylamine (dark chocolate).
   c. Food additives:
      1) Sodium nitrite;
      2) Monosodium glutamate (MSG); and
      3) Aspartame.

TREATMENT

1. Abortive therapy is *always* indicated because of the severe and disabling nature of the headaches; preventive therapy is only indicated when, despite effective abortive therapy, the headaches occur more often than three or four times a month.
2. The goal of abortive therapy is to provide *full* relief of headache and associated symptoms within 2 hours of initiation. Effective abortive therapy is important because of the pain and suffering migraine headaches entail and to prevent progression of the condition over time into chronic or transformed migraine.
3. As to the route of administration, abortive therapy should be directed to the intensity of the headache *at the time of therapy*. The reason for this is twofold:
   a. With increasing headache intensity, gastric emptying is impaired, delaying the absorption of oral medications; and
   b. Efficacy of therapy is determined by the speed of medication build-up in the system, with higher intensity headache requiring more effective therapy.
4. The triptans (selective serotonin 1B/D/F agonists) are first-line medications for the abortive therapy of migraine headache; seven are presently available but not all in every country:
   a. Almotriptan
   b. Eletriptan
   c. Frovatriptan
   d. Naratriptan
   e. Sumatriptan
   f. Zolmitriptan
5. All triptans are available in oral formulations; rizatriptan and zolmitriptan also as orally disintegrating tablets that dissolve in the mouth but are absorbed intestinally. Sumatriptan and zolmitriptan are available as nasal sprays as well and sumatriptan for subcutaneous (s.c.) injection, with an auto-injector.
6. The oral and orally disintegrating tablets are best administered at mild or mild-to-moderate headache intensity, to secure their absorption. They should be administered in their optimum doses, which should be repeated every 2 hours (for naratriptan every 4 hours), until the headache is *fully* relieved or the maximum daily dose is reached. The triptans should not be used within 24 hours of each other but if this is done, the maximum daily dose should not exceed that of one.

TABLE 11-1. ORAL TRIPTANS

Triptans	Tablet Sizes, mg	Optimum Doses, mg	Maximum Single Doses, mg	Maximum Daily Doses, mg
Almotriptan	6.25 and 12.5	12.5	12.5	25
Eletriptan	20 and 40	20	40	80
Frovatriptan	2.5	2.5	2.5	7.5
Naratriptan	1 and 2.5	2.5	2.5	5
Rizatriptan	5 and 10	10[a]	10[a]	30[a]
Sumatriptan	25, 50, and 100	50	100	200
Zolmitriptan	2.5 and 5	2.5	5	10

[a]In patients on propranolol 5 and 15 mg, respectively.

7. Table 11-1 presents the tablet sizes and optimum, maximum single, and maximum daily doses of the oral triptans.
8. Almotriptan, eletriptan, rizatriptan, sumatriptan, and zolmitriptan, in their optimum doses, have similar 2-hour efficacy rates. They also have similar recurrence rates of approximately one third, although almotriptan and eletriptan somewhat lower, which can, however, be reduced by two- to fourfold by pursuing therapy until headache is fully relieved, as opposed to leaving mild, residual headache behind.
9. Frovatriptan and naratriptan, in their optimum doses, due to a slower onset of action, have 2-hour efficacy rates that are approximately half that of the other triptans. However, they tend to be better tolerated, probably because of slower absorption, and have lower recurrence rates as a result of longer plasma-elimination half-lives.
10. The side effects of the triptans, when given orally, are generally mild and short lasting. Most common are numbness of the fingers and tightness of the throat; sometimes fatigue, lightheadedness, or nausea occurs. When a particular triptan cannot be tolerated or fails to provide relief, another should certainly be tried.
11. Although quite selective for the cranial circulation, the triptans are contraindicated in uncontrolled hypertension (HTN) and coronary artery disease. Rizatriptan, sumatriptan, and zolmitriptan are also contraindicated with the concomitant use of a monoamine-oxidase inhibitor. The concomitant use of propranolol requires a 50% reduction in rizatriptan dose because of interference with the breakdown of the triptan. Eletriptan should not be used within 72 hours of medications that are inhibitors of CYP3A4 activity (mycin antibiotics, antifungal and antiviral medications).
12. When oral medications fail to provide relief, usually impaired absorption is at fault. Rather than increasing the strength of the medication, it is generally more effective to alter the route of administration. Administration of a medication other than by mouth is also more effective once the headache has established itself, for example, when it is present on awakening in the morning or wakes the patient up out of sleep at night.
13. An effective nonoral route of administration of a medication is by nasal spray or rectal suppository.
   a. The nasal sprays that are available for the abortive therapy of migraine headache are:
      1) Sumatriptan (5 and 20 mg)
      2) Zolmitriptan (5 mg)
      3) Dihydroergotamine (2 mg)
   b. As rectal suppositories, the following medications can be used:
      1) Indomethacin (50 and 100 mg)
      2) Ergotamine with caffeine (Cafergot)
14. Dihydroergotamine and ergotamine are nonselective serotonin agonists, which means that they also interact with a number of other receptors. In this context, the

serotonin 2A and α-adrenergic receptors are particularly important, mediating coronary and peripheral vasoconstriction, respectively. Hence, they are also contraindicated, and more so than the triptans, in uncontrolled HTN and coronary artery disease.

15. The sumatriptan and zolmitriptan nasal sprays can, if necessary, be repeated after 2 hours, with a maximum of 40 and 10 mg/24 h, respectively. The sumatriptan nasal spray is used in the dose of 20 mg and the zolmitriptan nasal spray in that of 5 mg. The dihydroergotamine nasal spray is given only once in 24 hours, in a dose of four times 0.5 mg. Side effects of the nasal sprays are nasal congestion, nasal irritation, and a bad taste in the mouth.

16. The indomethacin suppository is given in a dose of 50 or 100 mg, if necessary, repeated after one half to 1 hour, with a maximum of 200 mg/24 h. Its most common side effect is orthostatic lightheadedness, due to a systemic vasodilator effect. The medication is contraindicated in peptic ulcer disease and bleeding disorders.

17. The Cafergot suppository contains 2 mg ergotamine in combination with 100 mg caffeine to improve its absorption. Nausea and vomiting are its most common side effects and, therefore, it is important to administer the medication with care. Patients are advised to take only one fourth or one third of a suppository at a time and repeat it, if necessary, every 30 minutes to 1 hour, with a maximum of two suppositories a day.

18. Injection is another route through which a medication can be administered for the abortive therapy of migraine headache. The two medications that are available for parenteral administration are:
    a. Dihydroergotamine (1 mg/mL)
    b. Sumatriptan (6 mg)

19. The dose of dihydroergotamine is 1 mg, which can be given by the s.c., intramuscular (IM), or intravenous (IV) route. It should *always* be given after an antinausea medication is administered, for example, 10 mg metoclopramide IM or IV, to prevent the occurrence or worsening of nausea and vomiting.

20. Sumatriptan is available with an auto-injector for easy self-administration by the patient. The injection is given s.c. in a dose of 6 mg, which can be repeated, if necessary, after 1 hour. However, it has been shown that the repeated injection does *not* increase the efficacy of the medication. Also, administration of sumatriptan by injection during the aura has been shown *not* to affect the ensuing headache. However, administration of the medication during the aura is safe, without effect on the intensity or duration of the aura symptoms. The most common side effects of the sumatriptan injection are a hot, tight, or tingling sensation, generally in the upper chest, anterior neck, and face, and lightheadedness.

21. When migraine headaches occur frequently (e.g., more than three or four times a month), when the headaches are intense or prolonged, and/or when abortive therapy is ineffective, preventive therapy is indicated.

22. The medications that, in randomized, double-blind, placebo-controlled studies, have been shown to be effective in migraine prevention are:
    a. Beta-blockers:
       1) Atenolol
       2) Bisoprolol
       3) Metoprolol
       4) Nadolol
       5) Propranolol
       6) Timolol
    b. Tricyclics:
       1) Amitriptyline
       2) Pizotifen
    c. Calcium-entry blockers:
       1) Flunarizine
       2) Verapamil
    d. Anticonvulsants:
       1) Divalproex sodium
       2) Topiramate

23. The beta-blockers effective in migraine prevention are those that lack partial agonist or intrinsic sympathomimetic activity. They increase peripheral vascular resistance by increasing blood vessel tone, thereby mitigating the process of migrainous vasodilation.

24. The tricyclics, amitriptyline and pizotifen, potentiate the effects of serotonin through pre- and postsynaptic mechanisms, respectively. In the central nervous system, serotonin inhibits the transmission of pain signals, resulting in an increase in pain threshold.

25. The calcium-entry blockers have also been shown to increase pain threshold, an effect that has been attributed to impairment of synaptic transmission, a calcium-dependent process. It is possible that they also interfere with the mechanism of neurogenic inflammation, which is calcium-dependent as well.

26. The mechanism of action of divalproex sodium and topiramate in migraine prevention may also be connected to inhibition of central pain transmission but through potentiating the γ-aminobutyric acid–ergic (GABA-ergic) inhibitory system.

27. The choice of preventive medication depends on the features of the headaches but also on the concomitant presence of other conditions.

28. When the frequency of the headaches is relatively low but the intensity high, the beta-blockers are generally most effective. Of those, propranolol tends to have most side effects, in particular fatigue, depression, insomnia, and impotence. These side effects can also occur with the other beta-blockers but do so generally less often.

29. When a particular medication out of the group of beta-blockers fails to provide relief or cannot be tolerated, another should certainly be tried. The starting dose should be low and should be gradually increased with intervals of at least 1 month. At the same time, side effects, in particular fatigue, as well as blood pressure (BP) and heart rate should be monitored. Fatigue can cause an increase in headache frequency, which can be addressed by lowering the dose.

30. The beta-blockers are contraindicated in sinus bradycardia, atrioventricular block, congestive heart failure, obstructive pulmonary disease (asthma), and diabetes mellitus.

31. When the headaches occur relatively frequently but are not very intense, amitriptyline and pizotifen are probably most effective, especially when the patient also experiences insomnia. The medications are long acting and can be taken once daily, preferably at bedtime, because of sedation. Patients who do not have insomnia tend not to tolerate them well because of drowsiness on awakening in the morning. In cases like this, a good alternative is flunarizine, which can also be given once daily at bedtime.

32. Apart from sedation, amitriptyline can cause dry mouth, constipation, and weight gain; pizotifen can cause weight gain and flunarizine occasionally causes depression. Amitriptyline is contraindicated in glaucoma, prostate hypertrophy, epilepsy, and cardiac disease; flunarizine and pizotifen do not have contraindications.

33. When the migraine headaches occur mostly during the night and wake the patient up out of sleep (nocturnal migraine), verapamil is the medication of choice. In its sustained-release form, it can be given twice daily; its most common side effects are constipation and hypotension. Verapamil is contraindicated in atrioventricular block and sick sinus syndrome because it slows down atrioventricular conduction.

34. The anticonvulsants, divalproex sodium and topiramate, are often not well tolerated. Divalproex sodium can cause nausea, tremor, weight gain, and hair loss and topiramate sedation, cognitive dysfunction, paresthesias, weight loss, and kidney stones. Divalproex sodium is contraindicated in liver disease or when liver function is abnormal.

35. It should always be attempted to treat the condition with a single medication first. However, if necessary, another medication can be added and a good combination is that of a beta-blocker with amitriptyline or pizotifen. Combinations that should

be used with care are those of a beta-blocker with verapamil (bradycardia) or flunarizine (depression).
36. The medications should be prescribed for at least 6 months, after which the dose is gradually decreased and the medication, if possible, discontinued.

MIGRAINE WITH AURA

BACKGROUND

1. Also known as classic migraine: headache preceded by transient focal neurologic symptoms, generally referred to as aura symptoms.
2. When the aura symptoms occur by themselves, not followed by headache, the condition is called isolated migraine aura or migraine aura without headache. In the older patient, this condition is an important differential diagnostic consideration in transient ischemic attack (TIA).
3. Occurrence in the general population:
   a. Lifetime prevalence: 5%; male-to-female ratio: 1 to 2;
   b. One-year prevalence: 3%; male-to-female ratio: 3 to 4.

PATHOPHYSIOLOGY

1. The aura symptoms are probably caused by a neurophysiologic phenomenon known as Leão spreading cortical depression, a wave of neuronal excitation that travels over the cerebral cortex at a slow rate and is followed by prolonged depression of cortical neuronal activity.
2. In the *sequential* concept of the pathogenesis of the migraine attack, the aura mechanism is considered to be the *cause* of the headache; in the *parallel* concept, the mechanisms of the migraine aura and headache are considered occurring parallel to each other, driven by the "migraine process."

PROGNOSIS

1. The occurrence of migraine aura symptoms, whether alone or followed by headache, does *not* represent a risk factor for stroke. Migraine in general does present such a risk factor but only of a minor nature and negligible from a clinical perspective. The condition is, therefore, *not* a contraindication for the use of oral contraceptives.
2. Migraine in general is rarely complicated by stroke (complicated migraine), usually consisting of ischemic infarction of an occipital lobe, resulting in homonymous hemianopia.

DIAGNOSIS

1. The migraine aura symptoms are invariably sensory in nature, usually visual but sometimes somatosensory.
2. The typical presentation of the visual migraine aura is the scintillating scotoma, also known as teichopsia or fortification spectra. Digitolingual paresthesias, also called cheiro-oral syndrome, represent the typical presentation of the somatosensory aura.
3. The aura symptoms usually last approximately 20 minutes, with a range from 10 to 30 minutes. When they last longer than 60 minutes, they are referred to

as prolonged aura, and when they last longer than 24 hours, they are called migraine aura status.

4. The scintillating scotoma usually begins near the center of vision as a twinkling star, which develops into a circle of bright and sometimes colorful, flickering zigzag lines. The circle opens up on the inside to form a semicircle or horseshoe, which further expands into the periphery of one visual field or the other. On the inside of the visual disturbance, a band of dimness follows in the wake of the crescent of flickering zigzag lines. The disturbance of vision ultimately disappears as it fades away in, or moves outside of, the visual field in which it developed.

5. The digitolingual paresthesias typically start in the fingers of one hand, extending upward into the arm, and, at a certain point, also involving the nose/mouth area on the same side. The progression of the somatosensory disturbance, similar to that of the scintillating scotoma, is slow and usually takes 10 to 30 minutes.

6. A progressing somatosensory disturbance similar to the digitolingual paresthesias of migraine can occur with stroke, although this is rare. What differentiates one from the other is the resolution of the disturbed sensation, to which the first–last rule applies: in migraine, what is involved first, resolves first, whereas in stroke, what is involved first resolves last.

7. When the aura symptoms are fixed in their lateralization, neurologic illness should be suspected, especially when occurring with contralateral headache. Occipital arteriovenous malformation is a notorious cause of symptomatic migraine with aura.

TREATMENT

1. Migraine with aura is treated as migraine in general, except that in its preventive therapy beta-blockers are avoided because they may aggravate the neurologic symptoms.

2. There is no specific therapy for the aura symptoms although re-breathing in a paper bag has been claimed helpful. With frequently occurring aura symptoms, with or without headache, preventive therapy with aspirin and/or a calcium-entry blocker can be considered.

NOCTURNAL MIGRAINE

BACKGROUND

Migraine variant in which the headaches develop predominantly at night.

PATHOPHYSIOLOGY

1. Headache is caused by arterial vasodilation in combination with neurogenic inflammation, probably in the extracranial circulation, preferentially involving the frontal branch of the superficial temporal artery, giving rise to the characteristically throbbing pain in the temple.

2. Associated autonomic and sensory symptoms are probably caused by activation of the sympathetic nervous system and ascending reticular arousal system, respectively, secondary to the pain of the headache.

PROGNOSIS

Headaches often do not respond to regular abortive and preventive antimigraine therapy. Therefore, recognition of this migraine variant is important because therapy can be very effective.

DIAGNOSIS

1. Headaches wake the patient up out of sleep at night, generally between 4 and 6 AM, or are present severely on awakening in the morning.
2. The patient tends to be older, that is, between age 40 and 60, and often has migraine headaches frequently, that is, several times per week.

TREATMENT

1. Abortive therapy is generally most effective with the sumatriptan 6-mg s.c. injection, which is available with an auto-injector for easy self-administration by the patient.
2. Preventive therapy is generally most effective with a calcium-entry blocker:
   a. Verapamil, 120 to 240 mg sustained-release (SR) twice daily; or
   b. Diltiazem, 120 or 240 mg extended release twice daily.

CLUSTER HEADACHE

BACKGROUND

1. Also known as migrainous neuralgia.
2. Population prevalence: 0.07%; male-to-female ratio: 14 to 1.

PATHOPHYSIOLOGY

1. Headache is caused by arterial vasodilation in combination with neurogenic inflammation, probably in the extracranial circulation, preferentially involving the ophthalmic artery, giving rise to the characteristically sharp, steady pain in and behind the eye.
2. Autonomic symptoms are probably caused by a localized shift in autonomic balance in favor of the parasympathetic and to the detriment of the sympathetic system, suggesting hypothalamic involvement.

PROGNOSIS

The episodic form may change into the chronic form and vice versa. The condition may start any time; however, this is usually in adulthood, and it may cease any time.

DIAGNOSIS

1. Unilateral headaches with fixed lateralization to the left or right, generally located in and behind the eye and described as sharp, steady in nature.
2. Headaches last for 30 to 120 minutes and occur daily or almost daily, once or twice per 24 hours, preferentially at night, often waking the patient up out of sleep between midnight and 2 AM.
3. Headaches can be associated with local autonomic symptoms involving the affected eye and/or ipsilateral nostril, such as tearing, reddening, congestion, and running. However, local autonomic symptoms are neither pathognomonic for the condition nor necessary for the diagnosis.
4. Headaches often associated with agitation, leading to rocking, pacing, head banging, and so forth.

TABLE 11-2. EFFICACY OF PREVENTIVE MEDICATIONS IN EPISODIC AND CHRONIC CLUSTER HEADACHE

Medications	Episodic Cluster Headache, %	Chronic Cluster Headache, %
Verapamil	73	60
Lithium	—	87
Prednisone	77	40

5. Headaches occur in episodes with remissions (85%) or chronically (15%). The chronic form can be primary (chronic from onset) or secondary (initially episodic).

TREATMENT

1. Common triggers of individual headaches are use of alcohol and daytime napping, activities that should be avoided when the condition is active.
2. Abortive therapy is most effective with:
   a. Sumatriptan, 6-mg s.c. injection;
   b. Oxygen, 100%, inhaled at a rate of 8 to 10 L/min; and
   c. Ergotamine, 2 mg sublingually.
3. Preventive therapy is most effective with:
   a. Verapamil;
   b. Prednisone; and
   c. Lithium.
4. Table 11-2 gives the efficacy of the preventive medications in episodic and chronic cluster headache, defined as more than 75% reduction in headache frequency.
5. If immediate headache prevention is required, a prednisone course generally provides relief within 24 to 48 hours. The starting dose is 60 mg/d, which should be given for 3 to 5 days, followed by a taper of 5 mg/d every 2 days.
6. Verapamil should be started along with the prednisone to prevent further occurrence of the headaches during and after the prednisone taper. The best results are obtained with the SR tablet, which should be given every 12 hours. The starting dosage is 120 mg SR twice daily, with an increase of 120 mg SR/d/wk. The result of the dose increase is usually evident in 3 to 5 days.
7. An electrocardiogram (ECG) to determine atrioventricular conduction should follow, within days, every dose increase beyond 480 mg SR/d. Prior to increasing the dose beyond 480 mg SR/d, an echocardiogram should be performed to rule out heart muscle disease.
8. The daily dose of SR verapamil required to obtain relief in episodic cluster headache ranges from 240 to 600 mg and from 240 to 960 mg in chronic cluster headache. If no relief is obtained at all, the diagnosis should be reconsidered.
9. If full relief of headaches cannot be obtained with verapamil or the required dose cannot be tolerated because of hypotension or constipation, lithium should be added to the maximum tolerated dose. A small dose of lithium in addition to the verapamil often suffices, that is, 150 to 300 mg twice daily.
10. Lithium used alone is particularly effective in chronic cluster headache but then doses of 900 to 1,200 mg/d are generally required.
11. Prednisone is contraindicated in HTN, diabetes mellitus, infectious illness, peptic ulcer disease, and diverticulosis. Its most common side effects are nausea, epigastric pain, fluid retention, agitation, and insomnia. Verapamil is contraindicated in atrioventricular block and sick sinus syndrome; constipation and hypotension are its most common side effects.
12. Lithium is contraindicated in electrolyte imbalance and when sodium restriction or diuretic therapy is required. Its most common side effects are nausea, tremor, and diarrhea. The serum level should be kept below 1.5 mEq/L; it should be determined regularly along with the electrolytes and kidney and thyroid functions. Symptoms of lithium toxicity range from tremor to convulsions.

EXERTIONAL HEADACHE

BACKGROUND

1. Headache brought on by exertion can be short- (seconds to minutes) or long-lasting (hours to days).
2. Long-lasting exertional headache resembles migraine headache in its presentation and is probably a variant thereof. It can occur by itself, especially in the younger patient, but can also be part of a migraine condition, with other triggers as well.
3. Short-lasting exertional headache is also known as cough headache, although coughing is generally not the only trigger; other triggers are sneezing, straining, and bending over. It may occur in the context of migraine or cluster headache but can also follow an upper or lower respiratory infection, triggered by repeated coughing or sneezing.

PATHOPHYSIOLOGY

1. Probably similar to migraine headache where it concerns long-lasting exertional headache, that is, caused by arterial vasodilation in combination with neurogenic inflammation in the extracranial circulation.
2. The short-lasting exertional headache is probably caused by perivascular inflammation, neurogenic in origin from vasodilation or vasodistention, involving intracranial venous structures (upper or lower respiratory infection) or extracranial arteries (migraine or cluster headache).

PROGNOSIS

1. Short-lasting exertional headache is generally limited in its occurrence and improves over time, especially when resulting from an (upper or lower respiratory) infection.
2. Long-lasting exertional headache in the younger patient may develop into a regular migraine condition in adulthood. When the headache occurs as part of a migraine condition, it often improves with effective preventive migraine therapy, especially when a beta-blocker or calcium-entry blocker is used.

DIAGNOSIS

Evident from the history; with short-lasting exertional headache, if etiology unclear, a posterior fossa lesion should be excluded with appropriate neuroimaging.

TREATMENT

1. Antiinflammatory medications are generally most effective:
   a. Short-lasting exertional headache can often be effectively relieved by a short course of prednisone, for example, 60 mg/d for 2 days, 40 mg/d for 2 days, and 20 mg/d for 2 days.
   b. Long-lasting exertional headache can often be prevented by taking a nonsteroidal antiinflammatory medication 30 minutes to 1 hour prior to the exertion (intercourse), for example, 50 mg indomethacin.
2. For long-term prevention of exertional headache, the beta-blockers and calcium-entry blockers used for migraine prevention can be used.

HYPNIC HEADACHE

BACKGROUND

Rare condition, possibly a variant of cluster headache (? bilateral cluster headache).

PATHOPHYSIOLOGY

Unknown, although possibly similar to cluster headache.

PROGNOSIS

Supposedly good.

DIAGNOSIS

Bilateral or global headaches waking the patient up out of sleep at night and lasting for 30 to 60 minutes.

TREATMENT

Lithium, 300 to 600 mg at bedtime.

PAROXYSMAL HEMICRANIA

BACKGROUND

1. Variant of cluster headache, identical in its presentation except for a higher frequency of the attacks and a shorter duration. However, it is treated differently, preferentially preventively with indomethacin, relieving the condition to the full extent.
2. Like cluster headache, it comes in an episodic and a chronic form.

PATHOPHYSIOLOGY

Unknown, although possibly similar to cluster headache.

PROGNOSIS

1. The condition can generally be very well controlled preventively. However, continuation of therapy may be required although, sometimes, at a lower dose than is initially necessary to relieve the headaches.
2. The long-term therapy with indomethacin needs to be monitored from a gastric as well as renal perspective, the former includes testing for the development of anemia (hemoglobin, ferritin).

DIAGNOSIS

1. Unilateral headaches with fixed lateralization to the left or right, generally located in and behind the eye and described as sharp, steady in nature.
2. Headaches last for 10 to 30 minutes and occur daily or almost daily, five to 15 times/24 h, also at night waking the patient up out of sleep.
3. Headaches can be associated with local autonomic symptoms involving the affected eye and/or ipsilateral nostril, such as tearing, reddening, congestion, and running. However, local autonomic symptoms are neither pathognomonic for the condition nor necessary for the diagnosis.
4. Headaches occur in episodes with remissions or chronically.

TREATMENT

1. For abortive therapy, the headaches are generally too short in duration.
2. For preventive therapy, indomethacin 25 to 50 mg four times daily, to be taken with meals and at bedtime with food as well to protect the stomach. If indomethacin cannot be tolerated or is contraindicated, the condition should be treated preventively like cluster headache.

STABBING HEADACHE

BACKGROUND

Also known as jabs-and-jolts or ice-pick headache, often occurring in conjunction with migraine or cluster headache. When occurring by themselves, the condition is referred to as jabs-and-jolts syndrome, which comes in an episodic and a chronic form.

PATHOPHYSIOLOGY

Unknown but probably vascular.

PROGNOSIS

Stabbing headaches are medically benign; when they occur in conjunction with another headache condition, they often improve with effective therapy of the condition associated with them; otherwise, they generally respond well to preventive therapy with a nonsteroidal antiinflammatory medication.

DIAGNOSIS

Short-lasting stabbing pains in the head or face; when occurring in the face, they need to be differentiated from trigeminal neuralgia.

TREATMENT

1. When the stabbing headaches occur sporadically, no therapy is required except for reassurance that the headaches are *not* indicative of serious neurologic illness.
2. When they occur frequently, therapy is generally most effective with daily intake of a nonsteroidal antiinflammatory medication, which can be a so-called selective cox-2 inhibitor. Particularly effective is indomethacin, 25 to 50 mg four times

daily, to be taken with meals and at bedtime with food as well to protect the stomach.

TRIGEMINAL NEURALGIA

BACKGROUND

Also known as tic douloureux; incidence: 4/100,000 population per year.

PATHOPHYSIOLOGY

1. In the elderly, it is probably due to compression of the trigeminal ganglion by a tortuous atherosclerotic artery, causing focal demyelination. In multiple sclerosis, it is probably caused by a demyelinating plaque at the trigeminal root entry zone.
2. Demyelination causes axonal hyperexcitability and damaged axons near each other become susceptible to chemical coupling. Synchronous discharge of hyperexcitable axons, activated by light mechanical stimulation and recruiting adjacent pain fibers, causes intense pain.

PROGNOSIS

Most patients can be treated effectively medically, especially early in the course of illness, also due to a tendency to spontaneous remission. If medical therapy is ineffective or poorly tolerated, surgery should be considered, especially late in the course of illness when spontaneous remission is less likely.

DIAGNOSIS

1. Short-lasting pains or volleys of such pains in one side of the face or mouth, restricted to one or more divisions of the trigeminal nerve, most often the maxillary division.
2. Trigger sites on the face, especially in the nasolabial fold, or in the mouth, which result in pain when stimulated. Mild numbness in the painful area may be present on neurologic examination.
3. Cranial magnetic resonance imaging (MRI) may reveal vascular compression of the trigeminal ganglion.

TREATMENT

1. Table 11-3 shows the medications that are used to treat trigeminal neuralgia.
2. Surgical therapeutic options are:
   a. Radiofrequency thermocoagulation;
   b. Microvascular decompression; and
   c. Stereotactic radiosurgery.

CHRONIC TENSION HEADACHE

BACKGROUND

1. Also known as chronic muscle-contraction or tension-type headache and a subcategory of chronic daily headache.

TABLE 11-3. MEDICATIONS USED TO TREAT TRIGEMINAL NEURALGIA

Medications	Start Doses	Maintenance Doses	Pretreatment Precautions	Important Side Effects
Carbamazepine	300 mg/d	1,500–2,000 mg/d	Hematology, electrolytes, ECG	Sedation, hyponatremia, leukopenia
Phenytoin	300 mg/d	300–400 mg/d	Hematology, ECG	Hirsutism, gingival hyperthrophy
Baclofen	15 mg/d	80 mg/d	None	Sedation
Lamotrigine	25 mg/d	300–600 mg/d	Kidney and liver function	Rash
Gabapentin	900 mg/d	2,400–3,600 mg/d	Kidney function	Sedation
Clonazepam	1.5 mg/d	6–8 mg/d	None	Sedation
Sodium valproate	500 mg/d	1,500–2,000 mg/d	Hematology, liver function	Weight gain, hair loss, nausea

ECG, electrocardiogram.

2. One-year prevalence (headache more than 15 d/mo) of 3%, accounting for half of daily headache in the general population.

PATHOPHYSIOLOGY

Sustained contraction of the craniocervical muscles, more likely caused by chronic fatigue than by chronic stress, anxiety, or depression.

PROGNOSIS

Over time, due to the secondary development of migraine or migraine-like headaches, may develop into tension-vascular headache (chronic tension headache coexistent with migraine headache).

DIAGNOSIS

1. Daily or almost-daily headaches, present all or most of the day; however, not in an intensity that they interfere with physical functioning and generally not associated with any other symptoms, except sometimes for mild photophobia and/or phonophobia.
2. The headaches may have been daily or almost daily from their onset (primary) or may have gradually become daily out of episodic tension headache, over time, with an increase in frequency and a progressive earlier occurrence during the day (secondary).
3. Headaches generally bilateral and diffuse in location, located across the forehead, on top or in the back of the head, described as tightness or pressure, and not associated with other symptoms, except sometimes for mild photophobia and/or phonophobia.
4. Headaches generally not associated with significant tightness of the neck and/or shoulder muscles, which is more common in migraine, especially when the headaches occur frequently.

TREATMENT

1. Although generally taken, use of analgesics abortively should be discouraged and use of muscle relaxants encouraged.
2. Use fast- and short-acting muscle relaxants abortively, such as:
   a. Carisoprodol, 350 mg;
   b. Chlorzoxazone, 500 mg;
   c. Metaxalone, 800 mg; and
   d. Methocarbamol, 500 mg.
3. Encourage rest and relaxation along with medication for abortive therapy.
4. For preventive therapy, using a heating pad daily on the neck and shoulder muscles can be helpful. Otherwise, physical therapy of the neck, shoulder, and upper-back muscles, with modalities such as heat, ultrasound, massage, stretching, myofascial release, and so forth.
5. Effective preventive medications are tricyclics, such as:
   a. Amitriptyline;
   b. Doxepin; and
   c. Imipramine.
6. Amitriptyline and doxepin are particularly helpful when there is also insomnia because the medications are sedating. Imipramine is less sedating and also otherwise better tolerated. It causes less weight gain and has less anticholinergic side effects, including dry mouth and constipation.
7. A good starting dose is 25 mg at bedtime, after which the dose is gradually increased until some dryness of the mouth develops. The dose of a tricyclic usually required to achieve a beneficial effect in tension headache lies between 25 and 75 mg/d.

TENSION-VASCULAR HEADACHE

BACKGROUND

1. Also know as chronic tension(-type) headache coexistent with migraine headache; it is a subcategory of chronic daily headache.
2. Accounts for half of daily headache in the general population and more than 90% of chronic daily headache in medical practice.
3. When developed out of (episodic) migraine, it is also know as chronic or transformed migraine.

PATHOPHYSIOLOGY

Sustained contraction of the craniocervical muscles with dilation and inflammation of extracranial arteries.

PROGNOSIS

A prospective diary study of almost 200 patients with chronic daily headache attending a headache practice showed 40% to improve 50% or more in terms of headache d/mo over the first 6 months of treatment The outcome was not dependent on gender, age at first consultation, or abrupt *versus* gradual onset of the daily headaches.

DIAGNOSIS

1. Daily headaches with severe migraine or migraine-like headaches, occurring 10 d/mo or less in approximately 60% of patients and more than 15 d/mo in approximately 25%.
2. In approximately 80%, the headaches are present on awakening or come on in the course of the morning. In approximately 25%, they are worst in the afternoon or evening. In approximately one third, the headaches wake the patients up out of sleep at night at least once per week.
3. The daily headaches are, at least twice per week, associated with nausea in approximately one third and with vomiting in approximately 10%. In approximately 50%, they are unilateral in location, often fixed to the right or left. The headaches are made worse particularly by physical activity, bending over, stress or tension, and menstruation.
4. The severe headaches have the same lateralization pattern as the daily headaches. They are associated, at least twice per month, with nausea in approximately 75% and with vomiting in approximately 40%.

TREATMENT

1. With frequent, if not daily, headache occurrence, the issue of overuse of vasoconstrictors, defined as intake that contributes to headache occurrence, needs to be addressed first.
2. Vasoconstrictors contribute to headache occurrence when they are taken at time intervals shorter than their duration of action. This allows the medications to build up in the system and to bring on headache whenever their effects wear off, a phenomenon known as rebound.
3. Caffeine is the most commonly involved vasoconstrictor in rebound headache. It remains in the system for up to 2 or 3 days and should not be used more often than 2 or 3 d/wk. A higher frequency of intake can be allowed for the shorter acting triptans, which have plasma-elimination half-lives of 2 to 4 hours. A lower frequency of intake has to be considered for the ergots, ergotamine and dihydroergotamine, because they induce vasoconstriction for 3 to 5 days.

4. Suspicion of rebound headache is based not only on the frequency of vasoconstrictor intake but also on *increasing* medication use over time, with *decreasing* efficacy. However, proof can only be obtained retrospectively, after withdrawal has been accomplished and headache occurrence is decreased.

5. Vasoconstrictor withdrawal is best accomplished abruptly; whether that is possible also depends on the kind and quantity of the medications taken along with the vasoconstrictors. When significant amounts of barbiturate-containing or opioid medications are used, withdrawal may require hospitalization for close monitoring of withdrawal symptoms and IV administration of alternative medications.

6. The withdrawal of a significant quantity of barbiturate-containing medication also requires a barbiturate taper to prevent seizure. The withdrawal of a significant amount of opioid medication requires expertise in addiction medicine and may have to be accomplished in a detoxification center. Otherwise, withdrawal from vasoconstrictors can generally be performed on an outpatient basis and several protocols have been developed to assist the patient with the withdrawal.

7. An outpatient protocol that I advocate makes use of a 3- or 6-day course of prednisone: 15 mg four times a day for 1 or 2 days, 10 mg four times a day for 1 or 2 days, and 5 mg four times a day for 1 or 2 days. If the patient exhibits prominent muscular symptoms, which is often the case, diazepam is added in a dosage of 2 to 5 mg four times a day to help to relax the muscles.

8. For patients whose outpatient attempt at withdrawal is unsuccessful because of inability to tolerate the withdrawal headache and/or accompanying nausea or vomiting and are admitted to the hospital, a similar protocol can be used. However, here metoclopramide is added as an antinausea medication, given IV in a dosage of 10 mg four times a day. It is important to start the metoclopramide immediately, that is, before the patient becomes sick, because once vomiting has developed, it is difficult to control even with IV administration of the medication. Instead of prednisone orally, dexamethasone can be given IV in a dosage of 4 mg four times per day, for several days. The diazepam can then be given every 6 hours but only as needed for severe headache and can be given IV. An alternative to diazepam IV is lorazepam IM in a dosage of 1 or 2 mg as needed every 6 hours.

9. For the daily headaches, the patients are allowed to use fast- but short-acting muscle relaxants, such as carisoprodol, chlorzoxazone, metaxalone, and methocarbamol. For the severe headaches, promethazine 50-mg suppositories can be helpful for the pain and accompanying nausea or vomiting. Once the headaches have become intermittent, effective abortive therapy should be provided for the severe headaches, preferably using specific antimigraine medications. It is important that this therapy is *consistently* effective, allowing the patient to wait until the pain is severe in intensity. This is the only way that patients can be prevented from falling back over time into a pattern of frequent vasoconstrictor intake.

10. With regard to preventive pharmacologic therapy, a particularly useful combination for patients with frequent *and* severe headaches is that of a tricyclic and a beta-blocker. Medications out of these two groups that have been demonstrated to be effective in the preventive therapy of tension or migraine headache should be given preference.

11. For those patients who continue to have frequent and severe headaches, despite being off vasoconstrictors and despite efforts at preventive therapy, there may be an indication for the use of long-acting formulations of opioids to relieve the pain and allow them to function more or less normally. The opioids that are available in long-acting formulations are:
    a. Fentanyl;
    b. Morphine sulfate; and
    c. Oxycodone.

12. The long-acting formulations of these opioids, however, generally work for a shorter period than the manufacturers indicate. The dose of the medications should be gradually increased until satisfactory pain control is achieved and the patient is back to a relatively normal level of functioning. Constipation is the most

common side effect of opioids and can often be effectively addressed with docusate, a stool softener, and/or magnesium.

POSTTRAUMATIC HEADACHE

BACKGROUND

1. Incidence of head injuries: approximately 200/100,000 population per year, predominantly caused by traffic collisions and, to a lesser extent, by falls and assaults.
2. Approximately one third of patients report persistent headaches 6 months after the head injury and approximately 25% after 1 year; approximately one third of patients are unable to work or go to school.

PATHOPHYSIOLOGY

1. The condition is related to neck injury rather than to head injury; in fact, it is inversely related to the intensity of the head injury, if present. Consequently, it is more likely associated with abnormalities on cervical radiography than on cranial CT scanning.
2. The neck injuries most likely to cause the condition are forceful forward and sidewise flexion.
3. Forceful forward flexion can be due to flexion injury (backward fall, hit in the back of the head) or extension–flexion injury (whiplash). It can be symmetric or asymmetric (hit in a side of the back of the head, head rotated at the time of injury).
4. Forceful sidewise flexion can be due to flexion injury (sidewise fall, hit in a side of the head) or flexion–flexion injury (sidewise whiplash injury).
5. Forceful flexion injury of the neck, forward or sidewise, causes acute muscle, ligament, and facet strain, as well as damage to the brain from forceful movement within the skull, causing axonal shearing.

PROGNOSIS

1. Settlement of litigation is associated with improvement of headaches in 8%, worsening in 8%, and no change in 84%.
2. Pharmacologic therapy with preventive antiheadache medications improves the condition in approximately two thirds of patients.

DIAGNOSIS

1. Headache frequency is monthly in 5%, weekly in 27%, and daily in 68%, with severe headaches occurring monthly in 39%, weekly in 32%, and daily in 29%.
2. The headaches are most commonly diagnosed as tension (36%) or tension-vascular (21%); less commonly, they resemble migraine (14%) or cluster headache (7%).
3. The condition is associated with insomnia in 76%, weight gain in 48% (decreased physical activity), and depression in 22%.

TREATMENT

Therapy depends on the actual headache presentation: chronic tension headache, tension-vascular headache, migraine headache, or cluster headache.

HEMICRANIA CONTINUA

BACKGROUND

Rare condition of daily continuous headache, unilateral in location and with fixed lateralization, fully relieved by preventive therapy with indomethacin.

PATHOPHYSIOLOGY

Unknown.

PROGNOSIS

1. Condition can generally be very well controlled preventively. However, continuation of therapy may be required although, sometimes, at a lower dose than is initially necessary to relieve the headache.
2. The long-term therapy with indomethacin needs to be monitored from a gastric as well as renal perspective, the former includes testing for development of anemia (hemoglobin, ferritin).

DIAGNOSIS

1. Continuous unilateral headache with fixed lateralization to the left or right.
2. Headache is relatively stable in intensity but dramatically relieved by nonsteroidal antiinflammatory medications used abortively, particularly aspirin.
3. Local autonomic symptoms involving the affected eye and/or ipsilateral nostril, such as tearing, reddening, congestion, and running, may be present but are *not* required for the diagnosis.

TREATMENT

1. Preventive therapy with indomethacin 25 to 50 mg, four times daily, to be taken with meals and at bedtime with food as well, relieves headache to the full extent.
2. Other nonsteroidal antiinflammatory medications used preventively can be effective as well but generally to a lesser extent.

HYPERTENSIVE HEADACHE

BACKGROUND

1. Headache and HTN are not uncommonly associated with each other; therefore, determination of BP is indispensable in the evaluation of the patient with headache.
2. HTN can cause headache by itself but can also aggravate a pre-existing headache condition, such as migraine.

PATHOPHYSIOLOGY

1. Acute hypertensive headache results from an abrupt increase in BP that remains within the range of cerebral autoregulation. As a result, neurologic functioning is

intact but the increased resistance created by the constricted small arteries and arterioles increases the transmural pressure in the larger cerebral arteries, which are sensitive to pain. These are the arteries at the base of the brain, mostly located in the posterior fossa, innervated by the cervical nerve roots and referring pain to the back of the head and neck.

2. Chronic hypertensive headache originates from the decrease in BP that occurs overnight, resulting in compensatory vasodilation. The headache abates as soon as the patient arises because the erect position increases the BP and causes compensatory constriction of the dilated blood vessels.

3. In hypertensive encephalopathy, the abrupt increase in BP exceeds the range of cerebral autoregulation. As a result, the tight endothelial junctions that constitute the blood–brain barrier are disrupted, allowing extravasation of plasma and erythrocytes. The resulting edema and petechiae disturb brain function and neurologic symptoms, often seizure, ensue.

PROGNOSIS

Good with effective BP control.

DIAGNOSIS

1. Four conditions involving headache and HTN can be distinguished:
   a. Acute hypertensive headache,
   b. Chronic hypertensive headache,
   c. Malignant HTN, and
   d. Hypertensive encephalopathy.
2. Of these conditions, the one that is not necessarily associated with headache and, in fact, often is not, is malignant HTN, due to the right shift in cerebral autoregulation that occurs with chronically elevated BP.
3. Acute or chronic HTN can be due to medication intake (decongestant, oral contraceptive, noradrenaline reuptake inhibitor, monoamine-oxidase inhibitor), renovascular disease, or pheochromocytoma.

TREATMENT

Numerous medical therapies are available for the effective control of acute and chronic HTN.

MENINGITIS

BACKGROUND

Incidence: 5/100,000 population per year; approximately one third viral (aseptic) and two thirds bacterial (septic).

PATHOPHYSIOLOGY

1. Headache is caused by infectious inflammation of the piaarachnoid.
2. Viral meningitis in approximately 80% caused by enteroviruses, transmitted by the fecal–oral route, and reaching the spinal fluid through the blood stream.
3. In approximately 50%, bacterial meningitis is caused by *Streptococcus pneumoniae* (adults) or *Neisseria meningitides* (children and adolescents; petechiae!); *Listeria*

monocytogenes (neonates), *Streptococcus* organisms (elderly), *Staphylococcus aureus*, and *Haemophilus influenzae* (young children) cause most of the rest.
4. The bacteria colonize the nasopharynx, penetrate the blood stream, and reach the blood–brain barrier to enter the spinal fluid and cause meningitis.

PROGNOSIS

In contrast to viral meningitis, bacterial meningitis can be associated with severe (neurologic) morbidity and mortality, which is the case in approximately 25%.

DIAGNOSIS

1. Headache, generalized in location and often severe in intensity, spanning hours to days, associated with fever, altered sensorium, and meningeal irritation.
2. Diagnosis is made through lumbar puncture (LP) and spinal fluid analysis, preceded by neuroimaging (CT scanning or MRI) if space-occupying lesion (abscess!) or hydrocephalus is suspected.
3. Spinal fluid analysis reveals an increased leucocyte count, higher in bacterial infection ($1,000–5,000/mm^3$) than in viral meningitis ($100–1,000/mm^3$), in bacterial meningitis neutrophilic and in viral meningitis after 24 hours, lymphocytic.
4. Spinal fluid pressure and protein content elevated, higher in bacterial than in viral meningitis, and glucose level normal in viral infection but usually less than 35 mg/dL in bacterial meningitis.
5. Causative agent is identified through:
   a. Spinal fluid gram stain and spinal fluid and blood cultures (bacterial meningitis); and
   b. Spinal fluid culture and antibody titer determinations in acute and convalescent serum (viral meningitis).

TREATMENT

1. Viral meningitis is treated with supportive therapy only; no specific antiviral therapy is available.
2. Bacterial meningitis is treated immediately and *before* definitive identification of the causative agent with:
   a. Ampicillin, 2 g IV every 4 hours; with
   b. Ceftriaxone, 2 to 3 g IV every 12 hours; or
   c. Cefotaxime, 2 g IV every 4 hours.
3. Once the identification and susceptibility of the bacteria are confirmed, antibiotic therapy is tailored to the specific etiology.
4. Antibiotic therapy can be combined with a corticosteroid to further improve outcome.

SUBARACHNOID HEMORRHAGE

BACKGROUND

1. Important diagnostic consideration in headache of very acute onset, regardless of intensity, because of the high morbidity and mortality associated with it.
2. Incidence: 10/100,000 population per year; mean age: 50.
3. Risk factors:
   a. Cigarette smoking
   b. HTN
   c. First-degree relative with subarachnoid hemorrhage

PATHOPHYSIOLOGY

1. Headache is caused by chemical inflammation of the piaarachnoid from blood in the subarachnoid space.
2. Bleeding into the subarachnoid space generally occurs from an aneurysm but occasionally from an arteriovenous malformation or as the result of a bleeding disorder.

PROGNOSIS

1. Twelve percent of patients die before receiving medical care.
2. Forty percent of hospitalized patients die within the first month.
3. One third of those who survive have major neurologic deficits.

DIAGNOSIS

1. Headache of very acute onset, often severe in intensity and associated with nausea and vomiting, sometimes also with (temporary) loss of consciousness, and with meningeal irritation on examination.
2. One third to one half of the patients have a history of similar acute-onset headaches in the days or weeks before the presenting hemorrhage occurs (sentinel headaches).
3. Cranial CT scanning is the preferred diagnostic test; it detects blood in the subarachnoid space in:
    a. Ninety percent to 95% within 24 hours;
    b. Eighty percent at 3 days;
    c. Seventy percent at 5 days;
    d. Fifty percent at 1 week; and
    e. Thirty percent at 2 weeks.
4. With clinical suspicion of a subarachnoid hemorrhage and negative findings on cranial CT scan, LP should be performed. However, it should not be performed until several hours after the onset of the headache to allow the development of xanthochromia. This is the yellow discoloration of spinal fluid after centrifugation that is diagnostic of subarachnoid hemorrhage.

TREATMENT

1. Surgical clipping or endovascular coiling of the aneurysm, resulting in obliteration by thrombosis.
2. Obliteration of the arteriovenous malformation by endovascular coiling and thrombosis or by gamma-knife radiation.

SUBDURAL HEMATOMA

BACKGROUND

1. Collection of (liquefied) blood between the dura and arachnoid, resulting from trauma to bridging veins. Acute subdural hematoma generally occurs in younger adults after major head injury. Chronic subdural hematoma affects the older adults (older than 50 years) after trivial, direct or indirect, head injury.
2. The incidence of chronic subdural hematoma is approximately 2/100,000 population per year, increasing sharply with advancing age to approximately 7/100,000 population per year for the age group, 70 to 79.
3. Apart from age, predisposing factors are:
    a. Anticoagulation;
    b. Alcoholism;

c. Epilepsy;
d. Bleeding disorder; and
e. Low spinal fluid pressure.

PATHOPHYSIOLOGY

1. Bleeding occurs from trauma to bridging veins, which are stretched and, thereby, more vulnerable as a result of generalized brain atrophy.
2. Headache, when present, is caused by stretching of meningeal blood vessels, which are sensitive to pain through nerve fibers originating from the mandibular nerve.

PROGNOSIS

1. Six-month mortality is approximately 30%, with neurologic status at the time of diagnosis being the most important prognostic factor.
2. Diagnosis is often delayed and, thereby, prognosis worsened because the condition is not suspected at the time of presentation: most common erroneous initial diagnoses are stroke and brain tumor.

DIAGNOSIS

1. Altered mental state (confusion, drowsiness, depression) is the most common presentation in the elderly (50%–70%).
2. Focal neurologic deficits, particularly hemiparesis, are present in approximately 60% of patients but are usually mild in comparison to the altered mental state and fluctuating in intensity.
3. Headache is often present but may be difficult to discern because of the altered mental state; seizure occurs in up to 60% of patients as the initial symptom.
4. Cranial CT scanning is the preferred diagnostic test; cranial MRI may be required in patients with isodense hematoma without midline shift.

TREATMENT

1. Surgical evacuation through twist drill or burr-hole craniostomy or craniotomy is the preferred therapy, although small hematomas may resolve spontaneously. Complications of surgical therapy are:
   a. Recurrent bleeding,
   b. Seizures, and
   c. Pneumocephalus.
2. Medically treated patients (small hematoma, frail condition) should be carefully monitored, with repeated neuroimaging upon clinical deterioration. Corticosteroids can be part of the medical management of the condition.

OPHTHALMIC ZOSTER

BACKGROUND

1. Also known as shingles, in this particular case affecting the ophthalmic nerve, the first division of the trigeminal nerve.
2. Lifetime prevalence: 10% to 20%; incidence: approximately 200/100,000 population per year.
3. The incidence increases with age to approximately 1,000/100,000 population per year over age 75.

PATHOPHYSIOLOGY

1. Reactivation of latent varicella-zoster virus in the trigeminal ganglion, resulting in a localized, cutaneous eruption in the ophthalmic dermatome.
2. The risk of reactivation increases with age due to declining virus-specific, cell-mediated immune response. The risk is also increased with:
   a. Neoplastic disease, especially lymphoproliferative cancers;
   b. Therapy with immunosuppressants, including corticosteroids; and
   c. Human immunodeficiency virus seropositivity.

PROGNOSIS

1. Specifically ophthalmic zoster is associated with ocular complications in approximately 50% of patients, that is, keratopathy, episcleritis, iritis, or stromal keratitis.
2. Increasing with advancing age, up to 70% of patients develop postherpetic neuropathy, that is, pain persisting for more than 30 days after onset of the rash or after cutaneous healing.

DIAGNOSIS

1. Abnormal skin sensations, ranging from itching to severe pain, in one side of the forehead and anterior vertex.
2. An erythematous maculopapular rash progresses to clusters of clear vesicles, which continue to form for 3 to 5 days and evolve through stages of pustulation, ulceration, and crusting.
3. Healing occurs over a period of 2 to 4 weeks, often resulting in scarring and permanent changes in pigmentation.

TREATMENT

1. Antiviral therapy should be initiated immediately to hasten cutaneous healing, decrease pain, and, most important, reduce the risk of ocular complications.
2. Only oral antiviral therapy is effective:
   a. Acyclovir, 800 mg every 4 hours;
   b. Famciclovir, 500 mg every 8 hours; or
   c. Valacyclovir, 1,000 mg every 8 hours.
3. Oral antiviral therapy is continued for 7 to 10 days and can be combined with corticosteroids, to further hasten healing and decrease pain.
4. Ophthalmologic consultation is indicated to evaluate for and follow-up on corneal involvement.
5. Therapy options for postherpetic neuropathy include:
   a. Opioids (short- and long-acting);
   b. Tricylics;
   c. Gabapentin;
   d. Capsaicin 0.025% to 0.075% cream; and
   e. Lidocaine 5% patch.

TEMPORAL ARTERITIS

BACKGROUND

1. Also known as cranial or giant cell arteritis, a chronic vasculitis affecting medium-sized arteries.

2. Incidence: approximately 20/100,000 population per year over age 50; male-to-female ratio: 1 to 2.
3. Incidence increases with age after 50 and peaks between 70 and 80 years.

PATHOPHYSIOLOGY

1. Granulomatous inflammation of the cranial arteries, particularly the temporal arteries, causing pain by inflammation and, possibly, vessel-wall ischemia.
2. Inflammation histologically characterized by degradation of the internal elastic lamina and occlusive luminal hyperplasia; giant cells are present in approximately 50% of patients.

PROGNOSIS

1. Permanent partial or complete loss of vision in one or both eyes occurs in up to 20% of patients and is often an early manifestation of the disease.
2. Visual loss is caused by ischemia of the optic nerve from involvement of the ophthalmic artery and/or its branches.

DIAGNOSIS

1. Headache occurs in approximately two thirds of patients and is generally gradual in onset, with temporal or occipital pain and scalp tenderness.
2. The affected arteries may be thickened, nodular, tender, or occasionally erythematous and the pulsations may be decreased or absent.
3. In approximately 50%, jaw claudication is present with pain on chewing and in approximately 15%, fever, usually low grade, which may be the presenting symptom.
4. Temporal artery biopsy is recommended in *all* patients, if possible before treatment is initiated.
5. If the temporal artery is abnormal on examination, only a small specimen needs to be removed. Otherwise, removal of a 3- to 5-cm segment is recommended, if negative also of the other side.
6. The sedimentation rate is at least 40 mm/h in approximately 80% of patients; however, the level of C-reactive protein is a more sensitive disease indicator.

TREATMENT

1. Prednisone, 40 to 60 mg/d, initiated *immediately* to prevent visual loss. Improvement occurs within days, and the dose is very gradually decreased after 2 to 4 weeks.
2. The therapy is guided by regular assessment of the clinical symptoms and the sedimentation rate or C-reactive protein level.

PSEUDOTUMOR CEREBRI

BACKGROUND

1. Also known as benign or idiopathic intracranial HTN, characterized by:
   a. Papilledema;
   b. Increased intracranial pressure (ICP) (above 200 to 250 mm H_2O) with normal spinal fluid composition, except, sometimes, for a low protein content; and
   c. Normal neuroimaging findings, except sometimes for small (slit-like) ventricles.

2. Incidence: approximately 1/100,000 population per year; male-to-female ratio: 1 to 8. Incidence in obese (more than 20% over ideal weight) women 20 to 44 years of age is approximately 19/100,000 population per year; peak incidence in the third decade.

PATHOPHYSIOLOGY

1. Decreased spinal fluid absorption causes generalized swelling of the brain, resulting in traction on the cerebral arteries and veins on the surface of the brain, which are sensitive to pain through nerve fibers originating from the ophthalmic nerve.
2. Spinal fluid is absorbed into the venous circulation by the endothelial cells of the arachnoid granulations, which is a (venous) pressure- and energy-dependent process.
3. Septic or aseptic thrombus and polycythemia (chronic respiratory insufficiency) can cause increased venous pressure, whereas hypothyroidism (obesity), anemia (iron deficiency), and corticosteroid withdrawal can cause compromised energy supply. Other causes of decreased spinal fluid absorption of unknown mechanism are tetracycline use and hypervitaminosis A (more than 100,000 U/d).

PROGNOSIS

Visual loss is the only serious complication of the condition, occurring in approximately 25% of patients.

DIAGNOSIS

1. Headache is the most common manifestation, present in approximately 95% of patients. It is generalized and tends to be worse upon awakening and increased with Valsalva maneuver.
2. Momentary visual blackouts, monocular or binocular, often with postural change, occur in approximately 70% of patients; double vision, usually from sixth nerve palsy, occurs in approximately 40%.
3. Visual-field defects are present in approximately 50% of patients, most commonly enlargement of the blind spot and constriction of peripheral vision.
4. Cranial MRI is the preferred neuroimaging method because it can demonstrate the presence of venous sinus thrombosis; empty sella is a nonspecific finding; enlarged ventricles exclude the diagnosis.
5. With normal neuroimaging findings, LP is performed; the pressure should be measured with the patient in the lateral decubitus position, legs straight and breathing easily.
6. Spinal fluid analysis should be performed, including VDRL test, as well as routine hematology and blood chemistry analysis.
7. Ophthalmologic examination should include:
   a. Visual acuity (best corrected)
   b. Pupillary function
   c. Visual field determination

TREATMENT

1. Medical therapy consists of:
   a. Weight loss, if appropriate; and
   b. Carbonic-anhydrase inhibitor, such as acetazolamide, to reduce spinal fluid production
2. Surgical therapy is indicated with severe headache and/or progressive loss of vision:
   a. Lumboperitoneal shunt

  b. Gastric bypass to facilitate weight loss
  c. Optic nerve-sheath decompression

LOW SPINAL FLUID PRESSURE HEADACHE

BACKGROUND

Postural headache associated with low spinal fluid pressure, usually resulting from LP performed for diagnostic or therapeutic purposes. Sometimes, it is due to craniospinal surgery or from the presence of a lumboperitoneal drain. It can also occur after trauma (trivial fall, exercise, coughing) as a result of tear of a nerve root sleeve or can be "spontaneous," due to rupture of a spinal meningeal cyst.

PATHOPHYSIOLOGY

1. Headache is caused by dilation of the cerebral veins and dural venous sinuses to compensate for the decreased spinal fluid volume resulting from the leak and by traction on these structures by the downward sagging of the brain upon assuming the erect position.
2. The structures are sensitive to pain through nerve fibers originating from the ophthalmic nerve, causing referred pain in the forehead and anterior vertex.

PROGNOSIS

Spontaneous resolution usually occurs within 2 weeks to several months.

DIAGNOSIS

1. Headache of recent onset, generalized and intense, postural in nature (e.g., occurring upon sitting or standing and relieved by lying down flat). It is *increased* in intensity by jugular vein compression and Valsalva maneuver, which can elicit the pain when the patient is supine.
2. LP reveals a spinal fluid pressure of 60 mm H_2O or less; the pressure can be so low that there is no spontaneous spinal fluid drainage. If this is the case, it is important to have the patient perform the Valsalva maneuver or aspirate gently to obtain spinal fluid.
3. The spinal fluid is often normal on analysis but the protein content and erythrocyte count can be elevated (meningeal hyperemia).
4. Gadolinium-enhanced cranial MRI reveals the meningeal hyperemia and, sometimes, subdural effusions.
5. Radionuclide cisternography, with 3 to 5 mCi of technetium-labeled, human serum albumin injected into the lumbar subarachnoid space, can be used to reveal the presence and site of the spinal fluid leak.

TREATMENT

1. Epidural blood patch;
2. Epidural saline infusion;
3. Oral caffeine;
4. Oral or IV fluids;
5. Carbon dioxide inhalation; and/or
6. Intrathecal saline infusion.

CEREBRAL VEIN THROMBOSIS

BACKGROUND

The condition affects all ages, its presentation and neuroimaging are diverse, and its potential for recovery is considerable. Therefore, it always needs to be on the mind of the physician evaluating a patient with neurologic illness.

PATHOPHYSIOLOGY

1. Septic thrombosis from infection of the nose area (carbuncle; *S aureus*), ethmoid or sphenoid sinusitis, dental abscess, otitis media.
2. In young women, during or after pregnancy or with the use of oral contraceptives.
3. Thrombocytemia and/or coagulation disorders.

PROGNOSIS

Outcome variable but much better than that for arterial thrombosis, especially with early treatment.

DIAGNOSIS

1. The onset of the condition is acute (less than 2 days) in approximately 30%, subacute (2 days to 1 month) in approximately 50%, and chronic in approximately 20%.
2. There are four main patterns of presentation, in order of decreasing frequency:
   a. Focal neurologic deficit and/or partial seizure, with headache or decreased level of consciousness;
   b. Increased ICP with headache, papilledema, and sixth nerve palsy;
   c. Subacute encephalopathy with decreased level of consciousness and, sometimes, seizure;
   d. Cavernous sinus thrombosis: painful third or sixth nerve palsy.
3. Diagnosis is based on neuroimaging:
   a. Cranial MRI is preferred, with increased signal of the thrombus on T_1- and T_2-weighted images.
   b. Cranial MR angiography shows loss of signal of the thrombosed vessel, due to absence of flow.
   c. Cranial CT scan with contrast shows "delta sign" in approximately one third of patients: filling defect in the torcular herophili.

TREATMENT

1. IV heparin (partial thromboplastin time 2–2.5 times control); or
2. Nadroparin s.c. (90 anti-Xa U/kg twice daily).

CAROTID ARTERY DISSECTION

BACKGROUND

Incidence: 2.5 to 3/100,000 population per year; peak: fifth decade.

PATHOPHYSIOLOGY

Intimal tear, often because of connective tissue disorder, allows blood, under arterial pressure, to enter the wall of the artery and form an intramural hematoma, which, in turn, causes:
1. Stenosis (subintimal dissection); or
2. Aneurysm (subadventitial dissection).

PROGNOSIS

1. Headache associated with dissection resolves within 1 week in approximately 90% of patients.
2. With regard to occurring stroke, approximately three fourths of patients make good functional recovery.

DIAGNOSIS

1. Most patients have at least two of the following three symptoms:
   a. Pain:
      1) Anterior neck (one fourth);
      2) Face/eye (50%); and/or
      3) Frontotemporal area (two thirds).
   b. Oculosympathetic palsy (less than 50%):
      1) Miosis; and
      2) Ptosis.
   c. Cerebral and/or retinal ischemia (50%–95%).
2. Cervical MR angiography is preferred, which can show the intramural hematoma, often crescent in shape and spiraling along the length of the artery.

TREATMENT

1. IV heparin followed by oral anticoagulation is recommended in *all* patients to prevent thromboembolic complications, unless contraindicated (for example, intracranial extension of the dissection).
2. Surgery should be reserved for patients who have persistent ischemic symptoms despite adequate anticoagulation:
   a. Ligation with bypass; or
   b. Percutaneous balloon angioplasty with stent placement.

BIBLIOGRAPHY

Adhiyaman V, Asghar M, Ganeshram KN, et al. Chronic subdural hematoma in the elderly. *Postgrad Med J* 2002;78:71–75.

Bates D, Ashford E, Dawson R, et al., for the Sumatriptan Aura Study Group. Subcutaneous sumatriptan during the migraine aura. *Neurology* 1994;44:1587–1592.

Bousser MG. Cerebral venous thrombosis: diagnosis and management. *J Neurol* 2000;247:252–258.

D'Alessandro R, Gamberini G, Benassi G, et al. Cluster headache in the Republic of San Marino. *Cephalalgia* 1986;6:159–162.

Diamond S, Baltes BJ. Chronic tension headache treated with amitriptyline: a double-blind study. *Headache* 1971;11:110–116.

Duckro PN, Greenberg M, Schultz KT, et al. Clinical features of chronic post-traumatic headache. *Headache Q* 1992;3:295–308.

Fields HL. Treatment of trigeminal neuralgia. *N Engl J Med* 1996;334:1125–1126.

Gabai IJ, Spierings ELH. Prophylactic treatment of cluster headache with verapamil. *Headache* 1989;29:167–168.

Gnann JW, Whitley RJ. Herpes zoster. *N Engl J Med* 2002;347:340–346.
Hadjikhani N, Sanchez del Rio M, Wu O, et al. Mechanisms of migraine aura revealed by functional MRI in human visual cortex. *Proc Natl Acad Sci U S A* 2001;98:4687–4692.
Kosmorsky G. Pseudotumor cerebri. *Neurosurg Clin N Am* 2001;36:775–797.
Lance JW, Curran DA, Anthony M. Investigations into the mechanism and treatment of chronic headache. *Med J Australia* 1965;52:909–914.
Lipton RB, Stewart WF, Diamond S, et al. Prevalence and burden of migraine in the United States: data from the American migraine study II. *Headache* 2001;41:646–657.
Morland TJ, Storli OV, Mogstad TE. Doxepin in the prophylactic treatment of mixed 'vascular' and tension headache. *Headache* 1979;19:382–383.
Packard RC. Posttraumatic headache: permanency and relationship to legal settlement. *Headache* 1992;32:496–500.
Rando TA, Fishman RA. Spontaneous intracranial hypotension: report of two cases and review of the literature. *Neurology* 1992;42:481–487.
Raskin NH. The hypnic headache syndrome. *Headache* 1988;28:534–536.
Rasmussen BK, Jensen R, Schroll M, et al. Epidemiology of headache in a general population: a prevalence study. *J Clin Epidemiol* 1991;44:1147–1157.
Rolak LA (ed). Immune and infectious diseases. In: Samuels M, Feske S, eds. *Office practice of neurology*. New York: Churchill Livingstone, 1996:350–447.
Russell BK, Olesen J. Migraine with aura and migraine without aura: an epidemiological study. *Cephalalgia* 1992;12:221–228.
Salvarani C, Cantini F, Boiardi L, et al. Polymyalgia rheumatica and giant-cell arteritis. *N Engl J Med* 2002;347:261–271.
Schievink WI. Intracranial aneurysms. *N Engl J Med* 1997;336:28–40.
Schievink WI. Spontaneous dissection of the carotid and vertebral arteries. *N Engl J Med* 2001;344:898–906.
Sheftell FD, O'Quinn S, Watson C, et al. Low migraine recurrence with naratriptan: clinical parameters related to recurrence. *Headache* 2000;40:103–110.
Sindrup SH, Jensen TS. Pharmacotherapy of trigeminal neuralgia. *Clin J Pain* 2002;18:22–27.
Sjaastad O, Spierings ELH. Hemicrania continua: another headache absolutely responsive to indomethacin. *Cephalalgia* 1984;4:65–70.
Spierings ELH. Acute and chronic hypertensive headache and hypertensive encephalopathy. *Cephalalgia* 2002;22:313–316.
Spierings ELH. Advances in migraine treatment: the triptans. *Neurologist* 2001;7:113–121.
Spierings ELH. Angiographic changes suggestive of vasospasm in migraine complicated by stroke. *Headache* 1990;30:727–728.
Spierings ELH. Daily migraine with visual aura associated with an occipital arteriovenous malformation. *Headache* 2001;41:193–197.
Spierings ELH. Eletriptan in acute migraine: a double-blind, placebo-controlled comparison to sumatriptan [letter]. *Neurology* 2000;55:735–736.
Spierings ELH. Episodic and chronic jabs and jolts syndrome. *Headache Q* 1990;1:299–302.
Spierings ELH. Episodic and chronic paroxysmal hemicrania. *Clin J Pain* 1992;8:44–48.
Spierings ELH. Flurries of migraine (with) aura and migraine aura status [letter]. *Headache* 2002;42:326–327.
Spierings ELH. Headache continuum: concept and supporting evidence from recent study of chronic daily headache. *Clin J Pain* 2001;17:337–340.
Spierings ELH. *Management of migraine*. Boston: Butterworth-Heinemann, 1996.
Spierings ELH. Pediatric and geriatric migraine. In: Samuels MA, Feske S, eds. *Office practice of neurology*. Philadelphia: Elsevier Science, 2003;1369–1373.
Spierings ELH. The aura-headache connection in migraine: a historical analysis. *Arch Neurol* 2004 *(in press)*.
Spierings ELH. The involvement of the autonomic nervous system in cluster headache. *Headache* 1980;20:218–219.

Spierings ELH, Gomez-Mancilla B, Grosz DE, et al. Oral almotriptan versus oral sumatriptan in the acute treatment of migraine: a double-blind, randomized, parallel-group, optimum-dose comparison. *Arch Neurol* 2001;58:944–950.

Spierings ELH, Schroevers M, Honkoop PC, et al. Development of chronic daily headache: a clinical study. *Headache* 1998;38:529–533.

Spierings ELH, Schroevers M, Honkoop PC, et al. Presentation of chronic daily headache: a clinical study. *Headache* 1998;38:191–196.

Waldenlind E, Ekbom K, Torhall J. MR-angiography during spontaneous attacks of cluster headache: a case report. *Headache* 1993;33:291–295.

Weiss HD, Stern BJ, Goldberg J. Post-traumatic migraine: chronic migraine precipitated by minor head or neck trauma. *Headache* 1991;31:451–546.

Yamaguchi M. Incidence of headache and severity of head injury. *Headache* 1992;32: 427–431.

12. STROKE AND CEREBROVASCULAR DISORDERS

Steven K. Feske

ARTERIAL ISCHEMIC STROKE AND TRANSIENT ISCHEMIC ATTACK

BACKGROUND

1. In the United States, stroke is the third leading cause of death and the most common cause of disability; hence, the optimal identification of those with stroke and those at risk and the optimal application of acute and preventive therapies are of major medical and economic importance.
2. Completed stroke and transient ischemic attack (TIA) have the same pathophysiology and are distinguished by the duration of ischemia, adequate to cause brain tissue necrosis in the case of stroke and brief enough to allow full recovery in the case of TIA.
3. TIA has been traditionally and arbitrarily defined clinically as focal brain ischemia with symptoms resolving completely within 24 hours. Sensitive neuroimaging with magnetic resonance imaging (MRI) has revealed that a large number of ischemic events with symptoms lasting many hours before complete resolution are, in fact, cerebral infarctions. This has led to the suggestion that the definition of TIA be changed to consider imaging data.

PATHOPHYSIOLOGY

1. Most cases of focal cerebral ischemia are caused by blockage of a cerebral artery. The most common causes of cerebrovascular occlusion are
   a. Embolism of thrombotic material from the heart or from another proximal source of clot formation, such as the aorta;
   b. Atherosclerosis in a large or medium artery, causing either stenosis and compromise of distal blood flow or artery-to-artery embolism to a distal branch; and
   c. Hypertrophy and ultimately luminal compromise of small penetrating vessels, usually under chronic exposure to hypertension (HTN), diabetes mellitus (DM), or other risk factors.
2. Less common causes of vascular occlusion include other arteriopathies, such as arterial dissection and arteritis, vasospasm, thrombophilia, and rarely, embolism of material other than thrombus, such as fat, air, tumor, amniotic fluid, or intravascular medical devices. Many disorders underlying stroke are listed in Table 12-1.

PROGNOSIS

The outcome of an individual ischemic event will depend on the location, extent, and duration of the ischemia, hence ultimately on the size and location of the completed stroke. The risk of a completed stroke in the weeks after a TIA depends on the mechanism of the TIA and the application of appropriate preventive therapies. When untreated, the average risk is high.

DIAGNOSIS

History

1. The history should attempt to distinguish stroke and TIA from potential mimickers such as migraine and focal seizures.

TABLE 12-1. SOME CAUSES OF STROKE

Atherosclerotic disease of large and medium arteries
Hyperlipidemia, HTN, DM, hyperhomocysteinemia, radiotherapy, pseudoxanthoma elasticum
Nonatherosclerotic disease of large and medium arteries
Arterial dissection, fibromuscular dysplasia, moyamoya disease, sarcoidosis, fungal and tuberculous vasculitis, varicella zoster vasculitis, systemic vasculitic syndromes, isolated CNS angiitis

Small-vessel disease
Lipohyalinosis, atherosclerosis, infections (syphilis, TB, cryptococcosis), vasculitis

Cardioembolism
HTN, cardiomyopathy, atrial fibrillation, valvular heart disease, paradoxical embolism, left atrial thrombus, ventricular mural thrombus after MI, bacterial endocarditis, nonbacterial thrombotic endocarditis (cancer, antiphospholipid antibody syndrome), left atrial myxoma

Prothrombotic states
Oral contraceptives, pregnancy and puerperium, antiphospholipid antibody syndrome, sickle cell disease, cancer, polycythemia vera, essential thrombocytosis, TTP, DIC, markedly elevated factor VIII, deficiency or dysfunction of protein C, protein S, or antithrombin III, activated protein C resistance (factor V Leiden genotype or acquired), dysfibrinogenemias, disorders of fibrinolysis

Drug abuse
Vasospasm, vasculitis, cardiac arrhythmias, endocarditis, mycotic aneurysm, injection of infected or thrombogenic material

Miscellaneous
CADASIL, Fabry disease, Sneddon syndrome, MELAS

TPP, thrombotic thrombocytopenic purpura; DIC, disseminated intravascular coagulation; CADASIL, cerebral autosomal dominant angiopathy with subcortical infarcts and leukoencephalopathy; MELAS, mitrochondrial encephalopathy with lactic acidosis and stroke-like episodes; CNS, central nervous system; TB, tuberculosis; MI, myocardial infarction; HTN, hypertension; DM, diabetes mellitus.

2. Onset is typically sudden, and symptoms vary according to the site of the ischemia.
3. History seeks underlying factors that suggest the pathophysiologic mechanism for the event:
   a. History of heart disease and peripheral arterial disease.
   b. History of atherosclerotic risk factors (HTN, DM, hypercholesterolemia, smoking, sedentary lifestyle, family history of atherosclerotic disease).
   c. History suggesting thrombophilia or trauma and neck, face, and head pain that might suggest arterial dissection; history of fever, chills, cardiac symptoms, or drug abuse that might suggest endocarditis.
4. When acute thrombolytic therapies are being considered, history should also elicit the precise time of symptom onset and any problems that might contraindicate such therapy.

Examination

1. The examiner should note the temperature, blood pressure (BP) and cardiac rhythm, the quality of carotid pulses and the presence of bruits, and the quality of heart sounds and presence of murmur.
2. The neurologic examination should define the neurologic deficits in a way that allows classification of the event into one of the clinical stroke syndromes. This will allow prediction of the vessel involved and the mechanism of vascular occlusion.

Major Stroke Syndromes

1. Middle cerebral artery (MCA) territory syndrome with contralateral gaze paresis, hemiparesis, and hemisensory loss, often with contralateral visual field loss, and cortical signs (aphasia with left hemispheric lesions; neglect with right).
2. MCA branch syndromes [i.e., partial MCA syndromes with nonfluent aphasia (Broca aphasia if perisylvian and transcortical motor aphasia if sparing the perisylvian area)] if involving anterior division branches and fluent aphasia (Wernicke aphasia if perisylvian and transcortical sensory aphasia if sparing the perisylvian area) if involving posterior division branches of the left MCA.
3. Anterior cerebral artery (ACA) syndrome with predominantly leg weakness and sensory deficits contralaterally and sparing of vision (bilateral frontal signs suggest a common origin of the two anterior cerebral arteries).
4. Posterior cerebral artery (PCA) syndrome with contralateral homonymous hemi- or quadrantanopsia, typically with intact motor and somatosensory function or with associated cortical deficits.
   a. Memory loss from medial temporal infarction
   b. Alexia without agraphia from dominant visual cortex and splenium of corpus callosum infarction
   c. Agnosias, such as color naming and recognition disorders and prosopagnosia (facial recognition disorder), from infarction of the inferior temporooccipital cortex
5. Mid-basilar artery syndrome implying atherosclerotic stenosis or occlusion of the mid-basilar artery with pontine (dysarthria, horizontal diplopia, vertigo, quadriparesis) and cerebellar dysfunction.
6. Top-of-the-basilar syndrome implying embolic occlusion of the distal basilar artery with midbrain (decreased arousal; vertical and horizontal diplopia; unequal and irregular, poorly reactive pupils), thalamic, and occipital dysfunction.
7. Lacunar syndromes suggesting primary occlusion of a small vessel [e.g., pure motor or pure sensory syndromes without visual loss or cortical findings (aphasia or neglect)] or an isolated hemiparesis with ataxia. Dysarthria is common when such lacunar infarcts are in the pons or the internal capsule.
8. Border-zone (watershed) infarcts occur when distal vascular flow is compromised from a proximal stenosis or from global loss of perfusion due to hypotension.
   a. Anteriorly, this most typically produces the man-in-a-barrel syndrome characterized by leg and proximal upper extremity weakness with relative sparing of the distal upper extremities from infarction of the ACA and MCA border zone in the high frontal convexity.
   b. Posteriorly, this may produce Balint syndrome (astereognosis, optic ataxia, ocular apraxia) from infarction of the MCA and PCA border zone in the parietooccipital region.

Neuroimaging

1. The goals of acute neuroimaging are
   a. To define the site and location of any established infarct when possible and the extent of ischemic tissue at risk,
   b. To identify the site of an acute vascular occlusion, and
   c. To identify hemorrhage or unexpected lesions mimicking acute cerebral infarction.
2. Computed tomography (CT) and CT angiography:
   a. Noncontrast CT will identify acute hemorrhage in most cases. It is insensitive for acute infarction when done within hours of stroke onset. However, subtle changes should be sought: dense MCA sign indicating a thrombus in the MCA stem, sylvian fissure dot sign indicating thrombus in the more distal MCA branches, or hypodensity, loss of gray–white differentiation, and sulcal effacement at the site o early infarction.
   b. CT angiography allows rapid anatomic evaluation of the cerebral vessels from the aortic arch through the neck and intracranially.

    c. CT perfusion techniques are now being developed to give acute information about infarct size and hypoperfused tissue at risk.

3. MRI and MRA:

    a. MRI is more sensitive than CT for early infarction. Acute infarction is best seen on diffusion-weighted imaging (DWI) sequences that reveal acute strokes as bright lesions within minutes of infarction. Correlation with low signal on apparent diffusion coefficient (ADC) maps can help to differentiate acute infarction from other causes of bright signal on DWI.

    b. MRA can define flow in the cerebral vessels from the aortic arch to the intracranial arteries.

    c. MRI perfusion techniques have been developed to define tissue at risk.

4. Conventional angiography:

    a. To define vascular pathology, conventional angiography is more sensitive and specific than either CTA or MRA, and it remains the gold standard for diagnostic vascular imaging; however, it is rarely indicated acutely except as part of planned acute interventional therapy.

5. Carotid duplex ultrasound:

    a. Carotid duplex ultrasound includes Doppler imaging of blood flow velocities and anatomic imaging by gray scale and color flow techniques.

    b. It is widely available, noninvasive, and, in good hands, reliably able to define many carotid lesions.

    c. Its greatest use is in the estimation of the degree of carotid stenosis and residual lumen diameter from atherosclerosis and the characterization of the atheroma. Doppler waveforms can also give indirect information about upstream and downstream stenoses that are outside of the field of carotid ultrasound.

6. Transcranial Doppler ultrasound (TCD):

    a. TCD allows imaging of the flow of the major vessels of the circle of Willis; the proximal middle, anterior, and posterior cerebral arteries; the ophthalmic artery; and the vertebral and basilar arteries. Information about direction and velocity of flow allows the examiner to identify sites of stenosis or vasospasm and to assess pathways of collateralization.

    b. High flow velocities suggest vascular narrowing, as from stenosis or vasospasm, or elevated flow, as in generalized high flow states, such as arteriovenous malformations or collateral flow in the setting of stenosis or occlusion at another site. Because ultrasound is safe and noninvasive, it can be used serially for repeated examinations in dynamic situations. Its most valuable application has been follow-up evaluation for cerebral vasospasm after subarachnoid hemorrhage (SAH).

Other Tests

1. Electrocardiogram (ECG), chest radiograph (CXR), glucose, electrolytes, blood urea nitrogen (BUN), creatinine, complete blood count (CBC) with platelets, and prothrombin time [(PT), international normalized ratio (INR)], and an activated partial thromboplastin time (aPTT) should be part of the initial evaluation to help determine the cause of the event and to provide information critical to the planning of acute therapy.

2. If fever or cardiac murmur is present, or if there are other reasons to suspect endocarditis, then erythrocyte sedimentation rate (ESR), blood cultures, and echocardiogram are important to pursue this diagnosis.

3. If there is reason to suspect drug abuse, toxicology screening is valuable.

4. In the postacute phase, echocardiography, cardiac rhythm monitoring, further definition of the cerebral vasculature if not completed acutely, and additional laboratory tests directed at stroke risk factors are indicated.

    a. All patients should have fasting serum glucose; total, low-density lipoprotein (LDL), and high-density lipoprotein (HDL) cholesterol; and triglycerides tested.

    b. Hyperhomocysteinemia has also been identified as a modifiable risk factor for atherosclerosis.

   c. Where aortic atheroma, valvular, or left atrial appendage visualization will alter secondary preventive therapy, transesophageal echocardiography should be considered, because the sensitivity of transthoracic echocardiography is low for lesions at these sites.

TREATMENT

Acute Therapy of Ischemic Stroke

Hemodynamic Considerations

1. Cerebral perfusion depends on the mean systemic arterial pressure (MAP) based on the basic hemodynamic relationship (CBF = MAP − CVP/CVR, where CBF = cerebral blood flow, CVP = cerebral venous pressure, and CVR = cerebrovascular resistance).
2. Areas of brain distal to narrowed or occluded arteries may be supplied by collateral vessels. When fully dilated (i.e., autoregulated to maximize CBF) flow in these vessels becomes passively dependent on the MAP. Therefore, it is desirable to maintain MAP high in the setting of acute stroke.
3. It is common for patients with acute stroke to have acute BP elevations on presentation.
   a. In general, this BP should not be lowered, unless
      1) BP lowering is necessary to fulfill criteria for safe thrombolysis (see Intravenous Thrombolysis and Tables 12-2 and 12-3 below), or unless acute medical issues demand it:
      2) Acute myocardial infarction
      3) Aortic dissection
      4) Hypertensive crisis with end-organ involvement [congestive heart failure (CHF), renal failure, hypertensive encephalopathy].
   b. No data define a threshold above which BP should be treated acutely outside of these complications; however, consensus guidelines from the American Stroke Association suggest that therapy should be withheld unless diastolic BP is above 120 or systolic BP is above 220 mm Hg.
   c. Patients with excessive BP elevation who are otherwise suitable for tissue plasminogen activator (TPA), should be treated acutely to achieve tolerable BP for therapy (systolic BP less than or equal to 185, diastolic BP less than or equal to 110). The antihypertensive goals and regimen used in the National Institute of Neurological Disorders and Stroke (NINDS) trial of intravenous (IV) TPA are shown in Table 12-2.

Metabolic Considerations

1. Patients should be monitored with pulse oximetry and given supplemental oxygen for desaturation less than 95%.
2. Both hyperthermia and hyperglycemia may increase the size of the ultimate infarct; therefore, patients should receive antipyretic medications and external cooling, if needed, to maintain normal body temperature and insulin to maintain glucose near normal.

Intravenous Thrombolysis

1. All patients who present within 3 hours of onset of stroke symptoms should be considered for IV thrombolytic therapy with TPA.
2. Indications and contraindications for IV thrombolysis are listed in Table 12-3.
3. For suitable patients, IV TPA should be given as soon as the essential evaluation can be completed. The dose of TPA is 0.9 mg/kg to a maximum total dose of 90 mg. Ten percent of this dose is given as a bolus over about 2 minutes. The remainder is infused over 1 hour. It is advised that emergency departments establish protocols for administration to speed up preparation and minimize errors.
4. BP should be controlled within recommended parameters for 24 hours after administration (see Table 12-2), and patients should be closely monitored for

TABLE 12-2. ACUTE ANTIHYPERTENSIVE THERAPY FOR ADMINISTRATION OF INTRAVENOUS TISSUE PLASMINOGEN ACTIVATOR

Monitor arterial BP during the first 24 h after starting treatment
- Every 15 min for 2 h after starting the infusion, then
- Every 30 min for 6 h, then
- Every 60 min for 24 h after starting treatment

If systolic BP is 180–230 mm Hg[a] or if diastolic BP is 105–120 mm Hg for two or more readings 5–10 min apart:
- Give IV labetalol 10 mg over 1–2 min. May repeat or double the dose every 10–20 min up to a total dose of 150 mg.
- Monitor BP every 15 min during labetalol treatment and observe for hypotension.

If systolic BP is greater than 230 mm Hg or if diastolic BP is 121–140 mm Hg for two or more readings 5–10 min apart:
- Give IV labetalol 10 mg over 1–2 min. May repeat or double the dose every 10–20 min up to a total dose of 150 mg.
- Monitor BP every 15 min during labetalol treatment and observe for hypotension.
- If no satisfactory response, infuse sodium nitroprusside (0.5 μg/kg/min).

If diastolic BP is greater than 140 mm Hg for two or more readings 5–10 min apart:
- Infuse sodium nitroprusside (0.5 μg/kg/min).
- Monitor BP every 15 min during infusion and observe for hypotension.

IV, intravenous; BP, blood pressure.
[a]Systolic BP greater than 185 for *pretreatment* therapy.
From the NINDS study of intravenous tissue plasminogen activator; *NEJM* 1995;333:1581.

evidence of hemorrhage with serial neurologic examinations and follow up CT scanning.
5. No adjunctive antiplatelet or anticoagulant medication should be given for 24 hours after IV thrombolysis.

Intraarterial Therapies
1. Where adequate facilities and expertise are available, emergency angiography allows for mechanical clot removal and delivery of intraarterial thrombolytic agents. Such therapies have been shown to promote early recanalization of occluded arteries and, in a single controlled study of patients with proximal MCA occlusion, clinical benefit when applied within 6 hours of symptom onset.
2. Proper concurrent use of heparins, antiplatelet agents, and induced HTN have not been established by systematic study, and at this time should be based on institutional protocols.

Acute Use of Antiplatelet Therapies and Anticoagulants
1. Acute use of aspirin and other antiplatelet agents has not been shown to decrease stroke size, although in very large trials, early institution of low-dose aspirin has slightly improved outcome probably by reducing the incidence of early recurrent events within approximately 2 weeks.
2. Early use of unfractionated heparin and low-molecular-weight heparins has been studied with variable results.
3. There appears to be some benefit in preventing early recurrent events in patients with carotid stenosis and atrial fibrillation.
4. Patients with prosthetic heart valves requiring anticoagulation and other cardiac lesions representing clear embolic risks are best placed on anticoagulants as early as this is judged to be safe.
5. Anecdotal data suggest that reperfusion into infracted tissue is more likely to cause hemorrhagic conversion when anticoagulants are given, when strokes are large,

TABLE 12-3. INDICATIONS AND CONTRAINDICATIONS FOR INTRAVENOUS TISSUE PLASMINOGEN ACTIVATOR FOR ACUTE ISCHEMIC STROKE

Indications
1. Acute ischemic stroke with disabling deficit
2. Onset time within 3 h
3. Head CT without well-established infarct, hemorrhage, or alternative explanation for focal neurologic deficit

Absolute contraindications
1. Hemorrhage on head CT; well-established infarct, or other diagnosis that contraindicates treatment (tumor, abscess, etc.)
2. Known CNS vascular malformation or tumor
3. Mild or rapidly improving deficit

Relative contraindications[a]
4. Bacterial endocarditis
5. Significant trauma within 3 mo
6. Stroke within 3 mo
7. History of intracranial hemorrhage or symptoms suspicious for subarachnoid hemorrhage
8. Major surgery within past 14 d or minor surgery within past 10 d, including liver and kidney biopsy, thoracocentesis, lumbar puncture
9. Arterial puncture at noncompressible site within 7 d
10. Pregnancy or early postpartum period
11. Gastrointestinal, urologic, or pulmonary hemorrhage within 21 d
12. Known bleeding diathesis or hemodialysis
13. PTT >40 s: INR >1.5; platelet count < 100,000 mm^3
14. SBP >185 or DBP >110 despite therapy to lower BP acutely
15. Seizure at onset of stroke[b]
16. Glucose <50 or >400[b]

CT, computed tomography; CNS, central nervous system; PTT, partial thromboplastin time; BP, blood pressure; INR, international normalized ratio; SBP, systolic blood pressure; DBP, diastolic blood pressure.
[a]These contraindications are taken from the National Institute of Neurological Disorders and Stroke (*NEJM* 1995;333:1581) study of intravenous plasminogen activator. In clinical practice where risk of permanent disability due to stroke is felt to be great, judgments may favor therapy.
[b]These relative contraindications are intended to prevent treatment of patients with focal deficits due to causes other than vascular occlusion. If the deficit persists after correction of the abnormal glucose, or ideally if rapid diagnosis of vascular occlusion can be made by CT angiography or magnetic resonance angiography, then treatment may be indicated.

when bolus doses of heparin are used, and when the level of anticoagulation is excessive. Therefore, care should be taken when anticoagulants are begun early after acute ischemic stroke.

Deep Vein Thrombosis Prophylaxis
1. Patients immobilized after acute strokes should be placed on low-dose subcutaneous heparin or low-molecular-weight heparin or be provided with pneumatic compression boots to minimize the risk of deep vein thrombosis (DVT).
2. Patients who cannot receive anticoagulants may benefit from aspirin for DVT prevention.

Hemicraniectomy
1. In patients with large hemispheric infarcts and malignant cerebral edema for whom medical therapy of the cerebral edema and mass effect may prove inadequate, hemicraniectomy, removal of a large segment of the overlying cranial bone and redundant dural patching, may directly relieve intracranial pressure (ICP) and

midline shift and herniation by allowing the swollen infarcted tissue to herniate through the surgical defect. This may greatly simplify medical therapy and increase survival after large strokes.

2. When this therapy is offered, it must be understood that, although it may be life-saving, the patient will survive with the disabling deficit resulting from the large infarction.

Secondary Prevention of Ischemic Stroke

Antiplatelet Therapies

Low-dose aspirin (81–650 mg/d), aspirin combined with dipyridamole [aspirin 25 mg/dipyridamole 200 mg twice a day (b.i.d.)], and clopidogrel (75 mg/d) have been shown to reduce the risk of recurrent events after stroke and TIA. Combining aspirin and clopidogrel may confer added benefit as has been shown for patients after coronary ischemic events, but data addressing this issue will have to await the publication of the MATCH trial now in progress. Aspirin is typically used in doses of 81 to 325 mg, although higher and lower doses have been shown effective. Lower doses confer less hemorrhagic risk.

Atrial Fibrillation

1. It has been demonstrated convincingly in many studies that warfarin reduces the risk of stroke in patients with atrial fibrillation and that strokes occurring in these patients tend to occur during lapses in their proper anticoagulation.
2. All patients with persistent or recurrent paroxysmal atrial fibrillation should be treated with warfarin with a goal INR of approximately 2 to 3, unless there are decided contraindications to its use.
3. Patients with lone atrial fibrillation (younger than 60 years, no prior stroke or TIA, normal ECG and echocardiogram, no HTN, no DM) are the sole exception. Such patients appear to have a risk of stroke comparable to that of the general population, and anticoagulation is not indicated for them for *primary* prevention.

Intracranial Arterial Stenosis

Symptomatic intracranial stenosis has not been studied adequately enough to support firm recommendations. The Warfarin in Asprin Symptomatic Intracranial Disease (WASID) study suggests that patients with symptoms thought to be due to stenosis of an intracranial large vessel have a reduced risk of recurrent stroke when treated with warfarin as compared to aspirin. However, this was a small retrospective study, and a large prospective look at this question is still under way. In patients with symptomatic intracranial stenoses who continue to have focal ischemic symptoms on warfarin, angioplasty and stenting have been successfully performed.

Valvular and Other Heart Disease

1. Patients with rheumatic and other valvular disease and evidence of embolic stroke or TIA may benefit from anticoagulation; however, the proper subsets of patients who should be treated with long-term anticoagulation have not been defined.
2. Patients with mechanical valve prostheses and increased embolic risk have a clear indication for anticoagulation. A goal INR range of 2.5 to 3.5 is recommended for most mechanical valves; bileaflet prosthetic valves in the aortic position with normal rhythm and left ventricular size and function may be anticoagulated to a goal of 2.0 to 3.0.
3. Patients with dilated cardiomyopathy have an increased risk of embolic stroke that is reduced with warfarin, but the threshold for anticoagulation has not been well defined. One large study found an increased risk with ejection fraction (EF) less than 0.35, progressive increases in risk with declining EF, and reduction of this risk with warfarin.
4. Clear standards for the treatment of cryptogenic stroke or TIA in the setting of a patent foramen ovale (PFO) have not been clarified. With PFO, risk of infarct appears to be increased in the presence of an accompanying atrial septal aneurysm.

Because of the high frequency of PFO in the healthy population, this is a difficult issue.

5. At this point, it seems reasonable to advise that all patients with stroke or TIA and PFO receive at a minimum antiplatelet agents, that those with identified venous side thrombus receive anticoagulation for at least 3 months, that those with hypercoagulable states be considered for long-term anticoagulation, and that those with recurrent events despite escalation to warfarin be considered for closure. Whether large size or the presence of atrial septal aneurysm alone justifies closure has not been established.

6. Closure can be accomplished by open surgery or by transvenous placement of various devices designed for this purpose.

Carotid Stenosis and Other Indications for Surgical Therapy

1. Patients with TIA or with partial strokes in the internal carotid artery (ICA) territory and with significant atherosclerotic carotid stenosis should be considered for carotid endarterectomy as soon as possible in the case of TIAs and as soon as it is deemed safe after partial territory strokes.

    a. The benefit of carotid endarterectomy in symptomatic patients with stenosis of 70% or greater has been clearly established in several trials. These early studies failed to show a benefit in patients with less than 30% stenosis. The North American Symptomatic Carotid Endarterectomy Trial (NASCET) study data suggest that those with stenosis of 30% to 69% have an intermediate risk and that in those with stenosis above 50%, a small surgical benefit accumulates statistical significance after 8 years.

    b. Primary prevention with carotid endarterectomy remains a difficult issue. One study shows, after 5 years of follow-up, a small benefit in favor of carotid endarterectomy in patients with stenosis of 60% or greater. This study enrolled few women and, unlike the studies of carotid endarterectomy in symptomatic patients, it did not find an increased risk of stroke and benefit of carotid endarterectomy with increasing degrees of stenosis above 60%. Therefore, it is difficult to give broad advice about thresholds for carotid endarterectomy in asymptomatic patients. With the available data, it is reasonable to recommend carotid endarterectomy in those with severe asymptomatic stenosis who are at low surgical risk.

2. There is increasing experience with angioplasty and stenting of stenotic carotid lesions, and this therapy is now being substituted for certain patients with significant lesions and high surgical risk.

Risk Factors for Atherosclerosis and Small-vessel Disease

1. Antihypertensive therapy:

    a. Hypertension is a major stroke risk factor even with mild elevations beneath the traditional conventionally defined normal thresholds. Both systolic and diastolic elevations increase risk. Therefore, all patients at risk should receive optimal BP control. Consensus treatment goals are shown in Table 12-4. Various agents might be used to accomplish this. The Heart Outcomes Prevention Evaluation (HOPE) trial suggests that angiotensin-converting enzyme inhibitors may confer a measure of stroke prevention beyond their BP-lowering effect.

2. Statins and cholesterol-lowering therapy:

    a. Elevation of LDL cholesterol and triglycerides and low HDL cholesterol are risk factors for atherosclerotic vascular disease, including stroke. The 3-hydroxy-3-methylglutaryl coenzyme A (HMG-CoA) reductase inhibitors (statins) have been shown to decrease LDL cholesterol and may lower triglycerides and elevate HDL cholesterol in some patients. These agents have been shown to lower the risk of atherosclerotic mortality and vascular events, including stroke. They may also confer benefits in addition to those of lipid lowering. Triglycerides may respond to glycemic control and fibrates, although statins may also contribute benefit. Niacin and fibrates are most effective in elevating HDL cholesterol, although these agents must be used with caution in diabetics. When combined

TABLE 12-4. TREATMENT GOALS FOR HYPERTENSION AND DYSLIPIDEMIA

Risk Factor	Treatment Goal for Secondary Prevention	
	ASA	ADA
HTN		
SBP, mm Hg	< 140 (135[a])	130
DBP, mm Hg	< 90 (85[a])	80
Dyslipidemia		
LDL, mg/dL	< 100	< 100
HDL, mg/dL	> 35	> 40
TC, mg/dL	< 200	
TG, mg/dL	< 200	< 150

ASA, American Stroke Association; ADA, American Diabetes Association; HTN, hypertension; SBP, systolic blood pressure; DBP, diastolic blood pressure; TC, total cholesterol; TG, triglycerides; LDL, low-density lipoprotein; HDL, high-density lipoprotein.
[a] If end organ damage is present.
From American Diabetes Association. Treatment of hypertension in adults with diabetes. *Diabetes Care* 2003;26[Suppl 1]:S80–82; and American Diabetes Association. Management of dyslipidemia in adults with diabetes. *Diabetes Care* 2003;26[Suppl 1]:S83–86, with permission.

with statins, niacin may cause hyperglycemia; fibrates may cause myositis. Consensus goals for treatment of hyperlipidemia are shown in Table 12-4.
3. Other risk factors:
   a. In all cases, weight loss, proper nutrition, moderation of alcohol use, smoking cessation, and regular physical exercise should be encouraged as first steps or concurrent steps in therapy of modifiable risk factors.
4. Hyperhomocysteinemia:
   a. Hyperhomocysteinemia contributes to stroke risk by two mechanisms: promoting atherosclerosis and promoting thrombosis. The importance of the latter mechanism cannot be determined in individual cases, and the best therapy is probably vitamin supplementation [e.g., folate, pyridoxine (B_6), and vitamin B_{12}] to lower the serum homocysteine level. The potential clinical benefit of vitamin therapy is under study using daily doses of vitamin B_{12} 500 μg, pyridoxine 25 mg, and folate 2 mg.

Other Arterial Lesions
1. Many arterial diseases other than atherosclerosis may lead to stroke. Many of these are listed in Table 12-1.
   a. The most common of these is arterial dissection. Arterial dissection is a common cause of stroke in young patients, so young age should raise suspicion. In addition, head or neck pain in the context of stroke suggests possible arterial dissection. Although many cases of dissection will be associated with trauma, many will not, or history will elicit minor trauma, such as coughing, that may have a questionable relationship to the dissection.
   b. Dissection of the carotid or vertebral arteries is most common and may cause symptoms by compromise of the vessel lumen and distal flow or by embolization from thrombus formed at the site of endothelial tear. The risk of the latter is probably decreased by anticoagulation, and a period of several months of anticoagulation is appropriate therapy until the lesion is stable, either with recanalization or with permanent closure of the dissected vessel. This therapeutic question is being studied systematically in an ongoing trial.

   c. Recurrent or multiple dissections should raise suspicion of underlying arterial disorders that predispose to dissection, such as fibromuscular dysplasia, type IV Ehlers–Danlos syndrome, or Marfan syndrome.
2. Headache or systemic illness, especially with elevated ESR or C-reactive protein, suggestive of a systemic vasculitic syndrome should suggest cerebrovascular vasculitis as a possible cause of a stroke or TIA.
   a. Large-vessel vasculitis as in giant cell arteritis (Takayasu arteritis or temporal arteritis) may cause territorial infarcts or retinal ischemia.
   b. Vasculitis of small and medium vessels usually causes small, deep infarcts typically with headache and often with recurrent events.
   c. Isolated central nervous system (CNS) vasculitis presents with these nonspecific features of cerebral vasculitis without systemic vasculitis. In such cases, cerebral angiography and ultimately brain and meningeal biopsy must be done to confirm a diagnostic suspicion.
   d. Biopsy is important to differentiate isolated CNS vasculitis from intravascular lymphoma or other mimicking disorders.
   e. Treatment of vasculitis usually requires immune suppression with corticosteroids. Primary CNS and some types of systemic vasculitis usually require more potent immune suppression with cyclophosphamide or other agents.

Thrombophilic States
1. The two most important thrombophilic states to consider when evaluating patients with arterial stroke are the thrombophilia of malignancy and the antiphospholipid antibody syndrome.
   a. Cancer, especially adenocarcinomas of the gastrointestinal tract, lungs, or breast, may induce a state of hypercoagulability characterized by activation of the thrombin generation and fibrinolytic systems. Patients may show laboratory evidence of this (elevated D-dimer and fibrin degradation products), however frank disseminated intravascular coagulation with consumption of fibrinogen, platelets, and clotting factors with prolongation of INR, aPTT, and thrombin time is uncommon.
   b. Strokes in such patients may be due to *in situ* thrombosis in cerebral vessels, embolization from cardiac lesions such as marantic endocarditis, or embolization from a venous source through a patent foramen ovale or other arteriovenous (AV) shunt. Anticoagulation may reduce thrombotic risk in such patients until more definitive therapy for the cancer can be given.
2. The major features of the antiphospholipid antibody syndrome are recurrent venous or arterial thrombotic events, thrombocytopenia, and, in women, recurrent second-trimester miscarriages. Other symptoms and signs are migraines, livedo reticularis, and rarely, chorea. Laboratory evidence is most commonly elevation of anticardiolipin antibodies at high titers [immunoglobulin G (IgG), IgM, or IgA], anti-β_2-glycoprotein antibodies, evidence of a circulating (lupus) anticoagulant on various functional tests of coagulation (e.g., Russell viper venom, modified aPTT, mixing study, platelet neutralization test for phospholipids dependence), thrombocytopenia, and positive antinuclear antibody (ANA), and false-positive rapid plasma reagin (RPR). Stroke is the most common manifestation of arterial thrombosis, and there is a tendency for a single patient to have recurrences in the same vascular bed (arterial or venous) as prior events. There is retrospective evidence that anticoagulation with warfarin at INR ranges above 2.6 to 3.0 is the most effective preventive therapy.
3. Other causes of thrombophilia include inherited and acquired deficiency or dysfunction of antithrombin III, protein C, and protein S, and factor V Leiden mutation, acquired activated protein C resistance, and the prothrombin *20210A* mutation. These states have been clearly linked to venous thrombosis. The association with arterial events such as stroke has been harder to confirm. Some studies of young stroke populations have found a statistical association. When these disorders are implicated by association with otherwise unexplained strokes and TIAs, then it is

reasonable to consider long-term antiplatelet therapy or anticoagulation; however, no systematic study of this issue guides clinical choice.

CEREBRAL VENOUS SINUS THROMBOSIS

BACKGROUND

Stroke may also occur because of occlusion of cerebral venous sinuses by thrombus. Although much less common than arterial occlusion, this is an important mechanism of stroke to keep in mind, especially in late pregnancy, the postpartum period, and in other thrombophilic states.

PATHOPHYSIOLOGY

Most venous sinus thromboses occur in the context of hypercoagulability, such as pregnancy or the puerperium, cancer, and the thrombophilias listed above (see Treatment, Thrombophilic States section of Arterial Ischemic Stroke and Transient Ischemic Attack). Trauma, adjacent tumor or inflammation, dural arteriovenous fistulas, or anatomic abnormalities may contribute in some cases. The infarcts that ensue are thought to be caused by the congestion of capillary blood flow that results from elevated venous pressures. Hemorrhagic conversion is common in venous infarcts.

PROGNOSIS

As with arterial strokes, prognosis depends on the size, location, and degree of hemorrhage, but venous strokes are typically less complete within the territory of the infarct, and in many cases, neurologic recovery is excellent.

DIAGNOSIS

History and Examination

As with arterial strokes, focal neurologic symptoms and signs are the most prominent findings. Women in late pregnancy or the postpartum period or patients with other evidence of thrombophilic states should raise suspicion. Bilateral signs, seizures, headache, papilledema, and other evidence of elevated ICP should all raise suspicion as well. Some patients with the pseudotumor cerebri syndrome alone have underlying venous sinus thrombosis.

Neuroimaging

1. Head CT may show hyperdensity in the region of a thrombosed venous sinus or at the site of a thrombosed cortical vein. With contrast, the surrounding dural wall of the superior sagittal sinus will enhance while the area of the thrombosis will not, creating the empty delta sign. In addition, a venous infarction may be visualized as hypodensity, swelling, or hemorrhage in the region of the affected sinuses, for example parasagittal (superior sinus thrombosis) or in the temporal lobe (transverse sinus thrombosis). These infarcts may cross boundaries of typical arterial territories providing a clue that they are due to venous occlusion. CT venography may show absence of contrast filling in thrombosed sinuses.
2. MRI may show signal intensities consistent with acute (isointense on T_1- and hypointense on T_2-weighted images) or subacute (bright on T_1- and T_2-weighted

images) thrombosis as well as features of venous infarction, often with hemorrhagic conversion. MR venography may show absence of flow in thrombosed sinuses.
3. Angiography is more specific than MR or CT venography, but where these are available, it is usually not needed to establish a diagnosis.

Lumbar Puncture

Findings on lumbar puncture (LP) are nonspecific. Cerebrospinal fluid pressure may be elevated. Protein may be elevated, there may be increased numbers of red and white blood cells.

Laboratory Tests

Laboratory tests may help reveal evidence of underlying thrombophilia, infection, or inflammation (see Thrombophilic States, above).

TREATMENT

1. Anticoagulation:
   a. Anticoagulation with heparin is indicated for most cases of venous sinus thrombosis. Patients with and patients without hemorrhage into venous infarcts appear to benefit. Duration of chronic anticoagulation with warfarin is not standardized, and decisions should be based on the reversibility of the underlying cause and the anatomic issues of recanalization and collateral flow.
2. Transvenous cannulation of the affected sinus with catheter-directed thrombolysis and mechanical removal of thrombus may be indicated when patients have severe deficits from involvement of the deep venous system or extensive involvement of superficial sinuses; however, there are no adequate controlled data to allow a general recommendation of this therapy.

HEMORRHAGIC STROKE

BACKGROUND

Intracranial hemorrhage accounts for about 15% of strokes. Consensus guidelines for diagnosis and management are available from the American Stroke Association.

PATHOPHYSIOLOGY

There are many causes of intracranial hemorrhage. Epidural and subdural hematomas are not usually classified as strokes, and they are not discussed here.
1. Catastrophic SAH is usually caused by rupture of an intracranial saccular aneurysm.
2. Intraparenchymal hemorrhage is most commonly due to long-standing hypertension. Such hypertensive hemorrhages are typically located in the basal ganglia, thalamus, pons, or cerebellum.
3. Lobar hemorrhages in elderly patients are often the outcome of underlying amyloid angiopathy.
4. Various cerebral vascular malformations may hemorrhage. These include arteriovenous malformations, dural arteriovenous fistulas, and cavernous malformations. Venous malformations and capillary telangiectasias rarely cause hemorrhage.

5. Coagulopathies, such as those from warfarin or thrombocytopenia in various hematologic and malignant disorders, may cause hemorrhages that are often multifocal.
6. Tumors may spontaneously hemorrhage, especially glioblastoma multiforme, oligodendrogliomas, and certain metastatic tumors, such as lung, melanoma, renal cell carcinoma, and choriocarcinoma.
7. Hematomas may occur in the context of drug abuse, especially of stimulants, such as cocaine, which cause marked increases in BP and, rarely, vasculitis.

PROGNOSIS

Prognosis varies greatly with the site and size of the hemorrhage and with the occurrence and management of complications.

DIAGNOSIS

1. SAH:
   a. All patients with thunderclap headache should be evaluated for possible SAH. In addition to the sudden severe headache, patients typically have stiff neck, photophobia, nausea, and vomiting, and they may have sudden loss of consciousness, which may be transient. The examiner should seek nuchal rigidity, subhyaloid retinal hemorrhages, and subtle neurologic deficits, especially cranial neuropathies.
   b. Sensitivity of head CT depends on the size of the SAH and the duration of time since its occurrence (Table 12-5). Yet, these estimates may be high, because in some studies, subtle changes were interpreted as positive, and no patients had mild headaches felt to be small warning leaks.
   c. Because a small but significant number of cases may be missed by CT, LP should be done to eliminate the diagnosis definitively. The findings of SAH on LP are red blood cells (RBCs) and xanthochromia. Although many ways to differentiate traumatic LP from true SAH have been proposed, such as declining number of RBCs, the opinion of the physician performing the LP, RBC crenation, and cytology for erythrophages, none of these methods is reliable.
   d. Xanthochromia is nearly 100% sensitive for up to 2 weeks, but only if spectrophotometry is used for detection. Also, it may take several hours for xanthochromia to develop.
   e. When the clinical context suggests SAH and CT and LP are not definitive, angiography should be done to look for an aneurysm. Patients should be classified by the Hunt and Hess grading system to facilitate therapeutic decisions (Table 12-6). After stabilization, patients should undergo four-vessel angiography to look for intracranial aneurysms.

TABLE 12-5. SENSITIVITY OF COMPUTED TOMOGRAPHY IN SUBARACHNOID HEMORRHAGE

Time after SAH of CT	Positive CT, %
2 d	96
5 d	85
1 wk	50
2 wk	30
3 wk	Almost nil

SAH, subarachnoid hemorrhage; CT, computed tomography.
From van Gijn J, van Dongen KJ. The time course of aneurysmal haemorrhage on computed tomograms. *Neuroradiology* 1982;23:153–156, with permission.

TABLE 12-6. HUNT AND HESS CLINICAL CLASSIFICATION OF PATIENTS WITH SUBARACHNOID HEMORRHAGE ACCORDING TO SURGICAL RISK

Grade I—Asymptomatic or minimal headache and slight nuchal rigidity
Grade II—Moderate to severe headache, nuchal rigidity, no neurologic deficit except cranial nerve palsies
Grade III—Drowsiness; confusion, mild focal deficit
Grade IV—Stupor, moderate or severe hemiparesis, possibly early decerebrate rigidity, vegetative disturbances
Grade V—Deep coma, decerebrate rigidity, moribund appearance
Grade VI—Dead

From Hunt WE, Hess RM. Surgical risk as related to time of intervention in the repair of intracranial aneurysms. *J Neurosurg* 1968;28:14–20, with permission.

2. Intraparenchymal hemorrhage:
   a. Intraparenchymal hemorrhage is reliably identified as a density on head CT and as a signal that varies in intensity with time on MRI.
   b. Gradient-echo MRI sequences are most sensitive for the residual hemosiderin of small old hemorrhages, and they may be useful in revealing amyloid angiopathy when it is suspected.
   c. Many patients with presumed amyloid angiopathy do not have evidence of multiple old hemorrhages on gradient-echo sequences.
   d. For classification and prognosis, the volume of the hemorrhage can be estimated by the formula $d^1 + d^2 + d^3/2$.*
   e. In addition to noting the size and location of the hemorrhage, the examiner should scrutinize the images for evidence of intraventricular extension, edema, midline shift, uncal, tonsillar, and transfalcine herniation, underlying vascular lesions, primary or secondary infarction, or tumor.
   f. When CT and MRI do not provide an adequate explanation of the cause of the hemorrhage and the patient is believed to be a surgical candidate, contrast angiography should be considered.

TREATMENT

General Principles

(See also Chapter 1, Neurologic Critical Care)
1. For all patients with intracranial hemorrhage, PT (INR), aPTT, and platelets should be checked. Prolonged PT and aPTT should be corrected immediately with fresh-frozen plasma. Two to six units are commonly needed, and adequate correction should be documented with repeated coagulation studies. Vitamin K is given to provide more prolonged correction of INR elevations. Vitamin K, 2 to 10 mg, may be given subcutaneously. IV administration of 0.5 to 2 mg is preferred for correction that is more rapid. The IV infusion rate should be less than 1 mg/min. Subcutaneous doses may be repeated over several days. When INR is elevated due to therapeutic warfarin, and the hemorrhage is mild enough and indication for warfarin strong enough that early reinstitution of anticoagulation is anticipated, low doses of vitamin K are advised to avoid later resistance to warfarin. Defibrinogenation is best corrected with cryoprecipitate. Heparin's effect is reversed with protamine sulfate 10 to 50 mg IV over 1 to 3 minutes (1.0–1.5 mg/1,000 U heparin, if given within 30 minutes of cessation of heparin infusion; 0.5 mg/1,000 U heparin, if given between 30 and 45 minutes of cessation of heparin infusion. The maximum dose is 100 mg; 50 mg in 10 minutes.) Patients receiving protamine sulfate should be observed closely for signs of hypersensitivity. Acutely, thrombocytopenia

*Volume of ellipse equals $4\pi/3$ $(d^1/2 + d^2/2 + d^3/2)$, hence, by simplification, approximately $d^1 + d^2 + d^3/2$.

(less than $100 \times 10^3/\mu L$) should be corrected with transfusion of platelets. More modest goals for ongoing correction of platelets may be necessary in disorders resistant to platelet transfusion.

2. Many patients with intracranial hemorrhage will have elevated BP. Those with SAH should have their BP normalized using IV agents such as labetalol, esmolol, or sodium nitroprusside.

   a. Labetalol is given by intermittent dosing (10–20 mg IV over 2 minutes; then 40–80 mg IV every 10 minutes until desired BP is achieved or 300 mg has been given; then repeat effective dose every 6–8 hours) or by continuous infusion (1–8 mg/min). Care should be taken to avoid excessive bradycardia. It should be converted to oral dosages of 200 to 400 mg every 6 to 12 hours.

   b. Esmolol is given as a loading dosage of 20 to 30 mg/min IV over 1 minute followed by a maintenance dosage starting at 2 to 12 mg/min and increasing by 2 to 3 mg/min every 10 minutes until desired BP is achieved (maximum dosage, 20 μg/min or 300 μg/kg/min).

   c. Sodium nitroprusside is given as a continuous infusion at 0.25 to 10 μg/kg/min. The initial dose should be low, to avoid the excessive abrupt lowering that some patients experience when the drug is started. Cyanide toxicity can occur with rapid and prolonged infusion. Metabolic acidosis, elevated lactate levels and lactate/pyruvate ratios, and increased mixed venous oxygen content suggest clinical toxicity. Cyanide levels increase with increasing infusion rate, and sustained infusion rates of more than 4 μg/kg/min risk toxicity. Symptoms of toxicity emerge at blood cyanide levels of 0.05 to 0.1 mg/dL. Thiocyanate levels vary with the cumulative dose. Toxic levels are not well established. Levels should remain below 1.75 μmol/L. Although levels may be useful to confirm diagnostic suspicion, diagnosis and a decision to proceed with therapy should be based on history of exposure and clinical findings.

   d. Hydralazine may be given IV 10 to 20 mg every 4 to 6 hours.

   e. Enaloprilat may be given IV 0.625 to 1.2 mg every 6 hours.

3. Patients with intraparenchymal hemorrhage should have their BP controlled without excessive reduction. Definitive optimal values have not been established, but systolic BPs less than 140 to 150 mm Hg are probably best, while avoiding problems of compromised CBF. Where elevated ICP is suspected, ICP monitoring allows measurement of the cerebral perfusion pressure (cerebral perfusion pressure = MAP − ICP). When the ICP is monitored, the cerebral perfusion pressure should be kept above 70 mm Hg. This is ideally achieved by lowering ICP to normal values with medical or surgical measures, but at times, it may require support of the MAP with vasopressors, such as

   a. Phenylephrine 2 to 10 μg/kg/min

   b. Dopamine 2 to 10 μg/kg/min, or

   c. Norepinephrine beginning at 0.05 to 0.2 μg/kg/min and titrating to the desired effect.

Subarachnoid Hemorrhage

General Care

1. All patients with SAH should have immediate neurosurgical consultation for consideration of early angiography and early aneurysm repair by open clipping or intraarterial coiling. Abnormalities of coagulation and platelets should be corrected promptly as described above. Patients should be monitored in an intensive care unit with nurses skilled in neurologic assessment and management. Patients should be placed on bed rest in a quiet room with adequate sensory stimulation, such as reading, radio, or family visitors. Frequent neurologic examinations should be done looking for changes in level of consciousness and new focal signs.

2. Adequate analgesics should be given, including

   a. Acetaminophen 325 to 1,000 mg,

   b. Oxycodone 5 to 10 mg every 4 hours

   c. Fentanyl 50 to 150 μg every 1 to 2 hours

   d. Morphine 1 to 20 mg every 2 to 3 hours

Fentanyl and morphine may be given by continuous infusion by dividing the total 24-hour dose needed by 24 to get the approximate infusion rate per hour. Mild sedation with benzodiazepines may be needed. Prophylactic anticonvulsants (e.g., phenytoin 20 mg/kg loading and 300 mg or more daily, as needed to maintain therapeutic levels) are given, because an early seizure may increase the risk of rebleeding. Stool softeners minimize straining that will transiently elevate ICP.

3. Adequate hydration should be given with normal saline. Serum sodium and urine volume should be monitored, since patients may develop renal salt wasting, syndrome of inappropriate secretion of antidiuretic hormone, or diabetes insipidus. Hyponatremia is common. There is evidence of both inappropriate secretion of antidiuretic hormone (ADH) with inadequate free water clearance as well as renal wasting of sodium, probably stimulated by atrial natriuretic factor or other plasma factors present in the setting of cerebral disease. Because it may be difficult to distinguish these two causes of hyponatremia clinically, because disordered ADH regulation and renal salt wasting may occur simultaneously, and because volume contraction and dehydration may increase the risk of cerebral vasospasm, hyponatremia in the setting of SAH should be treated with adequate sodium replacement and volume replacement and maintenance. Free water should be restricted.

Surgical Therapy

1. The definitive therapy of aneurysmal SAH is control of the ruptured aneurysm. As soon as the patient is stable, four-vessel angiography should be performed to define the ruptured aneurysm and any other aneurysms. If the ruptured aneurysm is surgically accessible and the patient is stable enough to undergo craniotomy, open surgical clipping of the aneurysm is the preferred therapy. When the aneurysm is not accessible or when other medical or neurologic issues contraindicate surgical clipping, thrombosis of the aneurysm with transarterial placement of coils may be done. Unruptured aneurysms may be treated at the time of the initial surgery or at a later date on the basis of surgical principles.

2. Other indications for which surgical intervention is indicated are mass effect from large hematomas requiring early surgical decompression and hydrocephalus that requires ventricular drainage. In most cases, hydrocephalus will resolve after the acute phase of illness, although some patients will need ventriculoperitoneal shunting for long-term drainage.

Cerebral Vasospasm

1. Nimodipine 60 mg is given by mouth or by nasogastric tube every 4 hours for 21 days to lower the risk of vasospasm.

2. Adequate hydration should be given with normal saline.

3. TCD is a safe and reliable study to follow up patients for evidence of cerebral vasospasm. A baseline study of the circle of Willis vessels should be done shortly after admission. Then, serial studies can be done during the period of risk in the first 2 to 3 weeks after hemorrhage. Volume expansion with colloid solutions such as albumin may be given.

4. After surgical control of the aneurysm has been achieved, then induced hypertension may minimize blood flow compromise in the setting of vasospasm. This may be achieved with volume expansion and vasopressor agents, such as phenylephrine ($10–1,000$ μg/min titrated to the desired effect). Clinical response will determine the level of elevation needed, usually systolic BP of 160 to 200 mm Hg adjusted to eliminate ischemic signs.

5. If patients have clinical and TCD evidence of persistent ischemia from vasospasm despite medical therapy, angiography should be done to confirm suspected vasospasm. Intraarterial therapy of refractory vasospasm with papaverine and balloon angioplasty should follow institutional protocols.

Intraparenchymal Hemorrhage

The major issues of therapy in patients with intracerebral hemorrhages are

1. Prevention of continued hemorrhage by early correction of coagulation and platelet abnormalities (see Treatment, General Principles, earlier),
2. Early control of elevated BP (see Treatment, General Principles, earlier),
3. Identification and control of urgent surgical issues such as threatening mass effect, intracranial hypertension (see Chapter 1, Neurologic Critical Care), and hydrocephalus, and ultimately
4. Definitive diagnosis of the cause of the hemorrhage and definitive treatment of the underlying cause.

BIBLIOGRAPHY

Acute Ischemic Stroke and Transient Ischemic Attack

Adams HP, Adams RJ, Brott T, et al. Guidelines for the early management of patients with ischemic stroke: a scientific statement from the Stroke Council of the American Stroke Association. *Stroke* 2003;34:1056–1083.

Adams HP, Brott TG, Crowell RM. Guidelines for the management of patients with acute ischemic stroke: a statement for healthcare professionals from a special writing group of the Stroke Council, American Heart Association. *Stroke* 1994;25:1901–1914.

Adams HP, Brott TG, Furlan AJ, et al. Guidelines for thrombolytic therapy for acute stroke: a supplement to the guidelines for the management of patients with acute ischemic stroke: a statement for healthcare professionals from a special writing group of the Stroke Council, American Heart Association. *Stroke* 1996;27:1711–1718.

American Diabetes Association. Management of dyslipidemia in adults with diabetes. *Diabetes Care* 2003;26[Suppl 1]:S83–S86.

American Diabetes Association. Treatment of hypertension in adults with diabetes. *Diabetes Care* 2003;26[Suppl 1]:S80–S82.

Antiplatelet Trialists; Collaboration. Secondary prevention of vascular disease by prolonged antiplatelet treatment. *Br Med J* 1988;296:320–331.

Barnett HJM, Taylor DW, Eliasziw M, et al. Benefit of carotid endarterectomy in patients with symptomatic moderate or severe stenosis. *N Engl J Med* 1998;339:1415–1425.

CAST (Chinese Acute Stroke Trial) Collaborative Group. CAST: randomized placebo-controlled trial of early aspirin use in 20,000 patients with acute ischaemic stroke. *Lancet* 1997;349:1641–1649.

Dagenais GR, Yusuf S, Bourassa MG, et al. Effects of ramipril on coronary events in high-risk persons: results of the Heart Outcomes Prevention Evaluation Study. *Circulation* 2001;104:522–526.

Executive Committee for the Asymptomatic Carotid Atherosclerosis Study. Endarterectomy for asymptomatic carotid artery stenosis. *JAMA* 1995;273:1421–1428.

Furlan A, Higashida R, Wechsler L, et al. Intra-arterial prourokinase for acute ischemic stroke: the PROACT II Study: a randomized controlled trial. *JAMA* 1999;282:2003–2011.

International Stroke Trial Collaborative Group. The International Stroke Trial (IST): a randomized trial of aspirin, subcutaneous heparin, both, or neither among 19,435 patients with acute ischemic stroke. *Lancet* 1997;349:1569–1581.

Johnston SC. Transient ischemic attacks. *N Engl J Med* 2002;347:1687–1692.

Khamashta MA, Cuadrado MJ, Mujic F, et al. The management of thrombosis in the antiphospholipid-antibody syndrome. *N Engl J Med* 1995;332:993–997.

Kopecky SL, Gersh BJ, McGoon MD, et al. The natural history of lone atrial fibrillation: a population-based study over three decades. *N Engl J Med* 1987;317:669–674.

Loh E, Sutton MSJ, Wun C-CC, et al. Ventricular dysfunction and the risk of stroke after myocardial infarction. *N Engl J Med* 1997;336:251–257.

Long-Term Intervention with Pravastatin in Ischaemic Disease (LIPID) Study Group. Prevention of cardiovascular events and death with pravastatin in patients with coronary heart disease and a broad range of initial cholesterol levels. *N Engl J Med* 1988;339:1349–1357.

Mas JL, Arquizan C, Lamy C, et al. Recurrent cerebrovascular events associated with patent foramen ovale, atrial septal aneurysm, or both. *N Engl J Med* 2001;345:1740–1746.

Moore PM. Diagnosis and management of isolated angiitis of the central nervous system. *Neurology* 1989;39:167–173.

National Institute of Neurological Disorders and Stroke rt-PA Stroke Study Group. Tissue plasminogen activator for acute ischemic stroke. *N Engl J Med* 1995; 333:1581–1587.

North American Symptomatic Carotid Endarterectomy Trial Collaborators. Beneficial effect of carotid endarterectomy in symptomatic patients with high-grade carotid stenosis. *N Engl J Med* 1991;325:445–453.

Powers WJ. Acute hypertension after stroke: the scientific basis for treatment decisions. *Neurology* 1993;43:461–467.

Powers WJ. Oral anticoagulation therapy for the prevention of stroke. *N Engl J Med* 2001;345:1493–1495.

Rosove MH, Brewer PMC. Antiphospholipid thrombosis: clinical course after the first thrombotic event in 70 patients. *Ann Intern Med* 1992;117:303–308.

Stein PD, Alpert JS, Dalen JE, et al. Antithrombotic therapy in patients with mechanical and biological prosthetic heart valves. *Chest* 1998;114:602S–610S.

Stroke Prevention in Atrial Fibrillation Investigators. Stroke Prevention in Atrial Fibrillation Study: final results. *Circulation* 1991;84:527–539.

Stroke prevention in Atrial Fibrillation Investigators. Warfarin versus aspirin for prevention of thromboembolism in atrial fibrillation: Stroke Prevention in Atrial Fibrillation II Study. *Lancet* 1994;343:687–691.

Task Force on Practice Guidelines (Committee on Management of Patients with Valvular Heart Disease. Guidelines for the management of patients with valvular disease. *Circulation* 1998;98:1949–1984.

Veterans Affairs Stroke Prevention in Nonrheumatic Atrial Fibrillation Investigators. Warfarin in the prevention of stroke associated with nonrheumatic atrial fibrillation. *N Engl J Med* 1992;327:1406–1412.

Wolf PA, Clagett GP, Easton JD, et al. Preventing ischemic stroke in patients with prior stroke and transient ischemic attack: a statement for healthcare professionals from the Stroke Council of the American Heart Association. *Stroke* 1999;30:1991–1994.

Cerebral Venous Sinus Thrombosis

Einhäupl KM, Villringer A, Meister W, et al. Heparin treatment in sinus venous thrombosis. *Lancet* 1991;338:597–600.

Hemorrhagic Stroke

Allen GS, Ahn HS, Preziosi TJ, et al. Cerebral arterial spasm—a controlled trial of nimodipine in patients with subarachnoid hemorrhage. *N Engl J Med* 1983;308:619–624.

Broderick JP, Adams HP, Barsan W, et al. Guidelines for the management of spontaneous intracerebral hemorrhage: a statement for Healthcare professionals from a writing group of the Stroke Council, American Heart Association. *Stroke* 1999;30:905–915.

van Gijn J, van Dongen KJ. The time course of aneurysmal haemorrhage on computed tomograms. *Neuroradiology* 1982;23:153–156.

Wolf PA, Cobb JL, D'Agostino. Epidemiology of stroke. In: Barnett HJM, et al., eds. *Stroke: pathophysiology, diagnosis, and management.* New York: Churchill Livingstone, 1992:6.

13. MOVEMENT DISORDERS

Lewis R. Sudarsky

PARKINSON DISEASE AND RELATED DISORDERS

BACKGROUND

1. Parkinson disease (PD) was described in 1817 by James Parkinson, when he observed the characteristic features of slowness, rigidity, rest tremor, and shuffling gait.
2. It is primarily a motor control disorder, although cognitive changes may develop in some patients over time.
3. PD is the second most common neurodegenerative disorder, affecting a half million people in the United States.
4. The disease is age related; it occurs infrequently before age 40.
5. Prevalence is roughly 1% at age 65 and 3.5% at age 85.
6. It is the most frequent reason for referral to a movement disorder specialist.

PATHOPHYSIOLOGY

1. PD results from loss of the dopamine innervation of the basal ganglia. Pathology shows deficiency of pigmented cells in the pars compacta of the substantia nigra; these cells contain neuromelanin and produce neurotransmitter dopamine. The dopamine projections to the caudate and putamen facilitate movement. When cell loss exceeds 60%, there is a critical deficiency of dopamine in the forebrain, resulting in motor symptoms.
2. The cause of the disease is not known.
   a. Some degenerating nigral neurons contain inclusions (Lewy bodies), which accumulate alpha synuclein protein and ubiquitin.
   b. While typical PD with onset after age 50 is not inherited, there are single gene mutations that cause a form of Parkinson. These genetic PD syndromes often have younger onset. Examples include the alpha synuclein mutations, and mutations of the parkin gene on chromosome 6. Studies of the hereditary forms of PD suggest there may be abnormalities in the ubiquitin proteolytic pathway, leading to protein aggregation.
   c. Toxin exposure (MPTP, rotenone) and oxidant stress have also been implicated in the pathogenesis.

PROGNOSIS

1. Dopamine cell loss in PD is progressive, beginning several years before clinical symptoms and continuing over 15 years or longer.
   a. The rate of progression is variable, and mobility can be supported with dopamine replacement therapy.
   b. Motor fluctuations develop in 40% to 50% of patients on levodopa at 5 years, 75% to 80% at 10 years. Some patients have accumulated substantial disability at 10 years, while others retain a stable levodopa response, good balance, and cognitive function.
   c. Dementia (10%–30%) and falls sometimes emerge as treatment-limiting issues in patients with longstanding PD.
2. The progression of the disease can be followed using clinical measures, such as the unified Parkinson disease rating scale (UPDRS, available at www.wemove.org), or through imaging measures of dopamine cell loss such as 18F-fluorodopa positive

emission tomography (PET) or beta-CIT single photon emission computed tomography (SPECT). The dopamine cells do not create a visible footprint on magnetic resonance imaging (MRI).

DIAGNOSIS

1. Diagnosis is based on clinical grounds; there are no laboratory tests. Onset is typically asymmetric. The cardinal clinical features are:
   a. Tremor at rest: typically a pill-rolling tremor of the hands, sometimes affecting the lower limbs or jaw.
   b. Bradykinesia: slowness of movement, difficulty initiating movement. This is the major source of disability, sometimes described by the patient as weakness or heaviness.
   c. Rigidity with cogwheeling: a physical sign, observed as the patient is passively moved. Cogwheeling is most easily appreciated at the wrist and neck.
   d. Flexed posture/shuffling gait: A flexed posture is characteristic of PD. Shuffling gait is also typical, but the least specific feature in differential diagnosis.
2. The most typical case begins asymmetrically in the limbs with a rest tremor. A diagnosis of PD is also based on a number of more impressionistic findings: loss of facial expression, hypophonic dysarthria, drooling, micrographia.
3. There is a degree of imprecision in clinical diagnosis. Ten percent to 15% of patients in a PD clinic will turn out to have a related disorder. Imbalance and falls occur later, after several years in PD; early occurrence should suggest an alternate diagnosis. Failure to respond to levodopa often indicates another diagnosis. The differential diagnosis of PD is reviewed in Table 13-1.
4. Several clues aid in the recognition of related neurodegenerative disorders:
   a. Multiple system atrophy (MSA):
      1) Manifestations:
         a) Progressive ataxia
         b) Signs of autonomic failure (prominent orthostatic hypotension, urogenital dysfunction)
      2) MSA is a synucleinopathy, with pathology involving the nigrostriatal system, the cerebellum, and the autonomic nervous system. It is a more aggressive disease with progression to death in 5 to 10 years, and a partial or waning response to dopaminergic treatment. Consensus criteria for a diagnosis of MSA are reviewed in Table 13-2.
   b. Diffuse Lewy body disease:
      1) Manifestations:
         a) Dementia, behavioral disorders
         b) Sleep disturbance
      2) Diffuse Lewy body disease is part of the PD spectrum, with pathology extending to other brainstem areas and neocortex.
   c. Progressive supranuclear palsy (PSP):
      1) Manifestations:
         a) Early imbalance or falls
         b) Axial dystonia
         c) Oculomotor abnormalities (particularly failure of conjugate downward gaze).
      2) In PSP, there is neurodegeneration of structures in the upper brainstem and diencephalon, with accumulation of neurfibrillary tau proteins.
   d. Corticobasal degeneration:
      1) Manifestations:
         a) Apraxia
         b) Cortical sensory loss
         c) "Alien limb" movements
      2) Corticobasal degeneration is also a tauopathy, with asymmetric onset. There is often focal cerebral volume loss on imaging.
5. Occasional patients will have an axial parkinsonian syndrome and gait disorder (lower body PD) related to cerebrovascular small-vessel disease. Secondary

TABLE 13-1. DIFFERENTIAL DIAGNOSIS OF PARKINSON DISEASE

Neurodegenerative disorders with atypical parkinsonism
  Progressive supranuclear palsy
  Multiple-system atrophy
    Shy–Drager syndrome
    Striatonigral degeneration
    Olivopontocerebellar atrophy
  Diffuse Lewy body disease
  Corticobasal degeneration
  Frontotemporal dementia with parkinsonism
  Alzheimer Parkinson overlap syndrome
  Parkinson–amyotrophic lateral sclerosis–dementia of Guam
  Huntington disease: rigid variant
  Hallervorden–Spatz disease
  Pure akinesia syndrome
  Primary progressive freezing gait

Secondary parkinsonism
  Toxic
    MPTP (methyl-4-phenyl-tetrahydropyridine)
    Manganese
    Carbon monoxide
  Drug-induced
    Neuroleptic drugs
    Metaclopramide, prochlorperazine
    Reserpine
  Vascular disease ("arteriosclerotic parkinsonism")
    Basal ganglia lacunes
    Binswanger disease
  Hydrocephalus
  Trauma
  Tumor
  Chronic hepatocerebral degeneration
  Wilson disease
  Infectious
    Postencephalitic parkinsonism
    Creutzfeldt–Jakob disease
    HIV/AIDS

parkinsonism from neuroleptic exposure (drug-induced parkinsonism) should always be considered as it is a treatable disorder. Drugs such as metoclopramide (Reglan), prochlorperazine (Compazine), and the atypical antipsychotics should not be overlooked. Neuroleptic drugs are highly tissue bound, and motor signs can persist 4 to 12 weeks after these drugs have been discontinued. Toxin-induced PD related to manganese, carbon monoxide, or MPTP should be considered when environmental exposures have occurred.

TREATMENT

We consider the therapy in three parts: 1) initial therapy of PD includes the initiation of dopaminergic medication and the "honeymoon period," lasting 3–6 years; 2) management of more advanced disease, including motor fluctuations and dyskinesias; and 3) management of mental status change. There is no algorithm, treatment should always be individualized.

Initial Therapy of Parkinson Disease

1. After confirmation of diagnosis, the next consideration is whether the patient has disability sufficient to warrant some form of dopamine replacement. Dopamine

TABLE 13-2. CONSENSUS CRITERIA FOR DIAGNOSIS OF MULTIPLE-SYSTEM ATROPHY

I. Autonomic and urinary dysfunction
  A. Autonomic and urinary features
    1. Orthostatic hypotension (20 mm Hg systolic and 10 mm Hg diastolic)
    2. Urinary incontinence or incomplete bladder emptying
  B. Criteria for autonomic failure or urinary dysfunction in MSA:
    Orthostatic fall in BP (by 30 mm Hg systolic or 15 mm Hg diastolic) or urinary incotinence (persistent, involuntary partial or total bladder emptying, accompanied by erectile dysfunction in men) or both
II. Parkinsonism
  A. Parkinsonian features
    1. Bradykinesia
    2. Rigidity
    3. Postural instability
    4. Tremor
  B. Criterion for parkinsonism in MSA:
    Bradykinesia plus at least one of items 2–4
III. Cerebellar dysfunction
  A. Cerebellar features
    1. Gait ataxia
    2. Ataxic dysarthria
    3. Limb ataxia
    4. Sustained gaze-evoked nystagmus
  B. Criterion for cerebellar dysfunction in MSA:
    Gait ataxia plus at least one of items 2–4

Possible MSA: one criterion plus two features from separate other domains. When the criterion is parkinsonism, a poor levodopa response qualifies as one feature.
Probable MSA: criterion for autonomic failure/urinary dysfunction plus poorly levodopa-responsive parkinsonism or cerebellar dysfunction
Definite MSA: pathologically confirmed by the presence of high-density glial cytoplasmic inclusions in association with a combination of degenerative changes in the nigrostriatal and olivopontocerebellar pathways

BP, blood pressure; MSA, multiple-system atrophy

replacement therapy is usually reserved for patients who have some difficulty in daily activities, difficulty with walking, or patients whose employment is compromised.

2. For patients with newly diagnosed PD, not yet requiring dopamine replacement, there is a range of therapeutic options:
  a. Selegiline: This drug is a monoamine oxidase B enzyme inhibitor, with mild symptomatic benefits in early PD. It can elevate mood and help with fatigue. In one large clinical trial, selegiline delayed the introduction of levodopa by a year. Most experts now agree that there are no direct disease-modifying effects (neuroprotective effects) of selegiline on dopamine cell loss. Five milligrams are usually sufficient, given once a day in the morning. No special diet is required at doses under 15 mg. Infrequent side effects include insomnia, nausea, and hypotension. The drug is not well tolerated by confused patients, and adverse interactions have been described with meperidine and selective serotonin reuptake inhibitor (SSRI) antidepressants.
  b. Amantadine: This older drug is an N-methyl D-aspartate (NMDA) glutamate receptor antagonist. It is often helpful, particularly with tremor in early symptomatic patients. In more advanced PD it can help reduce dyskinesia. The dose is 100 to 300 mg; side effects include livido reticularis and hallucination.
  c. Anticholinergic drugs: For younger patients with tremor as the major presenting symptom, trihexyphenidyl [Artane 2 mg three times a day (t.i.d.)], benztropine

[Cogentin 0.5 mg twice a day (b.i.d.)], or ethopropazine (Parsitan 50–100 mg t.i.d.) can be helpful. These drugs can cause or aggravate confusion, and are poorly tolerated in older patients. Other side effects include dry mouth and urinary retention.

   d. Neuroprotective options: There is presently no evidence that any of the drugs retard dopamine cell loss in PD, although several promising drugs are in clinical trials. Coenzyme Q (CoQ)–10 at 1,200 mg/d had some effect on progression of ADL scores in a small pilot study.

3. For patients whose PD has begun to affect their daily activities, and who have a degree of disability as a result, some form of dopamine replacement is indicated. The threshold for dopamine replacement therapy is somewhat subjective, as determined by the doctor and patient. The options include oral precursor loading with a levodopa compound, or the use of a synthetic, direct-acting dopamine agonist. Half of the patients with new PD can be successfully treated with a dopamine agonist as monotherapy for 3 to 5 years. Motor complications may be delayed, a particular advantage for younger patients. Levodopa remains the preferred initial therapy for older patients (older than 75 years), medically fragile patients, and those with cognitive and behavioral problems.

   a. Dopamine agonists (bromocriptine, pergolide, ropinirole, pramipexole):
   1) Advantages:
      a) Motor complications are delayed.
      b) Question of neuroprotection based on preclinical studies.
      c) Better outcome with surrogate markers (imaging) in randomized clinical trials.
   2) Disadvantages:
      a) Greater cost
      b) More adverse events
      c) Somnolence, sudden sleep attacks

   b. Levodopa preparations (sinemet, sinemet CR)
   1) Advantages:
      a) Easier to use, titrate
      b) Superior efficacy
      c) Better tolerated in frail, elderly patients and those with cognitive or behavioral changes
   2) Disadvantage: treatment-emergent side effects (fluctuations, dyskinesias)

   c. Carbidopa/levodopa (Sinemet): Mainstay of therapy for most patients with PD, and the drug with the best therapeutic index. Sinemet is a combination of levodopa with carbidopa, a peripheral DOPA decarboxylase inhibitor. At doses above 75 mg, carbidopa reduces the peripheral decarboxylation of levodopa, increases fourfold the central nervous system (CNS) delivery, and reduces nausea and hypotension. Sinemet comes in 25/100, 10/100, and 25/250 tablets. The usual initial dosage of levodopa is 50 to 100 mg b.i.d. to t.i.d., increasing as required to 300 to 600 mg. Side effects include nausea, hypotension, constipation, confusion and hallucination. No intravenous (IV) preparation is available for surgical patients, but sinemet tablets can be administered crushed by nasogastric (NG) tube.

   d. Sinemet CR (50/200 and 25/100): Carbidopa/levodopa in a polymer matrix designed to produce delayed enteric absorption and a 3- to 4-hour half-life. Absorption is incomplete, and onset of effect often takes 40 to 60 minutes. Some patients find this drug variable or unreliable.

   e. Benserazide/levodopa (Madopar 50/100): An alternative to carbidopa/levodopa, using a different decarboxylase inhibitor. It is sold primarily in Europe.

   f. Bromocriptine: An ergot-derived dopamine agonist used in initial therapy and adjunctive therapy of PD. Used alone, starting dosage should be small (2.5 mg; a half tablet b.i.d.), creeping up over weeks to a therapeutic target of 5 mg t.i.d. Doses as high as 30 to 60 mg may be required for monotherapy after the first year. Side effects include nausea, hypotension, confusion, hallucinations, leg edema, erythromelalgia; rarely pulmonary or retroperitoneal fibrosis.

g. Pergolide: An ergot dopamine agonist used as monotherapy for early PD, as well as adjunctive therapy for more advanced disease. Starting dosage is 0.05 mg t.i.d., titrating slowly to 0.5 mg t.i.d. or above. Side effects include nausea, hypotension, confusion, hallucinations, leg edema, erythromelalgia; rarely pulmonary or retroperitoneal fibrosis.

h. Ropinirole: A newer D2 and D3 dopamine agonist, unrelated to the ergot dopamine agonists. Used for initial monotherapy, or as adjunctive therapy of PD (with levodopa). There is a very large dynamic range, with doses as high as 27 mg/d and above. Initial titration begins at 0.25 mg t.i.d., proceeds slowly over 2 to 3 weeks to achieve 1 to 3 mg t.i.d; 16 mg/d or above often required for monotherapy after the first year. Adverse effects include nausea, somnolence, leg edema, confusion, and hallucinations. This drug is metabolized by CYP1A2 enzymes in the liver, and can interact with other medications that share this pathway. There are case reports of patients on pramipexole and ropinirole falling asleep while driving. Patients should not drive if somnolence is reported.

i. Pramipexole: A newer D2 and D3 dopamine agonist, unrelated to the ergot dopamine agonists. Used for initial monotherapy, or as adjunctive therapy of PD (with levodopa). Initial titration begins at 0.125 mg t.i.d., proceeds slowly over 2 to 3 weeks to achieve 0.5 to 0.75 mg t.i.d.; 3 mg/d or above are often required for monotherapy after the first year. Adverse effects include nausea, somnolence, leg edema, confusion, and hallucinations. There are case reports of patients on pramipexole and ropinirole falling asleep while driving. Patients should not drive if somnolence is reported.

j. Cabergoline: A newer ergot-derived dopamine agonist, which can be used as monotherapy for early PD, although not approved by the Food and Drug Administration (FDA) for this purpose in the United States. This drug has a long half-life, and can be given twice a week. Toxicity is similar to that for pergolide and bromocriptine.

4. For anorexia and nausea in patients on Sinemet, options include extra carbidopa (Lodosyn 25 mg). Patients with nausea often tolerate CR sinemet better, as the drug peaks more gradually. Addition of an antiemetic such as trimethobenzamine (Tigan) 25 mg t.i.d., or domperidone (Motilium) 10 mg prior to each dose, may be necessary to counter gastrointestinal (GI) side effects of dopamine agonists.

Management of More Advanced Disease

1. As PD progresses over time, patients may have difficulty maintaining a stable therapeutic response and independence in daily activities. Motor complications such as wearing off fluctuations, on–off fluctuations, and dyskinesias develop with increasing frequency in patients after 5 to 6 years of levodopa therapy. Gait freezing and falls may also develop over time, regardless of the choice of initial therapy.

2. Levodopa is a medication with a half-life of 90 to 120 minutes. Many patients with long-standing or advanced PD experience a wearing off of drug effect at 2 to 3 hours, as the bioavailability of the drug declines. With more advanced disease, motor fluctuations become more abrupt, erratic, and unpredictable. To extend the effect of levodopa, options include more frequent dosing, use of a longer acting levodopa preparation, and addition of a catechol-O-methyltransferase (COMT) enzyme inhibitor. The other major option is addition of a longer acting dopamine agonist as a second drug.

a. Entacapone (Comtan): Retards the enzymatic degradation of levodopa and dopamine, by a peripheral mechanism. It increases the central nervous system (CNS) delivery of levodopa, and improves the kinetics. (It is ineffective without levodopa.) Dose is 200 mg, given with each dose of levodopa. No dose titration necessary, although older patients often begin with 100 mg/dose. It increases on time in clinical trials by 15%. Side effects include discoloration of the urine, occasional diarrhea. It may increase dyskinesia.

b. Levodopa/carbidopa/entacapone (Stalevo): Newly approved drug that provides entacapone with levodopa/carbidopa in a fixed dose combination: 50/12.5/200,

100/25/200, and 150/37.5/200. It affords extra convenience, and simplifies the pill taking for patients on entacapone.
   c. Tolcapone (Tasmar): COMT inhibitor that is more potent than entacapone in clinical trials, and longer acting. The dosage is 100 to 200 mg t.i.d.. Side effects include serious, occasionally fatal hepatotoxicity, and not infrequent diarrhea. Because of a small number of cases of sudden hepatic failure, an informed consent process is required, and liver function tests (LFTs) must be monitored every 2 weeks for the first year of therapy, every 4 weeks for the next 6 months, and every 8 weeks thereafter.
3. Patients with troublesome dyskinesias will sometimes do better with a dopamine agonist as primary therapy, and a small dose of sinemet as needed to enhance the effect. Pergolide can be pushed to 6 to 10 mg/d, and ropinirole can be pushed to 24 to 30 mg. Supplemental use of amantadine can reduce dyskinesia in many patients. Functional neurosurgery [pallidotomy, deep brain stimulation (DBS)] is an option for patients with difficult motor fluctuations and disabling dyskinesias, and referral to a surgical program is sometimes appropriate. Surgical outcome is not good in patients with mental status changes, and surgery may exacerbate dysarthria.
4. Difficulty with gait initiation or freezing is a particularly frustrating problem. Freezing is sometimes overcome by visual cues, and some patients can use an inverted cane to step over. (A variation in this technique is the use of a laser pointer to provide a visual target for step initiation.) The problem does not always yield to increasing doses of dopaminergic medication, although this should be attempted. Postural instability and recurrent falls may become a problem after 5 to 10 years of PD. Such patients have difficulty standing from a chair and are easily displaced backward. The unfortunate reality is that drug treatment does not always improve balance. As patients are mobilized by medication, they may be at increased risk for falls. Surgery does not reliably improve "on" period gait freezing or falls. The best treatment for this problem is a physical therapy–based intervention to improve axial mobility and balance.
5. A degree of postural hypotension is common in PD because of autonomic involvement and the effects of medications. Decarboxylase inhibitors should be optimized, and selegiline should be discontinued. Some patients require supplemental mineralocorticoid (Florinef, 0.1–0.3 mg/d) and elastic hose. Midodrine (Proamitine, 2.5–5 mg t.i.d.) is occasionally required. Some patients require medication for bladder instability. GI motility is also a common problem in PD, and many require medication for constipation. Drooling results from a reduced rate of swallowing, and not from increased production of secretions. Nonetheless, reducing saliva is sometimes helpful. Options include injection of the parotid with botulinum toxin, or sublingual use of a drop of atropine 1.0% ophthalmic solution b.i.d.

Management of Mental Status Changes

1. Cognitive difficulty, behavioral disturbance, and sleep disorder are not emphasized in classic descriptions of PD, but each poses a common therapeutic problem. Delirium in PD is generally transient and reversible, related to medications. All antiparkinsonian medications have the potential to cause delirium, even transient psychosis. It is best to minimize the use of anticholinergic drugs, selegiline, and dopamine agonists in patients with mental status changes. The preferred strategy in such patients is to avoid polypharmacy and focus on the single drug with the best therapeutic index (carbidopa/levodopa). Use the lowest dose that provides adequate mobility.
   a. Clozapine (Clozaril): Clozapine in low dosage [12.5–75 mg at bedtime (hs)] has been useful when hallucinations, paranoid thinking, and nocturnal agitation persist on minimal levodopa. It can cause daytime sleepiness, but it does not appear to exacerbate motor symptoms of PD (tremor may actually improve). Patients must be monitored with weekly complete blood counts (CBCs) for leukopenia and agranulocytosis. The manufacturer maintains a national registry.
   b. Other atypical antipsychotics (quetiapine 25–150 mg, risperidone 0.5–3 mg, olanzapine 2.5–15 mg) are sometimes used in this context as they do not require

special monitoring. Again low doses are recommended. With time, these drugs accumulate, and motor symptoms may worsen. Sedation is the other major side effect. Older antipsychotics such as haloperidol and chlorpromazine should be avoided in PD.

2. Dementia occurs in 10% to 20% of patients with idiopathic PD. Episodic confusion (even off medication), slowness, and frontal behavioral features are most often observed. Many such patients have a transitional form of Lewy body disease. Cholinesterase inhibitors (donazepil, galantamine, rivastigmine) have a calming effect on these patients, and produce measurable (although modest) improvements in cognitive function.

3. Sleep disturbances are now recognized as an important issue in PD and are more frequent in patients with cognitive impairment. Some patients with PD awake rigid and uncomfortable, unable to turn in bed. These patients may require more nighttime medication. For other patients, disturbances in sleep state control may be aggravated by antiparkinsonian medications. Some patients experience daytime sleepiness, a frequent problem in patients on dopamine agonists; many have insomnia at night. Sleep is fragmented, and there may be reversal of the sleep–wake cycle. Judicious use of sleep medications or sedating antidepressants can sometimes break the cycle. Stimulant drugs like modafinil (Provigil 100–200 mg) methylphenidate (Ritalin 5–10 mg) and caffeine supplements have been used to counteract daytime sleepiness. Driving should be restricted in patients with PD who experience daytime sleepiness. A rapid eye movement (REM) sleep behavior disorder has been described in PD, with active nocturnal movements, such as talking, yelling, punching, kicking, jumping, or running out of bed. This syndrome may be improved by clonazepam (Klonepin 0.5–1.0 mg hs).

HYPERKINETIC MOVEMENT DISORDERS

Hyperkinetic movement disorders are grouped into physiologic descriptive categories: tremor, dystonia, chorea, athetosis, dyskinesia, myoclonus, and tic. In practical reality, the syndromes sometimes overlap. Tardive dyskinesia, for example, may take the form of a dystonia or a complex motor stereotypy resembling a tic. It is often possible to move beyond descriptive recognition to pathophysiologic or molecular diagnosis.

ESSENTIAL TREMOR AND ITS VARIANTS

BACKGROUND

1. Tremor can be defined as a repetitive, involuntary, rhythmic, shaking movement across a fixed axis, often about a joint.
2. Tremor at rest, as occurs in PD, can usually be distinguished from tremor with movement (action tremor). Tremor with movement can further be classified as enhanced physiologic tremor (sometimes amplified by medication or a metabolic disorder), essential tremor, and cerebellar tremor.
3. Medications that cause tremor are listed in Table 13-3.
4. Essential tremor is the commonest movement disorder, with a prevalence of 350/100,000 population, three times greater than that of PD, with which it is sometimes confused.
5. Task-specific tremors occur only with a particular movement, and not at other times. Primary writing tremor is an example.

TABLE 13-3. MEDICATIONS REPORTED TO INDUCE TREMOR

Thyroid hormone, synthroid
Epinepherine
Amphetamine, phenylepherine, and other sympathomimetics
Caffeine, theophyline, and other xanthenes
Nicotine
Lithium
Valproate
Phenothiazines and atypical antipsychotics
Tricyclic antidepressants
Methylbromide
Amiodarone
Cyclosporine, FK506
Monosodium glutamate
Corticosteroids (in high dose)
Insulin, oral hypoglycemic agents
Alcohol (withdrawal)
Metal intoxication (lead, arsenic, bismuth, mercury, manganese)

PATHOPHYSIOLOGY

1. The pathophysiology is not known.
2. Essential tremor has a central mechanism; functional imaging studies show increased activity in cerebellar outflow to the brainstem and thalamus. In many cases, essential tremor has a genetic basis, with an autosomal dominant pattern of inheritance.

PROGNOSIS

1. Onset varies widely from the teens to the 60's; it often runs a similar course within families.
2. Progression is slow over decades.

DIAGNOSIS

1. Essential tremor is a 4- to 10-/s action tremor, which may be large enough to interfere with activities of daily living.
   a. It most typically involves the upper limbs symmetrically and may involve the head or voice.
   b. There is both a postural and limb–kinetic tremor. Limb–kinetic tremor is multidirectional and it does not increase in amplitude as the target is approached (in distinction to cerebellar tremor).
   c. There is no dysmetria.
   d. Some patients with longstanding essential tremor have a bit of rest tremor admixed, but no bradykinesia.
   e. There are no current diagnostic tests or genetic markers; thyroid function should be checked, and copper studies as appropriate.
   f. Surface electromyogram (EMG) reveals a synchronous pattern of activation in antagonist muscles.
2. Enhanced physiologic tremor is usually rapid (8–12/s) and does not often achieve disabling amplitude, unless there is a problem with thyroid function or a medication.
   a. Essential head tremor can be confused with dystonic head tremor, which is directionally specific and is usually associated with a degree of torticollis.
   b. Lesions of the cerebellar outflow at a midbrain level produce a combination of a cerebellar postural tremor, rest tremor, and extrapyramidal rigidity (Holmes tremor).

3. Orthostatic tremor is a variant of essential tremor.
   a. Patients report discomfort or unsteadiness in the legs activated by standing, generally improved as they begin to walk. The tremor in the legs is rapid (16/s) and is not always visible, but it is palpable and can be demonstrated by surface EMG.
   b. Clonazepam is the drug of choice, but treatment of nonresponders is difficult.

TREATMENT

1. Not every patient with essential tremor will require pharmacologic treatment.
   a. Daily medication is usually reserved for patients with some degree of disability: difficulty with handwriting, drinking from a glass, or managing eating utensils.
   b. Patients who improve with alcohol will often respond to beta-blockers.
   c. In treating essential tremor, it is important to define the expected outcome. A 30% to 60% reduction of tremor amplitude is a good response.
   d. To achieve better reductions of tremor amplitude, patients may require neurosurgical treatment.
2. First-line agents:
   a. Propranolol (Inderal) is effective across a dose range of 40 to 240 mg. Starting dosage is 10 to 20 mg t.i.d. or 60 mg of the long-acting preparation. Contraindications include asthma, heart failure, and insulin-dependent diabetes. Side effects include hypotension, fatigue, depression, and sexual dysfunction. Other beta-blockers may be useful in particular patients, but do not offer better tremor control.
   b. Primidone (Mysoline) is the preferred therapy for patients with cardiovascular disease, and those with specific contraindications to beta-blockers. It is easier to use, particularly for fragile older patients with multiple medical problems. The usual dosage is 50 mg given at night or b.i.d.; starting dose is 25 mg to avoid sedation and nausea. There is incremental benefit up to 250 mg and above; anticonvulsant doses are not required. Primidone is metabolized by the liver, and it induces hepatic microsomal enzymes.
3. Second-line agents include some of the newer anticonvulsants (gabapentine, topiramate), benzodiazepines (clonazepam), mirtazapine, and methazolamide.
   a. Responses are less consistent, evidence for efficacy is difficult to establish, but each of these drugs has been helpful to some patients.
   b. Alternative therapies include botulinum toxin A and functional neurosurgery. Botox is particularly useful for head tremor.
4. Functional neurosurgery:
   a. Stereotactic thalamotomy or electrical DBS targeted at the ventral intermediate nucleus can produce reductions in tremor amplitude of greater than 80% in PD and essential tremor.
   b. Serious complications (intracranial hemorrhage, infection) occur in fewer than 5%.
   c. In comparison studies, patients prefer DBS to thalamotomy, although DBS is a costly option and minor problems with the leads and hardware are not infrequent.

DYSTONIA

BACKGROUND

1. Dystonia is defined as a syndrome of sustained or spasmodic muscle contraction, resulting in twisting movements and abnormal postures.
   a. Involuntary muscle spasms are either slow (tonic) or rapid, but they tend to be repetitive. Dystonia is traditionally classified as primary or secondary, generalized or focal.
   b. Dystonias of childhood onset are more likely to generalize, whereas most adult-onset dystonias remain regional or focal.

    c. The prevalence of primary childhood dystonia (idiopathic torsion dystonia or dystonia musculoram deformans) is 2 to 3/100,000 population. Focal dystonias probably exceed 30/100,000 as these disorders are not always recognized.

    d. Secondary dystonia occurs as a product of another neurologic disease.

PATHOPHYSIOLOGY

1. The pathophysiology of dystonia is not well understood. It is presumed to reflect a chemical and physiologic imbalance in the basal ganglia or upper brainstem. Dystonia is often a feature of well-characterized basal ganglia diseases, such as PD and Wilson disease. In primary dystonia due to the *DYT1* mutation, there is no neuropathology at the light microscope level. The disorder is caused by a GAG trinucleotide deletion on chromosome 9, a region coding for the protein torsin-A. Torsin-A is expressed in dopamine neurons, where it appears to function as a chaperone protein. Mutations in the genes for GTP cyclohydrolase 1 and tyrosine hydroxylase also produce dystonia. Both are involved in the metabolism of monoamine neurotransmitters. (On the other hand, hereditary myoclonus dystonia results from a sarcoglycan mutation.)

2. In the past 5 years, there has been an explosion of knowledge about the genetics of the primary dystonias. A number of genetic forms of the disorder have been identified; the most common are summarized in Table 13-4. The *DYT1* mutation is

TABLE 13-4. DIFFERENTIAL DIAGNOSIS OF DYSTONIA

Genetic Mutation	Protein Abnormality	Disease
Primary Dystonia		
DYT1	Torsin A	Idiopathic torsion dystonia (dystonia musculoram deformans)
DYT3		X-linked dystonia parkinsonism (Lubag)
DYT5	GTP cyclohydrolase-1	Dopa-responsive dystonia
DYT6		Mixed phenotype, (Amish, Menonite)
DYT7		Adult onset, cervical dystonia
DYT11	ϵ-Sarcoglycan	Myoclonus dystonia
DYT12		Rapid-onset parkinsonism/dystonia

Disease	Protein Abnormality
Secondary Dystonia	
Wilson disease	ATP7B
Hallervordean–Spatz syndrome	pantothenate kinase 2
Neuroacanthocytosis	
Lesch–Nyhan syndrome	
Familial calcification of the basal ganglia	
Parkinson and related disorders (MSA, PSP, CBD)	
Ceroid lipofuscinosis	
Dystonic lipidosis (with sea-blue histiocytes)	
Adult G_M1 gangliosidosis	
Mitochondrial encephalopathy (Leigh Leber)	
Juvenile striatal necrosis	
Cerebral palsy	

MSA, multiple-system atrophy; PSP, progressive supranuclear palsy; CBD, corticobasal degeneration.

autosomal dominant, with variable penetrance; the disorder is expressed in 30% of gene carriers. *DYT1* dystonia is most often found in the Ashkenazi Jewish population. It typically causes severe generalized dystonia of childhood onset, but mutations are sometimes seen in adult patients with a more restricted disorder. *DYT7* is expressed as hereditary torticollis.
3. The secondary dystonias are a diverse group of structural, metabolic, and neurodegenerative disorders. The common denominator appears to be damage to the basal ganglia. Examples include Wilson disease, Hallervorden–Spatz disease, juvenile striatal necrosis, and cerebral palsy.

PROGNOSIS

1. The prognosis in dystonia depends on etiology.
2. *DYT1* dystonia is typically a childhood-onset disorder, which can cause severe disability, but does not spread outside the motor system and does not shorten life expectancy.
3. Focal dystonias of adult onset typically remain regional or restricted and do not generalize. Spontaneous remissions sometimes occur in the first 2 years, but after the disorder is established it tends to persist.

DIAGNOSIS

1. Recognition of dystonia requires identification of the involuntary movements and abnormal postures as a neurologic disorder, as opposed to a musculoskeletal or psychological problem.
2. In a large number of patients, dystonia is initially misdiagnosed as psychogenic. The distinction between psychogenic and organic dystonia is one of the more difficult problems in neurology, as there are no laboratory tests. In contrast to a contracture, dystonia can usually be reduced, and the disorder will remit when the patient is asleep.
3. Imaging (head and/or spine) is often done to exclude a secondary cause.
4. Gene testing for *DYT1* is usually reserved for patients with some suspicion based on young onset or family history.

TREATMENT

Generalized Dystonia

1. Generalized dystonia is difficult to suppress with medication, although a variety of medications can produce partial symptomatic benefit.
    a. For most young-onset patients, a therapeutic trial of carbidopa/levodopa is warranted to exclude dopa-responsive dystonia. This disorder produces dystonia with diurnal variation and is exquisitely responsive to treatment. Lack of response to 400 to 600 mg of sinemet rules out the diagnosis.
2. Some patients benefit from a combination approach.
    a. Trihexyphenidyl (Artane): Begin at 2 mg bid (less for children); doses as high as 30 mg or above can be achieved in younger patients.
    b. Muscle relaxants (cyclobenzaprine, clonazepam, diazepam) can be helpful, although sedation is often a limiting issue.
    c. Carbamazepine (Tegretol) is sometimes helpful in generalized dystonias, particularly so in paroxysmal dystonia.
    d. Baclofen (Lioresal) is occasionally useful, particularly in cranial dystonias. It can also be administered as an intrathecal preparation through an implanted programmable pump for patients with severe generalized dystonia affecting the trunk and lower limbs.
    e. Tetrabenazine: This drug, not presently FDA-approved in the United States, is a dopamine-depleting agent. Beginning at 12.5 to 25 mg, the dosage can be advanced as needed to 50 mg t.i.d. or above. It is very effective, but can cause a parkinsonian syndrome.

3. In patients with severe dystonia who do not respond to these drugs alone or in combination, other options can be considered.
   a. Intrathecal baclofen and functional neurosurgery.
   b. Pallidotomy or DBS targeted at the pallidal or thalamic site has produced dramatic results in patients with primary generalized dystonia.

Focal Dystonia

1. Focal dystonia (torticollis, oromandibular dystonia, blepharospasm, writer's cramp) can be treated with intramuscular injection of botulinum toxin. There are several botulinum toxin preparations.
   a. Botulinum toxin A is a large peptide (molecular weight, 150,000), which acts presynaptically at the neuromuscular junction. The SNAP-25 protein is inactivated, blocking the release of acetylcholine. Effects persist for 2 to 4 months.
   b. Botulinum toxin B acts at the same synapse at a different site.
   c. There is a paradox in treating a disorder of CNS origin with a peripheral neuromuscular blocking agent, but the treatments are often effective.
   d. Results depend on targeting the active muscles, and best results are obtained with E MG guidance.
   e. A degree of resistance to botulinum toxin develops in roughly 20% of long-term patients, characterized by dose escalation and diminishing response. Half these patients have measurable antibodies to botulinum toxin. Switching to a different serotype is sometimes helpful.
2. Agents
   a. Botox (Oculinum) is a purified protein extract of botulinum toxin A. It is very potent, but has a good safety margin when given by intramuscular injection. Systemic side effects are rare when the dose is under 500 units. Doses in the range of 60 to 300 units are generally used to treat cervical dystonia. Twenty-five units per side is the usual dose for the orbital muscles in treating hemifacial spasm or blepharospasm.
   b. Dysport is another preparation of botulinus toxin A, widely used in Europe; 400 units of Dysport is equivalent to 100 units of Botox.
   c. Myobloc is a botulinum toxin B serotype. It comes prediluted and ready to use; 5,000 units of Myobloc is the equivalent of 100 units of Botox. Side effects (dry mouth, dysphagia) are more frequent, and the duration of action slightly less.

CHOREA, ATHETOSIS, AND DYSKINESIA

BACKGROUND

1. Chorea is characterized by irregular, brief, involuntary movements that flicker across the face, trunk, and limbs.
   a. Chorea, from the Greek, means dance. The movements are dance-like, but the choreography appears random and the movements are unpredictable. The gait has a particular marionette quality. An example is the chorea of Huntington disease (HD), a hereditary neurodegenerative disease described in Long Island in the 19th century.
   b. The prevalence is 6/100,000 population.
   c. Acute rheumatic chorea (Sydenham chorea) was described in the 19th century. An immunologic complication of streptococcal infection, it is less common in the antibiotic era.
2. The spectrum of choreic movement disorders includes hemiballismus, a large-amplitude, unilateral involuntary movement with flinging of the limbs on the affected side. It is caused by a small stroke in the region of the subthalamic nucleus. Athetosis is a slower, writhing involuntary movement. The athetosis of cerebral palsy is a good example. The term "dyskinesia" encompasses a variety of choreic and dystonic movements, frequently a side effect of medication. Dyskinesias are

usually repetitive and stereotyped, often involving the perioral area (lip smacking, tongue protrusion).

PATHOPHYSIOLOGY

1. All the disorders mentioned above produce an imbalance in the basal ganglia circuit, with underactivation of the striatal indirect pathway. The net result is decreased activity in the subthalamic nucleus and internal globus pallidus, reducing the basal ganglia output. In HD, the mutation on chromosome 4 is an expanded CAG trinucleotide repeat. The mutant protein has cumulative toxicity, resulting in neurodegeneration in mid adult life. The spiny projection neurons of the putamen, which use γ-aminobutyric acid (GABA) and enkephalin as their neurotransmitters, are most vulnerable. Ultimately a variety of neurotransmitters and intracellular messenger proteins are disturbed. There are also abnormalities of cellular energetics in the central nervous system in HD. There is recent evidence to suggest that the Huntington protein may function as a transcription factor.
2. *Tardive* means late; tardive dyskinesia occurs with chronic exposure to neuroleptic drugs. A minimum of 3 months is generally required. Involuntary movements are a consequence of chronic blockade of the D2 dopamine receptor, with up-regulation of receptor and its intracellular messengers. Through the D2 receptor, dopamine has an inhibitory effect on the striatal indirect pathway. The syndrome is much less common with the newer atypical antipsychotics.

PROGNOSIS

1. The prognosis depends on the etiology of the chorea.
2. In HD, typical age of onset is 35, with a large range (from younger than 10 to older than 60). There is an inverse correlation between number of CAG repeats and the age of onset.
3. Progression to loss of ambulation, dementia and death extends over 20 years.
4. Comorbid depression is common, and there is an increased risk for suicide in HD.
5. Tardive dyskinesia is sometimes reversible over a year if the onset is recent and the offending medication is promptly withdrawn. More often it is persistent and nonprogressive.

DIAGNOSIS

1. The differential diagnosis of choreic involuntary movements is broad, and includes a diverse group of disorders (Table 13-5). The common element is a disturbance in basal ganglia output.
2. The first step after recognition is to ascertain the family history and pertinent medication exposures.
3. In the absence of a family history or neuroleptic drug exposure, workup should include imaging. In HD there is a loss of mass in the caudate head.
4. Laboratory tests include an antinuclear antibody (ANA), antistreptolysin titer, and thick smear for acanthocytes.
5. If there is progressive chorea and a negative family history, consider HD genetic testing. In a surprising number of patients with HD, the family history is initially noninformative.

TREATMENT

1. For patients with chorea, treatment is best directed at the underlying disorder. Choreic movements can be severe and disabling, and suppression of involuntary movements with medication may be appropriate. Patients with HD often need primarily attention to depression, nutritional issues, and their caregivers and support system.
   a. Neuroleptics: Chorea can be decreased with conventional antipsychotic drugs such as haloperidol in low dose (0.5–2 mg). Larger doses are counterproductive, as they quickly accumulate and produce motor side effects.

TABLE 13-5. DIFFERENTIAL DIAGNOSIS OF CHOREA

Huntington disease
Benign hereditary chorea
Neuroacanthocytonsis
Dentatorubral–pallidoluysian atrophy
Familial calcification of the basal ganglia
Paroxysmal kinesiogenic choreoathetosis
Acquired hepatocerebral degeneration
Acute rheumatic chorea (Sydenham disease)
Systemic lupus erythematosis
Senile chorea
Encephalitis, HIV
Chorea gravidarum
Acute vascular hemichorea
Drug-induced dyskinesia:
    Neuroleptics
    Anticholinergic drugs
    Antihistamines
    Oral contraceptives
    Levodopa and dopamine agonists

   b. Atypical antipsychotics: Quetiapine (25–150 mg) and clozapine (12.5–75 mg) are often useful for agitation and behavioral problems in more advanced HD.
   c. Dopamine-depleting drugs: Reserpine and tetrabenazine can reduce choreic movements, but are not ideal for patients with HD, as they tend to aggravate or precipitate depression.
   d. Amantadine (100–300 mg): Amantadine is sometimes helpful to reduce chorea in HD, although the effects are modest.
   e. Benzodiazepines: Diazepam and clonazepam are sometimes useful as adjuncts in HD.
   f. Coenzyme Q (CoQ)–10: In one large clinical trial, CoQ at 600 mg/d was well tolerated in patients with HD, and there was a trend toward a slower decline in functional status over 30 months.
   g. Anticonvulsants (phenytoin, carbamazepine): These drugs are particularly effective for paroxysmal kinesiogenic choreoathetosis.
2. For tardive movement disorders, there is no ideal medication.
   a. Always reevaluate the need for neuroleptic drugs. If these medications are eliminated, some patients will resolve, although the dyskinesia can intensify over the short run.
   b. Suppressing the dyskinesia with increasing doses of neuroleptic is not recommended, as the long-term effect is to aggravate the underlying pathophysiology. Changing to a newer atypical antipsychotic may be helpful. Clozapine is sometimes successful when others fail. Dopamine-depleting agents may be useful, although side effects include hypotension and depression.

MYOCLONUS

BACKGROUND

1. Myoclonus is a brief, shock-like muscle jerk, generally less than 150 msec in duration, originating in the CNS.
2. It may be restricted in extent (focal, segmental) or more widespread (multifocal, generalized).

3. Myoclonus occurs in a variety of neurologic and metabolic disorders.
4. Asterixis, defined as a brief lapse of tonic muscle activation, is a related phenomenon.

DIAGNOSIS

1. Myoclonus can be classified by etiology or on the basis of its physiology.
2. The principal physiological distinction is between epileptic and nonepileptic myoclonus. Electroencephalogram (EEG) is helpful to distinguish.
3. Neurodegenerative dementias and prion disorders often exhibit myoclonus as a sign.
4. In hospitalized patients, myoclonus is common as a manifestation of a metabolic encephalopathy, as in renal failure, hyponatremia, or hypoglycemia. Evaluation should include glucose, electrolytes, calcium, magnesium, blood urea nitrogen, creatinine, and LFTs.
5. Medications and exogenous toxins can also produce myoclonus. Examples include bismuth, lithium, meperidine, levodopa, phenytoin, and the SSRI antidepressants.
6. A vexatious myoclonus is seen at times after cardiac arrest (postanoxic myoclonus).
7. Spinal myoclonus is typically regular (periodic) and restricted in expression. It reflects a disturbance of spinal segmental mechanisms, and can be seen after contrast myelography or spinal anesthesia.

TREATMENT

1. Therapy should be directed at the underlying encephalopathy, where possible. With cortical myoclonus, valproate and anticonvulsants that enhance GABA are particularly effective. For myoclonus unassociated with epilepsy or encephalopathy, clonazepam is usually the drug of choice. These agents should be tried empirically:
   a. Clonazepam: Effective in doses from 0.5 mg to 18 mg/d, in divided doses. Side effects include sedation, particularly at high dose, tolerance, and a withdrawal syndrome after chronic use.
   b. Valproate (Depakote): Particularly effective in epileptic myoclonus. Treat to achieve a therapeutic serum level (250–750 mg t.i.d.).
   c. Piracetam: This drug, not FDA-approved in the United States, is widely used for suppression of myoclonus in Europe. Usual dose range is 1,200 to 16,000 mg/d; it is well tolerated at up to 24 g/d.

TICS AND TOURETTE SYNDROME

BACKGROUND

1. A tic is a repetitive, stereotyped movement, longer in duration than a myoclonic jerk and more complex. It may appear be a caricature of a voluntary movement that has taken on a life of its own.
2. A tic has a subjective component: There is an urge to move, and a feeling of release after. It can be suppressed for a time by force of will, but the subjective discomfort will build up.
3. Some tics are simple, involving an isolated muscle group, others are complex.
4. Tics may involve vocalization. Tourette syndrome (TS) was described in 1885 by George Gilles de la Tourette, as he examined the movement disorders on the ward of the Salpetriere Hospital in Paris. The disorder appears to be genetic, with variable expression.

DIAGNOSIS

1. Diagnostic criteria specify multiple motor tics, at least one vocal tic, and onset before age 18. Tics wax and wane over time; old ones remit and new tics appear.

Echolalia and coprolalia (profane vocalization) occur in about 20%. Neurobehavioral disorders such as obsessive compulsive disorder (OCD) and attention deficit hyperactivity disorder (ADHD) occur in more than half of patients with TS.

2. Other related disorders include chronic tic disorder (multiple tics present for more than a year) and transient tic disorder. These tic disorders may be part of the Tourette spectrum. A family member may have just tics or just OCD. Tics also may be a secondary phenomenon, occurring with another neurologic disease such as encephalitis, tardive dyskinesia, HD, or dystonia.

TREATMENT

1. The main principle of therapeutics is to identify first the source of the patient's distress.
2. Behavioral disorders such as OCD and ADHD may respond to appropriate medication (fluoxitine, clomipramine, methylphenidate). If tic suppression is the treatment goal, options include the following:
   a. Clonidine (Catapres) is an α_2-adrenergic agonist. Begin at 0.1 mg/d, and advance to 1 to 2 mg/d; several months may be needed to see improvement. Sedation, fatigue, and hypotension are side effects. The drug should not be withdrawn rapidly, as rebound hypertension can occur.
   b. Guanfacine (Tenex): This drug is an α_2-adrenergic agonist, similar in mechanism to clonidine. Dose is 1 to 2 mg/d.
   c. Benzodiazepines such as clorazepate (Tranxene) 3.75 to 15 mg t.i.d. and clonazepam (Klonepin) 0.5 to 2 mg b.i.d. may reduce frequency of tics.
3. Neuroleptic drugs such as haloperidol and pimozide will ultimately work, but lower doses are preferred to minimize the risk of a tardive movement disorder.
   a. Risperidone (Risperdal): May be helpful (0.5–2 mg) for tic suppression and associated subjective distress. Once control is achieved, another agent such as clonidine or a benzodiazepine may be more successful:
   b. Haloperidol (Haldol): Starting dosage is 0.5 mg once or twice a day. Doses of 2 to 5 mg/d may be required. Higher doses should be avoided.
   c. Pimozide (Orap) This drug is a neuroleptic, marketed specifically for TS. Starting dose is 1 to 2 mg/d, doses of 6 to 16 mg/d may be needed.

RESTLESS LEGS SYNDROME

BACKGROUND

1. Restless legs syndrome (RLS) was described by Ekbom in the 1940's. The subjective discomfort and urge to move are the primary disturbance, and symptoms are relieved by walking. Patients describe a "creepy crawly" sensation in the legs and an inability to sit still.
2. The disorder is worse in the evening; periodic leg movements of sleep are often associated.
3. RLS is now recognized as common; in some cases there may be a family history.
4. The patient should be screened for associated disorders such as iron deficiency and peripheral neuropathy.

TREATMENT

1. Dopaminergic medication is the first line of treatment, if the discomfort is sufficient to warrant it.
   a. One hundred to 200 mg of Sinemet CR at bedtime may suppress symptoms.
   b. Newer dopamine agonists are quite effective at relatively low dosages: pramipexole 0.25 to 0.5 mg, ropinerole 0.5 to 2 mg hs.
   c. A second dose may be needed during the daytime for some patients.

2. Patients who fail dopaminergic drugs often respond to neurontin or low-dose opiates (tramadol 25–50 mg hs).

OTHER DISORDERS OF MOVEMENT

ATAXIA

BACKGROUND

1. Ataxia is easy to recognize, often difficult to diagnose, and nearly impossible to treat.
2. *Ataxia*, from the ancient Greek, means irregularity or disorderliness. We use the term to describe an incoordination of movement of cerebellar origin. The patient exhibits dysmetria (past pointing), difficulty with rapid alternating movements, and there may be intention tremor. There is usually a cerebellar dysarthria (irregular, sometimes poorly modulated speech) and an associated oculomotor disorder.
3. Gait ataxia is distinctive; the gait is wide-based with irregular stepping. The patient walks as if drunk.

PROGNOSIS

Prognosis in ataxia depends on the etiology of the disorder. Posterior fossa tumors, prion disease, and paraneoplastic degeneration are rapidly progressive (months to a few years), while some patients with pure cerebellar cortical degeneration and late onset remain ambulatory 15 or 20 years after diagnosis.

DIAGNOSIS

1. Ataxia can result from injury to the cerebellum through trauma, infection, or demyelinating or vascular disease. A group of neurodegenerative disorders also produces progressive ataxia. The symptomatic and metabolic ataxias are outside the scope of this chapter. The neurodegenerative ataxias divide in two large groups, hereditary and sporadic. These diseases are classified on the basis of their genetic and molecular markers. As noted by Anita Harding, older descriptive classifications have been problematic. A partial listing is included in Table 13-6. Hereditary ataxias have a combined prevalence of 5/100,000 population, roughly comparable to HD. A similar number of cases are sporadic. Full ascertainment of the family history is thus the most important initial step in evaluation.
2. The hereditary ataxias are classified as autosomal dominant, autosomal recessive, and maternal inheritance (mitochondrial). The dominantly inherited ataxias are difficult to diagnose from their clinical features in a single case, as there is a large overlap. Retinal pigmentary degeneration distinguishes SCA-7. SCA-3 (Machado–Joseph disease) patients can have significant dystonia or occasionally a parkinsonian syndrome. Some patients with SCA-6 have discrete episodes of vertigo, ataxia, or nausea, which is of interest as the mutation affects the *CACNA1A* calcium channel. (Point mutations in this gene cause episodic ataxia type 2 and familial hemiplegic migraine.) SCA-1, -2, -3, and -6 are CAG trinucleotide repeat disorders, resulting in an expanded polyglutamine tract in a widely expressed protein. DNA diagnostic testing is usually needed to make a diagnosis of any of these diseases, unless diagnosis has been confirmed in another family member.
3. Friedreich ataxia was described in 1861. The typical form has onset between ages 8 and 25, with ataxia, dysarthria, and a spinal disorder (sensory loss, absent reflexes, extensor plantar response). Associated features include pes cavus deformity,

TABLE 13-6. COMMON CAUSES OF ATAXIA

Hereditary ataxia
  A. Autosomal dominant
    SCA1   United States, Northern Europe
    SCA2   Cuba, Caribbean
    SCA3/Machado Joseph disease   Portugal, Azores, worldwide
    SCA6   Calcium channel
    SCA7   Retinal pigmentary degeneration
    DRPLA
    Episodic ataxia, types 1 and 2
  B. Autosomal recessive
    Friedreich ataxia
    Ataxia with vitamin E deficiency
    Ataxia telangectasia
  C. Mitochondrial

Sporadic ataxia
  Toxins: alcohol, phenytoin, cytosine arabinoside
  Hyperthermia
  Trauma
  Metabolic disorders
    Hypothyroidism
    Abeta lipoproteinemia
    Urea cycle disorders
  Paraneoplastic cerebellar degeneration
  Neurodegenerative ataxia
    Cerebellar MSA (olivopontocerebellar atrophy)
    Pure cerebellar cortical degeneration

MSA, multiple-system atrophy

---

scoliosis, and a hypertrophic cardiomyopathy. The disorder is autosomal recessive, the product of an expanded GAA trinucleotide repeat on chromosome 9. The frataxin protein is involved in mitochondrial metabolism. Patients have deficiencies of mitochondrial energetics and are vulnerable to oxidant stress. Iron accumulates in the mitochondria of myocardial cells. Availability of genetic testing has resulted in the appreciation of a wider spectrum of illness, including patients with late onset and those with retained spinal reflexes and a more restricted form of the disorder. Ataxia with vitamin E deficiency is similar to Friedreich in its clinical manifestations. This disorder is treatable, in that vitamin E replacement arrests the progression.

4. In cases of progressive ataxia with a negative family history (sporadic ataxia), the workup is focused on looking for a toxic, paraneoplastic, or treatable metabolic disorder. Evaluation should include imaging (to characterize the topography of cerebellar degeneration and to look for evidence of multiple system atrophy), thyroid stimulating hormone (TSH), vitamin E level, lipoprotein electrophoresis, lactate and pyruvate (for mitochondrial disorder), and search for antineuronal antibodies (anti-Yo, in particular). Genetic testing should be considered as well. As with HD, many patients with hereditary ataxia present without a family history. The cerebellar presentation of multiple system atrophy is known as olivopontocerebellar atrophy (OPCA) in the older literature. The disorder is distinguished by extrapyramidal and/or autonomic signs. There may be brainstem atrophy, increased signal in the putamen, or crossing fibers of the pons (cross sign) on MRI. A pure cerebellar cortical degeneration is characterized by more restricted clinical expression, and slower progression over decades.

TREATMENT

1. With Friedreich ataxia, therapy is focused on boosting mitochondrial function in an effort to improve cellular energetics and slow disease progression.
2. Modest neuroprotective benefits have been suggested in early clinical trials with CoQ and idebenone.
   a. CoQ: For neuroprotective therapy of Friedreich ataxia, CoQ is given 360 U/d with 2,000 U/d of vitamin E.
   b. Idebenone (investigational therapy; not approved or sold in the United States): a dose of 5 mg/kg/d has been used in clinical trials with pediatric patients. The recommended adult dose is 360 mg/d.
3. For all the other neurodegenerative ataxias, treatment is largely supportive. Symptomatic therapy of the ataxias has been relatively ineffective. The serotonin nerve terminal network in the cerebellar cortex has begun to attract interest as a point of therapeutic leverage. In efforts to enhance serotonergic tone in the cerebellar cortex, pilot studies have explored the response to trimethoprim, tetrahydrobiopterin, buspirone, and sertroline. While some patients report subjective improvements, it has been difficult to demonstrate benefit in randomized clinical trials. Part of the problem is that the neurodegenerative ataxias differ in how they prune the cerebellar circuit anatomy. Rehabilitation-based therapies are generally more successful than pharmacotherapy for ataxic symptoms.
   a. Buspirone (Buspar): Starting at 5 mg t.i.d. with dosages to 10 to 20 mg t.i.d. has been explored in patients with ataxia. Modest gains in gait and balance function have been observed by some patients, provided they are mildly affected and still ambulatory to begin with.
   b. Sertraline (Zoloft): Doses of 25 to 100 mg have been used in an effort to treat motor and affective/behavioral symptoms in ataxia patients.
   c. Primidone (Mysoline): Dosages of 25 to 100 mg b.i.d. have been used for cerebellar tremor, with variable success. Cerebellar outflow tremor may be disabling and severe, and is difficult to control with medications.

SPASTICITY

BACKGROUND

Spasticity is characterized by increased tone, hyperreflexia, and velocity dependent stiffness on passive movement. This is evident as "clasp knife" stiffness on examination of the limbs.

PATHOPHYSIOLOGY

Spasticity occurs with a disorder of upper motor neurons. The result is disinhibition of spinal segmental mechanisms, with increased activity in the muscle spindle and overactivation of alpha motor neurons.

DIAGNOSIS

1. Spasticity can be a consequence of cerebral or spinal pathology.
   a. Cerebral spasticity is most common with stroke, demyelinating disease, and birth injury (cerebral palsy).
   b. Spinal spasticity is usually the result of trauma or cervical spondylosis.
2. There are a number of clinical problems that occur as a consequence of spasticity. Some patients, particularly paraplegics, experience uncomfortable flexor spasms in the legs. Stiffness can restrict limb use in patients with partial function. Ambulatory patients can have difficulty with stiff-legged gait.

TREATMENT

1. Pharmacotherapy of spasticity is targeted at the intrusive positive symptoms (usually flexor spasm). These drugs will not help negative symptoms like muscle weakness, which is the principal functional limitation for many patients. At high dose, most spasticity drugs will increase weakness, so there is a therapeutic tradeoff. These drugs can be used in combination.

   a. Baclofen (Lioresal): a GABA-B agonist, which promotes inhibition in the spinal cord. The starting dosage is 10 mg b.i.d., which can be increased as tolerated to 80 to 120 mg in divided doses. Common side effects include sedation, dizziness, nausea, and weakness. Baclofen should not be given to seizure patients. Ambulatory patients do not usually tolerate doses over 60 mg. LFTs should be checked in the first 6 weeks. Intrathecal baclofen can be given through a programmable pump in patients with spasticity refractory to oral agents. Surgical implantation is required. Complications include infection, and pump malfunctions can result in serious overdose. (The protocol is available through Medtronics.)

   b. Diazepam (Valium) acts at a benzodiazepine-binding site that promotes GABA-mediated spinal inhibition. Starting dosage is 2 mg b.i.d. or t.i.d.. Some paraplegic patients benefit from doses as high as 40 to 60 mg/d, although sedation is often a limiting feature. Alcohol should be limited. Patients on long-term treatment with benzodiazepines develop dependence and can have a withdrawal syndrome.

   c. Tizanidine (Zanaflex) is an α_2 agonist, it increases presynaptic inhibition of motor neurons. Starting dose is 2 mg/d; it is titrated up over weeks by 4-mg increments as high as 8 to 12 mg t.i.d.. Side effects include weakness, hypotension, sedation, and dry mouth. LFTs should be checked in the first 6 weeks.

   d. Dantrolene (Dantrium) acts directly on skeletal muscle, interfering with the release of calcium from the sarcoplasmic reticulum. Initial dose is 25 mg/d, increased over 4 weeks to 200 to 400 mg. Weakness is a frequent and dose-related side effect. Dantrolene is most often used in nonambulatory patients with cerebral spasticity. It can cause serious hepatotoxicity, and should not be given to patients with known liver disease. LFTs should be monitored.

2. Botulinum toxin (Botox) is increasingly finding use in patients with spasticity. The principal advantages are its ability to target a particular muscle and the lack of systemic side effects. Disadvantages include expense and the need for repeated procedures to administer Botox three to four times a year. Botox can be used for a variety of spastic disorders characterized by stiff-legged gait, although the physiology of stiff-legged gait is complex and the application needs to be tailored. It should be used in the context of rehabilitation therapy, preferably by someone who can distinguish the various patterns and target muscles accordingly. Leg weakness and falls can result from overly vigorous application of Botox. Botox can sometimes help improve upper limb function, when stiffness constrains use of the arm in daily activities. It can also help with the bladder care of nonambulatory patients with adductor spasm.

STIFF MAN SYNDROME

BACKGROUND

1. Described by Moersch and Woltman in 1956, stiff man syndrome is an autoimmune disorder with involuntary stiffness of axial muscles and painful muscle spasm. It is rare, but is probably underdiagnosed.

2. Diagnostic criteria include slow progression of stiffness in the axial and proximal limb muscles, hyperlordosis and deformity of the spine, and episodic painful spasms precipitated by active or passive movement, sometimes triggered by sensory stimuli or emotional upset. Elemental neurologic exam is otherwise normal. Some patients have a peculiar stiff, wooden gait like the movie monster Frankenstein.

3. There is a therapeutic response to benzodiazepines, although large doses are often required to maintain benefit.

PATHOPHYSIOLOGY

Stiff man syndrome is an autoimmune disorder, and many patients have a personal or family history of other autoimmune diseases (thyroiditis, pernicious anemia, diabetes, vitiligo). Eighty percent have measurable antibodies to glutamic acid decarboxylase, or anti–islet cell antibodies. There appears to be a disturbance of GABA-mediated inhibition in the CNS. A variant of stiff man syndrome has been described in association with breast cancer.

TREATMENT

1. Benzodiazepines are the first line of treatment, but large doses are needed to maintain benefit.
   a. Diazepam may need to be given at 40 to 60 mg/d, and some patients require more than 100 mg/d.
   b. Baclofen has also been used to treat muscle spasm and stiffness in this syndrome. It can be given orally at doses up to 80 to 120 mg or intrathecally through a surgically implanted catheter and pump.
2. Immunotherapy is required to obtain control of symptoms in more severely affected patients. Prednisone and azothiaprine have been used.
3. Plasma exchange and IV immune globulin have also been effective as rescue therapy, but are not suitable for long-term treatment.

BIBLIOGRAPHY

Diederich NJ, Goetz CG, Drug-induced movement disorders. *Neurol Clin* 1998;16:125–139.

Gasser T, Bressman S, Durr A, et al. Molecular diagnosis of inherited movement disorders. *Mov Disord* 2003;18:3–18.

Gilman S, Low P, Quinn N, et al. Consensus statement on the diagnosis of multiple system atrophy. *J Neurol Sci* 1999;163:94–98.

Goetz CG, Koller WC, Poewe W, et al. Management of Parkinson's disease: an evidence based review. *Mov Disord* 2002;17[Suppl 4]:S1–S166.

Jankovic J, Brin M. Therapeutic uses of botulinum toxin. *N Engl J Med* 1991;324:1186–1194.

Kurlan R. Tourette's syndrome: current concepts. *Neurology* 1989;39:1625–1630.

Lang AE, Lozano AM. Parkinson's disease, I and II. *N Engl J Med* 1998;339:1044–1053, 1130–1143.

Marsden CD, Obeso JA. The functions of the basal ganglia and the paradox of stereotactic surgery in Parkinson's disease. *Brain* 1994;117:877–897.

Meige M, Feindel E. *Tics and their treatment.* New York: William Wood and Co., 1907. [Translated into English by S. A. K. Wilson.]

Tan E, Ashizawa T. Genetic testing in spinocerebellar ataxias: defining a clinical role. *Arch Neurol* 2001;58:191–195.

14. BEHAVIORAL NEUROLOGY AND DEMENTIA

Kirk R. Daffner and David A. Wolk

DISORDERS OF ATTENTION AND EXECUTIVE FUNCTIONS

BACKGROUND

Definitions

1. Attention involves a set of neural processes that allow a person to select which stimuli or thoughts will be the center of awareness, while filtering out potential distractors.
   a. Components of attention include arousal, orienting (shifting of the direction of sensory organs), selectivity (focusing on certain stimuli), the capacity to sustain processing (vigilance), and divide resources (during dual or multitasks).
   b. Disruption of attention is likely to undermine most cognitive functions.
2. Executive functions are complex cerebral processes that operate in nonroutine situations.
   a. They depend, in part, on appropriate attention and working memory (i.e., holding on-line and manipulating internalized representations that allow for the guiding of future behaviors).
   b. Executive functions include insight, judgment, and problem-solving skills.
   c. Executive functions consist of initiating context-appropriate behavioral responses while inhibiting unsuitable ones, maintaining and shifting cognitive sets, and monitoring and adjusting ongoing mental activity.
   d. Executive functions are most closely linked to a person's capacity to remain independent.

Presenting Syndromes

1. Acute confusional state (ACS):
   a. A disorder of higher cognitive function reflecting the loss of a normal coherent stream of thought or action.
   b. Its salient feature is a disruption of a patient's attentional matrix.
   c. "Delirium" is an alternative term for ACS that neurologists often reserve for agitated patients who exhibit autonomic instability and hallucinations.
2. Attention deficit hyperactivity disorder (ADHD):
   a. Defined by inappropriate levels of attention, impulsivity, or hyperactivity, which should manifest before age 7.
   b. Thirty percent to 60% of children with ADHD will continue to have symptoms in adulthood that can include inattention, disorganization, impulsivity, affective lability, learning problems, and impairment of executive functions (i.e., dysexecutive syndromes).
3. Dysexecutive syndromes:
   a. Cognitive: decreased planning, working memory, poor insight
   b. Behavioral: impulsivity, disinhibition, perseveration
   c. Motivational: apathy, abulia

PATHOPHYSIOLOGY

Neuroanatomic Components

1. Frontal–subcortical circuits:

   a. Frontal lobes→basal ganglia (caudate)→globus pallidus/substantia nigra→ thalamus (dorsal medial/ventral anterior)→frontal lobes.
   b. Disruption anywhere along these circuits can lead to similar behavioral outcomes.
   c. Topographically distinct circuits relate to the dorsolateral frontal cortex, the medial frontal cortex, and the orbital frontal cortex.
   d. Most often, the dorsolateral frontal circuit is associated with cognitive signs, the medial frontal circuit with altered motivation, and the orbital frontal circuit with lack of inhibition.
2. Ascending neurotransmitter systems:
   a. Norepinephrine (NE) from the locus ceruleus helps to mediate arousal and improves signal-to-noise ratio.
   b. Dopamine (DA) from the ventral tegmental area is necessary for functioning of prefrontal cortex and maintenance of appropriate behavioral engagement.
   c. Acetylcholine (ACh) from basal forebrain and brainstem reticular systems may modulate excitability of widespread regions of thalamus and cortex and influence overall information processing capacity.

Disorders

1. Attention and executive functions can be undermined by a wide range of medical, neurologic, and psychiatric conditions.
2. Common causes include the following:
   a. Toxic–metabolic encephalopathy (including side effects of medications)
   b. Multifocal injury (including cerebrovascular disease, closed head injury, multiple sclerosis)
   c. Developmental (e.g., ADHD)
   d. Degenerative diseases [including frontotemporal dementia (FTD), Alzheimer disease (AD), and Parkinson disease (PD)]
   e. Neuropsychiatric conditions (e.g., anxiety, depression, hypomania/mania, schizophrenia)
   f. Disorders of arousal and sleep (including sleep apnea and narcolepsy)

PROGNOSIS

Prognosis is variable and depends on the underlying conditions.

DIAGNOSIS

History (often very dependent on information derived from informants), mental status examination (MSE), including tests of complex attention/executive functions (e.g., word list generation, graphomotor sequencing, go–no go tasks), neuromedical assessment, toxic–metabolic screen.

TREATMENT

General Principles

1. Review medications. Eliminate nonessential medications, being particularly mindful of those with anticholinergic, sedative, or parkinsonian side effects.
2. Review and treat systemic/medical conditions (e.g., cardiac, pulmonary, renal, endocrine, pain, sleep).
3. Identify and treat neuropsychiatric conditions that may be contributing to impaired attention and executive functions (e.g., anxiety, depression, hypomania/mania, and psychosis).

TABLE 14-1. STIMULANT MEDICATIONS

Medication	Starting Dose	Dosing Range*
Short-acting		
Methylphenidate	5 mg b.i.d.–t.i.d.	Up to 60 mg/d
(Ritalin, Methylin)		
Dextroamphetamine	5 mg qd–b.i.d.	Up to 40 mg/d
(Dexedrine)		
Dextroamphetamine	5 mg qd–b.i.d.	Up to 40 mg/d
(DextroStat)		
Dexmethylphenidate	2.5 mg b.i.d.	Up to 20 mg/d
(Focalin)		
Amphetamine–dextroamphetamine	5 mg qd–b.i.d.	Up to 40 mg/d
(Adderall)		
Combined short- and intermediate-acting		
Methylphenidate	20 mg q AM	Up to 60 mg/d
(Ritalin-LA)		
Methylphenidate	20 mg q AM	Up to 60 mg/d
(Metadate CD)		
Dextroamphetamine	5–10 mg q AM	Up to 40 mg/d
(Dexedrine Spansule)		
Amphetamine–dextroamphetamine	10 mg q AM	Up to 30 mg/d
(Adderall XR)		
Methylphenidate	18 mg q AM	Up to 54 mg/d
(Concerta)		
Intermediate-acting		
Methylphenidate	20 mg q AM	Up to 60 mg/d
(Ritalin-SR)		
Methylphenidate	20 mg q AM	Up to 60 mg/d
(Metadate ER, Methylin ER)		
Pemoline	18.75–37.5 q AM	Up to 112.5 mg/d
(Cylert)		
Modafinil	100 mg qd–b.i.d.	Up to 400 mg/d
(Provigil)		

b.i.d., twice a day; t.i.d., three times a day.
*Some clinicians increase these medications to even higher doses, while carefully monitoring the clinical status of their patients. Modafinil has a different mechanism of action than stimulants.

Medications

Attentional Problems

1. Stimulant medications (Table 14-1): Food and Drug Administration (FDA) approval limited to ADHD and narcolepsy. Side effects can include insomnia, anorexia, exacerbation of tics, agitation, anxiety, psychotic symptoms, and seizures. Monitor blood pressure, especially in patients with hypertension. Avoid concomitant use of monoamine oxidase inhibitors (MAOIs). There are numerous medications currently available that vary in their pharmacokinetics, with short-acting, combined short- and intermediate-acting, and intermediate-acting preparations. Of note, pemoline has been associated with cases of fatal hepatic failure.
2. Modafinil (Provigil) has a different mechanism of action than stimulants and is approved for excessive daytime sleepiness related to narcolepsy. It may be helpful with inattention associated with fatigue and sleepiness.
3. Catecholamine "boosters":
   a. Atomoxetine (Strattera) is a selective norepinephrine reuptake inhibitor. Adult dose: begin 40 mg/d; increase to 80 to 100 mg/d as single daily or twice a

day (b.i.d.) dose. Potential side effects include gastrointestinal (GI) distress, increased blood pressure, sexual dysfunction, and urinary retention. It is less likely than stimulants to cause insomnia and is contraindicated in patients on MAOIs or with narrow angle glaucoma.

b. Bupropion (Wellbutrin; Wellbutrin SR; Wellbutrin XL): Neurochemical mechanisms not known, but probably works on both the NE and (DA systems, and in animals has stimulant effects. Increased risk of seizures, especially if more than 450 mg/d or more than 150 mg of immediate-acting formulation given at one time or the patient has bulimia. Start bupropion at 75 to 100 mg b.i.d.; increase up to 400 mg (in three divided doses), bupropion sustained-release (SR) 150 mg every morning and increase to b.i.d. (with ~8 hours between doses) up to 400 mg/d, or buproprion XL 150 mg every morning and increase to 300 mg (or rarely, 450 mg)/d. Contraindications include use of MAOIs and seizure disorders. Consider a concomitant antiepileptic drug if the patient does not have seizures but is at higher risk for them [e.g., history of traumatic brain injury and an abnormal electroencephalogram (EEG)]. Bupropion may be particularly helpful for inattentive patients with concomitant symptoms of depression. Of note, FDA approval of bupropion is limited to the treatment of depression and smoking cessation.

c. α_2-agonists: There are abundant α_2-receptors in the prefrontal cortex and studies have suggested that agonists may improve working memory and attentional focus. FDA approval of these agents is for the treatment of hypertension. Clonidine (Catapres) (0.1 mg/d, increase to b.i.d., up to 0.6 mg/d) and guanfacine (Tenex) (1 mg/d, increase up to 3 mg/d) only have FDA approval for the treatment of hypertention. Side effects include dry mouth, drowsiness, dizziness, constipation, and orthostatic hypotension. Guanfacine, a more selective α_2-agonist, tends to be less sedating.

d. Other (Table 14-2). Tricyclic antidepressants (TCAs) (e.g., nortriptyline, desipramine), selective serotonin reuptake inhibitors (SSRIs), or venlafaxine can be considered as primary or adjunctive therapies for inattention when patients exhibit concurrent problems with anxiety, depression, pain, or sleep disturbance.

Executive Dysfunction

1. See Treatment for Disorders of Attention and Executive Functions, earlier.

2. Dopamine agonists (DAs)/modulators (Table 14-3) may increase motivation, diminish apathy, and improve working memory or other executive functions. Evidence supports the notion that there is an optimal level of dopamine activity, with too little or too much leading to dysfunction.

a. FDA approval for most of these medications is limited to the treatment of PD. Clinicians can consider "empiric" treatment of dysexecutive symptoms with agents that enhance dopamine activity. In such circumstances it is crucial to closely monitor whether symptoms are improving and assess the impact of potential negative side effects.

b. Begin with the lowest dose possible and increase very slowly.

c. Patient response and side effects should be followed on a regular basis using items that can be measured or counted (e.g., days patient dressed without assistance, number of emotional outbursts in the prior week, body weight, standing blood pressure). Potential side effects of this class of medication include sedation, postural hypotension, hallucinations, GI symptoms (e.g., nausea), and peripheral edema. Amantadine (Symmetrel) is also associated with anticholinergic-like side effects.

d. We have had the most success with pramipexole.

e. Often, the medication dose used is lower than that typically prescribed for PD. However, in cases of profound abulia, some have used very high doses of these medications.

3. Cholinesterase inhibitors (Table 14-4) may augment cholinergic tone from basal forebrain to frontal cortex, with the potential to improve attention and executive functions.

TABLE 14-2. ANTIDEPRESSANT MEDICATIONS

Medication	Starting Dose	Dosing Range
SSRIs		
Fluoxetine (Prozac)	5–10 mg/d	Up to 80 mg/d
Sertraline (Zoloft)	12.5–25 mg/d	Up to 200 mg/d
Paroxetine (Paxil)	5–10 mg/d	Up to 60 mg/d
Citalopram (Celexa)	10–20 mg/d	Up to 100 mg/d
Escitalopram (Lexapro)	10–20 mg/d	Up to 60 mg/d
Fluvoxamine (Luvox)	12.5–25 mg/d	100–200 mg/d
5-HT$_2$ Antagonists		
Trazodone (Desyrel)	25–50 mg qhs	Up to 300 mg/d
Nefazodone (Serzone)	50 mg qhs	Up to 600 mg/d
TCAs		
Nortriptyline (Pamelor; Aventyl)	10 mg qhs	50–75 mg (therapeutic serum level: 50–150 ng/mL)
Desipramine (Norpramin)	10 mg b.i.d.–t.i.d.	Up to 150 mg (therapeutic serum level: 150–300 ng/mL)
Other		
Bupropion (Wellbutrin; Wellbutrin SR; Wellbutrin XL)	75–150 bupropion/d; 100–150 bupropion-SR/d; 150 buproprion XL/d	Up to 400 mg/d
Venlafaxine (Effexor; Effexor SR)	25 mg b.i.d.–t.i.d.	Up to 375 mg/d
Mirtazapine (Remeron)	15 mg qhs	Up to 90 mg/d

qhs, every night; b.i.d., twice a day; t.i.d., three times a day; SSRIs, selective serotonin reuptake inhibitors; TCAs, tricyclic antidepressants.

TABLE 14-3. DOPAMINERGIC AGENTS

Medication	Starting Dose	Daily Dose Range
Pramipexole (Mirapex)	0.125 mg qd–t.i.d.	0.375–4.5 mg
Pergolide (Permax)	0.05 mg	0.05–5 mg
Bromocriptine (Pariodel)	1.25 qd–b.i.d.	2.5–100 mg
Ropinirole (Requip)	0.25 qd–t.i.d.	0.25–24 mg
Amantadine (Symmetrel)	100 mg	100–300 mg
Selegiline (Eldepryl)	5 mg	5–10 mg

t.i.d., three times a day; b.i.d., twice a day.

TABLE 14-4. CHOLINESTERASE INHIBITORS

Medication	Starting Dose	Dosing Objective	Comment
Donepezil (Aricept)	5 mg	Increase to 10 mg after 4–6 wk	Once per day dosing
Rivastigmine (Exelon)	1.5 mg b.i.d.	Increase by 3 mg q 2–4 wk (as tolerated), up to 6 mg b.i.d.	? Impact of its butyl cholinesterase activity on ↓ AD disease progression
Galantamine (Reminyl)	4 mg b.i.d.	Increase by 8 mg/d ~q 4 wk up to 12 mg b.i.d.	? Impact of its modulation of nicotinic receptor on symptoms and ↓ AD disease progression
Huperzine A	50 μg b.i.d.	Up to 400 μg/d	(100 μg $\cong$ 5 mg of donepezil)

b.i.d., twice a day; AD, Alzheimer disease.

Apathy
1. Defined as a disorder of motivation. Presents with a decrease in goal directed behaviors that are appropriate to a patient's age and background, usually including a loss of independence in one or more Instrumental Activities of Daily Living (IADLs) such as shopping, driving, using public transportation, or handling finances. Patients with apathy are emotionally unresponsive and disengaged from their environment.
   a. Abulia can be viewed as a more extreme presentation of apathy with marked limitations in initiating purposeful behaviors.
   b. Akinesia reflects a disorder of movement, manifesting as a disinclination to initiate movements.
2. DA agonists (Table 14-3).
3. Stimulant medications (see Table 14-1).

Behavioral/Environmental

Depends on the severity of the impairments.
1. General principles:
   a. Organizational strategies/time-management techniques
   b. External support/guidance
   c. Increased structure (including cleaning and organizing the patient's living quarters (which may be squalid, if the patient has been living alone)
   d. Stable routines
   e. Concrete rewards and consequences in response to the patient's actions
   f. Planning for the patient's future
   g. Education and support of caregivers
2. Referrals:
   a. Occupational therapist/rehabilitation specialist to work on organizational techniques.
   b. Social worker to help ensure adequate safety, planning for the future, and necessary caregiver support.

DISORDERS OF AROUSAL AND WAKEFULNESS

BACKGROUND

An appropriate level of arousal is necessary, but not sufficient for awareness and the performance of specific cognitive tasks.

PATHOPHYSIOLOGY

1. Neuroanatomic components: reticular activating system, thalamus, bilateral cortical regions
2. Disorders: primary sleep disorders, cerebrovascular disease, closed head injury, medication side effects

PROGNOSIS

Prognosis is variable and depends on the underlying conditions.

DIAGNOSIS

1. History, emphasizing sleep–wake cycle, symptoms of apnea, periodic leg movements, and narcolepsy. Need to obtain information from patient's bed partner, including a history of snoring, apnea, jerky movements, or kicking off of covers.
2. Review of medications and systemic illnesses.
3. Sleep diary.
4. Consider formal sleep study.

TREATMENT

1. Medications: stimulant medications (see Table 14-1).
2. Improve sleep hygiene: Consistent bed and wake-up times; avoid caffeine after 12 noon; limit alcohol intake; avoid stressful activities before bedtime; avoid daytime naps; consistent exercise routine.
3. Simplify medical regimen if possible.

DISORDERS OF MEMORY

BACKGROUND

1. Although memory can be defined in terms of a variety of mental processes, the clinical focus is on explicit (declarative) memory. This involves the capacity to remember events that are related to a specific temporal or spatial context (episodic memory/new learning) or to recall information in more permanent stores without reference to the specific learning context (semantic memory/facts).
2. Amnestic syndrome is characterized by relatively well-preserved attention; antegrade memory loss; retrograde memory loss—events that occurred closest to the onset of memory loss are recalled least well (Ribot law).

PATHOPHYSIOLOGY

1. Neuroanatomic components: The limbic system and frontal lobes play a crucial role in episodic memory. The neurotransmitter, ACh, involved in pathways from basal forebrain to limbic structures, facilitates the process. In general, a rapid rate of forgetting (with loss of stored data and reduced ability even to "recognize" previously learned information when tested by multiple choice or true–false questions) strongly suggests impairment within the limbic system. Activation–retrieval difficulties, marked by preserved recognition in the setting of poor recall, may indicate problems with frontal network functioning.
2. Disorders:
   a. Degenerative dementias (see below)
   b. Other damage to limbic system or frontal networks [e.g., closed head injury, anoxia, Korsakoff syndrome, central nervous system (CNS) infection such as herpes, cerebrovascular disease]

PROGNOSIS

Variable and depends on the underlying conditions.

DIAGNOSIS

History, MSE, and neurologic examination: To detect more subtle memory disorders, the MSE should include tests appropriate to the patient's educational level and premorbid level of functioning.

TREATMENT

Medications

1. Cholinesterase inhibitors (Table 14-4):
   a. Increase the availability of ACh.
   b. Currently, FDA approval of the cholinesterase inhibitors is limited to the treatment of mild to moderate dementia of the Alzheimer type.
   c. Cholinesterase inhibitors have been shown to result in a modest improvement in cognitive function relative to placebo in a number of trials. In addition to improved cognitive functioning, there is evidence of reduced behavioral symptoms and delayed nursing home placement in patients with AD. There have been studies indicating their efficacy in treating patients with vascular dementia, mixed dementia, severe dementia of the Alzheimer type, and dementia with Lewy bodies.
   d. Clinicians can consider "empiric" treatment with cholinesterase inhibitors for other conditions with memory/cognitive disturbance. In such circumstances it is crucial to closely monitor whether symptoms are improving and be aware of the impact of potential negative side effects.
      1) Donepezil (Aricept) is a reversible acetylcholinesterase inhibitor that is dosed one time a day. In addition to acetylcholinesterase activity, rivastigmine (Exelon) inhibits butyl cholinesterase activity and galantamine (Reminyl) exhibits allosteric binding to nicotinic receptors. Both of these drugs currently are twice-a-day dosing and often require a slower titration period. As of yet, the data on head-to-head trials have been limited; thus, there is no clear indication for one agent over another. The once-a-day dosing of donepezil is appealing although the "second mechanisms" of galantamine and rivastigmine offer the possibility of additional benefits.
      2) Potential side effects of cholinesterase inhibitors include GI distress (e.g., nausea, anorexia, diarrhea, vomiting, weight loss), insomnia, vivid dreams, agitation, dizziness, and muscle cramps. Some patients have unacceptable side effects on one medication, but tolerate another. So it is worth considering switching to another agent prior to giving up on this class of drugs.
   e. Tacrine (Cognex), the first available agent, is rarely used because of its potential liver toxicity and short half-life.
   f. Huperzine A, an herbal acetylcholinesterase inhibitor, offers an alternative for patients who prefer a "natural" treatment. It has shown efficacy in trials both for AD and for ADHD, though it is not FDA-approved for any indication. It comes in tablets of 50 μg. A typical dosage is one pill twice a day. Up to four pills twice a day may be used if tolerated and necessary for optimal therapeutic benefit.
2. Herbal remedies:
   a. These have not been subject to the same scrutiny as medications that require FDA approval.
   b. Ginkgo biloba may have antioxidant properties, increase cerebral blood flow, inhibit platelet-activating factor and have mild stimulating effects. Some combination of these actions may be relevant to their potential efficacy in the treatment of dementia, and perhaps other disorders of cognitive impairment. Treatment has ranged from 120 to 360 mg in divided doses. One controlled study [using 40 mg three times a day (t.i.d.)] in patients with probable AD showed Ginkgo

to be beneficial, although there was a large dropout rate, making interpretation difficult.

3. Memantine, a chemical relative of amantadine, is a moderate-affinity, uncompetitive N-methyl D-aspartate (NMDA) receptor antagonist and weak booster of dopamine. It has a greater NMDA antagonist effect at high levels of receptor activation than at low ones. It comes in 10-mg tablets and the dose is up to 40 mg/d. Used for years in Europe, memantine has received approval (typically 10 mg b.i.d.) by the US FDA for moderate to severe dementia of the Alzheimer type. Studies support its potential efficacy in AD, vascular dementia, and mixed dementia. Although it may help protect against glutamate-induced excitotoxicity, symptomatic improvement of memory and cognition may result from improved signal-to-noise transmission across NMDA and possibly AMPA receptors. Combined treatment with cholinesterase inhibitors seems to be tolerated and may prove beneficial.

Behavioral/Environmental

1. Mnemonic devices
2. Increase depth of encoding
3. Rehearsal
4. External cueing to assist with retrieval
5. Use of written cues

BEHAVIORAL DYSREGULATION/OUTBURSTS

BACKGROUND

Agitation, aggression, and outbursts of intense emotional behavior are among the most socially undesirable and dangerous outcomes of neuropsychiatric disorders.

PATHOPHYSIOLOGY

1. Neuroanatomic components: Behavioral regulation is dependent on the appropriate functioning of limbic structures (e.g., hypothalamus, amygdala) and frontal networks (e.g., orbital frontal cortex). Many neurochemicals play an important modulatory role, including serotonin, ACh, γ-aminobutyric acid (GABA), norepinephrine, dopamine, and androgens.
2. Disorders: A wide range of disorders can be associated with behavioral outbursts, including delirium/ACS, dementia, cerebrovascular disease, closed head injury, and developmental disorders.

PROGNOSIS

Variable; depends on the underlying conditions.

DIAGNOSIS

History (including precipitating factors, medical and psychiatric history, baseline neurologic status), MSE, neuromedical evaluation, toxic–metabolic screen. Historic items to consider include physical, emotional, or sexual abuse; posttraumatic stress disorder (PTSD), antisocial or criminal behavior, traumatic brain injury, and the patient's work and home environments.

TREATMENT

General Principles

1. Evaluate and treat concurrent illnesses (e.g., toxic–metabolic state, infection, pain, constipation, sleep disturbance), especially in cognitively vulnerable patients (e.g., patients with dementia or mental retardation).

2. Identify and treat neuropsychiatric symptoms and disorders that may be contributing (e.g., depression, anxiety, hypomania/mania, thought disorder).
3. Simplify medical regimen, if possible.

Medications

1. Treatment depends on the urgency/acuteness of the situation.
   a. If a patient is wildly agitated and dangerous, consider intramuscular (IM) or intravenous (IV) haloperidol 5 mg with lorazepam 1 mg, or droperidol 5 to 10 mg with midazolam 2.5 to 5 mg; repeating as necessary until the patient is under control. (For older or cognitively disabled patients, much lower doses are appropriate, but the ratio of benzodiazepine to neuroleptic should be approximately the same.) The combination of a benzodiazepine with the neuroleptic potentiates sedation and antianxiety effects and tends to decrease extrapyramidal side effects.
   b. If the situation is less urgent, consider the interventions reviewed below.
   c. As with all treatments, the aim is to try to maximize efficacy and safety while minimizing untoward side effects.
   d. Behavioral strategies also should be instituted which may reduce or eliminate the need for medications.
2. Mood stabilizers:
   a. Antiepileptic drugs (AEDs) (Table 14-5) have been used for over three decades for their mood- and potentially behavior-stabilizing properties.
      1) Valproic acid, usually given as divalproex sodium (Depakote), is the only AED that has FDA approval for the treatment of mania.
      2) Carbamazepine (Tegretol) has a long history of use in the treatment of emotional outbursts and explosive behavior.
      3) Oxcarbazepine (Trileptal) probably has similar effects and does not have the risk of hematologic disorders and is less likely to have toxic side effects other than carbamazepine.

TABLE 14-5. ANTICONVULSANT MEDICATIONS AS POTENTIAL MOOD STABILIZERS

Medication	Starting Dose	Therapeutic Range	Comment
Valproic acid (Depakote)	125–250 mg qd to b.i.d.	75–125 μg/mL	Follow LFTs, CBC, platelets, weight gain, sedation, GI distress, tremor
Carbamazepine (Tegretol, Tegretol-XR, Carbatrol)	100 mg qd–b.i.d.	8–12 μg/mL	Follow LFTs, CBC, Na, sedation, ataxia, dizziness
Oxcarbazepine (Trileptal)	300 mg b.i.d.	Up to 2,400 mg/d in divided doses	Follow Na
Lamotrigine (Lamictal)	50 mg/d	300–500 mg/d in divided doses	Risk of rash (reduced by very slow dosage titration)
Gabapentin (Neurontin)	100–300 mg qhs	Up to 1,200 mg t.i.d.	Sedation
Topiramate (Topamax)	12.5–25 mg/d	Up to 400 mg/d in divided doses	Risk of cognitive side effects; monitor intraocular pressure because of glaucoma risk

b.i.d., twice a day; LFTs, liver function tests; CBC, complete blood count; GI, gastrointestinal; Na, sodium; qhs, at night.

      4) Other anticonvulsants have been studied using varying degrees of experimental control.

      5) In general, aim for doses and therapeutic levels similar to those appropriate for the treatment of epilepsy.

  b. Lithium should be used very cautiously in patients with gross brain disease. Begin with 300 mg daily or 150 mg b.i.d.. Increase slowly, by increments of no more than 300 mg/d. Lithium has a very low therapeutic index: Levels of 1.0 are needed for the best outcomes in primary bipolar disorder but a level of 2.0 will cause neurotoxic symptoms in most patients. Dehydration, diuretics, vomiting, or diarrhea can lead to a large rise in lithium levels; conditions that induce the kidney to conserve sodium also will increase the resorption of lithium from the renal tubules. Common side effects of long-term lithium use include hypothyroidism and nephrogenic diabetes insipidus. Both conditions can aggravate neurologic impairments. Kidney function should be monitored as least weekly during dosage adjustment and at least quarterly thereafter. Thyrotropin and T_4 should be checked every 3 to 6 months, and should be done again if the patient develops new symptoms compatible with hypothyroidism.

  c. Omega-3 fatty acids (fish oil) up to 9.6 g/d [total dosage of docosahexaenoic acid (DHA) plus eicosapentaenoic acid (EPA)] in up to three divided doses, may be a reasonable alternative, especially in patients resistant to taking traditional medications. They have been shown efficacious in a controlled clinical trial for treatment of bipolar disorder.

3. Beta-blockers:

  a. Propranolol (Inderal) 20 to 480 mg/d.

  b. Follow for signs of hypotension and bradycardia.

  c. Asthma is a relative contraindication. Improvement may not be noticeable for weeks.

4. Atypical neuroleptics (Table 14-6):

  a. Have FDA approval for the psychotic symptoms associated with schizophrenia, but are used widely to help in the treatment of nonpsychotic patients whose behaviors are potentially dangerous to themselves and others.

  b. All of the first generation atypical neuroleptics block D_2 dopamine and $5\text{-}HT_2$ serotonergic receptors and other dopamine and serotonin receptors to a degree that differs among the various drugs.

  c. These medications have differing impact on histaminic, α-adrenergic, and cholinergic receptors.

  d. Aripiprazole (Abilify), recently released, differs from the other atypical neuroleptics. Its principal pharmacologic action is dopamine partial agonism—it augments dopaminergic transmission when transmission is low, and decreases it when it is high.

  e. In general, potential side effects of neuroleptics include somnolence, dizziness, orthostatic hypotension, akathisia, extrapyramidal signs, dystonia, neuroleptic malignant syndrome, and tardive dyskinesia. Although the neurologic side effects are less frequent and less severe with the atypical neuroleptics, all of them can occur, and patients with pre-existing brain diseases and disorders are most vulnerable to getting them.

      1) Extrapyramidal side effects can be addressed with low doses of amantadine, pramipexole, or bromocriptine (see Table 14-3), while monitoring for aggravation of the underlying behavioral problems.

      2) Dystonia can be managed by parenteral anticholinergic agents (e.g., diphenhydramine 50 mg or benztropine 2 mg).

      3) Akathisia can be helped by propranolol 20 to 40 mg t.i.d.

5. Benzodiazepines (Table 14-7): An increase in GABA activity may reduce anxiety and have a calming effect. However, there is a risk of reducing inhibition, with a paradoxic increase in behavioral dyscontrol.

6. Buspirone, a 5-hydroxytryptamine 1A ($5\text{-}HT_{1A}$) agonist, may reduce aggressive behaviors. Begin 5 mg/d t.i.d. Increase up to 60 mg/d in divided doses. The effects are often delayed. Side effects tend to be minor and include headaches and

TABLE 14-6. ATYPICAL NEUROLEPTIC MEDICATIONS

Medication	Starting Dose	Dosing Range	Comment
Clozapine (Clozaril)	6.25–25 mg/d	25–300 mg b.i.d.	Minimal extrapyramidal effects. Risk of BM suppression (check frequent CBCs), seizures at higher doses. Patients with PD and psychosis may respond to very low doses.
Olanzapine (Zyprexa)	2.5–5.0 mg qhs	2.5–20 mg/d	Weight gain; glucose intolerance
Risperidone (Risperdal)	0.25–1.0 mg qd–b.i.d.	0.5–3 mg b.i.d.	Of the atypical neuroleptics, most likely to cause extrapyramidal effects. Possible ↑'d risk of stroke in elderly patients
Quetiapine (Seroquel)	25 mg qd–b.i.d.	25–600 mg/d	Weight gain; sedation
Ziprasidone (Geodon)	20 mg qd–b.i.d.	20–160 mg/d	↑'d QTc interval of unclear clinical significance; weight neutral
Aripiprazole (Abilify)	10–15 mg/d	15–30 mg/d	Weight neutral

b.i.d., twice a day; BM, bone marrow; CBC, complete blood counts; PD, Parkinson disease; qhs, at night.

TABLE 14-7. BENZODIAZEPINES

Medication	Initial Dose	Dosing Range
Lorazepam (Ativan)	0.25–1.0 mg t.i.d.	Up to 6 mg/d
Clonazepam (Klonopin)	0.25–0.5 mg t.i.d.	Up to 20 mg/d
Alprazolam (Xanax)	0.25–0.5 mg t.i.d.	Up to 4–5 mg/d; potential for rebound anxiety due to short half-life. Severe symptoms on abrupt withdrawal.
Oxazepam (Serax)	10 mg t.i.d.	Up to 120 mg/d
Diazepam (Valium)	1–2 mg t.i.d.	Up to 40 mg/d
Clorazepate (Tranxene)	3.75–15 mg/d	Up to 60 mg/d

t.i.d., three times a day.

nausea. Buspirone does not suppress respiratory drive, so it can be used in patients with lung disease.

7. SSRIs (see Table 14-2) may reduce irritability and behavioral outbursts, especially in patients with concomitant anxiety and dysphoria. SSRIs [e.g., citalopram (Celexa)] have been shown to reduce behavioral problems in demented elderly. They may be the most effective medication currently available to manage behavioral problems associated with FTD.
   a. In general, we suggest that for neurologic patients, SSRIs be started at doses that are lower than usual (e.g., 5 mg of fluoxetine, citalopram, or paroxetine; 12.5 mg of sertraline).
   b. Potential side effects of SSRIs include sexual dysfunction, increased apathy, restless leg syndrome/periodic leg movements, akathisia, agitation, and sleep disturbances. The last can include difficulty falling asleep and severe late afternoon sleepiness, sometimes requiring a nap to prevent a sleep attack.
   c. Although not well studied, clinicians have used a variety of treatments for SSRI-induced sexual dysfunction, including sildenafil (Viagra) (50–100 mg as needed), cyproheptadine (Periactin) (4–12 mg as needed), bupropion (Wellbutrin) (75–150 mg/d), amantadine (100–300 mg/d) or other dopaminergic agents (Table 14-3).

8. Trazodone (Desyrel) is a $5\text{-}HT_2$ antagonist; 25 to 300 mg/d has been used to help manage agitated patients. This medication is sedating and there is a small risk of priapism (~1/6,000).

9. Cholinesterase inhibitors (Table 14-4) have been shown to have beneficial effects on behavior and neuropsychiatric status in patients with probable AD.

Behavioral/Environmental

1. Safety: protect the patient from self-harm. Protect the caregivers from potentially injurious behaviors.
2. Reduce excessive environmental stimulation.
3. Establish a calm and "predictable" environment.
4. Improve sensory fidelity when feasible (e.g., glasses, hearing aids).
5. Improve sleep hygiene.
6. Ensure adequate fluids and nutritional intake.
7. Try to establish a modest exercise program.

OTHER NEUROPSYCHIATRIC CONDITIONS

Neurologists often care for patients who suffer from a range of neuropsychiatric conditions. They should be aware of diagnostic issues and be prepared to provide initial treatment. However, complicated patients (i.e., those with significant psychiatric history, those at high risk for violence or self-injury, or those resistant to first-line treatments) usually should be referred to qualified psychiatrists with special expertise in this area.

MAJOR DEPRESSION AND DYSTHYMIA

BACKGROUND

Major Depression

1. Characterized by depressed mood and loss of interest or pleasure occurring for most of the time during at least a 2-week period.

2. Key symptoms include weight loss (without dieting), sleep disturbance, psychomotor retardation or agitation, fatigue, feelings of worthlessness/guilt, problems with concentration/decision making, and/or recurrent thoughts of death.
3. These symptoms are associated with significant distress or impairment of daily functioning.
4. Cognitive problems tend to involve attention, executive function, and the activation–retrieval aspects of memory.
5. Clinically significant depression is common in neurologic patients either as a direct reflection of brain dysfunction/injury or as a reaction to associated disabilities.

Dysthymia

Reflects a chronically depressed mood that lasts more than 2 years and is associated with changes in appetite, alterations in sleep, fatigue, low self-esteem, diminished concentration, and hopelessness.

PROGNOSIS

Untreated depression is likely to further erode a patient's functional and cognitive status.

DIAGNOSIS

1. History.
2. MSE (including information about mood, energy level, libido, sleep, appetite, suicidal ideation/plans/attempts).
3. Formal inventories of mood (e.g., Beck Depression Inventory) are useful, but do not substitute for a sensitive clinical interview.

TREATMENT

Medications (Table 14-2)

1. SSRIs:
   a. Often the first medication initiated because of their relatively good side-effect profile/tolerability. They may also be helpful for patients suffering from dysthymia.
   b. SSRIs can cause/exacerbate apathy, which sometimes is mistaken for depression.
   c. SSRIs are often less effective than alternative therapies (e.g., bupropion, venlafaxine, stimulant medication) for patients who also exhibit diminished arousal/engagement/executive functioning.
   d. Abrupt discontinuation, especially of the shorter acting SSRIs (paroxetine, sertraline, fluvoxamine), can lead to flu-like symptoms (headache, nausea, malaise), paresthesias, dizziness, and rebound depression.
2. Tricyclic antidepressants (TCAs):
   a. A major issue is anticholinergic side effects, including dry mouth, urinary retention, sedation, constipation, exacerbation of glaucoma, and confusion, especially in cognitively vulnerable individuals.
   b. Heart block and short QT syndrome should be ruled out by electrocardiogram before initiating therapy.
   c. Secondary amine TCAs (e.g., desipramine, nortriptyline) have lower anticholinergic properties and cause less postural hypotension than tertiary amine TCAs (e.g., amitriptyline, imipramine).
   d. Blood levels of secondary TCAs are widely available and useful for therapeutic drug monitoring.
   e. If possible, TCAs should be tapered slowly to avoid symptoms of cholinergic rebound (e.g., GI distress, headache).

   f. Some would argue that TCAs are the most effective treatment for depressed patients with significant weight loss and sleep disturbance. They also may be particularly useful in depressed patients with pain, anxiety, or sleep problems. TCAs are less likely to suppress libido and inhibit orgasm than SSRIs.

   g. Both TCAs and SSRIs increase the risk of falling in elderly patients. With TCAs, it is often due to orthostatic hypotension, whereas with SSRIs the issue is one of mild motor impairment.

3. Venlafaxine (Effexor) is a selective serotonin–norepinephrine reuptake inhibitor that boosts both of these neurotransmitter systems. Potential side effects include insomnia, sedation, hypertension, sweating, and sexual dysfunction. Because of its relatively short half-life, clinicians need to be mindful of its "discontinuation syndrome" (dizziness, paresthesias, malaise, nausea, and headaches) and thus taper the medication slowly. One way to minimize this is to initiate an SSRI as the venlafaxine is tapered, then taper off the SSRI after venlafaxine has been eliminated.

4. Bupropion (Wellbutrin) (see Table 14-2).

5. MAOIs are effective antidepressants that also have antianxiety properties. They tend to be used in treatment-refractory cases of depression and should be prescribed by clinicians who have experience with this class of medication.

   a. Tranylcypromine (Parnate): initial dose 10 mg b.i.d. to t.i.d.; increase up to 30 to 60 mg/d. This medication also has stimulant effects.

   b. Phenelzine (Nardil): initial dose 15 mg b.i.d. to t.i.d.; increase up to 60 to 90 mg/d.

   c. Most serious side effects involve dangerous interaction with certain (tyramine containing) foods (e.g., red wine, beer, aged cheeses, fava beans) and medications (e.g., certain cold remedies, meperidine, antidepressants), which can precipitate a hypertensive crisis, stroke, or serotonin syndrome (altered mental status, fever, tremor, myoclonus, autonomic dysregulation, possibly leading to death). Patients should check with their physician before taking any new medications and should be warned specifically about over-the-counter (OTC) medications. There should be a delay (usually 2 weeks) between stopping an MAOI and initiating treatment with a variety of medications (e.g., TCAs, many SSRIs). Precautions also need to be taken in terms of delaying treatment with an MAOI after a patient has been on a range of other medications.

Caution

1. Antidepressants can precipitate mania/hypomania in vulnerable individuals. A mood-stabilizing medication often needs to be added.

2. Hypomania due to antidepressants may present with irritability, agitation, intense anxiety, disinhibition, or poor judgment, without euphoria. The possibility of antidepressant-related hypomania should always be considered when a patient's behavior deteriorates after an antidepressant has been started.

Psychotherapy

1. In combination with pharmacotherapy, psychotherapy tends to be the most effective strategy for treating depression.

2. It also provides neurologic patients with a needed avenue in which to work on adjusting to how their disease has impacted their lives.

ANXIETY

BACKGROUND

Common symptom in neurologic patients and has cognitive, somatic/affective, and behavioral components.

1. The cognitive experience is one of worry or fear.
2. Somatically, patients may feel inner shakiness or discomfort, muscle tension, shortness of breath, chest pressure, diaphoresis, or nausea.
3. Behaviorally, they may appear hyperactive and/or irritable, avoid exposure to certain stimuli, and repetitively seek reassurance.
4. Anxiety can undermine attention and executive functions.

DIAGNOSIS

1. History.
2. MSE.
   a. In assessing cognitively impaired patients, behavioral observations (e.g., patient's demeanor, movements, and facial expression) and reports from caregivers are essential.
   b. Inquire specifically about trauma and PTSD, obsessions and compulsions, and phobias.
3. Workup should include the identification of underlying medical/endocrinologic conditions (e.g., hyperthyroidism, hypercortisolism, hyperparathyroidism, partial seizures) or medications/drugs that can cause or exacerbate anxiety (e.g., sympathomimetics; caffeine, alcohol).

TREATMENT

Medications

Should be considered for patients whose anxiety is associated with significant distress, irritability, sleep disturbance, and/or disruption of daily living activities.
1. Benzodiazepines (Table 14-7) provide rapid relief of anxiety and are effective for the short-term management of these symptoms. These medications increase the risk of cognitive and behavioral impairment, especially in patients with frontal lobe dysfunction, and can exacerbate gait disturbance. Begin treatment with low doses and titrate until effective or untoward side effects develop. If patients are in need of longer term treatment for their anxiety, initiate an antidepressant (or buspirone), then taper off the benzodiazepine.
2. Antidepressants (Table 14-2): SSRIs especially are helpful for the treatment of anxiety. Therapeutic onset is slower than benzodiazepines. SSRIs (or in some cases TCAs) may be particularly appropriate in patients who have a mixture of anxiety and depression. In general, clinicians should initiate therapy with SSRIs at a lower dose than used for depression, as they may initially exacerbate anxiety.
3. Buspirone has the advantage of being associated with fewer side effects than benzodiazepines. However, often this medication is less effective and there can be a delay of up to several weeks before maximum response.
4. Atypical neuroleptics (Table 14-6) tend to be reserved for extremely anxious patients who also exhibit paranoid or delusional thoughts.

Psychotherapy/Behavioral

1. Consider psychosocial interventions (e.g., psychotherapy, counseling by treating clinicians, support groups, relaxation training) that are aimed at helping patients deal with the stressors that they face.
2. For some patients, anxiety can be significantly reduced when clinicians are able to fully address their questions and concerns.

PSYCHOSIS

BACKGROUND

Also known as thought disorder.

1. Can present with hallucinations, delusions (including paranoia), bizarre/disorganized behavior or speech, or highly unusual movements (e.g., posturing, immobility) not explained by a defined movement disorder.
2. More subtle manifestations of a thought disorder may include odd associations, vague speech, unusual beliefs that are intensely held, or inappropriate suspiciousness.
3. A thought disorder can be seen in patients suffering from delirium, toxic encephalopathy [e.g. secondary to drugs like amphetamines, phencyclidine (PCP), lysergic acid diethylamide (LSD)], temporolimbic seizure disorder (often with relatively preserved social behavior and executive functions), dementia, mood disorder (severe depression or mania), overwhelming stress (i.e., brief psychotic disorders), or schizophrenia-spectrum illnesses.

DIAGNOSIS

1. History (baseline psychiatric and cognitive status, precipitating events, drug history
2. MSE, neuromedical examination, toxic–metabolic screen, and often neuroimaging and electroencephalogram (EEG).

TREATMENT

1. Atypical neuroleptics (Table 14-6) are the mainstay of treatment.
2. These medications have their most immediate impact on agitation, irritability, and behavioral outbursts. Hallucinations, disorganized thinking, and delusions often take longer to resolve. Persistent delusions associated with schizophrenia tend to be more resistant to treatment.
3. The most effective treatment of patients with PD who exhibit disabling psychotic symptoms (e.g., hallucinations, delusions) is clozapine (at low doses), which does not tend to exacerbate motor symptoms.
   a. Given some of the dangerous side effects of clozapine, it is reasonable to begin treatment with another atypical neuroleptic (e.g., quetiapine, olanzapine).
   b. If increasing these medications to effective levels is prevented by the development of more severe parkinsonian symptoms then turn to clozapine.
4. Psychotic patients with concomitant mood disorders need additional treatment of their mania or depression (see Tables 14-2 and 14-5).
5. As noted above, in elderly demented patients, clinicians should initiate treatment with lower than usual doses.
6. In some cases, isolated visual hallucinations can sometimes be suppressed with ondansetron (Zofran), a 5-HT$_3$-antagonist (approved for the prevention of nausea)— from 1 mg to 8 mg, usually taken at bedtime if hallucinations are nocturnal; and in multiple doses if hallucinations occur around the clock.

DEMENTIA

DIAGNOSIS

1. The following diagnostic criteria are common to dementia of any type according to the *Diagnostic and Statistical Manual of Mental Disorders,* Fourth Edition (*DSM-IV*).

TABLE 14-8. CHARACTERISTICS OF DEMENTIA VERSUS DELIRIUM

	Dementia	Delirium
Onset	Months to years	Hours to days
Course	Steady	Fluctuating
Duration	Years	Days
Attention	Intact in mild/moderate stages	Altered (hypo- or hypervigilant)
Level of arousal	Normal	Fluctuating
Sleep–wake cycle	Usually normal	Often disturbed
Visual hallucinations	Infrequent	Frequent
Tremor	Infrequent	Frequent
Myoclonus	Infrequent	Frequent
Seizures	Uncommon	More common

TABLE 14-9. CAUSES OF DEMENTIA

Neurodegenerative
 Alzheimer disease
 Frontotemporal dementia
 Dementia with Lewy bodies
 Huntington disease
 Corticobasal degeneration
 Progressive supranuclear palsy
 Multisystem atrophy
 Argyrophilic brain disease
 Wilson disease
 Hallevorden–Spatz disease
 Mitochondial diseases
 Kuf disease
 Metachromatic leukodsytrophy
 Adrenoleukodystrophy

Inflammatory/Infectious
 Multiple sclerosis
 Syphilis
 Lyme
 HIV
 Creutzfeldt–Jakob disease
 Primary CNS vasculitis
 Vasculitis secondary to other autoimmune disorders (i.e., lupus)
 Sarcoid
 Chronic meningitis (i.e., tuberculosis, cryptococcus, etc.)
 Viral encephalitis (i.e., HSV)
 Whipple disease
 Systemic lupus erythematosus
 Sjögren syndrome

Vascular
 Vascular dementia
 Hypoxic/ischemic injury
 Post-CABG
 CADASIL (cerebral autosomal dominant arteriopathy with subcortical infarcts and leukoencephalopathy)

Metabolic/toxins
 Hypothyroid
 Vitamin B_{12}
 Thiamine deficiency (Wernicke–Korsakoff)
 Niacin deficiency (pellagra)
 Vitamin E deficiency
 Uremia/dialysis dementia
 Addison/Cushing
 Chronic hepatic encephalopathy
 Heavy metals
 Alcohol

Neoplastic
 Tumor (depends on location)
 Paraneoplastic limbic encephalitis (anti-Hu)
 Acute and chronic sequelae of brain radiation (acute and subacute encephalopathy, radiation necrosis, diffuse late brain injury)
 Chemotherapy
 Lymphomatoid granulomatosis

CNS, central nervous system; HSV, herpes simplex virus; CABG, coronary artery bypass graft; HIV, human immunodeficiency virus.
This list is not exhaustive, as any brain injury can result in dementia depending on location. Some diseases could be under multiple categories.

    a. The development of multiple cognitive deficits manifested by both:
      1) Memory impairment
      2) One (or more) of the following cognitive disturbances:
        a) Aphasia
        b) Apraxia
        c) Agnosia
        d) Disturbance of executive functioning
    b. The above cognitive deficits represent a decline from a previous level of functioning and cause significant impairment in social or occupational functioning.
    c. The deficits do not occur exclusively during the course of a delirium.
  2. Other diagnostic criteria are used for specific causes of dementia.
  3. Clinicians should be aware that not all dementias present with prominent memory deficits.
  4. As reflected in the *DSM-IV* criteria, delirium, acute confusional state, must be ruled out as the cause for the cognitive dysfunction seen in patients suspected of having dementia. Several clinical characteristics may help in this differentiation (see Table 14-8). Delirium has a multitude of etiologies, but is often a result of toxic–metabolic derangements or infections. Patients with dementia are particularly likely to develop delirium as a result of these perturbations.
  5. Table 14-9 lists many causes of dementia. This chapter will explore a select group of these causes.

NEURODEGENERATIVE DEMENTIAS

ALZHEIMER DISEASE

BACKGROUND

1. AD is the most common degenerative dementia and causes a progressive decline in cognitive function.
2. In most cases, an episodic memory deficit is the predominant initial complaint, but deficits in attention, visuospatial processing, naming/language, and executive functions may be present. Over time, the latter cognitive domains become progressively more involved and patients often reach the point where they are no longer able to perform their activities of daily living, recognize family members, and maintain continence. The memory deficit reflects impaired memory storage, as opposed to the encoding and retrieval difficulties that tend to be exhibited by patients with frontal networks impairment.
3. Psychiatric symptoms such as depression, apathy, agitation, and frank psychosis are common.
4. Atypical presentations with more focal brain region pathology do occasionally occur.
5. There are 15 million people worldwide with AD. In the United States, the prevalence increases from about 3% in people over 65 to 47% in those older than 85 years.

PATHOPHYSIOLOGY

Genetics

1. In 2% to 5% of cases, the disease is transmitted in an autosomal dominant fashion.
    a. Three known genetic mutations result in this mode of inheritance:
      1) Mutations of the amyloid precursor protein on chromosome 21 (hence the nearly invariable association of Alzheimer pathology with trisomy 21/Down syndrome)

     2) Presenilin 1 protein on chromosome 14

     3) Presenilin 2 protein on chromosome 1

  b. These mutations may result in increased accumulation of the β-amyloid (Aβ) 42 protein, thought to be the neurotoxic form of Aβ.

  c. The proteins encoded by presenilins 1 and 2 are likely involved in the cleavage of the amyloid precursor protein, from which Aβ is derived.

  d. Patients with autosomal dominant forms of AD often have an earlier age of onset, usually before age 60 and even as early as the 30's or 40's.

2. The remaining 95% of cases are considered sporadic, with the exception of a few described nondominant familial cases.

  a. These patients usually become symptomatic in their 60's or later.

  b. Multiple genetic and environmental factors may play a role in the development and timing of AD in the sporadic cases. The following may increase risk of clinical disease:

     1) Having a first-degree relative with AD,

     2) Having a history of stroke or head injury, and

     3) Being female all may increase an individual's risk of clinical disease.

     4) Another genetic risk factor in sporadic AD is the presence of the ϵ4 allele of the apolipoprotein gene on chromosome 19, which codes for a cholesterol-transporting protein that may be involved in the clearance of Aβ.

       a) Having at least one ϵ4 allele confers, perhaps, a threefold increased risk of AD in sporadic cases.

       b) Patients with the ϵ4 allele also tend to have an earlier age of onset.

       c) In contradistinction, the ϵ2 allele may reduce the risk of AD, serving a protective role.

Pathology

1. The main pathologic findings of AD are amyloid plaques, neurofibrillary tangles, and neuronal loss.

2. Amyloid plaques are an extracellular accumulation of Aβ. Neuritic plaques are amyloid plaques surrounded by dystrophic neuritic processes and may be neurotoxic. There is a modest correlation between plaque burden and disease severity.

3. Neurofibrillary tangles are intracellular, paired helical structures composed of hyperphosphorylated tau. Tangles seem to correlate well with disease severity and neuronal death. They are present in the hippocampus, amygdala, nucleus basalis of Meynert, locus ceruleus, dorsal raphe nucleus, and the neocortex (most prominently the posterior parietal and temporal association cortices).

Neurochemistry

1. There is reduction in the content of ACh and the activity of choline acetyltransferase as a result of basal forebrain degeneration.

2. This loss of ACh is associated with memory impairment making it a target for intervention.

3. The effectiveness of cholinesterase medications further supports the role of ACh depletion in the clinical phenomenology.

4. Other neurotransmitter systems are also impaired.

PROGNOSIS

1. The average course of the illness is 5 to 10 years after the onset of symptoms.

2. Most patients die from other medical conditions, including pneumonia or cardiac causes.

DIAGNOSIS

1. Except for "definite" AD, which is a pathologic diagnosis based on one of several consensually defined pathologic criteria, the diagnosis is clinical.

2. According to the National Institute of Neurological and Communicative Disorders and Stroke and Alzheimer Disease and Related Disorders Association (NINCDS-ADRDA) criteria, probable AD is defined as a progressive decline in memory and at least one other cognitive domain without another identifiable cause. These criteria have been shown to have a high sensitivity (around 90%), but a less impressive specificity (60%–70%). Several ancillary tests may be useful, particularly in the setting of atypical cases.

3. Magnetic resonance imaging (MRI) or computed tomography (CT) should be performed to rule out structural lesions or significant cerebrovascular disease. Medial temporal and posterior temporal and parietal atrophy may be seen.

4. Single photon emission computed tomography (SPECT)/positive emission tomography (PET) imaging may modestly increase sensitivity for the diagnosis of AD; bilateral hypoperfusion of the posterior temporal and parietal lobes is consistent with the diagnosis.

5. Some clinicians use cerebrospinal fluid (CSF) tau (increased) and Aβ (decreased) in atypical cases, but the diagnostic utility of these tests in this situation is unclear.

6. Detection of the $\epsilon4$ is not diagnostic, but may increase specificity in patients who meet clinical criteria.

TREATMENT

Potential Disease-modifying Agents

1. Alpha-tocopherol (vitamin E) is an antioxidant that inhibits free-radical formation and lipid peroxidation. In one trial, 2,000 IU/d was shown to delay clinical progression by 20 to 30 weeks, including time to placement in an institution and development of severe dementia. Caution should be used in patients taking anticoagulants and antiplatelet medication, as vitamin E may increase the risk of bleeding due to inhibition of platelet function. Some recommend lower doses in these instances.

2. Selegiline, an MAO inhibitor, has also been shown to slow clinical progression, but is less often used given its potential drug interactions and side-effect profile. The combination of vitamin E and selegiline does not seem to offer any extra benefit and is associated with increased side effects.

3. Ginkgo biloba has antioxidant, neurotrophic, and antiinflammatory properties. Data are mixed, but a meta-analysis and a large placebo-controlled trial suggest mild improved cognition relative to placebo. Further research is ongoing.

4. Antiinflammatory agents have been investigated given the probable contribution of inflammation to the pathogenesis of AD. Retrospective studies have suggested a decreased risk of AD, but data on benefit for patients already with the diagnosis are lacking.

5. Elevated homocysteine levels increase the risk of dementia, including clinical AD. High homocysteine has also been associated with mildly poorer cognitive function in normal elderly. Since treatment is relatively benign (B_{12}, B_6, and folic acid supplementation), vitamin supplementation is reasonable for patients with elevated homocysteine levels.

6. Future possibilities include the Aβ vaccine, passive immunization, inhibition of the γ- and β-secretases (involved in the processing of the amyloid precursor protein), neurotrophic factors, and novel cholinergic agonists.

Symptomatic Treatment

1. Cholinesterase inhibitors (see earlier and Table 14-4) have been shown to result in a modest improvement in cognitive function relative to placebo in a number of trials. In addition to improved cognitive functioning, there is evidence for reduced behavioral symptoms and delayed nursing home placement.

2. Memantine (see earlier) has demonstrated improved cognition over placebo in the treatment of moderate to severe AD in a 28-week trial. Potential disease modifying

effects of the medication due to its theoretic inhibition of glutamate mediated excitotoxic cell death merit further investigation.
3. Symptomatic treatment for neuropsychiatric symptoms and specific cognitive deficits should be pursued as outlined above.
4. Treat concurrent medical illnesses and chronic conditions (e.g., diabetes, hypertension) because patients with probable AD have diminished cognitive reserve.

MILD COGNITIVE IMPAIRMENT

BACKGROUND

1. Mild cognitive impairment (MCI) is thought to represent the transition from normal aging to dementia, in particular AD. This state (at least the amnestic form) is usually defined as an isolated memory impairment in the setting of preserved general cognitive and functional abilities.
2. Patients convert from MCI to AD at a rate of 10% to 15% per year compared to the 1% to 2% conversion of age-matched controls. A small proportion of patients, less than 20%, may not convert, and the MCI diagnosis does not always represent the early manifestation of a neurodegenerative process.
3. The epidemiology of MCI is uncertain given the heterogeneity of the definition used in various studies. One could argue that all patients with AD must have had a transitional MCI period.

PATHOPHYSIOLOGY

1. Most patients with MCI who have come to autopsy have been found to have neurofibrillary tangles in the hippocampus and entorhinal cortex. There are variable findings of amyloid plaques in the neocortex. These findings are consistent with the notion that MCI represents a transitional period to AD.
2. Less commonly, other diseases with medial temporal lobe pathology are found, perhaps explaining the incomplete conversion rate to AD.

PROGNOSIS

Rate of conversion to AD is described above. Hippocampal atrophy on MRI, poor performance on cued memory tasks, an ϵ4 allele, and elevated CSF tau may be predictive of more rapid conversion to AD.

DIAGNOSIS

1. The diagnosis is made on a clinical basis. Patients must present with memory complaints and have objective memory impairment compared with age- and education-matched norms, but perform well on other tests of general cognitive function and have no significant difficulty with activities of daily living.
2. Some have denoted the above as amnestic MCI, differentiating it from MCI in which a cognitive domain outside of memory is impaired or multiple domains are slightly impaired.
3. The latter patients are classified as nonamnestic MCI and may represent premorbid conditions for dementia types other than AD.

TREATMENT

1. There is no current consensus on treatment, but many trials are ongoing to evaluate both symptom amelioration (such as with cholinesterase inhibitors) and disease modification (vitamin E, ginkgo biloba, and nonsteroidal antiinflammatory drugs).

2. Risk/benefit ratios must be weighed in these patients, but antioxidant treatment with vitamin E and reduction of homocysteine levels (if elevated) are reasonable interventions.
3. A trial with a cholinesterase inhibitor could also be attempted depending on the patient's desire to treat his/her memory problem aggressively.
4. Further research is needed to determine appropriate management; this group of patients may potentially benefit from the novel disease-modifying interventions being developed.

FRONTOTEMPORAL DEMENTIA

BACKGROUND

1. At least three clinical syndromes have been described:
  a. Frontal variant of FTD:
    1) Marked primarily by changes in personality and behavior, a range of behavioral changes is seen, ranging from apathy to disinhibition. Patients may demonstrate inappropriate social behavior, such as making sexual gestures or comments, hyperphagia, utilization behavior, and abulia. Lack of insight and empathy are common features.
    2) Neuropsychologic tests of frontal lobe function are often impaired, especially attention and executive functions (sparing memory storage and visuospatial function), but may not be if the disease is primarily affecting the orbitomedial frontal lobes (most bedside frontal tests assess the function of the dorsolateral frontal lobes). Performance on testing is often marked by great variability, reflecting the underlying frontal impairment.
    3) Isolated frontal lobe or right frontotemporal atrophy may be present early in the course.
  b. Primary progressive (nonfluent) aphasia (PPA):
    1) Marked initially by selective impairment of speech production similar to a Broca aphasia.
    2) Patients produce phonemic paraphasic errors and have impaired production and comprehension of meaning based on syntax.
    3) They also may exhibit buccofacial apraxia ("show me how you would blow out a candle").
    4) Lexical fluency ("how many words can you think of that begin with 'F'") is impaired.
    5) Other cognitive domains remain relatively preserved and atrophy is usually limited to the dominant frontal and temporal perisylvian region in the early stages.
  c. Semantic dementia:
    1) In this form there is loss of semantics, or the meaning attached to words and objects.
    2) Patients are anomic and make frequent semantic paraphasic errors, often only able to produce the supraordinate category for an item ("animal" instead of "giraffe").
    3) Category fluency ("how many animals can you name in one minute?"), defining words, and the reading and writing of irregular words ("surface dyslexia") all may be impaired.
    4) Other cognitive domains remain relatively intact and atrophy is often limited to the left anterior and inferolateral temporal lobe early in the course.
2. Despite this syndromic classification, over time, features of all three types are present reflecting more diffuse frontal and temporal lobe involvement. The disease often presents in the fifth and sixth decades and may be as common as AD in this age group. In some cases, particularly when familial, features of parkinsonism and amyotrophic lateral sclerosis may be present.

PATHOPHYSIOLOGY

1. The pathology in FTD is varied. Involvement of the frontal and anterior temporal lobes is present with relative sparing of the occipital and posterior parietal and temporal lobes. The hippocampus is less involved than more anterior limbic structures (i.e., amygdala). The basal ganglia and substantia nigra also may be involved.
2. Pick body inclusions are seen in less than 20% of the cases (hence the change in name from Pick disease to FTD).
3. There may be severe gliosis with or without ballooned cells.
4. A nondescript histopathology with neuronal loss and microvacuolar changes also may be present.
5. The disease is often sporadic, but approximately 40% of cases are familial, less than half of which are autosomal dominant. Several of these families (with the frontal variant) have been found to have mutations in the tau protein on chromosome 17. Linkage to chromosome 17, but not to tau, and to other chromosomes also has been described.

PROGNOSIS

1. The estimated life span following diagnosis is 3 to 15 years.
2. Concomitant motor neuron or extrapyramidal disease may be an important factor in prognostication.

DIAGNOSIS

1. The diagnosis is clinical with a noted relatively high sensitivity and specificity, but prospective trials addressing this issue are lacking.
2. Spared-memory storage helps differentiate FTD from AD.
3. Structural imaging with MRI or CT may demonstrate focal atrophy.
4. SPECT has also proven to be useful in differentiating from AD, demonstrating bifrontal and bitemporal hypoperfusion in the frontal variant.

TREATMENT

1. There is some evidence that serotonin levels may be low in FTD and that treatment with SSRIs may improve behavioral symptoms (see Table 14-2).
2. Atypical neuroleptic agents may also be necessary for more severe behavioral manifestations (see Table 14-6).
3. Sparing of the cholinergic system in FTD likely underlies the lack of clear utility of acetylcholinesterase inhibitors.
4. As with other dementias, cognitive symptoms should be targeted and trials with various agents may be pursued.

DEMENTIA WITH LEWY BODIES

BACKGROUND

1. Dementia with Lewy bodies (DLB) may be the second most common form of neurodegenerative dementia.
2. It is characterized by fluctuations in cognition, visual hallucinations, and mild extrapyramidal features. The hallucinations tend to be well formed and are often of people or animals. Patients are disturbed to varying degrees as a result of the hallucinations.
3. Cognition tends to be mostly impaired in the realms of executive function, attention, speed of processing, and visuospatial abilities.
4. Memory is impaired at the level of encoding and retrieval.

5. Depression and rapid eye movement (REM) sleep behavior disorder are relatively common.
6. Marked exacerbation of extrapyramidal signs with neuroleptics and persistent parkinsonism after their withdrawal is suggestive of DLB in patients with dementia.
7. The clinical overlap with dementia associated with PD is substantial and distinguishing one from the other is often arbitrary.

PATHOPHYSIOLOGY

1. Cortical Lewy bodies (spheric, intracytoplasmic, eosinophilic, neuronal inclusions containing α-synuclein and ubiquitin proteins) are found on autopsy in these patients and likely contribute to dementia.
2. Lewy body pathology in the substantia nigra, locus ceruleus, and nucleus basalis also may result in some cognitive symptoms of DLB.
3. Additionally, Alzheimer pathology is common in these patients, 60% or more reaching pathologic criteria for AD.
4. The presence of an apolipoprotein ε4 allele may be a risk factor for DLB and is increased in prevalence in patients with PD and dementia as opposed to those PD patients without dementia.

PROGNOSIS

The course is similar, if not more rapid, than in AD with survival from 2 to 12 years.

DIAGNOSIS

1. Diagnosis is made clinically based on the above mentioned features. Having two of the three primary characteristics (fluctuations, visual hallucinations, and mild parkinsonism) is considered "probable" DLB.
2. By definition, parkinsonian features should not proceed the onset of the dementia by more than 12 months.
3. A structural imaging study should be performed to rule out other potential contributing processes, such as strokes.
4. SPECT and PET imaging may reveal occipital hypometabolism, which may help in differentiating DLB from AD.

TREATMENT

DLB is difficult to treat and requires a delicate balance of trying to improve motor symptoms without exacerbating confusion and hallucinations.
1. Motor symptoms: A trial with L-dopa or dopaminergic agonists (Table 14-3) is reasonable although it may result in increased hallucinations and confusion.
2. Depression: Treatment with SSRIs or bupropion (Table 14-2) may be effective. Electroconvulsive therapy (ECT) should be considered in severe, refractory cases.
3. Psychosis: Atypical neuroleptics, such as quetiapine, olanzapine, or clozapine (Table 14-6) should be used because they are less likely than typical neuroleptics to exacerbate extrapyramidal symptoms. Clozapine is the least likely to do so; but due to its side effect profile, should probably be reserved for use after treatment failure with another atypical neuroleptic. All of these agents may worsen fatigue and confusion. Anticholinergic medications may exacerbate confusion.
4. Cognition: Cholinesterase inhibitors may improve attention, processing speed, and behavioral symptoms (see Table 14-4). Rivastigmine has been studied the most rigorously, but the other cholinesterase inhibitors are likely to have similar efficacy. Theoretically, increasing ACh levels may worsen extrapyramidal symptoms, but clinically this has not proven problematic.

HUNTINGTON DISEASE

BACKGROUND

1. Huntington disease is an autosomal dominant disorder that is completely penetrant and causes progressive cognitive decline, marked extrapyramidal motor abnormalities, and psychiatric symptoms.
2. Impairment of executive functioning and attention is common.
3. Visuospatial deficits are also frequently seen.
4. Cognitive symptoms may proceed the motor symptoms.
5. Loss of voluntary motor control and the development of chorea (rapid involuntary movements around multiple joints) and other extrapyramidal symptoms are the hallmarks of the disease.
6. Depression is the most common psychiatric manifestation, but apathy, mania, anxiety, and delusional thinking can occur.
7. Patients tend to become symptomatic by midlife, but onset has been reported from early childhood to late life.
8. The disease is very rare occurring in 5 to 10/100,000.

PATHOPHYSIOLOGY

1. Huntington disease is due to a mutation of a gene on chromosome 4 for the protein huntingtin.
2. The disease results when a CAG trinucleotide repeat expands to more than 39 repeats (36–39 repeats is considered indeterminate).
3. Larger number of repeats are associated with earlier age of onset.
4. As expansion is most likely to occur in spermatogenesis, earlier onset cases tend to be transmitted through the father.
5. Degeneration occurs most prominently in the striatum, but there is also neuronal loss in the cortex and other deep grey nuclei.
6. Proteolytic products of the huntingtin protein containing polyglutamine repeats seem to be sequestered in cell nuclei and may interfere with cell regulation.

PROGNOSIS

1. Inevitably leads to death, usually 15 to 25 years after initial presentation.
2. Death is usually due to medical complications.
3. There is a relatively high rate of suicide.

DIAGNOSIS

1. The diagnosis should be considered in any patient presenting with chorea, particularly if there is concomitant cognitive decline or psychiatric symptoms.
2. A family history makes the diagnosis more obvious and genetic testing can be confirmatory.
3. Presymptomatic genetic testing is controversial and should involve genetic counseling.
4. MRI often reveals significant caudate atrophy later in the course of disease, but may appear normal early.

TREATMENT

1. There is currently no treatment to slow down the course of the illness.
2. Psychiatric and cognitive complaints should be treated symptomatically.
3. Chorea may respond to neuroleptic agents.

CORTICOBASAL DEGENERATION

BACKGROUND

1. Corticobasal degeneration (CBD) is marked by a progressive, asymmetric extrapyramidal motor disorder with cognitive decline referable to parietal and frontal lobe dysfunction.
2. An asymmetric rigid–akinetic parkinsonism or dystonia (usually of the upper limb) is prominent.
3. Severe apraxia (ideomotor, limb kinetic, and eye opening), cortical sensory loss, and the alien limb phenomenon (the limb "has a mind of its own"; up to 50% of patients manifest this) are other common features.
4. Orofacial apraxia, dysarthria, reflex myoclonus, supranuclear gaze palsy (horizontal as opposed to vertical, allowing differentiation from progressive supranuclear palsy [PSP]), and postural instability also may be seen.
5. Dementia is common at presentation, with prominent executive dysfunction in addition to apraxia.
6. Memory storage is usually preserved, but encoding and retrieval impairment is common. Slow speech production, nonfluent aphasia, and anarthria all may be present.
7. Depression and apathy are common neuropsychiatric features.
8. The onset of the disease is usually in the sixth decade, with the youngest reported case being 45 years old.

PATHOPHYSIOLOGY

1. Prominent atrophy of the frontal and parietal lobes is a hallmark of the disease, which is usually relatively symmetric by the time of death.
2. Degeneration of the substantia nigra pars compacta is also seen.
3. Microscopically, ballooned and achromatic neurons are a hallmark. These cells, as well as tau-positive inclusions, are seen in CBD, PSP, and FTD. There appears to be genetic, pathologic, and clinical overlap with FTD and PSP. There is one reported kindred with some members having clinically suspected FTD and others with CBD.

PROGNOSIS

The disease progresses to death in 5 to 10 years.

DIAGNOSIS

1. Diagnosis is difficult and made on a clinical basis with other studies being supportive.
2. MRI or CT findings can be normal early in the disease, but asymmetric posterior frontal and parietal atrophy is seen in most patients. As the disease further progresses, atrophy becomes more symmetric.
3. SPECT/PET imaging demonstrates decreased cerebral blood flow/glucose metabolism in regions found to be atrophic on MRI, as well as in the medial frontal and temporal cortical areas. Bilateral reduction of 18-fluorodopa uptake in the putamen and caudate is also consistent with the diagnosis.

TREATMENT

1. Treatment of motor dysfunction is difficult.
2. A few patients show modest improvement with carbidopa/levodopa.
3. Myoclonus may respond to clonazepam.
4. Botulinum toxin for painful dystonia is a consideration.
5. Treatment for neuropsychiatric and cognitive symptoms should be symptomatic.

6. Clinicians should be mindful that "typical" neuroleptics may worsen extrapyramidal symptoms.

NONNEURODEGENERATIVE DEMENTIA

VASCULAR DEMENTIA

BACKGROUND

1. Vascular dementia is a heterogeneous disease composed of multiple etiologies, including leukoariosis, small-vessel infarcts, multiple cortical strokes, or a single, strategically placed stroke.
2. As a result of the heterogeneity of etiology, there is concomitant clinical heterogeneity. Multiple lacunar infarcts or significant white matter disease (so-called Binswanger disease) result in apathy, frontal networks impairment, and corticospinal and bulbar signs. Large-vessel strokes cause syndromes specific to the site of the lesion, such as aphasia, agnosia, and so forth.
3. Vascular dementia is the second most common form of dementia (estimates vary from around 10% to more than 33%).
4. The prevalence of coexistent AD pathology (in more than 50% of cases diagnosed with vascular dementia) and the fact that vascular events seem to hasten the onset of clinical AD make estimates of the actual prevalence of vascular dementia problematic.

PATHOPHYSIOLOGY

1. The risk factors for vascular dementia are considered the same as those for stroke.
2. Leukoariosis is marked by white matter signal changes on MRI or CT and is associated pathologically with axon loss and demyelination.
3. Aging, hypertension, diabetes, and arteriosclerosis produce narrowing and tortuosity of deep white matter vessels. This narrowing likely results in poor vascular reserve and leukoariosis in the setting of episodic hypoperfusion. Disruption of white matter is thought to cause functional disconnection between gray matter structures.
4. Ischemia of deep gray structures also can contribute to cognitive dysfunction.
5. Cortical infarcts cause direct impairment of the cognitive function(s) subserved by those areas of cortex.

PROGNOSIS

1. The course is variable. The average time to death after diagnosis is about 4 years.
2. The causes of death include complications of dementia, stroke, and myocardial infarctions.

DIAGNOSIS

1. As defined by the National Institute of Neurological Disorders and Stroke and the Association Internationale pour la Recherche et l'Enseignement en Neuroscienses (NINDS-AIREN) criteria, probable vascular dementia requires cognitive decline in memory and two other domains interfering with the patient's activities of daily living.
2. The temporal course needs to suggest a vascular cause, including onset within 3 months after stroke, an abrupt onset, and/or a stepwise course.

3. Neuroimaging must support the diagnosis, with evidence of appropriately placed cortical strokes, subcortical strokes, or extensive white matter disease.
4. Other diagnostic criteria exist, but most have demonstrated relatively high specificity and low sensitivity.
5. Use of the Hachinski Ischemic Score can increase sensitivity, but is less useful in differentiating vascular dementia from mixed dementia.

TREATMENT

1. Preventive measures may play an important role in slowing down the course of disease, but no definitive studies have shown intervention with specific benefit in vascular dementia.
2. Because hypertension is a risk factor for both stroke and vascular dementia, adequate control should be a goal; reduction of blood pressure has been shown to protect against dementia in general.
3. Other stroke risk factors, including smoking, hyperlipidemia, homocysteine, and diabetes should also be managed as they are likely to be associated with vascular dementia.
4. The importance of risk reduction is made even more salient by the finding that stroke may hasten the onset of clinical AD.
5. The use of cholinesterase inhibitors (Table 14-4) in patients with vascular dementia or mixed dementia has been demonstrated to have a mild cognitive benefit.
6. A similar benefit has been seen with memantine (see Memory Disorders, Treatment, earlier).
7. Given the high association of depression after stroke, a trial with an antidepressant (see Table 14-2) is reasonable if there is any suspicion of a mood component.
8. Because frontal network impairment is a common neuropsychological finding, symptomatic treatment should be considered as outlined above.

NORMAL PRESSURE HYDROCEPHALUS

BACKGROUND

1. Normal pressure hydrocephalus (NPH) has classically been defined by the clinical triad of dementia, impairment of gait, and urinary incontinence.
2. Gait and cognitive findings generally occur early in the course while incontinence tends to occur later.
3. The dementia is characterized by impaired attention, concentration, and executive functioning.
4. Apathy can be a major feature.
5. NPH is most prevalent in the sixth and seventh decades, but can be seen at any age.
6. Overall prevalence is not well established.

PATHOPHYSIOLOGY

1. Normal pressure hydrocephalus results from greater production than absorption of CSF. This is most commonly thought to be due to insufficient absorption through the arachnoid granulations and villi.
2. Most cases are idiopathic, but many are secondary to such events as prior subarachnoid hemorrhage, meningitis, trauma, or elevated CSF protein.
3. Although intracranial pressure is "normal" by definition, transient elevations in pressure are believed to occur that result in ventricular enlargement. The frontal horns are often disproportionately enlarged, resulting in stretching of motor fibers to the legs and sphincters, which are located in this region. Compression of frontal white matter also likely accounts for the cognitive findings.

PROGNOSIS

1. If untreated, there is a risk of progression to an abulic/akinetic state.
2. Response to ventricular shunting is variable, but those patients with isolated gait difficulty or a shorter duration of dementia seem to have a higher likelihood for a good outcome.
3. More than 2 years of dementia or the presence of significant cerebrovascular disease predict poorer outcome.

DIAGNOSIS

1. Diagnosis can be difficult. Establishment of the appropriate clinical setting and evidence of hydrocephalus on CT or MRI are necessary.
2. Differentiation of hydrocephalus from hydrocephalus ex vacuo (i.e., atrophy, as seen in AD or with cerebrovascular disease) is not easy, but certain radiographic clues are helpful, such as less prominent cortical atrophy in NPH, disproportionate enlargement of the frontal and inferior horns, and prominent aqueductal flow on MRI.
3. Measurement of cerebral compliance with lumbar injections is another potential modality for diagnosis.
4. Radioisotope cisternography has also been used, but is relatively nonspecific.
5. A more traditional approach is a high-volume lumbar puncture (30 mL of CSF), which may produce transient improvement in cognition and gait, but false-negative results are possible.
6. Temporary lumbar drainage may prove a better test for the potential benefit of shunting, but shunting itself may be most helpful in establishing diagnosis.

TREATMENT

1. Surgical treatment is usually with ventriculoperitoneal shunt placement.
2. To decrease production of CSF, acetazolamide may be considered, but has not been established as effective in controlled trials.
3. Difficulties with attention, apathy, and executive functioning can be treated symptomatically, as outlined above.

DEMENTIA DUE TO INFECTIOUS PROCESSES

ACQUIRED IMMUNODEFICIENCY SYNDROME DEMENTIA

BACKGROUND

1. Acquired immunodeficiency syndrome (AIDS) dementia complex (ADC) is due to primary human immunodeficiency virus (HIV) infection and should be distinguished from cognitive impairment as a result of opportunistic infections.
2. Cognitive decline is noted to occur over 6 months or longer.
3. The dementia is characterized as being of the "subcortical type," involving impaired attention/concentration, psychomotor slowing, and memory loss at the level of encoding and retrieval.
4. Depression and/or apathy may be prominent.
5. As the disease progresses, patients may become increasingly withdrawn with mutism often present in the final stages.
6. Since the introduction of highly active antiretroviral therapy (HAART), the percentage of patients with AIDS developing ADC has dropped from 60% to 10%.
7. ADC is rarely the presenting complaint in AIDS.

PATHOPHYSIOLOGY

1. A high brain viral load is associated with development of dementia in populations, but is not necessarily high in any one individual.
2. Multinucleated macrophages and leukoencephalopathy are found on pathology. Subcortical gray structures are also prominently involved.
3. Cortical atrophy in the frontal and temporal lobes can occur with progression.
4. A major source of neuronal dysfunction or death is unlikely to be due to a direct infection of neurons, but rather local (toxic) environmental effects.
5. Neuronal apoptosis may be accelerated in AIDS.
6. The protective benefit of HIV therapy that poorly penetrates the CNS suggests that the pathophysiology of dementia is initiated systemically.

PROGNOSIS

1. Without treatment, time from diagnosis to death is approximately 6 months.
2. With antiretroviral treatment, this time may be extended.

DIAGNOSIS

1. The diagnosis is made on the basis of clinical findings in patients with HIV.
2. Testing for HIV should be pursued in patients with the appropriate cognitive profile, particularly young patients or patients with risk factors for HIV infection.
3. MRI is important to help rule out opportunistic infections, such as toxoplasmosis and progressive multifocal leukoencephalopathy, as well as primary CNS lymphoma.
4. In patients with ADC without opportunistic infections, MRI may show ill-defined, increased white matter signal on T_2-weighted images and diffuse cerebral atrophy.
5. Early subcortical hypermetabolism and later cortical/subcortical hypometabolism has been seen with PET.
6. MR spectroscopy has demonstrated increased sensitivity compared to conventional MRI in preliminary studies.
7. CSF should be examined to rule out cryptococcal meningitis, cytomegalovirus (CMV), and neurosyphilis. CSF biomarkers, including viral load, may prove useful.

TREATMENT

1. Treatment should be aimed at reducing the plasma viral load.
2. HAART therapy should be used to this end.
3. It is unclear which particular combinations of antiretrovirals are most effective in the treatment of ADC.
4. The nucleoside analogs penetrate the blood–brain barrier more effectively than other antiretrovirals.
5. Azidothymidine (AZT) has been studied most rigorously and does result in neurocognitive improvement.
6. Selegiline may have a neuroprotective effect in these patients.
7. Symptomatic treatment of cognitive dysfunction should be pursued.

NEUROSYPHILIS

BACKGROUND

1. Syphilis is a sexually transmitted disease caused by *Treponema pallidum*.
2. Tertiary syphilis, which occurs in 30% of untreated patients, may produce dementia.
3. Meningovascular syphilis (usually 2 to 10 years after infection) can produce both dementia and strokes through arteritic occlusion of blood vessels.

4. General paresis, which is a chronic low-grade encephalitis often occurring 15 to 30 years after initial infection, produces slow intellectual decline.
5. Almost any neuropsychiatric symptom may be present, including psychosis, grandiosity, mania, and depression.
6. A significant minority (20%–40%) have only dementia. Poor attention and memory (on the basis of encoding and retrieval impairment) are common features.
7. Reduced speech output and anomia may occur.
8. Pseudobulbar palsy may be another prominent feature.
9. Signs and symptoms of other manifestations of tertiary syphilis are often present, including tabes dorsalis, Argyll–Robertson pupils, and optic atrophy.

PATHOPHYSIOLOGY

1. General paresis is thought to be due to direct CNS infection.
2. Atrophy is most pronounced in the frontal and temporal cortices.
3. Cortical organization is disturbed with neuronal loss and astrocytic and microglial proliferation.
4. Inflammatory infiltrates around penetrating blood vessels may be seen.
5. The disease tends to be more aggressive in patients with HIV, presumably due to their impaired immune system.

PROGNOSIS

1. About half of patients will demonstrate improvement with treatment.
2. Arrest of further progression in those who do not improve is another potential outcome.

DIAGNOSIS

1. Any patient with signs or symptoms suspicious for the diagnosis should have serologic testing.
2. The rapid plasma reagin (RPR) serology provides an initial screen, but is associated with false-positive results (false-negative results occur less commonly).
3. A positive test should be followed by a treponemal serologic test, such as the fluorescent treponema antibody (FTA), to confirm the diagnosis.
4. If tertiary syphilis is suspected, CSF should be obtained.
5. An elevated protein level, pleocytosis, and a positive VDRL test are expected, but if at least one is present, treatment should be pursued.

TREATMENT

1. The treatment of choice is penicillin G at 4 million units every 4 hours for 10 days.
2. For patients who have a penicillin allergy, amoxicillin, doxycycline, and ceftriaxone are alternatives, but of less known efficacy.
3. CSF should be examined every 3 to 6 months for gradual return to normal protein and cell count, as well as disappearance of or stable reduction in titer of VDRL test.
4. Due to an increased treatment failure rate in patients with HIV, some have recommended additional treatment with weekly intramuscular benzathine penicillin for 3 weeks or doxycycline 200 mg twice a day (b.i.d.) for 30 days after initial treatment. Prophylactic measures in HIV-positive patients need further study. These patients should be carefully monitored for relapse for up to 2 years after treatment.

PRION DISEASE

BACKGROUND

1. These disorders represent a collection of neurodegenerative diseases caused by abnormal accumulation of the prion protein.

2. They can occur sporadically, as in Creutzfeldt–Jakob disease (CJD; 85% of cases), or in families, as in fatal familial insomnia (FFI), Gerstmann–Straüssler–Scheinker syndrome (GSSS), and familial Creutzfeldt–Jakob disease.
3. A small percentage of cases have been acquired iatrogenically from pooled human growth hormone, corneal transplants, and incompletely sterilized surgical equipment.

Creutzfeldt–Jakob Disease

1. The classic clinical triad is of dementia, myoclonus, and ataxia.
2. Often, a rapidly progressive dementia precedes the onset of progressive pyramidal, extrapyramidal, and cerebellar abnormalities.
3. Rare variants present with more prominent visuospatial abnormalities (Heidenhain variant) and ataxia (Brownwell–Oppenheimer variant).
4. This disease usually presents in the fifth through seventh decades and has an annual incidence of less than 1 per million.

New Variant Creutzfeldt–Jakob Disease

1. New variant Creutzfeldt–Jakob disease (nvCJD) has been seen primarily in the United Kingdom and is thought to be the human transmitted form of bovine spongiform encephalopathy (mad cow disease).
2. The course is more indolent than sporadic CJD and marked by more prominent early neuropsychiatric symptoms.
3. The average age of onset is in the second decade and the youngest reported case was of a 12-year-old.

Gerstmann–Straüssler–Scheinker Syndrome

1. GSSS is a familial disease with a prominent spinocerebellar ataxia and decreased reflexes.
2. Dementia, motor neuron disease, and extrapyramidal disease is variably present.
3. Patients usually present in their 30's or later.

Fatal Familial Insomnia

1. This prion disease is marked by severe insomnia, dysautonomia, and ataxia.
2. Extrapyramidal and pyramidal signs may occur, with dementia being less prominent.

PATHOPHYSIOLOGY

1. Disease-causing prions are abnormal isoforms of the human prion protein, which cause the normal form to fold into the abnormal isoform leading to accumulation of the abnormal protein.
2. The different clinical syndromes are a reflection of differences in the location and form of the histopathology.
3. Sporadic CJD demonstrates spongiform changes, gliosis, and neuronal loss in the grey matter. Unlike sporadic CJD, in GSSS there are many protein amyloid plaques.
4. Dense prion protein plaques surrounded by a halo of spongiform change (florid plaques) are unique to nvCJD.
5. FFI has few spongiform changes, but is marked by gliosis of the thalamus, inferior olives, and cerebellum.

PROGNOSIS

1. The median and mean survival for sporadic CJD are 4 and 7 months, respectively, with up to 90% of patients dying within the first year.
2. nvCJD has a somewhat longer course, with a median survival of 14.5 months.
3. The course for GSSS can be up to 10 years.

DIAGNOSIS

1. CJD:
   a. Diagnosis is made on the basis of clinical findings.
   b. In one third to two thirds of patients, the classic EEG finding of 1- to 2-Hz generalized, triphasic periodic sharp waves will be present.
   c. MRI has also proven useful with fluid-attenuated inversion recovery (FLAIR) and diffusion-weighted imaging.
   d. Hyperintensities in the cortex, basal ganglia, thalamus, and cerebellum have been described.
   e. In the appropriate clinical context, the 14-3-3 protein detected in the CSF has a high sensitivity and specificity for CJD.
   f. Brain biopsy is definitive.
2. nvCJD:
   a. Diagnostic criteria are relatively sensitive.
   b. Probable cases require at least 6 months of a progressive psychiatric disorder and at least four of five clinical symptoms, including ataxia, dementia, extrapyramidal movement disorder, persistent dysesthesias, and early psychiatric symptoms.
   c. The EEG should not show the classic pattern of sporadic CJD.
   d. MRI should be consistent with the diagnosis. T_2-weighted, FLAIR, and diffusion-weighted imaging often show increased signal in the pulvinar and/or dorsomedial thalamic nuclei.
   e. Tonsil biopsy holds promise in detection of nvCJD.
3. GSSS and FFI:
   a. May be diagnosed clinically with attention to family history.
   b. MRI findings are often normal in FFI, but PET may show thalamic and cingulate hypometabolism.
   c. Genotyping can also be pursued.

TREATMENT

1. There is no current treatment available.
2. Symptomatic treatment may be pursued, but there is little data supporting any particular agent.

VITAMIN DEFICIENCY STATES/TOXINS

B_{12} DEFICIENCY

BACKGROUND

1. Deficiency of vitamin B_{12} can result in cognitive and psychiatric complaints. These can range from mild memory impairment to severe dementia and neuropsychiatric symptoms.
2. Myelopathy (subacute combined degeneration of the spinal cord) and large-fiber peripheral neuropathy are also common nervous system abnormalities.

3. The hematologic manifestation of B_{12} deficiency, macrocytic anemia with hyper-segmented neutrophil nuclei, is not always present in the setting of neurologic symptoms.
4. The epidemiology is not well established, but some studies have shown as many as 15% of the elderly have deficiency.
5. Patients with HIV and AIDS, as well as malnourished populations and vegans, are thought to have a high prevalence.

PATHOPHYSIOLOGY

1. The most common cause of B_{12} deficiency is pernicious anemia.
2. Other potential etiologies include dietary deficiency, gastric resection (loss of intrinsic factor), or disease of the ileum (portion of the bowel in which absorption takes place).
3. B_{12} is a cofactor in two enzymatic reactions, the conversion of homocysteine to methionine and the conversion of methyl malonyl–coenzyme a (CoA) to succinyl-CoA.
4. The hematologic effect is thought to be due to the impact of B_{12} deficiency on the quantity of 5,10-methylene tetrahydrofolate, important in purine synthesis.
5. The cause of CNS dysfunction with deficiency is unclear, but it is thought to be due to impaired myelin synthesis.
6. However, in the spinal cord there is evidence of both the degeneration of myelin and axons.
7. Demyelination is seen in the cerebral white matter.

PROGNOSIS

1. If untreated, low B_{12} levels can produce progressive myelopathy, encephalopathy, and anemia.
2. At least partial resolution of cognitive deficits and perhaps white matter changes are possible.

DIAGNOSIS

1. Diagnosis is based on detection of a low serum B_{12} level.
2. However, low-normal values may be associated with the deficiency state and measurement of homocysteine and methylmalonic acid should be obtained.
3. Increased levels of either suggest relative B_{12} deficiency.
4. MRI of the spine may reveal posterior column T_2-weighted signal hyperintensities.
5. Cerebral white matter may also show T_2-weighted hyperintensities.

TREATMENT

1. Treatment is with cyanocobalamin 1,000 μg intramuscular (IM) for 5 days.
2. If the cause of deficiency cannot be corrected, monthly injections or high oral doses (1 mg/d) are necessary.
3. Various associated cognitive deficits can be treated symptomatically.

KORSAKOFF SYNDROME

BACKGROUND

1. Korsakoff syndrome often follows Wernicke encephalopathy and is most commonly associated with chronic alcohol use.
2. Wernicke encephalopathy is marked by relatively acute onset of a confusional state with the presence of ataxia, ophthalmoplegia, and nystagmus.

3. Korsakoff syndrome is most notable for anterograde and retrograde memory deficits out of proportion to impairment of other cognitive domains. However, frontal executive impairment and apathy are often present, as is confabulation.
4. Epidemiologic studies have suggested a low occurrence of the disease.

PATHOPHYSIOLOGY

1. Thiamine (vitamin B_1) deficiency is thought to underlie the disorder.
2. Alcoholics are particularly disposed to the syndrome due to poor dietary intake and impaired absorption of thiamine.
3. Other forms of malnutrition or malabsorption can also cause the disorder.
4. Periventricular lesions with petechial hemorrhage are found in the regions of the third and fourth ventricles.
5. Midbrain and cerebellar lesions explain some of the clinical manifestations of Wernicke encephalopathy.
6. The memory deficits of the Korsakoff syndrome are thought to relate to damage to the anterior thalamic nucleus and/or the mamillary bodies.
7. Dorsomedial thalamus injury may contribute to executive function impairment.
8. Thiamine is thought important in glucose metabolism and energy production.
9. The higher energy demands of the lesioned periventricular structures may makes them susceptible to thiamine deficiency.

PROGNOSIS

Most patients do not improve or recover over time.

DIAGNOSIS

1. The diagnosis is largely clinical.
2. A history of alcohol abuse, malnutrition, and Wernicke encephalopathy strongly suggest the diagnosis in a patient with predominant memory findings.
3. MRI may reveal periventricular lesions or mamillary body atrophy.

TREATMENT

1. Thiamine replacement with 100 mg/d IV or IM may reverse signs and symptoms of Wernicke encephalopathy and prevent further deterioration.
2. Cholinesterase inhibitors have had mixed results, but should probably be tried (see Table 14-4).

EXPOSURE TO HEAVY METALS

BACKGROUND

1. Exposure to several metallic agents can result in dementia, often with associated peripheral nervous system and systemic illness.
2. Lead, mercury, manganese, arsenic, thallium, aluminum, gold, tin, bismuth, nickel, and cadmium have been associated with impairment of intellectual function.
3. These toxins also tend to produce extrapyramidal and cerebellar signs and symptoms.

PATHOPHYSIOLOGY

These agents likely interfere with cellular metabolism and produce structural brain damage.

PROGNOSIS

Once structural injury has occurred, recovery is unlikely, but progression can be halted.

DIAGNOSIS

1. Diagnosis is based on the clinical features and potential for exposure.
2. Several of these exposures have specific findings that are highly suggestive of the diagnosis; for example, Mees lines in arsenic poisoning, basophilic stippling with lead exposure, and alopecia with thallium poisoning.
3. Serum or urine tests for heavy metals provide more definitive diagnosis.

TREATMENT

1. Removal of the exposure is crucial.
2. Treatment with chelation, usually with ethylenediaminetetraacetic acid (EDTA) or penicillamine may also be helpful and result in some recovery.
3. Symptomatic treatment of cognitive deficits is warranted.

ACKNOWLEDGMENT

We thank Dr. Barry Fogel for his thoughtful comments.

BIBLIOGRAPHY

American Psychiatric Association. *Diagnostic and Statistical Manual of Mental Disorder,* Fourth Edition. Washington DC: American Psychiatric Association, 1994.

Barrett ES. The use of anticonvulsants in aggression and violence. *Psychopharmacol Bull* 1993;29:75–81.

Chiarello RJ, Cole JO. The use of psychostimulants in general psychiatry: a reconstruction. *Arch Gen Psychiatry* 1987;44:286–295.

Cummings JL, Benson DF. *Dementia: a clinical approach.* Boston: Butterworth-Heineman, 1992.

Cummings JL. *Clinical neuropsychiatry.* Boston: Grune & Stratton, 1985.

Cummings JL. Frontal-subcortical circuits and human behavior. *Arch Neurol* 1993;50:873–880.

Doody RS, Stevens JC, Beck C, et al. Practice parameter: management of dementia (an evidence-based review)—report of the Quality Standards Subcommittee of the American Academy of Neurology. *Neurology* 2001;56:1154–1166.

Erkinjuntti T, Kurz A, Gauthier S, et al. Efficacy of galantamine in probable vascular dementia and Alzheimer's disease combined with cerebrovascular disease: a randomized trial. *Lancet* 2002;359:1283–1290.

Evans DA, Funkenstein HH, Albert MS, et al. Prevalence of Alzheimer's disease in a community population of older persons: higher than previously reported. *JAMA* 1989;262:2551–2556.

Fogel BS, Schiffer RB, Rao SM, eds. *Neuropsychiatry.* Baltimore: Williams & Wilkins, 1996.

Frye MA, Ketter TA, Kimbrell TA, et al. A placebo-controlled study of lamotrigine and gabapentin monotherapy in refractory mood disorders. *J Clin Psychopharmacol,* 2000;20:607–614.

Goldman-Rakic PS. Circuitry of primate prefrontal cortex and regulation of behavior by representational memory. In: Plum F, Mountcastle VB, Geiger ST, eds. *The handbook of physiology, section 1: the nervous system, vol. V., higher functions of the brain, part 1.* Bethesda: American Physiological Society, 1987.

Greenhill LL, Osman BB, eds. *Ritalin: theory and practice,* 2nd ed. Larchmont, NY: Mary Ann Liebert, 2000.

Growden JH, Rosser MN. *The dementias.* Boston, Butterworth-Heineman, 1998.

Hachinski VC, Lassen NA, Marshall J. Multi-infarct dementia: a cause of mental deterioration in the elderly. *Lancet* 1974;2:207–210.

Hardy J, Selkoe DJ. The amyloid hypothesis of Alzheimer's disease: progress and problems on the road to therapeutics. *Science* 2002;297:353–356.

Heilman KM, Valenstein E, eds. *Clinical neuropsychology,* 3rd ed. New York: Oxford University Press, 1993.

Knopman DS, DeKosky ST, Cummings JL, et al. Practice parameter: diagnosis of dementia (an evidence-based review)—report of the Quality Standards Subcommittee of the American Academy of Neurology. *Neurology* 2001;56:1143–1153.

Marin RS. Apathy: a neuropsychiatric syndrome. *J Neuropsychiatry Clin Neurosci* 1991;3:243–254.

Mayeux R, Sano M. Treatment of Alzheimer's disease. *N Engl J Med* 1999;341:1670–1679.

Mayeux R, Saunders AM, Shea S, et al. Utility of the apolipoprotein in the diagnosis of Alzheimer's disease. *N Engl J Med* 1998;338:506–511.

McDowell S, Whyte J, D'Esposito M. Differential effect of a dopaminergic agonist on prefrontal function in traumatic brain injury patients. *Brain* 1998;121:1155–1164.

McKeith IG, Galasko D, Kosaka K, et al. Consensus guidelines for the clinical and pathologic diagnosis of dementia with Lewy bodies (DLB): report of the consortium on DLB international workshop. *Neurology* 1996;47:1113–1124.

McKhann G, Drachman D, Folstein M, et al. Clinical diagnosis of Alzheimer's disease: report of the NINCDS-ADRDA Work Group under the auspices of the Department of Health and Human Services Task Force on Alzheimer's Disease. *Neurology* 1984;34:939–944.

Mesulam MM, ed. *Principles of behavioral and cognitive neurology.* 2nd ed. New York: Oxford University Press, 2000.

Morris J, Storandt M, Miller JP, et al. Mild cognitive impairment represents early-stage Alzheimer disease. *Arch Neurol* 2001;58:397–405.

Muller U, von Cramon DY. The therapeutic potential of bromocriptine in neuropsychological rehabilitation of patients with acquired brain damage. *Prog Neuro-Psychopharmacol Biol Psychiatry* 1994;18:1103–1120.

Petersen RC, Doody R, Kurz A, et al. Current concepts in mild cognitive impairment. *Arch Neurol* 2001;58:1985–1992.

Petersen RC, Stevens JC, Ganguli M, et al. Practice parameter: early detection of dementia: mild cognitive impairment (an evidenced-based review): report of the Quality Standards Subcommittee of the American Academy of Neurology. *Neurology* 2001;56:1133–1142.

Post RM, Weiss SR, Chuang DM. Mechanisms of actions of anticonvulsants in affective disorders: comparisons with lithium. *J Clin Psychopharmacol* 1992;12[Suppl 1]:23S–35S.

Raskind MA, Peskind ER, Wessel T, et al. Galantamine in AD: a 6-month randomized, placebo-controlled trial with a 6-month extension. *Neurology* 2000;54:2261–2268.

Ratey J, Greenberg MS, Bemporad JR, et al. Unrecognized ADHD in adults. *J Child and Adolesc Psychiatry* 1994;2:267–275.

Reisberg B, Doody R, Stoffler A, et al. Memantine in moderate-to-severe Alzheimer's disease. *N Engl J Med* 2003;348:1333–1341.

Rogers SL, Farlow MR, Doody RS, et al. A 24-week, double-blind, placebo-controlled trial of donepezil in patients with Alzheimer's disease. *Neurology* 1998;50:136–145.

Roman GC, Tatemichi TC, Erkinjuntti T, et al. Vascular dementia: diagnostic criteria for research studies-report of the NINDS-AIREN International Workshop. *Neurology* 1993;43:250–260.

Rosler M, Anand R, Cicin-Sain A, et al. Efficacy and safety of rivastigmine in patients with Alzheimer's disease: international randomized controlled trial. *BMJ* 1999;318:633–640.

Royall DR. Executive dyscontrol: an important factor affecting the level of care received by older retirees. *J Am Geriatr Soc* 1998;46:1519–1524.

Schatzberg AF, Cole JO, DeBattista C. *Manual of clinical psychopharmacology,* 4th ed. Washington DC: American Psychiatric Publishing, 2003.

Seshadri S, Beiser A, Selhub J, et al. Plasma homocysteine as a risk factor for dementia and Alzheimer's disease. *N Engl J Med* 2002;346:476–483.

Shader RI, Greenblatt DJ. Use of benzodiazepines in anxiety disorders. *N Engl J Med* 1993;328:1398–1405.

Silver J, Yudofsky S. Propanolol for aggression: literature review and clinical guidelines. *International Drug Therapy Newsletter* 1985;20:9–12.

Snowden DA, Greiner LH, Mortimer JA, et al. Brain infarction and the clinical expression of Alzheimer disease: the Nun Study. *JAMA* 1997;277:813–817.

Stoll AL, Severus WE, Freeman WE, et al. Omega 3 fatty acids in bipolar disorders: a preliminary double-blind, placebo-controlled trial. *Arch Gen Psychiatry* 1999;56:407–412.

Stoppe G, Brandt CA, Staedt JH. Behavioural problems associated with dementia: the role of newer antipsychotics. *Drugs Aging* 1999;14:41–54.

Vermeer SE, Prins ND, den Heiher T, et al. Silent brain infarcts and the risk of dementia and cognitive decline. *N Engl J Med* 2003;348:1215–1222.

15. NEUROOPHTHALMOLOGY

Donald C. Bienfang

DISORDERS LIMITED TO LID POSITION

LID PTOSIS

BACKGROUND

Slight asymmetries of lid position are common; usually the patient is the best source of information regarding their importance.

PATHOPHYSIOLOGY

The major muscle holding the lid up is the levator palpebrae innervated by the third cranial nerve; a minor muscle is Mueller muscle innervated by the sympathetic nervous system.

PROGNOSIS

Prognosis is a function of cause.

DIAGNOSIS

1. Most acquired cases of upper lid ptosis that come to the attention of a neurologist will raise the question of a partial third nerve palsy or myasthenia gravis or the relatively slight ptosis of Horner syndrome.
2. If these entities have been ruled out by examination and appropriate testing, most seemingly "new" cases of upper lid ptosis will in fact prove to be old if photographs are reviewed.
3. Local trauma, ocular surface injury, and chronic use of topical steroids are other causes.

TREATMENT

1. Mild and severe lid ptosis of any etiology can be helped by surgical procedures that lift the lid.
   a. Volume 4 of Albert and Jakobiec's text describes how to do this.
   b. Some caution must be exercised because there is a risk that in myopathies the ptosis may be the first expression of what later will involve other eye muscles.
   c. If the surgical procedure leaves the patient with a partial inability to close the lid and the patient loses the protective Bell reaction later, a corneal ulcer may develop.
   d. This is particularly common in cases of chronic progressive ophthalmoplegia.
2. In some cases "lid crutches" fitted to the back of a pair of glasses by a skilled optician can be helpful.
3. Taping of the lid to the forehead is often unsuccessful.

LID RETRACTION

BACKGROUND

This entity is often confused with exophthalmos, which it mimics.

PATHOPHYSIOLOGY

1. The two major mechanisms for causing this appearance are overstimulation of the sympathetic fibers to Mueller muscle and scarring of the levator palpebrae muscle or the lid itself.
2. Ptosis of the lid of the opposite side and weakness of the ipsilateral superior rectus are other causes.

PROGNOSIS

This is a function of etiology.

DIAGNOSIS

Almost all cases of acquired upper lid retraction are due to thyroid eye disease.

TREATMENT

1. An ophthalmic plastic surgeon can weaken the small sympathetically driven Mueller muscle to correct this problem (see Volume 4 of Albert and Jakobiec's text).
2. In cases of thyroid lid retraction, an equally successful and simpler procedure is to create a small laterally placed adhesion between the upper and lower lids. This is done by abrading equal lengths of the lid margin of the upper and lower lid and then bringing them into anatomic apposition by means of a suture that passes through both lid margins in a mattress stitch fashion. It should be left in place 2 to 3 weeks and then removed.
3. Although one might expect that successful treatment of the thyroid would eliminate this problem, unfortunately this is not always the case.

ASYMMETRIC PUPILS

BACKGROUND

In the absence of any other neurologic findings, especially in the absence of any related to the eye, most pupil asymmetries will turn out to have a local or no obvious cause.

PATHOPHYSIOLOGY

Since the pupil is innervated by both the sympathetic system (which dilates the pupil) and the parasympathetic (which constricts via the third cranial nerve), the opportunity for pupillary abnormalities being present as part of a variety of neurologic conditions is rich.

PROGNOSIS

Abnormally small pupils rarely cause much problem for the patient unless there is a cataract present. Large pupils result in glare from light.

DIAGNOSIS

Although asymmetric pupils are a common problem for the neurologist, many such cases are not an expression of any serious pathology. A simple general principle can be applied to determine which cases are worrisome and which pupil is abnormal: the large one or the small one. Simply stated, the abnormal pupil is the one that does not move normally. It either does not dilate in the dark or does not constrict in the light.

TREATMENT

1. Small pupils such as seen in Horner syndrome cause little problem to the patient and can be ignored.
2. The droopy lid of Horner can be fixed surgically if necessary.
3. Dilated pupils as seen in Adie pupil, third cranial nerve palsies, and as an effect of drugs or trauma are more of a visual problem.
   a. If the pupillary sphincter is responsive, a drug such as pilocarpine can be used to make the pupil smaller. Unfortunately, this is not without its dangers. Pilocarpine is an uncomfortable drug to the patient and can cause retinal detachment. The lowest possible dosage that is effective should be used. Commercially this is 0.5%. It may have to be used two to three times a day to maintain miosis.
   b. Another solution is the fitting of a contact lens that has a painted ring at the periphery artificially, thus making a small aperture.

DEGENERATIVE MYOPATHIES

BACKGROUND

Slowly progressive often with a suggestive family history, this group of entities expresses itself in many parts of the body in addition to the eye. The pupil is spared.

PATHOPHYSIOLOGY

This seems to be a disorder of the mitochondria giving rise to the "ragged red fibers" seen pathologically.

PROGNOSIS

These entities usually have a steady downhill course over a prolonged period.

DIAGNOSIS

The diagnosis depends on characteristic clinical, biopsy, and electrophysiologic findings.

TREATMENT

1. Degenerative myopathies of the ocular muscles such as chronic progressive ophthalmoplegia are largely not treatable in any way that would restore normal eye movement. A special caution must be exercised since these conditions often present first with lid ptosis before there are other expressions.
2. If a surgical procedure is done to lift the lid and later the patient loses Bell reaction because the superior rectus loses function and then later develops a weakness of orbicularis function, a corneal ulcer may develop. (Treatment for this is discussed in the section on seventh nerve palsies.) This is such a frequent sequence of events that the experienced ophthalmologist learns to recognize that a corneal ulcer is a common first clue that a patient has chronic progressive external ophtalmoplegia (CPEO).
3. Because lid ptosis is so disfiguring and disturbing visually, lid crutches in this condition are the best solution. Once the extraocular muscle weakness has reached a steady state, prism glasses can be given to allow single binocular vision in most

cases. Prisms are especially effective in this condition since there is little or no eye movement.

MYASTHENIA GRAVIS

BACKGROUND

The subject of myasthenia gravis as it affects the eye is so similar to generalized myasthenia that the reader is referred to this subject, which is covered elsewhere in this book.

TREATMENT

1. The challenge of ocular myasthenia is its fluctuation in a given patient. This makes prism fitting and surgery therapeutic solutions only at a stage that can be considered stable. Given the nature of the disease, this decision may be difficult and hazardous.
2. A particular problem with the use of prisms in this condition and many of those described in this chapter is that the double vision may vary greatly depending on the direction of gaze. One can often only hope to get the patient visually aligned in straight-ahead and down positions; even this may require two sets of glasses.
   a. A device that artificially blurs the vision in one eye is often the easiest solution; however, this need not be a patch, which calls attention to the patient.
   b. Adequate blurring without as much cosmetic disfigurement can be accomplished by "frosting" one lens of a pair of glasses. Clear nail polish applied to a lens and then patted with the finger before it dries is an inexpensive solution.
3. One might think that lid ptosis by occluding one eye should be a good solution. Patients differ on this: A droopy lid is very disfiguring. Many patients prefer to have the lid propped up by a crutch or with tape even though they have double vision as a result.
4. The systemic therapy of myasthenia gravis that seems to be mainly affecting the eyes should be no different from the therapy of generalized myasthenia gravis and therefore is outside of the scope of this chapter. However, it should be obvious that if the ocular problem can be dealt with easily by the patient, systemic therapy will probably be limited to those therapies that are more easily tolerated, such as cholinesterase inhibitors.

TRAUMA

BACKGROUND

Direct mechanical trauma to the orbit can result in a bewilderingly complex array of eye movement disorders. The principles of management share many features.

PATHOPHYSIOLOGY

1. It is in this group of entities that detailed computed tomography (CT) imaging of the orbital walls and contents is indispensable.

2. One has to rapidly make some decisions about the cause of any muscle dysfunction. As time passes, scarring becomes an issue that will complicate later repairs; thus, any problems such as entrapment of muscle in fractures and muscle disinsertions from the globe need to be surgically dealt with early on.
3. Hemorrhage or inflammation of the muscle itself or the same two entities around the muscle can be treated by expectation and dealt with later.

PROGNOSIS

The prognosis depends entirely on the cause.

DIAGNOSIS

This is usually straightforward given the history.

TREATMENT

1. When a final status has been reached, combinations of muscle surgery with appropriate prism fine tuning can have as their goal at least some degree of single vision in the straight-ahead and down gaze positions.
   a. These are the most important areas for adults to have single vision and should be the first goal of all therapies.
   b. If this cannot be achieved, a patch, usually on the eye with the worse motility, may be the only solution.
2. Iatrogenic trauma to eye muscles is also common after cataract, retina, and sinus surgery. A large proportion of these seem to be restrictive myopathies and appropriate recessions of the affected muscles are usually in order.

MYOPATHY OF GRAVES DISEASE

TREATMENT

1. This entity is usually very responsive to a combination of muscle recession operations and prism.
2. The muscles most commonly affected are the inferior rectus and the medial rectus, in that order.
3. The muscle becomes inelastic and stiff and does not allow the eye to move as if the muscles had become leather straps.
4. Surgery should be delayed until the active phase of the orbitopathy has passed.

MOTOR AXON DISEASE

THIRD CRANIAL NERVE PALSIES

BACKGROUND

Seen in the context of aging, diabetes, tumor, and aneurysm, an evaluation as to cause is more important with this nerve than with cranial nerve IV or VI.

PATHOPHYSIOLOGY

1. Partial third nerve palsies only imply that the cause has not completely destroyed the nerve; it should not be reassuring.
2. In a complete palsy, sparing of the pupil is reassuring, although rare exceptions occur.

PROGNOSIS

1. If tumor or aneurysm is the cause, the prognosis is poor, especially if the paralysis has been present for a long time and if aberrant regeneration has begun.
2. Pupil-sparing palsies in which the cause is believed to be vasculopathic have a better prognosis, although several months may pass before resolution.

DIAGNOSIS

It is not the purpose of this text to provide a complete evaluation of third nerve palsies. But because myopathies, myasthenia, and a number of other conditions can deceive the physician, it is wise to evaluate these patients in whom a third nerve palsy is suspected with special caution.

TREATMENT

1. A well-established, complete third nerve palsy is such a challenging entity for correction by prism or surgery that it is often wise not to hold out much hope for the patient.
   a. The first and most hoped for therapy is time.
   b. During this time, it is probably best that a patch, if necessary, be alternated on a daily basis between the two eyes.
   c. Most idiopathic third cranial nerve palsies will express most of their resolution within the first 2 to 3 months.
   d. Surgeons often wait 6 months before considering surgery.
2. The surgical repair of paralytic ocular muscle palsies for the most part depends on the presence of some tone in the weak muscle and another functioning muscle whose tone can be grafted to the tone of the dysfunctional muscle. The only muscle available for transplantation is the superior oblique, which may have its insertion moved close to that of the superior rectus.
   a. In a complete third nerve palsy, there simply is not enough to work with. These are cases in which adjustable sutures are mandated. The lid ptosis that some patients consider so cosmetically unacceptable can usually be helped by appropriate surgery, but the double vision now exposed remains a challenge. Reports of successful outcomes are at the case report level and are not to be routinely expected.
   b. If the third nerve palsy is partial, there may be options for the usual combinations of surgery and prism again with a goal of at least single vision in straight ahead and in straight ahead down positions.
   c. Later on, if aberrant regeneration emerges, the situation becomes even more complex.

FOURTH CRANIAL NERVE PALSIES

BACKGROUND

In contrast to third cranial nerve palsies, fourth cranial nerve palsies can usually be helped by a number of maneuvers.

PATHOPHYSIOLOGY

Most acquired cases are caused by head trauma or are idiopathic. Congenital fourth nerve palsies are common and often unrecognized by the patient.

PROGNOSIS

Again, there is often considerable or complete spontaneous recovery of idiopathic palsies in 2 to 3 months. The prognosis in traumatic cases is not as good; in these cases the palsies may be bilateral.

DIAGNOSIS

1. The affected eye elevates on adduction. Head tilt to the shoulder with the higher eye on adduction makes the hypertropia worse but to the opposite side makes it better. The patient sees a horizontal line as two lines that come closer together at one end pointing like an arrow to the affected eye.
2. Diplopia down and to one side is the position of greatest double vision.
3. The first clue to a symmetric bilateral fourth nerve palsy is that the patient prefers a chin-down position to a head tilt. Otherwise the diagnosis of a bilateral fourth nerve palsy can be challenging.

TREATMENT

1. The patient may have already discovered that tilting the head to the side opposite the weak muscle solves many of the double-vision problems.
   a. For many partial fourth nerve palsies, the major problem for the patient is some vertical double vision in down gaze. A separate pair of reading glasses with a vertical prism may be all that is needed.
   b. If the vertical deviation is beyond what can be solved by prism (usually when the total prism power would have to be in the teens), muscle surgery may be necessary. The fourth cranial nerve is very long and if the axon damage is close to the cell body, the regenerating axons may take several months to reach the muscle.
2. Commonly, the ipsilateral antagonist, the inferior oblique, is surgically weakened. This operation simultaneously addresses the torsional problem and the hyperdeviation. In some cases of fourth nerve palsies, weakening of the inferior oblique is not enough. This is a particular problem in long-standing fourth nerve palsies. In those cases, depending on the measurements in the various fields of gaze, surgery on the contralateral muscles that control vertical movements, the superior rectus and inferior rectus and even the ipsilateral vertical movers may be necessary.

SIXTH CRANIAL NERVE PALSIES

BACKGROUND

Because of the straightforward nature of this problem it provides an excellent example of the difference in therapy of a muscle weakness versus the therapy of a muscle paralysis.

PATHOPHYSIOLOGY

The unusual length of this nerve in isolation from other brainstem structures multiplies the potential causes of its dysfunction.

PROGNOSIS

Prognosis depends on the cause but if this is a mononeuropathy and likely to be ischemic in etiology, recovery often can be expected in 2 to 3 months.

DIAGNOSIS

1. If the lateral rectus muscle is completely paralyzed, the eye will abduct only as far as the midline. This is accomplished by the relaxation of the medial rectus plus the normal elastic forces within the orbit.
2. Reaching the midline is not evidence of any active contraction of the lateral rectus. Later, the eye will not even reach the midline as the medial rectus contracts.

TREATMENT

1. If there is no evidence of active lateral rectus function, there is no procedure one can do on that muscle to make it function better. The only solution is to bring in muscle tone from other muscles, usually the superior and inferior rectus muscle of the same side, using a muscle-sharing procedure.
   a. The medial rectus muscle can be weakened by means of a recession and chemo-denervation with Botox (5 units) but this alone will not be enough to straighten the eye. Some active tone must be supplied by a functioning muscle to counteract the tone in the medial rectus.
   b. The analysis can be complicated by medial rectus contraction even though there is some lateral rectus tone.
   c. To discover this situation, perform a test in which the eye is grasped by some device and active contraction against this hold by the lateral rectus with the eye in the adducted position is demonstrated.
2. If there is tone in the lateral rectus as evidenced by abduction beyond the midline or by active pulling on the forceps when the eye is adducted and the patient is asked to abduct, tightening by means of shortening the muscle but leaving its insertion on the globe unchanged will move the position of the eye laterally into alignment with the fellow eye.
   a. Experienced eye muscle surgeons have a rough idea how much tightening to do along with weakening of the medial rectus by means of recessing the insertion on the globe in order to achieve alignment.
   b. The weakening of the medial rectus can be done in such a way that the muscle insertion location can be adjusted after the effect of anesthetic is over, the adjustable suture technique.
3. Surgery is not usually considered until all hope of spontaneous recovery has passed, usually 6 months.
   a. As a sixth nerve palsy recovers, there is usually a period during which the patient has single vision in part of the horizontal field of gaze and diplopia in the rest. During this period partial taping of the lens to block vision in the eye with the weak muscle may be useful.
   b. Most people who deal with these problems encourage patients to exercise the paretic eye muscle. This is done by alternately patching one eye on 1 day and the other eye on the next.
   c. Again as with the third and fourth, in milder cases a prism in the glasses may suffice.

SEVENTH (FACIAL MOTOR) CRANIAL NERVE PALSY

BACKGROUND

This condition is commonly seen in any center with an active neurosurgical service.

PATHOPHYSIOLOGY

The seventh nerve is vulnerable to inflammation- (e.g., Lyme disease), trauma-, and tumor- induced damage.

PROGNOSIS

There are two overriding principles that govern this condition.

1. If the paralysis of motor function is not associated with any anesthesia of the cornea, it becomes much less likely that there will be any scarring and loss of vision.
2. The second principle is that surgical closure of the lids should be done sooner rather than later. A common mistake is to wait until advanced ulceration or even scarring has developed before performing a tarsorrhaphy. Trying to play catch up often results in permanent damage to the eye.

DIAGNOSIS

Seeing how well the patient can close the eye most easily makes diagnosis.

TREATMENT

1. Mild cases in which there is some ability to close the lids, there is a good Bell reaction, and the ultimate prognosis for recovery is good may be treated with intense daytime lubrication, either drops (usually the most viscous one can obtain) or, better yet, ointment.
2. In general, patching of the eye is disappointing.
   a. The ability of an eye to open under even the firmest of patches is remarkable. Under such a circumstance one not only has an open lid but the added possibility of the patch rubbing against the corneal surface.
   b. If the patient or a friend is skilled and motivated, the use of tape, frequently attended to and changed after thorough cleaning of the skin of the lids, can keep the lid closed.
3. A surgical lid closure should be done early in most cases that are likely to last for more than a few weeks.
   a. Often is it enough to bring the lateral lid margins together allowing just enough of an aperture medially to allow inspection of the eye and especially the cornea. A common technique is to abrade the lid margins and bring them in apposition to one another with a heavy suture on a bolster. The suture can be removed in a couple of weeks. An advantage of this is that the tarsorrhaphy can be gradually taken down as the condition improves. A disadvantage is that the lid margin and lashes are often permanently scarred in an unpleasant way. Also this technique is less useful if the medial portions of the lids must also be closed. There is more pull at this level and the skin bridge that forms between the lids can stretch out to create an unsightly band across the interpalpebral fissure.
   b. A stronger bond using less of the lid margin can be created by splitting the lid on the gray line for just 1 or 2 mm of depth. The two raw surfaces from the upper and lower lids can be brought together with an absorbable mattress suture. This bond is very strong, uses only a small amount of lid margin to be effective, and can be used medially as well as laterally.
4. Another approach is the insertion of gold weights into the upper lid, the use of springs, and reinnervation of the facial musculature by nerve grafting. These techniques are best handled by an experienced plastic surgeon.
5. If the corneal exposure has evolved to the point of frank ulceration, a soft contact lens in addition to lid closure may be necessary as a temporary aid to healing. Even so, a scar is likely.

MULTIPLE CRANIAL NERVES

BACKGROUND

It is incumbent for the physician faced with such a patient to carry out an especially thorough search of serious etiologies.

PATHOPHYSIOLOGY

Depending on the location, in most cases something of considerable size or capable of considerable spread is necessary to cause such an entity.

PROGNOSIS

1. Hopefully removal of the offending agent will alleviate the problem.
2. The next best hope is that there will be enough balance between opposing groups (III vs. VI) that the eye will be in a almost straight-ahead position barring complete ptosis of the upper lid, which makes the whole issue mute. In general these situations are complex and different from case to case; thus, therapy may be unique for each case.
3. This is an entity that is sadly often detected too late for effective therapy.

MUCORMYCOSIS

PROGNOSIS

This grave condition has a poor prognosis, especially once it is apparent that the infection has spread beyond the sinuses.

TREATMENT

1. Consultation with ear, nose, and throat (ENT) and infectious disease specialists will be necessary. Often a biopsy, *not a culture*, of the nasal tissue will be necessary to confirm the diagnosis.
2. Amphotericin B with doses beginning at 0.25 mg/kg and advancing to up to 1.0 mg/kg will be necessary combined with débridement perhaps including exenteration will be necessary.

INTERNUCLEAR OPHTHALMOPLEGIA

BACKGROUND

Although there are exceptions, most of which are case reports, the two major causes of this condition are multiple sclerosis (MS) and stroke; another situation is the occasional patient whose symptoms mimic this condition but has myasthenia gravis.

PATHOPHYSIOLOGY

1. The problem with this condition is that it looks deceptively like a medial rectus weakness, but it is not.
2. In contrast to a medial rectus weakness, these patients' eyes can often fuse the two images in the primary positions allowing them to look straight ahead without double vision and to read in down gaze successfully.

PROGNOSIS

Prognosis depends on etiology.

DIAGNOSIS

Weakness of medial rectus coordination with the lateral rectus is sometimes expressed only by a "sliding in" of the eye on adduction on lateral gaze with or without nystagmus of the abducting eye.

TREATMENT

1. The strabismus therapies that might be applicable to a weakness of an individual muscle do not always work in this condition. Fortunately there is often no real need to do anything.
   a. Prism added to glasses is often enough to bring the images into alignment in the important two directions of gaze mentioned above (straight ahead and straight down).
   b. It is not usually possible to achieve normalization of eye movement that will allow single vision in all fields.
   c. Reportedly, surgery designed to affect alignment in one field without disturbing alignment in others (often involving a posterior fixation suture) has been successful, but these are anecdotal reports. The most I have been able to accomplish is to reduce the amount of head turn needed for single vision.
2. If the cause of the internucleurophthalmoplegia (INO) is not correctable (e.g., myasthenia gravis or a treatable tumor), it is often best just to comfort the patient with the knowledge that they can usually attain single vision although in a limited field of gaze with either prism or a head turn.

SKEW DEVIATIONS

BACKGROUND

Skew deviations almost always accompany some other more disabling disorder of function of the pons (e.g., dizziness or loss of balance) that makes the presence of a skew less important.

PATHOPHYSIOLOGY

This ocular deviation can be generated from lesions almost the entire length of the brainstem but it is the vestibular system in these areas that is dysfunctional.

PROGNOSIS

Prognosis depends on cause and is therefore uncertain.

DIAGNOSIS

1. Skew deviations are a type of vertical diplopia that is more apparent at the extremes of lateral gaze than in the primary positions. For this reason, they are easily confused with fourth nerve palsies and inferior oblique palsies.
2. The double vision may in many cases be ignored by the patients as they learn to move their heads when looking at something rather than moving their eyes.

TREATMENT

1. A small amount of residual hypertropia that does interfere with vision in the more primary positions can be dealt with by prism. Rarely is the deviation of such an angle that muscle surgery is needed.
2. In such cases, however, a resection (tightening) of the inferior rectus muscle of the hyperdeviating eye can be helpful.
3. In cases of central and peripheral disorders of the vestibular system where there is some double vision it is usually less of a problem than the nystagmus which will be dealt with in a later section.

GAZE PARALYSIS

PATHOPHYSIOLOGY

Patients with this condition will not have double vision. Since in most cases, the patients will be able to reach the midline by relaxation of the gaze direction that is functional, they may need to therapy at all. Learning to turn the head may be enough, particularly for horizontal gaze palsies. Patients with vertical gaze palsies are more disabled. The person who cannot look down has trouble reading and the one who cannot look up has a sore neck. There are solutions that work well for these situations if one remembers that all the solutions sacrifice some part of the intact field of gaze in the attempt to help the dysfunctional field.

PROGNOSIS

Prognosis depends on the potential for elimination of the cause and viability of the remaining nervous tissue.

DIAGNOSIS

Diagnosis should be straightforward. The only issue is what part of the brain is not functioning since gaze palsies can be generated from multiple sites.

TREATMENT

1. For those unable to look down, placing base-down prisms of appropriate strength into the reading glasses is helpful. In general, it is less important for adults to look up, but in the same way, base-up prisms in distance glasses can be helpful for those patients. For those unable to look to the right, prisms in both lenses with base to the left will be helpful and visa versa for those unable to look left.
2. What can be done with prism can also be attempted surgically. Appropriate resections or recessions of yoke muscles will move the two eyes so that the needed direction of gaze is more easily attainable. Unfortunately surgery is less precise

and less predictable than prism. If the surgery is not perfectly balanced between the two eyes double vision may be generated.

ACQUIRED NYSTAGMUS AND RELATED CONDITIONS

BACKGROUND

With a tremendous number of possible causes and clinical situations, nystagmus is almost always part of a complex neurologic disorder of the brainstem.

PATHOPHYSIOLOGY

In general, nystagmus and related conditions such as bobbing disturb vision in direct proportion to the amplitude of the movement. Most commonly, the central vestibular system is in some manner disturbed.

PROGNOSIS

The prognosis is variable but generally poor for spontaneous recovery.

DIAGNOSIS

The characteristic to-and-fro motion is so different from normal eye movements that little confusion should occur.

TREATMENT

1. If the nystagmus is limited to one eye, it can be ignored or the patient can wear a patch. The same is true if the nystagmus is only troublesome in a field of gaze other than the primary ones, straight ahead or straight down. The trouble with nystagmus is that there are no simple or even reliable solutions.
2. There is one entity that can be responsive to therapy, neuromyotonia. This is a momentary contraction of an individual muscle.
   a. A common example is orbicularis myokymia in which individual fascicles of the orbicularis muscle contract for a moment. Patients with orbicularis myokymia should have their parotid glands palpated since tumors in this region can give this symptom. More commonly, however, it is a stress and fatigue symptom.
   b. Superior oblique myokymia is another common expression of neuromyotonia and has similar causes.
   c. Finally, one of the other extraocular muscles can be involved, particularly after its nerve has been irradiated.
   d. One consistent feature of myokymia and neuromyotonia is that the twitching is brought out by sustained use of the muscle such as in the case of the orbicularis squeezing the lids together. The second feature is that the muscle usually can be demonstrated to be a little deficient in its function.
   e. All three conditions are commonly responsive to gabapentin or Tegretol.
   f. Combined surgical weakening of the superior oblique and inferior oblique muscle of an eye with superior oblique myokymia can be helpful in cases not responsive to drugs.
3. There are two special and rare types of nystagmus that do respond to therapy. Periodic alternating nystagmus is responsive to Baclofen and familial periodic nystagmus with ataxia may be responsive to Diamox.

4. If the nystagmus is present in both eyes but is absent in one direction of gaze but that direction is not a useful one, there are muscle operations which can attempt to move the resting and nystagmus free direction of gaze from an eccentric position to a more useful, usually straight ahead position. These are variations on the so-called Kestenbaum procedure. They can be applied to one or more commonly both eyes. The challenge again is to be so skilled or fortunate that things end up equal in the two eyes so that nystagmus is not replaced by diplopia.

5. One might think that Botox would be a good solution. In certain cases success has been reported. But the results are often disappointing. The effect is temporary but more troublesome is the tendency for Botox to spread to muscles one does not wish to weaken, with resultant complicated diplopia and even more troublesome, upper lid ptosis.

6. Various central nervous system–active drugs have been reported to be helpful in nystagmus (not myokymia) in anecdotal cases. Gabapentin is a good example. Sadly, the results are not reliable and often large doses with the attendant side effects may be required.

AMAUROSIS FUGAX

BACKGROUND

There are so many potential causes for this symptom that a differential would be beyond the scope of this book.

PATHOPHYSIOLOGY

One would assume that most but not all cases imply some temporary reduction in blood flow to the eye.

PROGNOSIS

Depends on presumed etiology. Especially in younger patients for whom a full workup has failed to lead to a diagnosis, often the symptom seems to disappear. For older patients it can be a warning sign of impending stroke.

DIAGNOSIS

To direct the evaluation, careful attention must be paid to the duration of the attacks, associated symptoms at the time of the attacks, frequency of the attacks, how much vision is lost, and precipitating causes.

TREATMENT

1. The therapy depends on the etiology.
2. Evaluation for clotting disorders (usually there is a family history), narrowing of the carotid arteries, and embolic sources (especially the valves of the heart) usually covers most cases. Depending on the findings, surgery to remove the source of the problem or anticoagulation is indicated.
3. Many cases fail to yield an identifiable pathology, and the treating physician may wish to choose some form of antiplatelet therapy, such as aspirin or Plavix.

ANTERIOR ISCHEMIC OPTIC NEUROPATHY

GIANT CELL ARTERITIS

BACKGROUND

This ancient condition seems for the most part to be restricted to elderly Europeans. Patients with polymyalgia rheumatica are at especial risk.

PATHOPHYSIOLOGY

A giant cell inflammation of media of medium sized arteries narrows the lumen and leads to ischemia. The cause of this inflammation is unclear.

PROGNOSIS

This is an acute illness. Most of the damage in untreated cases occurs early in the course of the disease.

DIAGNOSIS

1. A sudden loss of vision usually first in one eye sometimes preceded by amaurosis fugax with the finding of a pallid swelling of the nerve head and perhaps a splinter hemorrhage at the edge of the nerve head is characteristic of this condition.
2. If it is followed by vision loss in the fellow eye with the same findings the diagnosis is almost assured.
3. Anemia, an elevated erythrocyte sedimentation rate (ESR), and a positive superficial temporal artery biopsy are other findings.

TREATMENT

1. There are two emergency situations in which high doses of oral or even intravenous (IV) glucocorticosteroids are indicated:
   a. The first is when the patient with giant cell arteritis (GCA) is experiencing amaurosis fugax.
   b. The second is when such a patient has already recently lost vision from GCA.
   c. Based on the fact that the ESR usually goes back to more normal levels in about 3 days after intensive steroid therapy, a logical schedule is 3 days of 1 g/d of methylprednisolone followed by oral prednisone at the usual levels for treatment of GCA.
2. If there appears to be no imminent threat to vision or stroke threat, oral prednisone can be started. There never has been a good study to establish an appropriate dosage but somewhere around 1 mg/kg of body weight of prednisone per day is probably adequate.
   a. A biopsy must always be done to establish the diagnosis. The window for doing the biopsy is about 4 days after starting the prednisone, although positive biopsies have been reported months into the therapy.
   b. Unfortunately for the patient, the prednisone therapy with all its unpleasant side effects must be prolonged. The eye and the brainstem, the two most frequently attacked tissues, remain vulnerable for about 2 months; therefore, a high dosage must be continued for that period.
   c. After 2 months, a slow taper may be started. A major problem at this stage is deciding how fast to taper and whether at some level the disease has reactivated to a dangerous level. It is probably better to return to higher doses on the basis of patient symptoms than to depend on the ESR. Complete normalization of the

ESR is not common in GCA, and if you try to achieve a normal ESR it will prolong high doses of therapy beyond what is necessary.

3. Since GCA is a disease of many months' duration, I believe starting at 2 months from the onset of therapy a slow taper aiming at the goal of no treatment by 9 months to 1 year from the onset. This remains a rule of thumb, however, and individual cases may be treated differently.

4. Alternate-day therapy with steroids and other immune-modulating drugs is not effective in the treatment of this condition.

NONARTERITIC ANTERIOR ISCHEMIC OPTIC NEUROPATHY

BACKGROUND

Most cases are seen in older men with some vasculopathic predisposition especially hypertension. Most patients will have a small or absent optic nerve cup in the other eye.

PATHOPHYSIOLOGY

The best evidence at this time suggests that there is an occlusion of small feeder vessels to the optic nerve head. This seems to start a pathologic cascade that is aided by the already anatomically "crowded" nerve head.

PROGNOSIS

1. The affected eye has roughly a one third chance of getting better, getting worse, or staying the same.
2. In a small percentage of cases, the other eye will be affected months to years later.

DIAGNOSIS

This condition mimics the anterior ischemic optic neuropathy of GCA except that the amount of vision loss is usually much less and the associated symptoms and signs of GCA that suggest a systemic illness are missing.

TREATMENT

1. There is no convincing evidence that any therapy is helpful in this condition.
2. Based on some similarities between this condition and glaucoma, if the patient has an elevated intraocular pressure, topical medications that normalize the pressure may be indicated.
3. Other therapies such as levodopa 25 to 100 mg three times a day (t.i.d.) have also been proposed but need confirmation.
4. Optic nerve sheath decompression is not helpful.

DIABETIC ANTERIOR ISCHEMIC OPTIC NEUROPATHY (AION)

BACKGROUND

A diabetic has a mild form of anterior ischemic optic neuropathy.

PATHOPHYSIOLOGY

The pathophysiology is unclear.

PROGNOSIS

This entity has a good prognosis without therapy.

DIAGNOSIS

While this entity is similar to other types of AION, the patient is more likely a juvenile diabetic whose diabetes is under good control or is yet to be diagnosed.

TREATMENT

This entity has a good prognosis without therapy.

COMPRESSIVE AND INTRINSIC OPTIC NEUROPATHIES DUE TO TUMOR AND ANEURYSM

PATHOPHYSIOLOGY

Most of the dysfunctions caused by these entities are due to direct compression but in some cases, interruption of blood supply plays a part.

PROGNOSIS

Duration of the insult and age of the patient are important variables.

DIAGNOSIS

This is an area where neuroimaging has made a major contribution.

TREATMENT

1. Obviously the main therapeutic approach is to remove the offending lesion.
    a. One issue that needs to be decided is whether a tumor is infiltrating the optic nerve or just compressing it. A decision must be made because while the latter can be treated by treating the tumor, the former may require direct radiation to the nerve with the increased risk of radiation-induced optic neuropathy.
    b. An even more controversial situation is that of optic nerve glioma of childhood. An argument can be made that resection of the involved nerve may in the long term protect the uninvolved nerve and/or the chiasm. But surgery in this area is hazardous and one may find that further vision is lost apparently from the surgery itself.
2. Another example is meningioma.
    a. When this does not directly involve the optic nerve or its sheaths but is compressing the nerve from the outside, surgical excision with radiation for tumor not resectable is a common approach. However, if there is direct involvement of the nerve sheaths surgery is often complicated by more vision loss.
    b. Radiation of such tumors has some benefit but the effect is often temporary and one must factor in that often these tumors are so slow growing that no therapy is a reasonable option.

LEBER HEREDITARY OPTIC NEUROPATHY (LHON)

BACKGROUND

This is one of the gene mutation diseases.

PATHOPHYSIOLOGY

Ninety percent of cases of this condition are due to gene mutations at loci 11778, 3460, or 14484. The hereditary pattern is matrilineal.

PROGNOSIS

Unfortunately, improvement of vision is a rare occurrence.

DIAGNOSIS

A male with a positive family history who presents with progressive optic atrophy in both eyes associated with telangiectatic blood vessels on and near the disc in the early phases is characteristic.

TREATMENT

1. Claims for successful therapies must be tempered by the fact that spontaneous improvement may be seen in this condition without therapy.
2. Assuming that a nerve already damaged by LHON is more vulnerable to toxins, advice about avoiding smoking, alcohol and other toxins is probably well-founded.
3. Therapies aimed at improving nerve function have been disappointing. They range from steroid use, surgical decompression, coenzyme Q10, succinate, vitamin K, vitamin C, thiamine, and vitamin B_2.

RADIATION-INDUCED OPTIC NEUROPATHY

BACKGROUND

1. Most of these cases will be seen in patients treated with radiation for tumor near the optic nerves.
2. When radiation is the only treatment, this form of optic neuropathy usually does not appear before a year has passed. However, the concomitant use of some chemotherapeutic agents can accelerate the process.

PATHOPHYSIOLOGY

The best guess at this time is that the radiation induces a vasculitis.

PROGNOSIS

Although prognosis is poor, there are exceptions.

DIAGNOSIS

The diagnosis is usually one of exclusion of recurrence of the tumor originally treated.

TREATMENT

1. Many consider this condition, which may occur a year or more after radiation to the optic nerve, as untreatable.
2. There are advocates, however, for the following regimen. It should be emphasized that if this arduous course is to be taken it should be initiated early in the disease process.
   a. Hyperbaric oxygen for at least 20 sessions for 90 minutes at 2.4 atmospheres pressure is the only treatment that has ever been thought to be effective.
   b. IV Solu-Medrol 1 g/d for 3 days followed by a 2-week oral taper may be used at the same time.
   c. Trental 400 mg two or three times a day is also advocated by some in addition to the above.

RETROGENICULATE VISUAL FIELD LOSS

BACKGROUND

Most of these patients have suffered from stroke or tumor.

PATHOPHYSIOLOGY

Interruption of the visual radiations is necessary.

PROGNOSIS

Largely depends on the cause but age of the patient and duration of the process are also important.

DIAGNOSIS

Visual fields locate the site of the damage.

TREATMENT

1. If a patient loses the right half of the visual field in both eyes, it is tempting to try prism with the base to the right, to move the field that cannot be seen into a functioning part of the visual field.
   a. Most patients do not adapt well to this therapy, although there is the occasional exception.
   b. The prism power would be from 20 to 40 prism diopter.
   c. A more recent modification involves putting the prism in only the upper or lower half of the lens. This may be more tolerable.
2. Patients with a left homonymous hemianopia have trouble finding the beginning of the next line when they are reading. A ruler or a piece of string placed at the left edge of the print is helpful to them.
3. Those with a right homonymous hemianopia may find themselves mistakenly moving from one line to line above or below. Using the index finger to focus attention on a single line is helpful.

RETROBULBAR OPTIC NEURITIS

BACKGROUND

This is a common cause of monocular loss of vision in a young person, especially females.

PATHOPHYSIOLOGY

There is an inflammation within the optic nerve.

PROGNOSIS

Most cases will improve without treatment; however, normal vision may not return. Complaints of decreased contrast and decreased color vision are common.

DIAGNOSIS

1. While a clinician may strongly suspect that the patient presenting with the relatively sudden onset of loss of vision, a relative afferent pupil light defect, pain on eye movement, and a normal fundus exam has retrobulbar optic neuritis, I believe that this diagnosis should be supported by a neuroradiologic study which if it doesn't support the diagnosis with confirmatory imaging changes in the nerve at least does not suggest an alternative diagnosis. Cases of tumor compression of the nerve can fool even the experienced clinician.
2. Once convinced of the diagnosis, the next decision relates to MS. Without a magnetic resonance imaging (MRI) of the brain and spinal cord, this decision can be difficult. One can question the patient about previous neurologic episodes, but it is hard to know what to do with that episode of numbness and tingling of a limb that happened a few years ago, went away after a couple of weeks, and was attributed to a "pinched nerve." If the MRI shows three or more white matter lesions larger than 3 mm, oriented and located properly, the patient has about a 50% chance of developing MS in the next 5 years. Without these lesions the chance is 16%. A major problem in many centers is that the radiologist may "overread" the MRI and call any tiny white spot "possible MS." This is a situation where one must personally look at the MRI.

TREATMENT

1. Retrobulbar neuritis in patients with the aforementioned MRI findings treated first with 10 days of IV methylprednisolone at a dose of 1 g/d, followed by oral steroids at a dosage of 1 mg/kg for 11 days with a 4-day taper (20 mg, 10 mg, 0 mg, 10 mg), will resolve more rapidly than when not treated. Treated patients will be less likely to have any clinical signs of MS for the next 2 years. However, starting at 2 years, MS expression in the treated and nontreated groups will start to approach each other. However, once-weekly Avonex after completing the steroid course will significantly reduce the clinical and MRI expression of new MS lesions. Betaseron and Rebif are considered higher dose interferons than Avonex. The choice of which of these three to give depends on patient tolerance for the route of administration and the clinical severity of the disease. However much of this has not been subjected to well-controlled clinical trials. Copaxone is a different type of drug and is more easily tolerated (as is Avonex) than Betaseron and Rebif and it may have some neuroprotective effect. But further studies need to be done comparing all these drugs.

2. While the above corticosteroid treatment schedule will shorten the course of the optic neuritis in patients *without supportive MRI findings* it will not improve the long-term visual result over those patients who are not so treated.
3. Oral steroids in modest doses will relieve the pain of retrobulbar neuritis. However, there is a danger: Optic neuritis treatment trial showed that oral steroids actually increased the recurrence rate of optic neuritis.

SWOLLEN DISC

BACKGROUND

Some causes of "swollen disc" are considered elsewhere (AION, LHON). Other causes either require no therapy (e.g., hyperopia, disc drusen, disc anomalies). Still others have disc swelling as an incidental finding when the problem is obvious (e.g., systemic hypertension, ocular hypotony).

PAPILLEDEMA DUE TO RAISED INTRACRANIAL PRESSURE

BACKGROUND

Raised, congested ("choked"), bilateral optic nerves lacking spontaneous venous pulsations, surrounded by hemorrhages and linear folds in the retina suggest this entity.

PATHOPHYSIOLOGY

This has been the subject of much debate over the years. There are proponents of a direct effect of the cerebrospinal fluid pressure on the nerve and also proponents of a vascular intermediary.

PROGNOSIS

1. This depends on duration and the severity of the papilledema itself.
2. Certain associated findings indicate a poor prognosis for vision loss in cases of papilledema. The major one is systemic hypertension. Others are high-grade disc edema, peripapillary subretinal hemorrhages, vision loss at presentation, old age, myopia opticociliary shunt vessels, and glaucoma.

DIAGNOSIS

1. A lumbar puncture is the definitive diagnostic test.
2. Often papilledema alone is a sign that indicates the direction of an evaluation and thus the treatment.
3. If there is an underlying mass lesion as a cause for the raised intracranial pressure (ICP), it should be treated.
4. If the raised ICP may be due to a medication such as tetracycline, vitamin A, cortisone or its cessation, nalidixic acid, nitrofurantoin, or lithium these drugs should be stopped.

5. If the elevated ICP is due to sarcoidosis, steroids are indicated.
6. Often the diagnosis in a young obese woman is pseudotumor cerebri. In these cases, weight loss, Diamox, repeated lumbar punctures, and shunt surgery are options.
7. Often papilledema itself does not need to be treated. Treatment of the underlying cause is enough. The main reasons for more aggressive treatment are severity of headache and loss of vision (usually constriction of the visual field).

TREATMENT

1. There are methods for treating papilledema directly. This is often an issue in pseudotumor cerebri.
2. Diamox may be used to lower ICP. Some use up to 4 g/d. A particularly well-tolerated form is 500-mg sustained-release capsules.
3. Shunting procedures are also effective by ventriculoperitoneal or lumboperitoneal shunt or optic nerve sheath decompression.
4. In cases in which there is coexistent systemic hypertension and raised ICP, caution must be used in lowering the systemic blood pressure. A sudden drop in blood pressure may cause vision loss.

PAPILLITIS

BACKGROUND

There are many causes. The diagnosis may be difficult because it depends on good evidence that the cause of the unilateral disc swelling is truly inflammation.

PATHOPHYSIOLOGY

This seems to be straightforward enough.

PROGNOSIS

Depends on etiology.

DIAGNOSIS

1. When one encounters inflammatory swelling of the optic nerve head, the differential becomes much wider than with retrobulbar optic neuritis.
2. The nerve head should be swollen and usually has dilated capillaries. Presence of white blood cells in the vitreous over the swollen nerves is a very helpful confirmatory finding.
3. In papillitis, MS is only one of several entities to consider. Sarcoidosis and systemic lupus are also common conditions that create this entity.
4. An elevated ESR with papillitis is thought by some to be an indication for steroid therapy.

TREATMENT

Most causes are sensitive to systemic steroid therapy.

TOXIC OPTIC NEUROPATHIES

BACKGROUND

For most cases one will encounter there will be a history of excessive use of some stimulant. In modern times it may be difficult to decide which of several potential drugs is at fault.

PATHOPHYSIOLOGY

Depends on the agent and even then often hard to understand.

PROGNOSIS

Prognosis depends on etiology but even when the etiology is identified it is often difficult for the individual patient to give up use of the offending agent.

DIAGNOSIS

Some cases are straightforward for others the diagnosis is considered when presented with a patient who has slowly progressive loss of optic nerve function in both eyes.

TREATMENT

1. The first therapy is to remove the offending agent. The second therapy is to make up for metabolic deficiencies (e.g. vitamin B) with supplementation. Therapies combining the two in the hope that some additional agent will help treat a toxic neuropathy (e.g., tobacco/alcohol neuropathy) have often been disappointing. However, cessation of smoking and alcohol is beneficial. Some advocate intramuscular injections of hydroxocobalamin.
2. In the early phases of methanol and ethylene glycol poisoning, administration of ethanol helps to block the metabolism of the toxin.. Bicarbonate aids in the treatment of the acidosis and dialysis speeds elimination of the toxin. It is often difficult with these two toxins to institute effective therapy before permanent damage is done.

TRAUMATIC OPTIC NEUROPATHIES

BACKGROUND

This entity is usually considered when vision loss after head trauma is not explained by the examination of the eye.

PATHOPHYSIOLOGY

Except for the obvious cases, this is often obscure. Those cases in which the vision is lost immediately must have a different pathophysiology than those that have sight after the trauma only to lose it later; however, this is unclear.

PROGNOSIS

Since many cases improve seemingly without any effective therapy, the prognosis should always be hopeful.

DIAGNOSIS

In this entity, high-quality neuroradiologic imaging is a necessity. It is often surprising how little head trauma is necessary to cause this entity. In unilateral cases, there should be a relative afferent pupillary light defect.

TREATMENT

1. If a compressive lesion (fragment of bone or hematoma) can be demonstrated, an argument can be made for surgical repair or decompression.
2. If it can be demonstrated that an orbital hematoma is compressing the optic nerve, a lateral canthotomy may be helpful.
3. If there is a sense that there is some swelling around the optic nerve that could be compromising its function, an argument can be made for systemic steroids for a few days.
4. If there is blood in the optic nerve sheath or under the periosteum around the nerve, this can be drained.
5. Most cases of traumatic optic neuropathy lack these features. Attempts to extend the logic of the treatment of spinal cord trauma with large doses of IV steroids to the anatomically very different optic nerve has not convincingly proved useful when compared with no treatment, and the same applies to decompressive surgery on the optic canal if there is no identifiable deformity. These two therapies seem to do no better than no therapy in which case spontaneous recovery is often also observed.

PROLONGATION OF IMAGES—IMAGE SMEAR

BACKGROUND

1. The patient will describe that when he looks at an object and then looks away there is a comet-like trail of the image as the eye moves.
2. Another different but similar presentation is clear-cut preservation of an image after one looks away from it—palinopsia.

PATHOPHYSIOLOGY

1. Most patients with smear will have no identifiable etiology for it. One must presume that some suppressive mechanism has been eliminated.
2. Most patients with palinopsia have had a stroke in the visual radiations.

PROGNOSIS

For the idiopathic cases the prognosis is good. For those cases caused by drugs the drug must be eliminated.

TREATMENT

1. Certain drugs seem to cause image smear in some patients—Clomid, Trazodone, and Serzone.
2. Even after these medicines are stopped, it may take weeks or months before the symptom resolves.

ILLUSIONS

BACKGROUND

The public and some physicians tend to view patients with this symptom with some suspicion. While this suspicion is often justified, there can be real organic reasons for this complaint.

PATHOPHYSIOLOGY

Unfortunately the underlying physiology is poorly understood.

PROGNOSIS

This depends on the cause but in general it is good without treatment.

DIAGNOSIS

1. While formed and unformed illusions can be seen with disorders of the visual system from the retina to the occipital pole and their treatment naturally relates to therapy for the underlying disorder, there is one category that deserves special mention.
   a. Rather stereotyped illusions are common in the early days after strokes affecting the visual radiations.
   b. They are a special case because many patients so affected are very worried by these and because they literally think they are losing their mind and so fail to mention them to anyone.
   c. The physician should ask about their presence, explain that they are temporary and commonly seen in this condition.
2. Illusions are part of what are called positive visual phenomena, a term that includes palinopsia.

TREATMENT

1. There are occasional reports of these phenomena being reduced by treatment with anticonvulsant drugs.
2. Prolongation of the positive scotomas of migraine is a rare but annoying symptom. It may be responsive to anti-seizure medication such as Depakote.

NONPHYSIOLOGIC LOSS OF VISION

HYSTERIA

BACKGROUND

One of the first psychiatric disorders to receive modern attention, it still remains a prominent part of any neurologic practice.

PATHOPHYSIOLOGY

It still seems to be more common in younger women.

PROGNOSIS

Even without any form of treatment symptoms seem to disappear with time in most cases.

DIAGNOSIS

I will use this term to refer to patients who are not conscious of their loss of vision being nonorganic.

TREATMENT

One might be tempted to turn to the psychiatrist for help with this problem. This is not always necessary. Many cases of this condition are caused by temporary stresses that will pass and with this passage the symptom will go away also.

MALINGERING

BACKGROUND

This condition has probably been present since the dawn of humanity. In modern times, there is almost always a lawyer lurking in the background somewhere.

PATHOPHYSIOLOGY

Greed seems to be at the heart of most cases.

PROGNOSIS

Sadly, patients with this condition will never have enough reward to make them happy.

DIAGNOSIS

I will use this term to refer to people who are consciously pretending to have loss of vision usually for some tangible gain.

TREATMENT

A diagnostic test is also therapeutic. A carefully worded sentence that indicates you doubt the veracity of their claim printed in type smaller than they allege to be able to read, which is presented with other sentences in writing large enough for them to read, will quickly clear the office of this type of pest.

BIBLIOGRAPHY

Albert DM, Jakobiec FA, eds. *Principles and practice of ophthalmology,* vol. 4. Philadelphia: WB Saunders, 1994.

Arnold A. Treatment of anterior ischemic optic neuropathy. *Semin Ophthalmol* 2002;17:39–46.

Barnett JH, Bernstein EF, Callow AD, et al. The Amaurosis Fugax Study Group: amaurosis fugax (transient monocular blindness): a consensus statement. In: Bernstein EF, ed. *Amaurosis fugax.* New York: Springer-Verlag, 1988.

Beck RW, Trobe JD. Optic Neuritis Study Group: the Optic Neuritis Treatment Trial: putting the results in perspective. *Opthalmology* 1995:15:131–135.

Beck RW, Trobe JD. Optic Neuritis Study Group: what have we learned from the Optic Neuritis Treatment Trial? *Ophthalmolology* 1995;102:1504–1508.

Bienfang DC. Neuroophthalmology of the pupil and accomodation. In: Albert DM, Jakobiec FA, eds. *Principles and practice of ophthalmology*, vol. 4. Philadelphia: WB Saunders, 1994: 2470–2482.

Bienfang DC, Kurtz D. Management of functional visual loss. *J Am Optom Assoc* 1998;69:12–21.

Borruat FX, Schatz NJ, Glaser JS, et al. Radiation Optic Neuropathy: report of cases, role of hyperbaric oxygen therapy, and literature review. *Neuro-ophthalmol* 1996;16:255–266.

Capo H, Guyton DL. Ipsilateral hypotropia after cataract surgery. *Ophthalmology* 1996;103:721–730.

Donahue SP, Lavin PJM, Mahoney B, et al. Skew deviation and inferior oblique palsy. *Am J Ophthalmol* 2001;132:751–756.

Gottlob I, Catalano RA, Reinecke RD. Surgical management of oculomotor palsy. *Am J Ophthalmol* 1991;111:71–76.

Helveston EM, Grossman RD. Extraocular muscle lacerations. *Am J Ophthalmol* 1976;81:754–760.

Helveston EM. The relationship of extraocular muscle problems to floor fractures. *Trans Am Acad Ophthalmol Otolaryngol* 1977;83:660–662.

Kitchens J, Kinder J, Oetting T. The drawstring temporary tarsorrhaphy technique. *Arch Ophthalmol* 2002;120:187–190.

Kohn R, Hepler R. Management of Limited rhino-orbital mucormycosis without exenteration. *Opthalmology* 1985;92:1440–1444.

Leigh RJ, Zee DS, eds. *The neurology of eye movements,* 2nd ed. Philadelphia: FA Davis Co, 1991.

Leigh RJ, Zee DS. Diagnosis of central disorders of ocular motility. In: Leigh RJ, Zee DS, eds. *The neurology of eye movements,* 2nd ed. Philadelphia: FA Davis Co, 1991:407.

Levin LA, Beck RW, Joseph MP, et al. The treatment of traumatic optic neuropathy. *Ophthalmology* 1999;106:1268–1277.

Liu GT, Glaser JS, Schatz NJ, et al. Visual morbidity in giant cell arteritis. clinical characteristics and prognosis for vision. *Ophthalmology* 1994;101:1779–1785.

Mashima Y, Hiida Y, Oguchi Y. Remission of Leber's hereditary optic neuropathy with idebenone. *Lancet* 1992;340:328–369.

McCord CD. *Eyelid surgery: principles and techniques.* Philadelphia: Lippincott–Raven, 1995.

Miller NR, Newman NJ. *Walsh and Hoyt's clinical neuro-ophthalmology,* 5th ed. Philadelphia: Williams & Wilkins, 1998.

Regillo CD, Brown GC, Savino PJ, et al. Diabetic papillopathy: patient characteristics and fundus findings. *Arch Ophthalmol* 1995;113:889–895.

Repka MX, Lam GC, Morrison NA. The efficacy of botulinum neurotoxin a for the treatment of complete and partially recovered chronic sixth nerve palsy. *J Pediatr Ophthalmol Strabis* 1994;31:79–83.

Rizzo JF and Lessell S. Tobacco amblyopia. *Am J Ophthalmol* 1993;116:84–87.

Rosenbaum JT, Simpson J, Neuwelt CM. successful treatment of optic neuropathy in association with systemic lupus erythematosis using intravenous cyclophosphamide. *Br J Ophthalmol* 1997;81:130–132.

Rossi PW, Kheyfets S, Reding MJ. Fresnel prisms improve visual perception in stroke patients with homonymous hemianopia or unilateral visual neglect. *Neurology* 1990;40:1597–1599.

Rothrock JF. Successful treatment of persistant migraine aura with divalproex sodium. *Neurology* 1997;48:261–262.

Rush JA. Pseudotumor cerebri. *Mayo Clin Proc* 1980;55:541–546.

Sedwick L, Boghen D, Moster M. How to handle the pressure or too much of a good thing. *Surv Ophthalmol* 1996;40:307–311.

Shorr N, Christenbury JD , Goldberg RA. Management of ptosis in chronic progressive ophthalmoplegia. *Ophthalmic Plast Reconstr Surg* 1987;3:141–145.

Spoor TC, Garrity JA, Ramocki JM. *Atlas of neuro-opthalmic surgery.* Blue Bell, PA: Field and Wood, 1992.

Swash M. Visual perseverations in temporal lobe epilepsy. *J Neurol Neurosurg Psychiatry* 1979;42:569–571.

Von Noorden GK, Helveston EM. Strabismus: A Decision Making Approach. Mosby, 1994.

Wright KW. *Color atlas of ophthalmic surgery: strabismus.* Philadelphia: JB Lippincott Co, 1991.

16. TOXIC AND METABOLIC DISORDERS

Martin A. Samuels

HEPATIC (PORTOSYSTEMIC) ENCEPHALOPATHY

BACKGROUND

1. Hepatic encephalopathy is the most common term used to describe the neurologic manifestations of the failure of the liver to perform its normal detoxification tasks.
2. The clinical categories of hepatic encephalopathy are:
   a. Acute hepatic encephalopathy
   b. Chronic recurrent hepatic encephalopathy
   c. Chronic progressive hepatic encephalopathy
      1) Wilson disease
      2) Acquired non-Wilsonian hepatocerebral degeneration

PATHOPHYSIOLOGY

1. The *sine qua non* for the development of hepatic encephalopathy is shunting of blood from the portal circulation to the systemic circulation with inadequate exposure to a functioning liver.
2. This may occur because of endogenous liver disease (e.g., hepatitis, cirrhosis), portosystemic shunts (intrahepatic or extrahepatic), or both.
3. Clinical and experimental evidence support two major mechanisms underlying the neurologic effects of portosystemic shunting of blood.
   a. Endogenous benzodiazepine-like substances are incompletely metabolized by the liver and thus reach the brain to bind to γ-aminobutyric acid (GABA) receptors, resulting in excessive inhibition of neuronal function thereby creating an encephalopathy. The benefit of the benzodiazepine antagonist, flumazenil, may be explained by this mechanism.
   b. Ammonia that is inadequately detoxified by the hepatic urea cycle reaches the brain where it is metabolized by the glutamate–glutamine system in astrocytes. When this system becomes saturated, ammonia reaches neurons where it is directly toxic, thereby producing the encephalopathy. The typical astrocytic change seen in all forms of liver disease (Alzheimer type II gliosis) may be due to the up-regulation of the glutamate–glutamine detoxification system that is compartmentalized to these cells. The fact that the encephalopathy may improve with lowering of the serum ammonia is taken as evidence that this mechanism is important.

PROGNOSIS

1. Hepatic encephalopathy may be acute, recurrent, subacute, or chronic.
2. The prognosis depends on the underlying cause.

DIAGNOSIS

1. The major clinical manifestations of hepatic encephalopathy are:
   a. Alteration of the level of consciousness including confusion with or without agitation (delirium), drowsiness, stupor, and coma.
   b. Movement disorders, the most frequent of which are asterixis, myoclonus, and tremor.

   c. Symptoms and signs of corticospinal tract disease are common (i.e., leg weakness, spasticity, increased tendon reflexes, and Babinski signs) and occasionally are the sole manifestation of hepatic encephalopathy (hepatic paraplegia).

   d. Extrapyramidal symptoms and signs (i.e., rigidity, bradykinesia, and dysarthria) are common, particularly in the chronic hepatocerebral degenerations.

2. Hepatic encephalopathy should be considered in any patient with an unexplained encephalopathy who might have liver disease, portosystemic shunting, or both. There is no single diagnostic test that is perfectly sensitive and specific but the diagnosis is more likely when:

   a. The blood ammonia is elevated. Arterial ammonia may be slightly better correlated with clinical state than venous ammonia but both are unreliable.

   b. High-intensity signal in the basal ganglia (particularly the putamen and globus pallidus) on T_1-weighted magnetic resonance imaging (MRI). This signal may represent deposition of paramagnetic substances (e.g., manganese and copper), although the precise reason for this deposition is usually unknown.

   c. High-amplitude triphasic sharp waves may be seen on the electroencephalogram (EEG). Although not specific for hepatic encephalopathy, the finding suggests a metabolic cause.

TREATMENT

1. Reduce sedating drugs to a minimum.

2. Correct fluid and electrolyte disturbances.

3. Treat any concomitant infection.

4. Reduce protein load by:

   a. Searching for and treating any gastrointestinal (GI) hemorrhage.

   b. Prescribing a low-protein diet, but providing enough calories to prevent proteolysis. Each liter of 10% dextrose in water provides 400 kcal. If nasogastric feeding is possible, 10% dextrose in water and lipids may be given to provide about 25 kcal/kg/d. The diet should be supplemented with vitamins (folate 1 mg/d, vitamin K 10 mg/d, and multivitamins).

   c. Administering cathartics to help eliminate whatever protein remains in the bowel. Magnesium citrate 20 mL or sorbitol, 50 g in 200 mL water may be administered via nasogastric tube or by mouth.

   d. Administering lactulose (a synthetic disaccharide that cannot be digested in the upper GI tract) will allow large-bowel bacteria to metabolize the sugar, thus producing hydrogen ions that will convert ammonia (NH_3) to ammonium (NH_4) that is not neurotoxic and is eliminated in the stool. Lactulose 30 to 50 mL (0.65 g/mL) may be administered by mouth, by nasogastric tube, or by retention enema three times a day.

   e. Flumazenil (Romazicon) [0.2 mg/min intravenous (IV)] may have a temporary beneficial effect on the encephalopathy.

   f. Hepatic transplantation may be life-saving for patients with hepatic failure and may reverse some or all of the neurologic manifestation of hepatic encephalopathy. In general, the longer the encephalopathy has been present, the lower the chance that it will be improved with liver transplantation.

HYPEROSMOLALITY AND HYPERTONICITY

BACKGROUND

1. Hyperosmolality is defined as a serum osmolality of greater than 325 mOsm/L.

2. Osmolality may be measured directly or may be estimated using the following formula: $2(Na^+ + K^+)$ + glucose/18 + blood urea nitrogen (BUN)/2.8.
3. Effective osmolality is called tonicity.

PATHOPHYSIOLOGY

1. As can readily be seen from the determinants of osmolality, in most clinical settings, hyperosmolality is due to hypernatremia, hyperglycemia, azotemia, or the iatrogenic addition of extrinsic osmoles (e.g., mannitol, glycerol).
2. *Hypernatremia* is defined as a serum sodium (Na) concentration of greater than 145 mEq/L. In all tissues other than the nervous system, hypernatremia leads to attraction of intracellular water leading to cell shrinkage. The nervous system is unique in that it is capable of generating solute (e.g., idiogenic osmoles) such as glutamine, taurine, and urea to minimize cell shrinkage. When hypernatremia is prolonged or unusually severe (serum Na over 160 mEq/L) these mechanisms fail leading to encephalopathy. When hypernatremia occurs, thirst increases and antidiuretic hormone (ADH) is released, leading to renal retention of pure water thereby lowering serum Na toward normal. Hypernatremia is thus due to a defect in thirst, inadequate release or effect of ADH, loss of hypotonic fluid, or retention of Na.
3. *Hyperglycemia* is nearly always due to diabetes mellitus either caused by inadequate insulin production or end-organ insulin resistance. In neurologic patients, this is often precipitated by the therapeutic use of glucocorticoids.
4. *Azotemia* is due to renal failure or inadequate renal perfusion (prerenal azotemia).
5. *Hyperosmolar* agents such as mannitol or glycerol are often used in neurologic patients and may result in hyperosmolality.

PROGNOSIS

1. Hyperosmolality usually produces a generalized encephalopathy without localizing or lateralizing features, but an underlying focal lesion (e.g., stroke, multiple sclerosis, neoplasm) could become symptomatic under the metabolic stress of a hyperosmolar state.
2. The prognosis of the hyperosmolality itself is good, but the long-term outlook depends on the cause.
3. For unknown reasons, hyperosmolality alone, particularly when due to hyperglycemia, may lead to continuous partial seizures, even when careful studies fail to uncover any underlying lesion. These seizures generally respond promptly to lowering of the serum glucose.

DIAGNOSIS

1. The diagnosis is made by calculating and/or measuring the serum osmolality using the formula $2(Na^+ + K^+)$ + glucose/18 + BUN/2.8 or by directly measuring osmolality.
2. The difference between the measured and calculated osmolality is termed the "osmolal gap," which should be less than 10 mOsm/L in normal circumstances.
3. The presence of large amounts of lipid (e.g., hyperlipidemia) or proteins (e.g., myeloma) may cause a factitiously low measurement of the serum Na, but does not interfere with measured osmolality, thereby causing an increase in the osmolal gap.
4. In the absence of hyperlipidemia or hyperproteinemia, an increased osmolal gap reflects the presence of solute such as alcohol or ethylene glycol or therapeutic substances such as mannitol, sorbitol, or glycerol.

TREATMENT

1. Calculate the water losses using the following approach:
   a. Calculate the normal total body water (NTBW) as follows:
   b. Body weight (in kilogram) × 0.6 = NTBW

    c. Calculate the total body Na (TBS) as follows:
    d. NTBW × 140 mEq/L = TBS
    e. Calculate the patient's body water (PBW) as follows:
    f. TBS/patient's serum Na = PBW
    g. Calculate the patient's water deficit (PWD) as follows: NTBW × PBW = PWD
2. Replace the water losses so that the serum Na falls no faster than 2 mEq/L/h using:
    a. Normal saline in hypovolemic patients (i.e., those with azotemia and/or hypotension).
    b. Pure water in hypervolemic patients.
    c. Renal dialysis if there is acute or chronic renal failure.
3. Insulin is administered (with frequent blood sugar testing) if there is hyperglycemia.
    a. Intramuscular (IM) and subcutaneous insulin may be unpredictably absorbed, particularly in hypovolemic patients because of poor tissue perfusion.
    b. Rapid-acting insulin 0.1 U/kg by IV push followed by 0.05 U/kg/h by continuous IV infusion is usually sufficient to reduce the blood sugar adequately and safely.

HYPONATREMIA

BACKGROUND

Hyponatremia is defined as a serum Na of less than 125 mEq/L.

PATHOPHYSIOLOGY

1. Hypotonicity is always associated with hyponatremia, but hyponatremia may be isotonic (e.g., infusion of salt-poor solutions, hyperlipidemia, or hyperproteinemia); hypertonic (e.g., hyperglycemia, mannitol); or hypotonic (impairment of free water excretion or an enormous free water load, as in psychogenic water drinking).
2. Tonicity (effective osmolality) is calculated using the formula $2(Na^+ + K^+) +$ glucose/18 + BUN/2.8 and osmolality is measured in the clinical laboratory. The difference between the calculated and measured osmolarity (the osmolal gap) should not exceed 10 mOsm/L (see section on treatment of hypernatremia, above).

PROGNOSIS

1. The prognosis of hyponatremia depends on the rate and magnitude of the fall in serum Na and its cause.
2. In acute hyponatremia (a few hours or less), seizures and severe cerebral edema may be rapidly life-threatening at serum Na levels as high as 125 mEq/L whereas patients may tolerate very low serum Na levels (even below 110 mEq/L) if the process develops slowly. Rapid correction of acute hyponatremia may be lifesaving whereas rapid correction of chronic hyponatremia may be dangerous. Nervous system cells compensate for chronic hyponatremia by excreting solute to avoid water retention. If upon this substrate serum Na rapidly rises, brain cells can rapidly shrink causing osmotic demyelination (formerly known as central pontine myelinolysis).
3. The cause of hypotonic hyponatremia is best determined by dividing all possibilities into three categories on the basis of the clinical estimate of the state of the extracellular fluid space. Blood pressure and heart rate with orthostatic measurements, the

degree of engorgement of the neck veins, and the presence or absence of the third heart sound (S_3) allow all patients with hypotonic hyponatremia to be categorized into three types:
  a. Hypovolemic (reduced effective blood volume): hypotension, tachycardia with orthostatic worsening
  b. Hypervolemic (edematous states)
  c. Isovolemic (retention of free water)

DIAGNOSIS

1. The diagnosis is made with a measurement of the serum Na followed by an assessment of extracellular volume.
2. The major diagnoses in each category are:
   a. Hypovolemic hyponatremia
      1) Gastrointestinal Na losses
      2) Hemorrhage
      3) Renal salt wasting (including cerebral salt wasting syndrome)
      4) Diuretic excess
      5) Adrenal insufficiency
   b. Hypervolemic hyponatremia
      1) Congestive heart failure
      2) Hepatic failure with ascites
      3) Nephrotic syndrome
   c. Isovolemic hyponatremia
      1) Syndrome of inappropriate secretion of antidiuretic hormone (SIADH)
      2) Psychogenic water drinking
      3) Acute and chronic renal failure
      4) Resetting of the osmostat (the sick cell syndrome)

TREATMENT

1. Hypertonic hyponatremia:
   a. Treat the underlying disorder (e.g., hyperglycemia, exposure to mannitol).
   b. Replace only estimated salt losses.
2. Isotonic hyponatremia:
   a. No fluid treatment for pseudohyponatremia disorders (e.g., hyperlipidemia, hyperproteinemia).
   b. Reduce Na-poor solutions if possible (dextrose; mannitol).
3. Hypotonic hyponatremia:
   a. Hypovolemic hypotonic hyponatremia
      1) Replace volume with isotonic saline.
      2) Treat underlying renal, adrenal, gastroenterologic conditions.
      3) Recognize and treat causes of cerebral salt wasting (e.g., intracerebral or subarachnoid hemorrhage).
   b. Hypervolumic hypotonic hyponatremia
      1) Free water restriction.
      2) Treat underlying edematous disorders (congestive heart failure, liver failure, nephrotic syndrome).
   c. Isovolemic hypotonic hyponatremia
      1) Chronic, slowly developing
         a) Water restriction.
         b) Antagonize ADH with lithium or demeclocycline if water restriction fails.
      2) Acute (less than 48 hours) rapidly developing
         a) Three percent saline (containing 513 mEq/L of Na) 300 to 500 mL IV over 1 hour will correct at about 1 mEq/L/h for 4 hours; then slow correction rate to less than 10 mEq/L/24 hours.
         b) Free water restriction or normal (0.9%) saline.

HYPOKALEMIA

BACKGROUND

Hypokalemia is defined as a serum potassium (K) level below 3.5 mEq/L.

PATHOPHYSIOLOGY

1. Serum potassium may be low because of abnormal intracellular or extracellular potassium balance or because of excessive potassium losses (renal or extrarenal).
2. Hypokalemia due to excessive cellular potassium uptake may be due to:
   a. Insulin
   b. Catecholamines
   c. β_2 adrenergic agonists
   d. Hypokalemic periodic paralysis
   e. Alkalosis
   f. Hypothermia
3. Extrarenal potassium loss (urine K^+ less than 20 mEq/d) may be caused by:
   a. Diarrhea (low serum bicarbonate)
   b. Cathartics; sweating (normal serum bicarbonate)
   c. Vomiting (high serum bicarbonate)
4. Renal potassium loss (urine K^+ more than 20 mEq/d) may be due to:
   a. Hyperreninemia
   b. Hyperaldosteronism
   c. Renal tubular acidosis
   d. Diuretic use
   e. Hypomagnesemia

PROGNOSIS

Severe hypokalemia (serum potassium less than 1.5 mEq/L) may be life threatening due to cardiac arrhythmia and severe muscle weakness.

DIAGNOSIS

1. The diagnosis of hypokalemia is made with a serum potassium measurement.
2. Urinary potassium measurement may help determine whether the potassium loss is renal or extrarenal but it should be borne in mind that such measurements are only valid in the face of a normal dietary and urinary Na as Na restriction may result in some masking of renal potassium wastage.
3. The measured serum sodium bicarbonate, plasma renin, plasma aldosterone, and urinary chloride levels and blood pressure may also help in the differential diagnosis of the cause of hypokalemia.

TREATMENT

1. Correct potassium balance problems, if possible (e.g., reduce β_2 adrenergic agonists)
2. Dietary sodium restriction (less than 80 mEq/d) will reduce renal potassium losses
3. Oral potassium chloride (KCl) for mild hypokalemia (30–35 mEq/d)
4. For moderate (1.5–3.0 mEq/L) or severe (less than 1.5 mEq/L) hypokalemia, especially with cardiac arrhythmias and/or severe muscle weakness, IV KCl may be administered at the rate of 15 mEq over 15 minutes with continuous cardiac monitoring, aiming for a 1mEq/L increase in the serum potassium. Thereafter, the rate should be slowed to less than 5 mEq/h of a solution of KCl no more concentrated than 60 mEq/L.

HYPERKALEMIA

BACKGROUND

Hyperkalemia is defined as a serum potassium concentration of greater than 5 mEq/L.

PATHOPHYSIOLOGY

1. Hyperkalemia may be seen in circumstances that cause an excess of whole body potassium or not.
2. The common causes of hyperkalemia without an excess of potassium are:
   a. Muscle injury (e.g., trauma, persistent seizures, muscle infarction)
   b. β_2 adrenergic antagonists (e.g., propranolol)
   c. Insulin resistance
   d. Metabolic acidosis
   e. Digitalis poisoning
   f. Depolarizing muscle relaxants (e.g., succinyl choline)
   g. Hyperkalemic periodic paralysis (muscle sodium channel mutation)
3. Common causes of hyperkalemia caused by whole-body potassium excess include:
   a. Addison disease
   b. Aldosterone deficiency [e.g., hyporeninemia; angiotensin-converting enzyme (ACE) inhibitor therapy; nonsteroidal antiinflammatory drugs (NSAIDs), heparin]
   c. Aldosterone resistance (e.g., renal failure, renal tubular disorders, potassium-sparing diuretics)

PROGNOSIS

1. The first sign of hyperkalemia is usually peaking of the T wave of the electrocardiogram (ECG), which usually occurs with a potassium level of about 6.0 mEq/L. As the potassium rises, the QRS complex widens, followed by reduction in its amplitude and then disappearance of the T wave.
2. Muscle weakness usually develops when the potassium is greater than 8 mEq/L.

DIAGNOSIS

1. Hyperkalemia may be suspected when the characteristic ECG pattern is seen, particularly when combined with weakness, sometimes with paresthesias.
2. The diagnosis is confirmed with measurement of the serum potassium.

TREATMENT

1. If hyperkalemia is considered life threatening because it is producing ECG changes and/or severe muscle weakness, one should treat by protecting the heart against life-threatening arrhythmias, promoting redistribution of potassium into cells, and enhancing potassium removal.
2. Cardiac protection: calcium gluconate 10% solution, 20 mL IV push.
3. Redistribution into cells:
   a. Glucose 50 g/h IV
   b. Insulin 5 units IV push every 15 minutes
   c. Albuterol 10 to 20 mg by inhaler
4. Enhance removal of potassium:
   a. Sodium polystyrene sulfonate (Kayexalate) 15 to 60 g with sorbitol by mouth (p.o.) or 50 to 100 g with retention enema

b. Hemodialysis
c. Loop diuretics
   1) Furosemide 40 to 240 mg IV over 30 minutes
   2) Ethacrynic acid 50 to 100 mg IV over 30 minutes
   3) Bumetanide 1 to 8 mg IV over 30 minutes

VITAMIN DEFICIENCY, DEPENDENCY, AND TOXICITY

VITAMIN A

BACKGROUND

1. Vitamin A deficiency is an important cause of blindness in large parts of the world but is rare in economically developed countries.
2. Vitamin A intoxication is seen in people who engage in megavitamin therapy.

PATHOPHYSIOLOGY

In many developing countries, general malnutrition is the major cause of vitamin A deficiency whereas in developed countries it is usually related to malabsorption or an unconventional diet.

PROGNOSIS

1. If treated early, the neurologic manifestations are usually completely reversible.
2. Once blindness has occurred, little can be done to reverse the visual loss.

DIAGNOSIS

1. Night blindness and dry eyes are probably the earliest symptoms of vitamin A deficiency.
2. Dry pruritic skin is also an early symptom of this deficiency.

TREATMENT

1. Vitamin A 1,000 units daily for 6 months and restoration of a normal diet for early disease.
2. Vitamin A up to 100,000 units daily for 6 months with restoration of a normal diet may be needed for moderate or advanced symptoms. Long-term use of vitamin A is not advisable as it may produce hypercoagulable state with consequent increased intracranial pressure (ICP) (pseudotumor cerebri) possibly caused by cerebral venous thrombosis. Treatment consists of discontinuation of the vitamin A.

VITAMIN B_1 (THIAMINE) DEFICIENCY

BACKGROUND

1. Vitamin B_1 (thiamine) deficiency occurs in parts of the world where polished rice is a major dietary staple or in people who are malnourished for any reason.
2. In developed countries, it is strongly linked to alcoholism.

PATHOPHYSIOLOGY

Thiamine is the coenzyme in thiamine pyrophosphate catalysis of decarboxylation of pyruvic acid and α-ketoglutaric acid.

PROGNOSIS

Treatment of Wernicke encephalopathy [the central nervous system (CNS) disease caused by thiamine deficiency] is usually quite successful, but the longer treatment is delayed the greater the probability of irreversible brain disease.

DIAGNOSIS

1. Thiamine deficiency should be assumed to be present in all malnourished people including, but not limited to, those with alcoholism.
2. The full triad of Wernicke encephalopathy (i.e., mental change, ataxia, and eye findings) is present in only a minority of those people later found to have Wernicke encephalopathy by pathologic study.
3. Measurement of 24-hour urine thiamine excretion is available and red blood cell transketolase may be measured.
4. For confirmation of the diagnosis, MRI may show lesions characteristic of Wernicke encephalopathy (i.e., small mamillary bodies and/or hypothalamic peri-third ventricular necrosis).

TREATMENT

1. Thiamine 100 mg IV push followed by:
2. Thiamine 25 daily for several months and restoration of a normal diet.

VITAMIN B₂ (RIBOFLAVIN) DEFICIENCY

BACKGROUND

Riboflavin deficiency is caused by general malnutrition or malabsorption.

PATHOPHYSIOLOGY

Riboflavin is a coenzyme in the flavoprotein enzyme system.

PROGNOSIS

Treatment is usually successful unless the disease is far advanced.

DIAGNOSIS

1. The clinical syndrome of cheilosis, angular stomatitis, visual loss, night blindness, glossitis, and burning feet in a susceptible person suggests the diagnosis.
2. Urinary 24-hour riboflavin excretion measurements are available (less than 50 μ/24 hours) but are rarely used except in problematic diagnostic dilemmas.

TREATMENT

1. Riboflavin 5 mg p.o. three times a day (t.i.d.).
2. Vitamin A replacement may help in relieving riboflavin induced ocular symptoms (see Treatment section of Vitamin A, above).
3. Restoration of a normal diet.

NIACIN (NICOTINIC ACID AND NICOTINAMIDE) DEFICIENCY

BACKGROUND

Niacin deficiency (pellagra) is usually associated with general malnutrition, often with alcoholism.

PATHOPHYSIOLOGY

Niacin is the coenzyme for nicotinamide dinucleotide codehydrogenase for the metabolism of alcohol, lactate and L-hydroxybutyrate.

PROGNOSIS

Untreated pellagra is lethal, but if recognized during life will usually respond favorably to therapy.

DIAGNOSIS

1. The characteristic triad of dermatitis (sun sensitivity followed by hyperpigmentation), diarrhea, and mental symptoms (usually a disorder of attention and/or mood followed by confusion, drowsiness, stupor, and coma) suggests the diagnosis in the setting of malnutrition.
2. The diagnosis can be confirmed with a 24-hour urinary niacin excretion of less than 3 mg/24 hours.

TREATMENT

1. Niacin or nicotinamide 50 mg p.o. ten times daily for 3 weeks.
2. In patients unable to take oral feedings, nicotinamide may be given IV 100 mg/d for 5 to 7 days.
3. Resumption of a normal diet is important for long-term recovery.
4. If pyridoxine deficiency is also deemed to be present (e.g., isoniazid therapy), vitamin B_6 (pyridoxine) must also be replaced as it is required for the normal conversion of tryptophan to niacin.

VITAMIN B_6 (PYRIDOXINE) DEFICIENCY, DEPENDENCY, AND TOXICITY

BACKGROUND

1. Pyridoxine deficiency is rarely seen in developed countries except in people who are taking isoniazid, an antituberculosis drug that is an antagonist of pyridoxine.
2. Cycloserine, hydralazine, and penicillamine also may lead to pyridoxine deficiency.
3. Pyridoxine toxicity is seen in people who take more than the recommended daily allowance of 2 mg because of perceived health benefits of megavitamin therapy.

PATHOPHYSIOLOGY

Pyridoxine is a cofactor in the conversion of tryptophan to 5-hydroxytryptophan and the conversion of homocysteine to cystathionine.

PROGNOSIS

Treatment usually results in complete resolution of the complaints.

DIAGNOSIS

1. Pyridoxine deficiency causes a generalized sensory and motor neuropathy.
2. Pyridoxine dependency is a rare autosomal recessive condition that leads to neonatal seizures.
3. Pyridoxine overuse also causes a peripheral neuropathy.
   a. Long-term low-dose (about 50 mg/d) exposure to pyridoxine leads to a small-fiber neuropathy.
   b. Shorter exposure to very high doses (over 100 mg/d) may produce a primary sensory neuronopathy that is less likely to improve with cessation of exposure to the vitamin.

TREATMENT

1. Pyridoxine deficiency caused by:
   a. Malnutrition: 50 mg/d p.o. for several weeks followed by 2 mg/d and resumption of a normal diet.
   b. Pyridoxine antagonists: 50 mg/d *only* while taking the antagonist.
2. Pyridoxine dependency: 10 mg IV push to terminate neonatal seizures and then 75 mg/d for life.
3. Pyridoxine toxicity: discontinue pyridoxine supplementation.

VITAMIN B$_{12}$ (COBALAMIN) DEFICIENCY

BACKGROUND

1. Vitamin B$_{12}$ deficiency may result from inadequate dietary intake, but this is rare as the daily requirement is small (2 μg/d) and the body stores are high (4 mg or about a 7-year supply).
2. Vegans who assiduously avoid animal protein may become cobalamin-deficient but this process requires many years.
3. More commonly, cobalamin deficiency is caused by failure to mobilize vitamin B$_{12}$ from the GI tract because of insufficient intrinsic factor, most often caused by autoimmune gastritis (pernicious anemia).
   a. Aging alone may lead to enough gastric parietal cell atrophy to cause intrinsic factor deficiency and consequent vitamin B$_{12}$ deficiency.
   b. In rare circumstances, the ingested cobalamin may be consumed before absorption by a parasite (the fish tapeworm *Diphyllobothrium latum*) or be inaccessible to cells because of a genetically determined deficiency in one of the cobalamin-carrying proteins (transcobalamin I and II).
   c. Human immunodeficiency virus (HIV) may lead to abnormal cobalamin function by an unknown mechanism, possibly involving abnormal transmethylation.

PATHOPHYSIOLOGY

1. Cobalamin is bound to salivary R protein. In the duodenum, pancreatic enzymes digest the R protein allowing cobalamin to be bound to intrinsic factor that is synthesized in gastric parietal cells. The cobalamin-intrinsic factor dimer is absorbed by specific receptors in the microvilli of the distal ileum. The newly absorbed cobalamin enters the portal circulation bound to transcobalamin II. Transcobalamin I is bound to previously absorbed cobalamin.
2. Inside cells, cobalamin is converted to its two active forms, methylcobalamin and adenosylcobalamin.
   a. Methylcobalamin is the coenzyme for the enzyme methionine synthetase (also known as methyl transferase), which catalyzes the conversion of homocysteine to methionine. Cobalamin is then remethylated to methylcobalamin by a methyl group donated by methyl tetrahydrofolate (serum folate). By this process, the

demethylated folate may participate in the formation of thymidylate, which is required for DNA synthesis. These interlocking reactions account for the fact that many of the clinical manifestations of vitamin B_{12} and folate deficiencies are similar.
   b. Cobalamin also participates in an important metabolic pathway that is independent of folate. In mitochondria, adenosylcobalamin acts as a coenzyme for the enzyme methyl malonyl coenzyme A (CoA) mutase that catalyzes the conversion of methyl malonyl CoA to succinyl CoA. Thus homocysteine and methylmalonic acid act as biologic markers for the intracellular effectiveness of cobalamin's two coenzymes.

PROGNOSIS

1. The clinical features of the cobalamin deficiency syndrome are dominated by a demyelinating process of the CNS affecting the lateral and posterior columns of the spinal cord (subacute combined degeneration), the white matter of the brain, and the optic nerves. A peripheral neuropathy may also be present.
2. Patients usually present with upper extremity paresthesias followed by stiffness of the legs, slowness of thinking, and reduced visual acuity. For unknown reasons, the optic neuropathy or mental change may dominate the clinical picture in some patients.
3. Most of the manifestations of the disease are reversible with appropriate therapy, but far-advanced disease may not completely respond.
4. Exposure to nitrous oxide may precipitate an acute presentation of cobalamin deficiency (anesthesia paresthetica) as it is a blocker of methyl transferase, one of the enzymes for which cobalamin is a coenzyme.

DIAGNOSIS

1. Hypersegmented (i.e., greater than five lobes) polymorphonuclear leukocytes are often seen on the peripheral blood smear.
2. Bone marrow may show megaloblasts (i.e., red blood cell precursors with a relatively immature nucleus compared to the cytoplasm).
3. Vitamin B_{12} levels are usually low:
   a. When less then 100 pg/mL, cobalamin deficiency is likely.
   b. When between 100 and 180 pg/mL, cobalamin deficiency is possible.
   c. When over 180 pg/mL cobalamin deficiency is unlikely.
4. Serum methylmalonic acid is the most specific test for intracellular cobalamin failure. Levels above 0.5 μmol/L suggest intracellular cobalamin failure.
5. The Schilling test may be useful to determine the cause of vitamin B_{12} deficiency.
   a. Phase I is aimed at determining whether the patient can absorb crystalline vitamin B_{12}.
   b. Phase II identifies those who are vitamin B_{12}–deficient because of intrinsic factor deficiency.
   c. The food Schilling test, in which radiolabeled vitamin B_{12} is attached to egg albumin, is used to identify those patients who are unable to extract vitamin B_{12} from food because of an inadequately acidic environment.
6. Anti–intrinsic factor antibodies are specific but insensitive for autoimmune gastritis.
7. Anti–parietal cell antibodies are sensitive but not specific for autoimmune gastritis.

TREATMENT

1. Cyanocobalamin 1,000 μg IM daily for 1 week, followed by weekly injections for 1 month, followed by monthly injections for life.
2. Cyanocobalamin 1 mg/d p.o. may be effective, but methylmalonic acid levels should be monitored to ensure that the treatment is having the expected metabolic effect.
3. Discontinue any exposure to nitrous oxide.

VITAMIN B$_9$ (FOLATE)

BACKGROUND

1. Folate is synthesized by plants and microorganisms. Its major dietary source is green leafy vegetables.
2. The daily requirement is 50 μg except in pregnant and lactating women when it is increased approximately tenfold.
3. Folate is ingested as a polyglutamate, which is metabolized to pteroylmonoglutamate and absorbed in the jejunum. In the bowel mucosal cells, it is reduced to tetrahydrofolate and methylated to methyl-tetrahydrofolate (serum folate).
4. Only about a 12-week supply of folate is stored in the body, so folate deficiency may become rapidly evident with malnutrition.

PATHOPHYSIOLOGY

1. Folate interacts intimately with vitamin B$_{12}$ (cobalamin). Serum folate (methyl-tetrahydrofolate) is the methyl donor that reconstitutes cobalamin into methyl-cobalamin in the conversion of homocysteine to methionine. Thus, homocysteine levels are a reflection of the effectiveness of both folate and vitamin B$_{12}$ in the methyltransferase (methionine synthetase) reaction.
2. Once demethylated, tetrahydrofolate undergoes polyglutamation and is converted to 5,10-methylene tetrahydrofolate, which, catalyzed by thymidylate synthase, generates deoxythymidine monophosphate for the synthesis of the thymidine needed for DNA synthesis.
3. Vitamin B$_{12}$ deficiency causes release of folate from cells and interferes with its utilization, thereby leading to an elevated serum folate level (the folate trap).
4. When vitamin B$_{12}$ is repleted, the folate level may precipitously fall, leading to a folate-deficiency state unmasked by the cobalamin therapy.

PROGNOSIS

1. Pure folate deficiency is rare as it is usually associated with generalized malnutrition, but it may be seen when folate inhibitors are used (e.g., methotrexate and sulfonamides are inhibitors of dihydrofolate reductase and phenytoin interferes with folate absorption).
2. It is clear that folate deficiency during gestation causes neural tube defects.
3. In adults, pure folate deficiency probably causes a sensory–motor polyneuropathy. In most cases, folate repletion leads to reversal of the neurologic deficits and adequate provision of folate during pregnancy reduces the risk of neural tube defects.

DIAGNOSIS

1. The blood and bone marrow changes of folate deficiency are indistinguishable from those caused by vitamin B$_{12}$ deficiency.
2. A serum folate level is specific but not particularly sensitive.
3. If the serum folate level is normal, but folate deficiency is suspected on clinical grounds, a red blood cell folate level should be obtained because it reflects the average intracellular folate level over the life span of the red blood cell and therefore is not unduly affected by recent dietary intake.

TREATMENT

1. Folic acid 1 mg/d p.o.
2. Resumption of a normal diet.
3. For patients on folate antagonists, folinic acid (leucovorin, citrovorum factor) 15 mg p.o. every 6 hours for 10 doses starting 24 hours after the dose of methotrexate is given. If folate deficiency develops from phenytoin, another antiepileptic drug

should be chosen, because folate replacement may reduce the antiepileptic efficacy of phenytoin.

VITAMIN C (ASCORBIC ACID)

BACKGROUND

Vitamin C deficiency (scurvy) is rare in developed countries, occurring almost exclusively in generally malnourished people who are poor, elderly, alcoholic, or adherents of unusual diets.

PATHOLOGY

1. Ascorbic acid is found in citrus fruits, green vegetables, and tomatoes and is absorbed from the small intestine via a transport system.
2. It has multiple functions, including acting as an antioxidant, a promoter of iron absorption, and a cofactor in the conversion of dopamine to norepinephrine and the synthesis of carnitine.
3. Consuming less than 10 mg of ascorbic acid daily will result in deficiency in a few months.

PROGNOSIS

1. Vitamin C deficiency (scurvy) is characterized by symptoms and signs of abnormal connective tissue such as perifollicular hemorrhages and bleeding from the gums. Neurologic symptoms include weakness, fatigue, depression, and confusion.
2. Treatment usually results in complete remission of the clinical syndrome.
3. Megadoses of vitamin C (i.e., greater than 2 g/d) may result in GI bleeding and oxalate kidney stones, but no hypervitaminosis C syndrome of the nervous system is known.

DIAGNOSIS

A plasma level of vitamin C of less than 11 μmol/L is considered abnormal, but most patients with clinical scurvy with neurologic impairment have an undetectable plasma vitamin C level.

TREATMENT

Vitamin C (ascorbic acid) 100 mg q.i.d. for 1 week followed by 100 mg t.i.d. for 1 month and resumption of a normal diet.

VITAMIN D

BACKGROUND

1. Vitamin D (1,25-dihydroxycholecalciferal; vitamin D_3) is the least classic of the vitamins in that it can be synthesized in the skin in adequate amounts for metabolic needs provided there is adequate sun exposure.
2. Vitamin D deficiency or resistance is the cause of rickets in the growing skeleton and osteomalacia in adults.

PATHOPHYSIOLOGY

1. Ultraviolet radiation converts provitamin D_3 (dihydrocholesterol) to vitamin D_3 in the skin.
2. In the liver, vitamin D_3 is converted to hydroxylated D_3 and then in the liver a final hydroxylation step is performed to yield the biologically active vitamin D (1,25 dihydroxyvitamin D_3).

PROGNOSIS

1. Vitamin D metabolism is intimately linked with numerous disorders of calcium and phosphate metabolism. The precise prognosis varies depending on the cause of the disorder.
2. In vitamin D deficiency related to intestinal malabsorption in adults, the symptoms may be expected to dramatically improve with vitamin D repletion.

DIAGNOSIS

1. Vitamin D deficiency causes a syndrome of pain and proximal muscle weakness. It is suspected when a painful myopathic syndrome is encountered in a patient who is at risk for osteomalacia (e.g., inadequate exposure to sunlight; antiepileptic drug treatment; hepatic and/or renal failure; inadequate dietary vitamin D).
2. Vitamin D levels can be measured in the serum to confirm the diagnosis.

TREATMENT

1. For dietary deficiency or inadequate exposure to sunlight: vitamin D_2 (ergocalciferol) or vitamin D_3 (cholecalciferol) 800 to 4,000 IU (0.02–0.1 mg) daily for 8 weeks, followed by 400 IU/d until the cause (e.g., inadequate exposure to light or inadequate diet) is resolved.
2. For tetany: calcium gluconate 10% 10 to 20 mg IV.
3. For patients on antiepileptic drugs: add 1,000 IU/d and monitor serum calcium and 1,25-hydroxyvitamin D_3 levels.

VITAMIN E (TOCOPHEROL)

BACKGROUND

1. Vitamin E is a family of fat-soluble tocopherols, which is never deficient for dietary reasons.
2. All vitamin E deficiency is due to severe malabsorption or genetic disorders that affect the transport or receptors for vitamin E.

PATHOPHYSIOLOGY

1. Of the eight naturally occurring tocopherols, RRR-α-tocopherol is the most biologically active.
2. It is taken up by the liver as chylomicrons, incorporated into very-low-density lipoprotein, and stored in brain, fat, and muscle.
3. Abetalipoproteinemia causes severe vitamin E deficiency by reducing both absorption and transport capacity.

PROGNOSIS

1. Vitamin E deficiency and resistance is manifested in the nervous system as a spinocerebellar degeneration, sometimes with features of myopathy, progressive external ophthalmoplegia, and pigmentary retinopathy.

2. Response to treatment depends on the precise cause, but early symptoms may respond well to vitamin E treatment.

DIAGNOSIS

1. Serum tocopherol may be measured.
2. An α-tocopherol level of less than 5 μg/mL or less than 0.8 mg of tocopherol per gram of total lipid are considered diagnostic abnormalities.

TREATMENT

1. For patients with pure vitamin E deficiency: α-tocopherol 800 to 1,200 mg/d
2. For patients with abetalipoproteinemia, α-tocopherol 5,000 to 7,000 mg/d

VITAMIN K

BACKGROUND

Vitamin K is a family of fat-soluble quinones that are involved in the coagulation cascade.

PATHOPHYSIOLOGY

1. Vitamin K_1 (phylloquinone) is found in vegetables, particularly leafy vegetables (e.g., spinach), and vitamin K_2 (menaquinone) is synthesized by gut flora.
2. The fat-absorption mechanisms mediated by the pancreas allow for absorption of vitamin K after which it may be stored in the liver and transported bound to lipoproteins.
3. Vitamin K is a cofactor necessary for the binding of calcium to a number of proteins involved with coagulation, including prothrombin.
4. Vitamin K deficiency may lead to bleeding including the predisposition for intracerebral, intraventricular, subarachnoid, subdural, and epidural hemorrhages.

PROGNOSIS

Treatment with vitamin K will rapidly reverse the coagulation abnormalities, but the prognosis depends on the location and extent of any hemorrhages that occurred prior to treatment.

DIAGNOSIS

1. A prolonged prothrombin time in a susceptible person (i.e., a patent with known fat malabsorption, use of antibiotics that sterilize the bowel, use of warfarin, or in infancy) suggest vitamin K deficiency.
2. Vitamin K levels may also be obtained in problematic cases.

TREATMENT

Vitamin K 10 mg IV followed by 1 to 2 mg/d p.o. or 1 to 2 mg/wk parenterally until the underlying cause is resolved.

HEAVY-METAL POISONING

LEAD

BACKGROUND

1. Lead toxicity is an important cause of intellectual impairment.
2. Despite dramatic lowering of children's blood lead levels in recent years as a result of stringent public health policy in developed countries, low levels of lead toxicity are still a cause of long-term neuropsychological problems.

PATHOPHYSIOLOGY

1. The most common cause of lead poisoning in children is residential remodeling. Inorganic lead is present in paints (both interior paints, which still line the walls of many older buildings, and modern exterior paints).
2. The organic lead compound tetraethyl lead is a gasoline additive, which is present in high concentrations in the atmosphere around tanks used to store gasoline and in dirt collected from urban areas near heavily traveled intersections and expressways.

PROGNOSIS

1. Encephalopathy:
   a. Epidemiology:
      1) Lead encephalopathy occurs in children who ingest large amounts of lead salts.
      2) It occurs only rarely in adults and only in those exposed to tetraethyl lead, which is lipid-soluble and reaches high levels in the CNS.
      3) In children, it is usually accompanied by pica, and it is most common between the ages of 1 and 3 years.
      4) Lead encephalopathy is more common in summer than in winter.
   b. Signs and symptoms:
      1) The usual symptoms of lead encephalopathy are personality change, lethargy, and irritability progressing to somnolence and ataxia, and finally, seizures, coma, and death.
      2) In children, acute episodes of lead encephalopathy may recur, superimposed on a state of chronic lead intoxication.
   c. Prognosis: The mortality of acute lead encephalopathy is less than 5% in the best of hands, but 40% of victims are left with permanent and significant residual neurologic deficits, which may include dementia, ataxia, spasticity, and seizures.
2. Lead colic is the most common manifestation of lead poisoning in adults.
   a. The patient is anorectic and constipated, and often has nausea and vomiting. There is abdominal pain but no tenderness. Characteristically, the patient presses on the abdomen to relieve the discomfort.
   b. Lead colic generally accompanies lead encephalopathy in children.
3. Neuromuscular form:
   a. Slowing of motor nerve conduction velocity is an early sign of lead poisoning in children, but symptomatic neuropathy is rare.
   b. In adults, however, symptomatic neuropathy is common in lead poisoning.
   c. Typically, lead neuropathy is predominantly motor, but paresthesias and sensory changes may occur.
   d. Extensors are weakened before flexors, and the most used muscle groups (usually the extensors of the wrist) are involved earliest.
4. It is likely that chronic low-level lead exposure in children causes an attention deficit disorder with hyperactivity.

DIAGNOSIS

1. Physical examination: The only characteristic physical finding of lead poisoning is the presence of lead lines around the gum margins. These occur in a minority of patients and only in patients with poor dental hygiene.
2. Blood smear: In chronic lead exposure, there is usually a microcytic anemia that may be superimposed on an iron deficiency anemia. Basophilic stippling is seen in a minority of cases, and the bone marrow may show ringed sideroblasts.
3. Urine: There is proximal renal tubular dysfunction associated with lead toxicity, with glycosuria, phosphaturia, and aminoaciduria.
4. Radiographs: Lead lines may be seen in the long bones. In children who have recently ingested lead-containing paint, radiopaque flecks may be seen in the abdomen.
5. Laboratory evidence of increased body lead burden:
    a. The serum lead level is the most useful screening test, although it does not reflect that total-body lead burden accurately.
        1) Lead levels that are measured on capillary blood (obtained from a finger stick) are subject to contamination by lead on the skin. Consequently, a cleanly obtained venous specimen is preferred.
        2) The 24-hour urinary lead excretion test has the same limitations as the serum lead level test. Lead levels of greater than 10 μg/dL (0.483 μmol/L) are of concern, but there is some evidence that any level of lead could be associated with long-term neurobehavioral problems.
    b. An ethylenediaminetetraacetic acid (EDTA) test measures total body lead burden more accurately than does a single serum or urinary level test.
        1) This test is dangerous in children with high lead burdens because EDTA may mobilize lead from the tissues and precipitate encephalopathy. Therefore, it should not be performed in a child who has a serum lead level higher than 70 μg/dL or who has symptoms of early encephalopathy.
        2) The test is performed by administering calcium EDTA in one or three doses of 25 mg/kg IV at 8-hour intervals. A 24-hour urine specimen is collected, and the total lead excreted in 24 hours is measured.
        3) A positive test consists of greater than 500 mg of lead excreted per 24 hours or greater than 1 mg of lead excreted per 24 hours per milligram of EDTA administered.
    c. Several tests measure the toxic effects of lead on porphyrin metabolism. These tests are generally the most sensitive measures of lead toxicity.
        1) Δ-aminolevulinic acid (δ-ALA) dehydratase activity in erythrocytes is the most sensitive test of lead poisoning, but it is not readily available.
        2) Urinary or serum δ-ALA levels higher than 20 mg/dL are indicative of lead toxicity.
        3) Urinary coproporphyrin excretion greater than 150 mg/24 hours is indicative of lead toxicity.
        4) Erythrocytic protoporphyrin (EP) levels higher than 190 μg/dL of whole blood are diagnostic of lead poisoning in the absence of either iron deficiency or erythropoietic protoporphyria, both of which may also elevate EP levels.

TREATMENT

1. Encephalopathy:
    a. For lead encephalopathy caused by the ingestion of inorganic lead, chelation therapy with EDTA and dimercaprol or British anti-Lewisite (BAL), is instituted immediately.
        1) The immediate medical needs of the patient, which may include seizure control and protection of the airway, are managed first.
        2) A urine flow of 350 to 500 mL/m^2/d is established. Overhydration, especially with free water, endangers the patient with increased ICP and should be avoided.
        3) Dimercaprol is given at a dose of 500 mg/m^2/d by deep IM injection in divided

doses every 4 hours for children younger than 10 years of age. The adult dose is 3 mg/kg/d in divided doses every 4 hours.

4) Beginning 4 hours after the initial dimercaprol injection, simultaneous injections of dimercaprol and EDTA are given in separate sites. The dose for EDTA is 1,500 mg/m^2/d IM in divided doses every 4 hours for children younger than 10, and 12.5 mg/kg/d for adults. In adults, EDTA may be administered as a continuous IV infusion of a solution of EDTA in 5% dextrose in water at a concentration no greater than 0.5%. The maximum adult dose is 7.5 g/d.

5) The usual course of therapy is 5 days.

6) Because of the danger of vomiting with dimercaprol, food is withheld for the first 3 days and then is given only if the patient is fully alert and without GI upset. Iron therapy is not administered simultaneously with dimercaprol. Electrolytes, including calcium and phosphate levels, are measured daily. SIADH frequently accompanies encephalopathy.

7) Increased ICP is managed with osmotic agents. The role of steroids is unclear. There is some evidence of an adverse interaction of EDTA and steroids, so some experts avoid their concurrent use.

b. Side effects of chelation therapy:

1) Dimercaprol may produce lacrimation, blepharospasm, paresthesias, nausea, vomiting, tachycardia, and hypertension. Its use is contraindicated in the presence of glucose 6-phosphate dehydrogenase deficiency.

2) EDTA may produce renal injury, cardiac conduction abnormalities, and electrolyte disorders. Renal function, calcium, and electrolytes are followed daily, and urine output is carefully monitored and maintained.

3) The IM injection of EDTA is painful. It is commonly mixed with procaine at a final concentration of 5%.

2. Lead colic and lead neuropathy in adults:

a. These conditions require immediate attention but are not emergencies. The cornerstone of therapy is removal of the patient from the offending environment and elimination of sources of future lead exposure.

b. In patients who are very symptomatic and in those with serum lead levels of 100 μg/dL or greater (or EP levels higher than 190 μg/dL, whole blood), a course of chelation therapy with dimercaprol plus EDTA is given and followed with a course of oral penicillamine or succimer.

c. In mildly symptomatic patients without markedly elevated serum lead or erythrocytic protoporphyrin levels, a course of oral penicillamine or succimer is probably adequate.

d. Lead colic responds acutely to calcium gluconate, 1 g IV, repeated as necessary.

3. Long-term therapy:

a. A 5-day course of dimercaprol plus EDTA usually removes about 50% of the soft-tissue stores of lead and reduces the serum lead level by a corresponding amount.

1) After chelation therapy is stopped, however, lead may be mobilized from bone, again raising the soft-tissue and serum lead concentrations. Consequently, the serum lead should be checked every few days after completion of a course of chelation therapy, and another course given if the serum lead rises about 80 μg/dL.

2) Some patients may require three or four courses of chelation therapy.

b. Succimer (dimercaptosuccinic acid) may be used for the oral therapy of lead intoxication.

1) The drug is administered at a dose of 30 mg/kg/d or 1,050 mg/m^2 in three divided doses for 5 days. The dose is then reduced to 20 mg/kg/d or 700 mg/m^2 in two divided doses for 14 more days.

2) It is important to treat concurrent iron deficiency.

3) Adverse effects can include GI upset, allergic rashes, and elevated liver enzymes.

4) The drug has an unpleasant odor, which reduces patient compliance. The capsules may be opened and the drug sprinkled into juice or a food vehicle.

    c. Penicillamine is not generally used in lead poisoning, and its precise role is not well defined. It was widely used prior to the introduction of succimer to promote the further excretion of lead following a course of dimercaprol plus EDTA. Its use now is reserved for patients who require oral chelation therapy but who cannot tolerate succimer.

        1) It is administered orally at a dosage of 600 mg/m^2/d in a single dose. It should be administered on an empty stomach, at least 2 hours apart from meals. The therapy must be continued for 3 to 6 months.

        2) Toxic reactions to penicillamine include nephrotic syndrome, optic neuritis, and blood dyscrasias.

4. Tetraethyl lead can be absorbed through the respiratory tract and, unlike inorganic lead salts, can produce encephalopathy in adults.

    a. The usual treatment is chelation therapy with dimercaprol plus EDTA, although there is not strong evidence of its effectiveness.

    b. Serum lead levels and EP concentrations are not helpful in monitoring treatment of acute poisoning with tetraethyl lead.

    c. Both diagnosis and therapy must be based on clinical findings.

5. Asymptomatic lead exposure in children:

    a. Children at high risk for lead poisoning should be screened with serum lead levels every 6 months.

    b. Management is based on the serum lead level.

        1) Serum lead levels less than 10 μg/dL require only continued routine screening.

        2) Serum lead levels of 10 to 20 μg/dL may require more frequent screening and discussion with the family about eliminating potential sources of environmental lead.

        3) Serum lead levels of 20 to 45 μg/dL demand an evaluation of the patient's medical status, with particular attention to nutrition and possible anemia or iron deficiency, and vigorous efforts to remove the patient from environmental lead exposure. A course of oral chelation therapy with succimer should be considered.

        4) Serum lead levels of 45 to 69 μg/dL require a full medical evaluation, removal from the source of exposure, and immediate chelation therapy with succimer or EDTA.

        5) Serum lead levels of 70 μg/dL or greater require immediate inpatient chelation therapy with EDTA plus dimercaprol.

MERCURY

BACKGROUND

Mercury toxicity may occur because of exposure to elemental mercury vapor, inorganic mercury, or organic mercury, such as methylmercury.

PATHOPHYSIOLOGY

1. Mercury salts and mercury vapor are potential environmental toxins in the chemical, paint, and paper industries, especially in chlorine production.

    a. Mercury vapor and dust are absorbed through the skin and lungs, and ingested mercury salts are absorbed from the gut.

    b. Elemental liquid mercury is poorly absorbed from the GI tract unless it is finely divided.

2. Organic mercury compounds pose the greatest threat to the nervous system.

    a. Phenolic and methoxy methyl mercury are degraded to inorganic mercury in the body and are metabolized as inorganic mercury salts.

    b. Alkyl mercury, primarily methyl and ethyl mercury, is produced as a waste product in the plastics and agricultural fungicide industries. It is well absorbed through skin and is highly lipid-soluble, reaching high concentrations in the CNS.

PROGNOSIS

1. Acute mercury poisoning from a brief exposure to a large amount of mercury produces stomatitis and a metallic taste; a sensation of constriction of the throat; ulcers on the tongue and palate; GI upset with nausea, vomiting, and bloody diarrhea; abdominal pain; acute renal failure; and circulatory collapse. The neurologic manifestations include lethargy, excitement, hyperreflexia, and tremor.
2. Chronic inorganic mercury poisoning produces stomatitis and a metallic taste, loss of appetite, a blue line along the gingival margin, hypertrophied gums, tremor, chorea, ataxia, nephrotic syndrome, and erythrism (a syndrome of personality change, shyness, and irritability). Pink disease, or acrodynia, occurs in children. It is characterized by irritability, insomnia, stomatitis, loss of teeth, hypertension, and erythema.
3. Organic mercury intoxication produces fatigue, apathy, memory loss, emotional instability, ataxia, dysarthria, tremor, dysphagia, paresthesia, and characteristically, constriction of the visual fields. This may progress to seizures, coma, and death. Organic mercury also crosses the placenta and can produce retardation and paralysis in the offspring of asymptomatic mothers. Renal lesions with proximal tubular dysfunction also occur.

DIAGNOSIS

1. Mercury poisoning must be diagnosed by the history of exposure and the clinical picture.
2. Whole-blood levels of mercury are normally <10 μg/L. A level of greater than 50 μg/L is considered toxic.

TREATMENT

1. The aims of therapy are to remove unabsorbed mercury from the GI tract, chelate mercury that has already been absorbed, and prevent acute renal failure.
2. Emesis or gastric lavage is used to empty the stomach, which is then rinsed with a proteinaceous solution (egg white, albumin, or skim milk) or charcoal. Because of the locally corrosive nature of mercury salts, the trachea is intubated if the patient is not fully alert.
3. Sodium formaldehyde sulfoxylate may decrease mercury absorption by chemically reducing mercuric salts to the less-soluble form of metallic mercury. Two hundred fifty milliliters of a 5% solution may be instilled into the duodenum.
4. Dimercaprol can be given at a dosage of 4 to 5 mg/kg IM every 4 hours, with no dose exceeding 300 mg. After the first 24 hours, the frequency of doses is reduced to every 6 hours for 2 to 3 days, and then 8 hours for the remainder of a 10-day course. N-acetyl-D,L-penicillamine may be the best chelating agent for mercury compounds, but it is not generally available.
5. IV fluids are administered to maintain urine flow, and mannitol, 1 g/kg IV, is given if the patient is oliguric. Dialysis may be necessary if the kidneys have failed and the patient is severely intoxicated. Electrolyte management might be difficult due to the diuresis induced by mercury salts, with sodium and potassium losses as well as volume depletion.
6. Inorganic mercury poisoning is most often a chronic process. There is an enterohepatic circulation of alkyl mercury, so excretion may be promoted by binding the mercury compound in the small intestine with an unabsorbable resin. Cholestyramine, 16 to 24 g/d in divided doses, may be given together with enough of an osmotic cathartic (e.g., sorbitol) to prevent constipation. The dosage of cholestyramine in children has not been established.

ARSENIC

BACKGROUND

1. Organic arsenicals were once used as a treatment for syphilis and as diuretics, but they are no longer in clinical use.
2. Most toxicity is now due to intentional ingestion for the purpose of murder or suicide.

PATHOPHYSIOLOGY

1. The primary cause of arsenic poisoning today is pesticide ingestion, either accidentally in children and agricultural workers or intentionally through suicide or homicide.
2. Arsenic-containing rat poison is no longer in widespread use, but it might still be stored in some homes and farms.
3. Occasionally, iatrogenic poisoning occurs from arsenic-containing antiparasitic agents used in the treatment of trypanosomiasis (e.g., tryparsamide, carbarsone, and senite).

PROGNOSIS

1. Acute poisoning:
   a. Acutely, arsenic produces capillary endothelial damage with leakage, especially in the splanchnic circulation. Nausea, vomiting, abdominal pains, and muscle cramps also occur.
   b. With somewhat larger doses, intravascular hemolysis can occur, which may lead to acute renal failure. Abnormalities are present on the ECG, and stomatitis appears.
   c. With lethal doses, a sequence of shock, coma, and death occurs in 20 to 48 hours.
2. Chronic poisoning:
   a. GI symptoms are less prominent than with acute poisoning, but weight loss, anorexia, nausea, and diarrhea or constipation may occur.
   b. Neurologic toxicity may be manifested by a sensorimotor neuropathy, excessive salivation and sweating, and encephalopathy.
   c. The encephalopathy, in its early stages, consists of fatigue, drowsiness, headache, and confusion, but it may progress to seizures, coma, and death.
   d. Rarely, there may be increased cerebrospinal fluid (CSF) protein and a mild pleocytosis along with fever, so the picture might be mistaken for an infectious process.
   e. Dermatologic signs can be diagnostic, with characteristic arsenical keratoses and transverse lines in the nails (Mees lines).
   f. Hepatic and renal damage may occur.

DIAGNOSIS

1. Acute arsenic intoxication must be recognized by a history of ingestion and by the clinical presentation. In acute intoxication, the urinary arsenic excretion may be extremely high.
2. Chronic arsenic poisoning:
   a. Chronic arsenic poisoning is suggested by the clinical picture, especially the dermatologic manifestations.
   b. The upper limits of normal urinary arsenic excretion are not sharply defined, but levels higher than 0.1 mg/L are suggestive of abnormally high exposure. Concentrations of arsenic in the nails or hair that are greater than 0.1 mg/kg are indicative, but not diagnostic, of arsenic poisoning.
   c. Individuals who are chronically exposed to arsenic may harbor large amounts in their tissues and excrete large amounts without developing symptoms of toxicity.

d. With chronic arsenic ingestion, there is increased urinary coproporphyrinogen III but normal urinary α-ALA excretion.

TREATMENT

1. Removal from exposure and elimination of unabsorbed arsenic from the GI tract by the use of emesis or gastric lavage and osmotic cathartics are the initial steps.
2. Dimercaprol is an effective chelating agent for arsenic.
   a. The usual course consists of 4 to 5 mg/kg/IM every 4 hours for 24 hours, followed by the same dose every 6 hours for 2 to 3 days, followed by tapering doses to complete a 10-day course.
   b. Neuropathy may require months to resolve.
3. Fluid and electrolyte disturbances must be rapidly repaired, and intravascular volume must be protected with electrolyte and albumin solutions. Pressors may be required in cases of acute poisoning.
4. The abdominal pain of acute arsenic poisoning may be severe and require large doses of narcotics.

THALLIUM

BACKGROUND

Thallium was once used as a treatment for several human diseases including syphilis, gout, and tuberculosis, but is no longer in any pharmaceuticals.

PATHOPHYSIOLOGY

1. Thallium is the primary ingredient of some depilatories and rat poisons. Poisoning usually occurs as a result of accidental ingestion of these materials.
2. The thallous ion is similar in size to potassium, allowing it to interfere with potassium dependent reactions.

PROGNOSIS

1. Alopecia is the hallmark of thallium intoxication.
2. Neurologic manifestations are prominent: ataxia, chorea, restlessness, and hallucinations, progressing to coma and death.
3. Blindness, facial paralysis, and peripheral neuropathy may occur. Nausea, vomiting, constipation, and liver and renal damage may also occur.

DIAGNOSIS

1. Normal urine thallium levels are less than 0.3 μg/L.
2. Alopecia may occur with urine levels above 20 μg/L and major neurologic effects occur with level above 50 μg/L.

TREATMENT

1. Removal from exposure and elimination of unabsorbed thallium from the GI tract with emesis or gastric lavage and catharsis are the primary modes of therapy.
2. Prussian blue (potassium ferric hexacyanoferrate) may be introduced by tube into the duodenum and may decrease thallium absorption. The dose is 250 mg/kg given over 24 hours in two to four divided doses.

CARBON MONOXIDE POISONING

BACKGROUND

Carbon monoxide is the most common cause of death by poisoning, either because of accidental exposure (e.g., smoke) or because of intentional exposure for the purpose of murder or suicide.

PATHOPHYSIOLOGY

1. The acute manifestations of carbon monoxide inhalation are those of hypoxia without cyanosis.
   a. The textbook "cherry-red" appearance is uncommon.
   b. The earliest neurologic dysfunction is lethargy, which may progress to coma.
   c. Retinal hemorrhages may occur.
   d. As hypoxia becomes more severe, brainstem functions fail.
   e. Cardiac ischemia and acute myocardial infarction may occur.
2. The patient might recover completely from the acute episode, if rescued in time, or be left with residual neurologic dysfunction.
   a. Characteristically, the basal ganglia are the most vulnerable structures (particularly the globus pallidus).
   b. The patient might also recover completely from the acute intoxication only to succumb to a massive subacute demyelination of the cerebral white matter that begins 1 to 3 weeks after exposure.

PROGNOSIS

The outcome depends on the length of the exposure.

DIAGNOSIS

1. The history is usually sufficient to give the diagnosis. The cherry-red appearance might also give a clue. Generally, if the patient has inhaled smoke or flame, rather than air contaminated by carbon monoxide, the damage to the respiratory epithelium by heat or oxides of nitrogen is of more immediate concern than carbon monoxide poisoning.
2. Many blood gas laboratories can measure carbon monoxide saturation of blood. (Note that venous blood is adequate for carbon monoxide determinations.)
   a. In the absence of lung disease or a right-to-left shunt, SaO_2, while the patient is breathing 100% oxygen, will give an estimate of the carbon monoxide saturation.
   b. The PaO_2 is of no use in estimating carbon monoxide saturation because it will not be affected by the combination of hemoglobin with carbon monoxide.

TREATMENT

1. The primary therapy for carbon monoxide intoxication is to remove the patient from exposure as rapidly as possible and to administer 100% oxygen.
   a. Any patient with symptoms of hypoxia or carbon monoxide saturation greater than about 40% should be observed in the hospital for at least 48 hours and maintained on supplemental oxygen until the carbon monoxide concentration falls below 20%.
   b. For severely poisoned patients, hyperbaric oxygen administration or exchange transfusion may be of benefit.
2. Any maneuvers that reduce the tissue demand for oxygen should be undertaken.
   a. Patients are kept at rest and tranquilized if they are hyperactive from encephalopathy or other causes.
   b. Hyperthermia is treated vigorously.

3. Fire victims frequently inhale both carbon monoxide and cyanide (a product of combustion of many plastics and synthetic materials). Although methemoglobin-forming agents such as amyl nitrite and sodium nitrite are routinely used to treat cyanide poisoning, they reduce the oxygen-carrying capacity of the blood and should probably be avoided when carbon monoxide levels are high.
4. Residual movement disorders are common after severe carbon monoxide poisoning.
   a. Choreoathetosis, myoclonus, and a parkinsonian syndrome can occur. These disorders are treated symptomatically in the same manner as movement disorders of other causes (see Chapter 13).
   b. For parkinsonism associated with carbon monoxide intoxication, direct-acting dopamine agonists (bromocriptine, pramipexole, pergolide) may be more effective than L-dopa.
5. There is no known treatment for or specific means of preventing the delayed massive demyelination that sometimes follows carbon monoxide poisoning.

ACETYLCHOLINESTERASE INHIBITOR POISONING

BACKGROUND

Acetylcholinesterase (AChE) (the enzyme that catalyzes the hydrolysis of acetylcholine at cholinergic synapses) is blocked either competitively or irreversibly by many naturally occurring substances, agents used for chemical warfare and insecticides.

PATHOPHYSIOLOGY

1. The usual source of AChE inhibitors is organophosphorus insecticides. Acute poisoning may occur through ingestion, inhalation, or absorption through the skin.
2. Chronic poisoning produces chronic peripheral neuropathy. Its only treatment is discontinuation of exposure to the toxin.

PROGNOSIS

1. Acute AChE inhibitor poisoning causes a combination of local effects, systemic muscarinic and nicotinic effects, and CNS toxicity.
2. Local effects:
   a. Inhalation exposure produces symptoms referable to the eyes, mucous membranes of the nose and pharynx, and the bronchial smooth muscle. Pupillary constriction, conjunctival congestion, watery nasal discharge, wheezing, and increased respiratory secretions are all prominent.
   b. Ingestion of AChE inhibitors produces anorexia, nausea, vomiting, abdominal cramps, and diarrhea.
   c. Skin exposure produces localized swelling and muscle fasciculations.
3. Muscarinic effects include salivation, sweating, lacrimation, bradycardia, and hypotension. Severe poisoning produces involuntary urination and defecation.
4. Nicotinic effects referable to the neuromuscular junction include muscle fatigue, weakness, and fasciculations that progress to paralysis. The most immediate life-threatening effect of AChE inhibitor intoxication is respiratory paralysis, which is especially dangerous when combined with bronchospasm and copious bronchial secretions.
5. CNS toxicity is manifested by confusion, ataxia, dysarthria, and diminished deep tendon reflexes, which may progress to seizures and coma.

DIAGNOSIS

1. The clinical presentation and a history of exposure are the key elements to diagnosis.
2. Some clinical laboratories assay AChE activity in plasma and erythrocytes. Although the normal range for AChE activity is broad, patients with significant systemic AChE inhibitor toxicity all have extremely low levels.

TREATMENT

1. Exposure is terminated by removal of the patient from contaminated air, washing the skin copiously with water, or gastric lavage as indicated.
2. The airway must be protected, especially if gastric lavage is required, and respiratory assistance must be provided if necessary. Frequent suctioning of respiratory secretions is required.
3. Circulatory collapse is treated with maintenance of fluid volume and pressors as necessary.
4. Seizures are treated by the usual methods (see Chapter 2).
5. Muscarinic effects can be blocked with atropine in large doses.
   a. Therapy should begin with 2 mg IV and then be repeated every 3 to 5 minutes until muscarinic symptoms disappear and bradycardia is reversed.
   b. If the patient is alert, doses of atropine may then be given p.o. as required. IV doses will need to be repeated every few hours in comatose patients.
6. Reversal of peripheral AChE may be achieved with pralidoxime for the proportion of the enzyme that has not "irreversibly" bound the inhibitor.
   a. The initial dose for adults is 1 g, infused IV over 2 or more minutes.
   b. If improvement is not noted within 20 minutes, the dose is repeated.
   c. The earlier pralidoxime is administered in the course of intoxication, the greater its effect. It may need to be repeated every 8 to 12 hours.
   d. Pralidoxime does not reach CNS AChE, and compounds that do so are not generally available.

ALCOHOL

BACKGROUND

1. Alcohol accounts for the most neurologic toxicity of any drug or toxin.
2. Since alcoholism is often associated with malnutrition, the neurologic complications of alcoholism are a mixture of those caused by the direct effects of alcohol (and/or its metabolites) and the neurologic complications of malnutrition.

PATHOPHYSIOLOGY

1. Pharmacokinetics of ethyl alcohol:
   a. Ethanol is completely absorbed from the GI tract within 2 hours. It is absorbed less rapidly if there is food in the stomach at the time of ingestion.
   b. Ethanol is metabolized by the liver, and it is more rapidly metabolized in those who drink regularly and heavily than in occasional drinkers.
   c. The rate of ethanol metabolism is approximately 7 to 10 g/h, which represents about 1 oz of 90-proof spirits or 10 oz. of beer per hour.
   d. The lethal blood level of alcohol is about 5,000 mg/L. In a 70-kg man, this represents about 1 pt of 90-proof spirits distributed throughout total body weight.
   e. The toxicity from a dose of ethanol depends on the maximum blood ethanol level,

the rapidity with which that level is obtained, the patient's prior experience with alcohol, and the presence of other drugs.

PROGNOSIS

1. Acute alcohol intoxication is completely reversible.
2. Chronic alcohol toxicity may be associated with irreversible loss of neurologic function either because of the direct effects of alcohol and/or the effects of malnutrition.

DIAGNOSIS

1. The history suggests alcohol as the possible cause of a neurologic problem.
2. Acute alcohol toxicity may be confirmed with a blood level of more than 100 mg/dL but tolerance may develop such that people may be asymptomatic with levels as high as 800 mg/dL.

TREATMENT

1. Alcohol intoxication:
   a. In mild intoxication, the most important aspect of management is to see that patients can get home safely, without endangering themselves and others by attempting to drive. Analeptics, such as caffeine, amphetamines, and theophylline, do not help "sober up" the patient or improve driving performance.
   b. Moderate intoxication with alcohol poses no danger to patients if they are merely observed until ready to make their own way home. If there has been ingestion within the preceding 2 hours, emesis, gastric lavage, and catharsis may be used to prevent further absorption. As with mild intoxication, analeptics are of no use.
   c. The chief danger in severe ethanol intoxication is respiratory depression. As long as adequate supportive care is provided before significant hypoxia occurs, the outlook is excellent. Within 24 hours, the alcohol will be metabolized.
      1) The blood alcohol level may be measured directly or estimated by measuring the serum osmolality. Each 100 mg/L of blood ethanol raises the serum osmolarity by approximately 2 mOsm/L.
      2) Tracheal intubation and respiratory support are provided at the earliest sign of respiratory depression. Respiratory support should be continued until the patient is fully awake.
      3) Gastric lavage is performed if there is a possibility of alcohol or other drug ingestion within the preceding 2 hours. If the patient is not fully awake, the trachea is protected with a cuffed endotracheal tube before gastric lavage is undertaken.
      4) Frequently, life-threatening ethanol ingestion is accompanied by ingestion of other CNS depressants. This possibility should be considered if the patient's mental status is depressed out of proportion to the blood ethanol level or if unexpected neurologic signs are present.
      5) Fluids are given to maintain adequate blood pressure and urine output, but there is no need to induce a forced diuresis.
      6) If the patient is suspected of being a chronic alcoholic or having severe liver disease, blood is drawn for determination of glucose and electrolytes. Thiamine 50 mg IV and dextrose 50 g IV are administered in the event of complicating Wernicke encephalopathy or hypoglycemia.
      7) Chronic alcoholics are frequently potassium-depleted and may require replacement with KCl. Acid–base balance is maintained, and alcoholic ketoacidosis is either ruled out or treated appropriately with IV glucose and fluids.
      8) If the blood ethanol level is extremely high (more than 7,000 mg/L) peritoneal dialysis or hemodialysis may be justified to reduce the ethanol level rapidly.
      9) Although fructose administration hastens ethanol metabolism, its risk does not justify the benefit obtained.

2. Alcohol withdrawal:
  a. Mild withdrawal syndrome:
    1) Clinical manifestations of mild ethanol withdrawal are anxiety, weakness, tremulousness, sweating, and tachycardia.
    2) In the absence of other intercurrent illness, such as coronary artery disease or infection, these patients may be treated at home if the social situation is appropriate.
    3) Patients are given thiamine, 50 mg IM, and a prescription for multivitamins if they are malnourished. They are instructed to maintain adequate hydration and food intake during the period of withdrawal.
    4) A benzodiazepine tranquilizer minimizes the symptoms of withdrawal.
      a) In general, one may begin with chlordiazepoxide, 25 to 50 mg p.o. every 4 hours, for the first 48 to 72 hours, and then taper the dosage over 5 to 7 days.
      b) Diazepam is equally effective. The initial dosage is 5 to 10 mg p.o. every 4 to 6 hours.
  b. Moderate and severe withdrawal syndromes:
    1) Patients who are febrile, irrational, hallucinating, or extremely agitated must be hospitalized until the severe manifestations of ethanol withdrawal have resolved.
    2) These patients frequently are dehydrated, and total body potassium is depleted. Those deficits are replaced with appropriate electrolyte solutions. Vascular collapse may occur, but it usually responds to rigorous volume replacement.
    3) Ethanol withdrawal is often precipitated by an intercurrent illness, often infection. Such illnesses must be detected and treated appropriately.
    4) Chronic alcoholics are subject to bleeding disorders from liver disease or thrombocytopenia. Consequently, acetaminophen, 600 mg or 1.2 g p.o. or per rectum, is preferred to aspirin for the treatment of hyperthermia.
    5) The patient is usually magnesium-depleted. There is no good evidence that replacing magnesium has any effect on the course of the withdrawal syndrome, but many physicians elect to administer magnesium if the patient is admitted early in the course of withdrawal. Magnesium sulfate may be given in 50% solution, 1 to 2 mL IM, or the same amount may be mixed with IV electrolyte solutions.
    6) Severe liver disease may result in hypoglycemia, and starvation may result in ketoacidosis. Consequently, glucose is administered early, either as a bolus of 25 to 50 g (if the patient is comatose) or as a dextrose-plus-electrolyte solution.
    7) Thiamine, 50 mg IV or 50 mg IM, is always administered to chronic alcoholics prior to glucose because of the risk of Wernicke encephalopathy.
  c. Tranquilization:
    1) The benzodiazepines are the preferred drugs for sedation in alcohol withdrawal.
    2) Diazepam and chlordiazepoxide are essentially identical in their therapeutic effect when used in equipotent doses.
      a) Both have a prolonged duration of action (12–36 hours), are well absorbed p.o., are erratically absorbed when administered IM, and have a rapid and predictable effect when given IV.
      b) The primary danger from both drugs is excessive CNS depression after repeated doses, due to the cumulative effect of successive doses given within 24 hours of each other. Respiratory arrest may occur occasionally with rapid IV injection of either drug, but the risk is minimized with small doses.
      c) Diazepam can be administered IV in 2.5-mg or 5-mg doses every 5 minutes until the patient is calm, and then 5 to 10 mg p.o. or by slow IV injection every 2 to 6 hours as necessary.

d) Chlordiazepoxide can be used in an identical manner; chlordiazepoxide, 12.5 mg, being equivalent to diazepam, 2.5 mg.

3) The most important aspects of managing alcohol withdrawal with IV benzodiazepines are frequent observation of the patient to prevent cumulative toxicity and avoidance of large doses (diazepam, approximately 5 mg, lorazepan 2 mg, or chlordiazepoxide, approximately 25 mg) in any one IV injection. It is essential that each patient be individually titrated with tranquilizer and repeatedly reevaluated rather than being put on a fixed-dosage schedule.

d. Withdrawal seizures:

1) Ethanol withdrawal seizures occur between 12 and 30 hours after cessation of regular ethanol ingestion, are generalized major motor convulsions, and are usually brief and one or two in number. They can be prolonged, however, and status epilepticus may occur.

2) The interictal EEG is normal, and except for periods of drug withdrawal, the patient is not predisposed to unprovoked seizures.

3) The diagnosis of ethanol withdrawal seizure can be made only if the seizure fits the typical clinical pattern and there is no other possible cause. Seizures from other causes are likely to be precipitated by ethanol withdrawal and should be treated appropriately (see Chapter 2).

4) Phenytoin:

a) Phenytoin may partially protect against ethanol withdrawal seizures.

b) Assuming patients have not been taking an antiepileptic, they can be given a 1-g loading dose, either IV as a single dose infused over 20 to 30 minutes or p.o. divided into two or three doses given 1 to 2 hours apart. Then patients are maintained on 300 mg/d p.o. or IV for 3 days, and the dose is tapered over about 1 week after the risk of withdrawal seizures has passed.

c) Ethanol withdrawal seizures are not an indication for long-term anticonvulsant therapy.

d) Experts differ over the indications for phenytoin prophylaxis of withdrawal seizures. Some would administer phenytoin to all patients seen during the first 24 hours of withdrawal from heavy ethanol use. Others would limit its use to those with a history of withdrawal seizures or with an underlying seizure disorder.

5) If a patient is seen after a withdrawal seizure has occurred, it is reasonable merely to observe the patient without therapy as long as other causes (particularly head trauma, subdural hematoma, metabolic derangement, and CNS infection) for the seizure have been ruled out. The probability is high that the seizure either will not recur or, if it does recur, will be brief. Some would argue that the risk involved in phenytoin use is sufficiently low that it should be used in this situation until the patient is out of danger.

6) If the patient is allergic to phenytoin, carbamazepine is the alternative. Barbiturates should be avoided, as they may potentiate the respiratory depressant effects of benzodiazepines used to treat withdrawal symptoms.

WERNICKE ENCEPHALOPATHY

BACKGROUND

Wernicke encephalopathy is a thiamine-deficiency disease that occurs in chronic alcoholics or patients with chronic malnutrition.

PATHOPHYSIOLOGY

1. It has an acute onset, and its cardinal manifestations are confusion and memory loss, nystagmus, extraocular movement deficits (most often unilateral or bilateral sixth nerve palsies), and ataxia, occurring in any combination.
2. Drowsiness, stupor, and even coma may occur.

PROGNOSIS

1. With prompt treatment, the ocular abnormalities usually clear within days, but about one fourth of patients will be left with Korsakoff psychosis, in which the ability to form new memories is impaired far out of proportion to other higher cortical functions.
2. Any patient with an appropriate predisposition who has any sign of ataxia, confusion, or extraocular movement abnormality should be treated for Wernicke encephalopathy.

DIAGNOSIS

1. The diagnosis is often obvious clinically, but it can be confirmed with erythrocyte transketolase levels or thiamine levels.
2. The blood sample must be drawn before the administration of thiamine to be diagnostic.

TREATMENT

1. The treatment is parenteral thiamine. The dosage required is not known, but it is customary to give 50 to 100 mg IV or IM immediately and then 50 mg/d p.o. or IM for 3 days thereafter. Except for extremely rare immediate hypersensitivity reactions to commercial thiamine preparations, the drug causes no toxicity.
2. Prophylaxis:
   a. The administration of glucose before thiamine in a severely thiamine-deficient patient may precipitate Wernicke encephalopathy. It is therefore recommended that thiamine be given before glucose in any patient in whom thiamine deficiency is a possibility, including patients with coma of unknown cause.
   b. Patients at risk for Wernicke encephalopathy should be treated with multivitamins, including vitamin B complex, along with thiamine.

OPIATE ABUSE

OPIATE OVERDOSAGE

BACKGROUND

1. Opiates are the pharmacologically active alkaloids that may be extracted from the poppy.
2. Commonly used opiates include opium (paregoric) morphine, hydromorphone, oxymorphone, oxycodone, levorphanol, hydrocodone, and codeine.

PATHOPHYSIOLOGY

1. Depressed mental status, respiratory depression, and pinpoint pupils are the typical symptoms of acute opiate poisoning.

2. The body temperature may be subnormal, the blood pressure may be low, and the limbs and jaw are generally flaccid.
3. With very high doses, convulsions and pulmonary edema may occur.

PROGNOSIS

1. If treated promptly, the neurologic effects of opiate intoxication are completely reversible.
2. Long-term complications are caused by hypoxemia, which is secondary to respiratory depression.

DIAGNOSIS

1. The history suggests the use of opiates.
2. Depressed consciousness with very small fixed pupils support the diagnosis and opiate levels confirm it.

TREATMENT

1. Patients who are cyanotic, have a respiratory rate below ten/minute, or cannot protect their own airway are intubated with an orotracheal or nasotracheal tube and given respiratory assistance with positive pressure ventilation.
2. Naloxone (Narcan) an opiate antagonist, is given in 0.4-mg increments by rapid IV injection until the patient is breathing normally or until a total of 10 mg has been given, at which point the diagnosis must be called into question.
   a. The duration of action of naloxone is only 1 to 4 hours, depending on the dose, which is shorter than the duration of commonly available opiates. Therefore, after the action of an opiate is reversed with naloxone, patients require close observation in the event that they relapse into coma. Repeated doses of naloxone may be required, especially in methadone intoxication, because of the long duration of action of methadone (24–36 hours).
   b. Paradoxically, opiate addicts are more sensitive to narcotic antagonists than are patients who are not tolerant of opiates. Therefore, narcotic antagonists are administered in small IV doses (naloxone, 0.4 mg) repeated every 2 to 3 minutes until the desired effect is achieved or until a total of 10 mg has been given.
      1) When given to opiate addicts, narcotic antagonists may precipitate severe acute withdrawal within minutes of IV injection if given in sufficient doses.
      2) Once the antagonist is administered, the withdrawal syndrome will be extremely resistant to reversal by the administration of opiates until the effect of the antagonists has waned.
   c. In narcotic addicts, one should not attempt to reverse all of the narcotic effects immediately with naloxone. Rather, the aim is to return patients' spontaneous respirations and restore level of consciousness to the point where they can protect their own airway and make spontaneous postural adjustments in bed.
   d. Narcotic antagonists, including naloxone, have an emetic effect. Therefore, in comatose patients, the trachea is protected by a cuffed endotracheal tube.

OPIATE WITHDRAWAL

BACKGROUND

Opiate withdrawal symptoms peak at 24 to 72 hours after the first dose but may last as long as 7 to 10 days.

PATHOPHYSIOLOGY

The withdrawal syndrome is mediated by endogenous opiate receptors, which had up-regulated during the period of opiate usage.

PROGNOSIS

The withdrawal syndrome is unpleasant but not life threatening.

DIAGNOSIS

Irritability, anxiety, lacrimation, and yawning often joined by signs of overactivity of the sympathetic nervous system (tachycardia, tremor, dilated pupils, sweating) suggest the diagnosis in a patient with history of opiate use.

TREATMENT

1. Although many of the symptoms of opiate withdrawal are dramatic, the only potentially dangerous manifestation is dehydration due to nausea, vomiting, sweating, and diarrhea, combined with failure to take in oral fluids. Consequently, the essential aspect of management of severe narcotic withdrawal is the administration of appropriate electrolyte solutions to maintain intravascular volume and electrolyte balance.
2. At any point in the course of the syndrome, as long as a narcotic antagonist has been administered, the symptoms may be rapidly relieved by narcotic administration. For example, morphine sulfate may be administered by IV injection in small incremental doses of 2 to 5 mg every 3 to 5 minutes until the desired effect is achieved.
3. Clonidine, an α-adrenergic agonist and antihypertensive agent, administered as a single dose of 5 μg/kg, will alleviate the symptoms of opiate withdrawal. The patient may then be treated with a 2-week course of clonidine, beginning with a dosage of 0.1 mg every 4 to 6 hours, as necessary to prevent withdrawal symptoms; the dose is adjusted to a maximum of 1.2 mg/d or until oversedation or hypotension supervenes.
4. Methadone 20 mg p.o. once or twice daily blunts the withdrawal syndrome. The methadone may be tapered as the symptoms recede.

BARBITURATE INTOXICATION

BACKGROUND

Barbiturates do not occur naturally, so exposure is always due to the use of sedative and antiepileptic drugs.

PATHOPHYSIOLOGY

Barbiturates bind to part of the GABA receptor, which controls a chloride channel, which in turn leads to hyperpolarization of neuronal cell membranes, leading to inhibition in the CNS.

PROGNOSIS

Barbiturates do no direct damage to the nervous system, so every patient who reaches medical attention before the development of CNS damage from hypoxia or shock has the potential to recover completely with adequate supportive therapy.

DIAGNOSIS

1. A classification of the level of barbiturate intoxication is useful in determining the prognosis:
   a. Class 0: patients who are asleep but can be aroused to purposeful activity.
   b. Class I: patient who are unconscious but withdraw from noxious stimuli and whose muscle stretch reflexes are intact (the corneal reflex may be depressed).
   c. Class II: patients who are unconscious and do not respond to painful stimuli, but who retain muscle stretch reflexes and have no respiratory or circulatory depression.
   d. Class III: patients who are unconscious with loss of some or all reflexes, but with spontaneous respirations and normal blood pressure.
   e. Class IV: patients with respiratory depression, cyanosis, or shock.
2. A complete history of the events surrounding the ingestion is obtained. In particular, the ingestion of alcohol, other sedatives, or tranquilizers along with barbiturates is common, accounting for neurologic depression that is out of proportion to the dose or serum level of barbiturate taken.
3. The initial laboratory evaluation of patients in classes III and IV should include:
   a. Hemogram [hematocrit, white blood cell (WBC) count, and differential]
   b. Creatinine, BUN, or both
   c. Electrolytes
   d. Glucose
   e. Chest radiograph
   f. Urinalysis
   g. Arterial blood gases
   h. A screen of the serum and urine for toxic substances
4. Serum barbiturate levels are helpful, but they must be interpreted in the context of the clinical situation.
   a. A high barbiturate level confirms the diagnosis of barbiturate intoxication.
   b. Prognostically, the serum level correlates with the duration of coma. However, the usual method of measuring barbiturates does not distinguish between the different varieties of barbiturates, so the level must be interpreted with a knowledge of the compound ingested.
   c. The drug level may not correlate with the clinical status of the patient in several situations:
      1) In mixed ingestions, the patient's nervous system may be more depressed than would be predicted from the barbiturate level.
      2) Patients who take barbiturates habitually, either therapeutically or as drugs of abuse, can tolerate much higher levels of barbiturates than those who have tolerance for the drug.
      3) CNS stimulants (analeptic agents) may temporarily elevate a patient's mental status.

TREATMENT

1. Supportive therapy:
   a. The lowest mortality reported (8%) was achieved at a Scandinavian center that used only supportive measures in the treatment of barbiturate intoxication.
   b. Respiration:
      1) Patients in class IV require immediate endotracheal intubation and respiratory assistance.
      2) Patients in classes 0 to III require a cuffed endotracheal tube if gastric lavage is to be undertaken, if the cough reflex is absent, or if there is any doubt as to the adequacy of respirations.
   c. Cardiovascular: Hypotension occurs in barbiturate poisoning from decreased intravascular volume, from hypoxia with acidosis, and, at extremely high doses, from the direct myocardial depressant effects of barbiturates. The decreased intravascular volume is caused by dehydration and the escape of fluid from the capillaries because of increased capillary permeability, which results from both

barbiturate toxicity and hypoxia. The venous pooling of blood that follows may impair cardiac output further.

   1) The chief therapy of hypotension consists of correction of hypoxia, if it exists, and replacement of vascular volume. A central venous pressure (CVP) line is placed, and volume-expanding solutions are infused at about 20 mL/min until the CVP reaches 2 to 6 cm H_2O.

   a) The initial liter of volume replacement may be in the form of a 5% albumin solution because it will not only expand intravascular volume rapidly but will also bind some of the circulating barbiturates. However, this latter effect is significant only for long-acting and intermediate-acting compounds.

   b) An isotonic electrolyte solution may be used after the initial liter of albumin is infused.

   2) Pressors may be required in patients with severe intoxication in which the blood pressure does not respond to volume replacement. In general, the pressor chosen is infused at a rate that is sufficient to maintain systolic blood pressure at about 90 mm Hg, but the urine output is the ultimate guide. In cases of ingestion of long-acting and intermediate-acting barbiturates, which are excreted primarily in the urine, dopamine is the pressor of choice.

   d. Other supportive measures:

   1) Frequent turning, attention to skin care, and other supportive measures are necessary for comatose patients.

   2) Frequent suctioning of intubated patients, pulmonary physical therapy, and prompt antibiotic treatment of respiratory infections are also required.

2. Removal of unabsorbed drug from the GI tract is helpful only if the patient is seen within 3 hours of ingestion. The only exceptions are the rare patients who ingest large amounts of barbiturates and develop a resultant ileus. Because of their intestinal hypomotility, these patients retain unabsorbed drug in the gut for many hours.

   a. Emesis should be induced only in patients with mild ingestion who are awake and able to protect their own airways from aspiration.

   b. Gastric lavage may be undertaken inpatients who are seen within 3 hours of ingestion, but it should be performed only with a cuffed endotracheal tube in place.

   c. After the stomach is evacuated, if bowel sounds are present, an osmotic cathartic ay be administered.

   1) Sorbitol, 50 g mixed with about 200 mL of water, or magnesium citrate, 200 mL of the standard commercial solution, may be used.

   2) Activated charcoal will bind barbiturates and may be given along with the cathartic; the usual dose is 30 g.

3. Removal of absorbed barbiturate from the body:

   a. Both forced diuresis and, in the case of the phenobarbital, alkalinization of the urine hasten excretion of barbiturates. However, these methods pose risks of volume and sodium overload and have failed to improve outcome. Therefore, they are not generally recommended.

   b. Hemodialysis is more effective for removing intermediate and long-acting barbiturates than short-acting compounds. The indications for its use are:

   1) Renal or hepatic insufficiency severe enough to prevent the elimination of the drug.

   2) Shock or prolonged coma that does not respond to conservative management.

   3) Ingestion of a lethal dose of drug (3 g of a short-acting or 5 g of a long-acting barbiturate).

   4) A serum drug level predictive of prolonged coma (approximately 3.5 mg/dL for short-acting barbiturates or 8 mg/dL for phenobarbital).

4. Complications of barbiturate intoxication result primarily from prolonged coma, but pneumonia and bladder infections are encountered frequently. Acute renal failure due to acute tubular necrosis or to nontraumatic rhabdomyolysis can also occur.

5. Psychiatric evaluation and care are provided to all patients who ingest overdoses of drugs intentionally.

6. Barbiturate withdrawal:
  a. Acute barbiturate withdrawal presents a clinical picture that is strikingly similar to that of alcohol withdrawal, with tremor, delirium, and seizures being prominent. In contrast to ethanol withdrawal, the seizures associated with withdrawal from short-acting barbiturates are often severe.
  b. IV barbiturate is the treatment of choice.
   1) Pentobarbital may be given in 25-mg increments every 5 to 10 minutes until symptoms abate.
   2) Diazepam is generally effective, but the combination of barbiturate and diazepam frequently produces respiratory depression.
  c. After the acute symptoms are under control, the patient may be withdrawn from barbiturates gradually. As with ethanol withdrawal, careful attention is directed to fluid and electrolyte balance, antipyresis, and prevention of infectious complications.
7. Poisoning with nonbarbiturate CNS depressants:
  a. The basic therapy of acute intoxication with all CNS depressants is similar to that of barbiturate intoxication. The respiratory and cardiovascular systems must be stabilized, unabsorbed drug is removed by lavage and catharsis, and the elimination of the drug from the body is speeded by whatever techniques are feasible for each drug.
  b. Individual drugs:
   1) Glutethimide:
    a) Glutethimide (Doriden) overdose carries high mortality. The characteristic fluctuating course is probably caused by delayed absorption of drug as a result of paralytic ileus. The signs are similar to those of barbiturate intoxication, except that the drug also possesses anticholinergic activity, producing dilated pupils.
    b) Treatment is primarily supportive, and elimination of the drug may be hastened by forced diuresis. Hemodialysis against a lipid-containing dialysate should be used if the patient has renal failure, fails to respond to conservative measures, or has ingested a potentially lethal dose (more than 10 g total or blood level higher than 3 mg/dL).
   2) Chloral hydrate and ethchlorvynol:
    a) Chloral hydrate (Noctec) and ethchlorvynol (Placidyl) intoxications resemble barbiturate intoxication, except that chloral hydrate may produce constricted pupils.
    b) Treatment is identical to that for barbiturate overdose. Hemodialysis is effective in eliminating both drugs and should be used with the same indications as for barbiturate overdose.
   3) Benzodiazepines:
    a) Diazepam and chlordiazepoxide taken alone p.o. generally do not produce life-threatening intoxication in medically sound patients. Respiratory depression is of significance only in patients with intrinsic lung disease or in cases of mixed ingestions.
    b) Treatment of benzodiazepine intoxication consists of eliminating unabsorbed drug from the GI tract and supporting these patients until they awaken.

STIMULANTS (AMPHETAMINES, COCAINE, PHENCYCLIDINE)

BACKGROUND

Stimulant drugs are usually ingested for recreational purposes or for weight loss (appetite suppression).

PATHOPHYSIOLOGY

1. Stimulant drugs work by increasing the effective concentrations of catecholamines at synapses in the CNS.
2. This may occur by release of preformed catecholamine in synaptic vesicles (amphetamine, phencyclidine) and/or by blocking reuptake of released catecholamine in the synapse (cocaine).

PROGNOSIS

1. Acute stimulant toxicity produces psychosis, hyperpyrexia, hypertension, dilated pupils, vomiting, and diarrhea.
2. Life-threatening effects of severe intoxication include cardiac arrhythmias, intracerebral hemorrhage, seizures, coma, and respiratory arrest.

TREATMENT

1. Sedation with neuroleptics controls psychotic manifestations. Haloperidol 1 to 2 mg IV or chlorpromazine 50 mg IM, may be given initially and every 30 minutes until the patient is calm. Oral therapy with atypical neuroleptic drugs may then be used. Risperdal 2 to 4 mg p.o. q.d. or olanzapine 5 to 10 mg q.d. are reasonable choices.
2. Hyperpyrexia can be controlled with a cooling blanket and vigorous wetting with towels soaked in tepid water.
3. Arrhythmias are treated with appropriate drugs.
4. Seizures are short-term problems if no irreversible CNS damage occurs from hypoxia or cardiac arrest. They should be treated with the usual measures (see Chapter 2).
5. Unabsorbed drug is removed with emesis, lavage, catharsis, or all three, as appropriate. Lavage may be of benefit even several hours after ingestion.
6. Acidification of the urine hastens the excretion of amphetamines and should be used in the event of severe intoxication. Ammonium chloride may be administered p.o. or IV at a total dosage of 8 to 12 g/d, and the urine pH is checked frequently. Ammonium chloride is contraindicated in shock, systemic acidosis of any cause, hepatic failure, or portosystemic shunting.
7. Severe hypertension is best treated with an alpha-blocking agent, such as phentolamine (Regitine). Moderate hypertension responds to chlorpromazine.

ANTICHOLINERGIC AND POLYCYCLIC ANTIDEPRESSANT TOXICITY

BACKGROUND

Many anticholinergic drugs were derived from nature (e.g., belladonna), but nearly all clinical toxicity is the result of exposure to drugs that are primarily anticholinergic (e.g., scopolamine) and have anticholinergic side effects (e.g., polycyclic antidepressants).

PATHOPHYSIOLOGY

Anticholinergic drugs work by competitively or noncompetitively binding the muscarinic and/or nicotinic acetylcholine receptors.

PROGNOSIS

1. The acute toxic effects of anticholinergic drugs are hyperpyrexia, dilated pupils, hypertension, tachycardia, and dryness of the skin and mucous membranes.
2. The life-threatening manifestations are coma, seizures, cardiac arrhythmias, and cardiac conduction defects.

DIAGNOSIS

The diagnosis is made with a history of anticholinergic drug use and the characteristic clinical syndrome.

TREATMENT

1. The initial emergency treatment is the same as for any overdose: stabilization of respiratory and cardiac status and elimination of unabsorbed drug from the GI tract.
2. Cardiac conduction defects and arrhythmias are prominent in tricyclic intoxication. The patient should be on a cardiac monitor, a temporary transvenous pacemaker should be readily available, and the patient should be placed in an intensive or coronary care unit. Lidocaine is effective for ventricular arrhythmias. Propranolol should be used with extreme care if a conduction defect is present.
3. Hyperpyrexia can be controlled with a cooling blanket or by vigorous rubdowns with towels soaked in tepid water. Chlorpromazine may increase the effectiveness of hypothermic methods.
4. Severe hypertension responds to the administration of an alpha-blocker such as phentolamine.
5. Physostigmine is reported to antagonize the CNS toxicity of tricyclics and other anticholinergics.
   a. Physostigmine injection may serve as a diagnostic test to confirm anticholinergic ingestion.
      1) Physostigmine, 1 mg is injected subcutaneously, IM, or slowly IV, which will produce peripheral cholinergic signs within 30 minutes if no anticholinergics have been ingested.
      2) These signs include bradycardia, salivation, lacrimation, and papillary constriction.
      3) In a patient who has ingested anticholinergics, the injection will produce no significant effect.
   b. For the treatment of anticholinergic overdose: 1-mg doses of physostigmine are injected IM or slowly IV at 20-minute intervals until 4 mg has been administered or cholinergic signs appear.
   c. Indications:
      1) Physostigmine is most effective against the toxic delirium of anticholinergic overdose. It will occasionally awaken a comatose patient.
      2) However, physostigmine is itself toxic, so its use should be reserved for patients with life-threatening complications of tricyclic overdose, respiratory depression, intractable seizures, or severe hypertension.
   d. Side effects:
      1) If excessive physostigmine is administered, cholinergic side effects may in themselves exert harmful effects.
      2) Excessive respiratory secretions, salivation, and bronchospasm can interfere with pulmonary function. Vomiting, abdominal cramps, and diarrhea can also occur. Excessive cholinergic effects may be counteracted with atropine (see Treatment of Acetylcholinesterase Inhibitor Poisoning, above). Physostigmine at toxic doses or administered rapidly IV can cause seizures.
   e. The duration of action of physostigmine is only 1 to 2 hours, whereas tricyclics persist over 24 hours. Therefore, the patient must be monitored and repeated doses are administered as necessary.

SALICYLATE INTOXICATION

BACKGROUND

1. Salicylates are the medications that most frequently produce clinically significant intoxication. The most common source is aspirin, but sodium salicylate and oil of wintergreen are also common causes.
   a. Aspirin: Adult aspirin tablets contain 325 mg of aspirin, whereas children's tablets contain 8 g/mg. Some so-called extrastrength aspirin tablets contain as much as 750 mg.
   b. Oil of wintergreen contains methyl salicylate in a concentration of about 0.7 g/mL. It is highly toxic, and 1 or 2 tsp can be a fatal dose for a small child.
2. The toxic dose of salicylate is about 250 mg/kg in a healthy person. Lower doses of both methyl salicylate and aspirin can be intoxicating in a person who is dehydrated or in renal failure.

PATHOPHYSIOLOGY

1. Salicylates are well absorbed from the GI tract, over 50% of a therapeutic dose being absorbed within 1 hour of ingestion. Poisoning has occurred from oil of wintergreen from cutaneous absorption.
2. Once absorbed, aspirin is rapidly hydrolyzed to salicylic acid.
3. Salicylic acid is variably bound to albumin. At toxic levels, the serum albumin binding sites are 100% saturated.
4. Salicylic acid is excreted both unchanged and as its glucuronidated product in the urine. Salicylic acid has a pK_a of about 3, so it can be "trapped" in the alkaline solution. Thus, alkalinization of the urine can increase salicylic acid excretion by as much as fivefold.

PROGNOSIS

1. CNS abnormalities dominate the clinical picture.
   a. The earliest signs are tinnitus and impaired hearing.
   b. Agitation progressing to delirium, stupor, and coma results from severe intoxication.
   c. Seizures can occur as a direct effect of salicylate toxicity or as a secondary manifestation of hypoglycemia or effective hypocalcemia.
   d. Salicylates in toxic doses stimulate respiration and produce hyperpnea, usually with tachypnea and respiratory alkalosis.
   e. With extremely high doses, respiratory depression occurs.
2. Metabolic derangements:
   a. Salicylates interfere with carbohydrate metabolism.
      1) Hypoglycemia may occur in young children.
      2) The brain uses glucose inefficiently and may experience a "relative hypoglycemia" even with a normal blood glucose level.
      3) The organic aciduria, with or without glycosuria, produces an osmotic diuresis, which in turn produces dehydration.
      4) The respiratory alkalosis, when prolonged, has secondary effects on electrolyte metabolism.
         a) There is renal sodium and potassium wasting. The hypokalemia renders the metabolic acidosis unresponsive to alkali therapy until the potassium is repleted.
         b) The respiratory alkalosis produces decreased unbound serum calcium levels, which can lead to tetany and seizures.
      5) SIADH has been reported in association with salicylate poisoning.
3. Effects on blood clotting:

a. Salicylate in toxic concentrations exerts an antiprothrombin effect, with prolongation of the prothrombin time (PT) and diminished factor VII activity.
b. Salicylates interfere with platelet function, even in nontoxic doses.
c. Salicylates are locally irritating to the gastric mucosa and can lead to GI hemorrhage.

DIAGNOSIS

1. Salicylate intoxication occurs frequently in three groups:
   a. Children younger than 5 years, as a result of accidental ingestion.
   b. Adolescents and young adults, as a result of intentional ingestion.
   c. Unintentional overdose in patients taking salicylates for rheumatic disease.
2. The diagnosis is obvious with an adequate history of ingestion: however, it is frequently masked by chronic therapeutic overdose if the physician is unaware that the patient is taking salicylates.
3. The diagnosis is considered in patients with mental status changes, hyperpnea, and respiratory alkalosis, with or without superimposed metabolic acidosis.
4. Serum salicylate levels confirm the diagnosis.
   a. A level higher than 30 mg/dL may produce early symptoms of salicylism; mental changes and hyperpnea occur at levels higher than 40 mg/dL.
   b. With chronic ingestion, blood levels correlate poorly with the clinical status of the patient but will nevertheless serve to make or to rule out the diagnosis.
5. The ferric chloride test serves as a rapid screening test for the presence of salicylic acid.
   a. A few drops of a 10% solution of ferric chloride are added to 3 to 5 mL of acidified urine. A purple color indicates a positive result.
   b. The test is extremely sensitive, so a positive result is not diagnostic of salicylate intoxication.
   c. Ferric chloride reacts only with salicylic acid, not with aspirin. Therefore, it cannot be used to test for the presence of aspirin in gastric contents.
   d. Phenothiazines react with ferric chloride, but they tend to give a pink rather than a purple color.
   e. Acetoacetic acid, present in ketosis, will react with ferric chloride. Its presence may be excluded, however, if the urine is boiled and acidified before the ferric chloride is added.
6. The initial laboratory evaluation of a patient with salicylate intoxication should include the following:
   a. Serum salicylate level is of prognostic importance and gives a baseline value with which to judge the effects of therapy.
   b. Patients with intentional overdoses should have blood or urine (or both) screened for the presence of other toxic substances.
   c. Complete blood count (CBC), including platelet count.
   d. Stool and gastric contents are tested for the presence of occult blood.
   e. Arterial blood gases and pH.
   f. BUN (or creatinine), electrolytes, calcium and phosphorus.
   g. Liver function tests, including aspartate aminotransferase, lactate dehydrogenase (LDH), alkaline phosphatase, total bilirubin, total protein, and albumin levels.
   h. PT and partial thromboplastin time.
   i. Chest radiograph.
   j. ECG, giving particular attention to signs of hypokalemia or hypocalcemia.
   k. Urinalysis with specific gravity. If the serum sodium is low and SIADH is a possibility, urine sodium concentration and osmolality are measured.

TREATMENT

1. Routine emergency measures for the treatment of drug intoxications:
   a. Protect the airway and support respiration, if necessary.
   b. Empty the GI tract of unabsorbed drug.

   1) Forced emesis is used if the patient is alert.
   2) Gastric lavage is performed after tracheal intubation with a cuffed endotracheal tube if patients are stuporous, in coma, or unable to protect their own airways.
   3) Activated charcoal is given as 200 to 300 mL of a thick suspension to bind unabsorbed salicylates.
   4) Cathartics are administered after the charcoal has been given.
2. Fluid and electrolyte management is used to treat shock, to maintain urine output, and to restore electrolyte and acid–base balance.
3. Alkalinization of the urine by the infusion of sodium bicarbonate hastens the excretion of salicylic acid. However, in practice, the technique has no value.
   a. In elderly patients and those with abnormal heart function, the risks of increased sodium load are not justified by the expected benefits of alkalinization of the urine.
   b. In patients with metabolic acidosis, the urine cannot be alkalinized except with massive and dangerous quantities of alkali.
   c. In patients with respiratory alkalosis and alkalemia, the administration of alkali is contraindicated.
4. Hypoglycemia:
   a. In young children, after blood has been drawn, 50% mg dextrose in water (D/W) (0.5 mL/kg IV) is administered immediately.
   b. Only glucose-containing fluids are used for maintenance.
5. Hemorrhagic complications:
   a. In severe salicylate poisoning, vitamin K, 50 mg IV, is given after an initial PT has been measured. The vitamin K is repeated as necessary to maintain a normal PT.
   b. If bleeding occurs or if the PT is found to be longer than twice the control value, fresh-frozen plasma or concentrates of clotting factors (Konyne) are given.
   c. Platelet transfusion might be required to achieve control of hemorrhage because the patient's own platelets will have a disordered function.
   d. In comatose patients, antacids and histamine antagonists may be given by nasogastric tube in an effort to prevent gastric hemorrhage.
6. Tetany may be treated with the IV infusion of calcium gluconate in 1-g doses, repeated as often as necessary.
7. Seizures:
   a. Hypoglycemia and hypocalcemia are treated appropriately. Other metabolic causes of seizures, such as hyponatremia and hypoxia, must also be considered.
   b. Seizures that occur as a direct toxic effect of salicylate are a poor prognostic sign, generally indicating the necessity for hemodialysis to hasten elimination of the salicylate. Diazepam, given IV, or muscle paralysis and respiratory support may be used for the temporary control of seizures until the salicylate level is lowered.
8. Fever can be treated with tepid water baths.
9. Methods to hasten the elimination of salicylates:
   a. Forced diuresis is of little benefit, and the patient should not be subjected to a larger fluid load than necessary to achieve a reasonable urine output.
   b. Alkalinization of the urine has no practical use in salicylate poisoning.
   c. Peritoneal dialysis is about as efficient as the normal kidney in eliminating salicylate from the blood. Its primary use is in the setting of renal failure. The addition of albumin to the dialysis solution hastens the elimination of salicylate, but there is no evidence that its benefits outweighs the expense and added complexity of the dialysis.
   d. Hemodialysis is the most efficient means available for the elimination of salicylate. The generally accepted indications for hemodialysis are:
      1) Salicylate level higher than 70 mg/dL or known absorption greater than 5 g/kg.
      2) Profound coma with respiratory failure.
      3) Severe metabolic acidosis.

4) Renal failure.
5) Failure to respond to conservative therapy.

HYPERTHERMIA

BACKGROUND

Hyperthermia is a common cause of neurologic dysfunction. It is particularly dangerous and may even be lethal in the summer months.

PATHOPHYSIOLOGY

1. Rises in body temperature may be due to excessive heat gain, insufficient heal loss, or both.
2. Excessive heat gain:
   a. Exercise
   b. High ambient temperatures
   c. Increased metabolic rate
   d. Release of pyrogen (e.g., by infection)
   e. Neuroleptic malignant syndrome
3. Defective heat loss:
   a. Excessively warm clothing
   b. Increased humidity
   c. Low wind velocity
   d. Advanced age
   e. Anticholinergic drugs (e.g., phenothiazines, tricyclic antidepressants)
   f. Sympathetic autonomic failure with decreased or absent sweating due to:
      1) Elevated body temperatures
      2) Spinal cord transection above T-1

PROGNOSIS

1. Heat cramps: Muscle or abdominal cramps associated with exercise are commonly seen.
2. Heat exhaustion (heat prostration, exertional heat injury) is marked by moderately elevated body temperatures (i.e., 39.5°C to 42.0°C) and a neurologic syndrome characterized by headache, piloerection, hyperventilation, nausea, vomiting, unsteady gait, and confusion. Sweating remains intact in patients with heat exhaustion, so the skin is wet and cool.
3. Heat stroke:
   a. When body temperatures rise high enough, CNS mechanisms for control of heat loss might fail. When this occurs, there is a very rapid further rise in body temperature, which is a life-threatening medical emergency.
   b. Such patients might be diaphoretic or have hot, dry skin (sweating having failed) and elevated body temperatures (higher than 41°C, ranging as high as 43°C).
   c. The level of consciousness becomes deranged, often quite suddenly, so that patients can deteriorate rapidly from confusion or delirium to deep coma, often with seizures.
   d. Cerebral edema occurs, which can lead to widespread cerebral ischemia and eventually brain death.
   e. Other abnormalities include circulatory failure, disseminated intravascular coagulation, severe dehydration, and hepatic necrosis. Electrolyte abnormalities, most commonly respiratory alkalosis and hypokalemia, are common.

DIAGNOSIS

The diagnosis is made in a patient in compatible history and physical examination and elevated body temperature.

TREATMENT

1. Heat cramps: Rest and oral electrolyte replacement are usually adequate.
2. Heat exhaustion:
   a. Patients should be admitted to the hospital for treatment because some may progress to heat stroke.
   b. Rest and parenteral rehydration are usually adequate to reverse the syndrome.
3. Heat stroke:
   a. Surface cooling should be started immediately. The most effective means is to use evaporative cooling by spraying the naked patient with tepid water and using a powerful fan to maintain a flow of air over the patient's body. Alternatively, immersion in ice or cold water may be used.
   b. IV fluids should be administered with care, as typically the patient is normovolemic but has redistributed fluid to peripheral, vasodilated tissues. With cooling, fluid will redistribute and cardiac output will be restored.
   c. A bladder catheter should be placed and urinary output carefully monitored.
   d. Isoproterenol via constant infusion (1 μg/min) may be used to increase cardiac output.
   e. Avoid α-adrenergic drugs (e.g., norepinephrine), which produce vasoconstriction and thus retard heat loss.
   f. Avoid anticholinergic drugs (e.g., atropine), which retard the return of sweating.
   g. Monitoring of ICP using a dural bolt might be necessary if consciousness does not return promptly.
   h. Treat increased ICP as outlined in Chapter 1.
   i. Seizures may be treated with phenytoin or phenobarbital as outlined in Chapter 6.
   j. If disseminated intravascular coagulation develops, heparin, 1,000 U/h by constant infusion, may be used.

NEUROLEPTIC MALIGNANT SYNDROME

BACKGROUND

1. Neuroleptic malignant syndrome (NMS) is characterized by hyperthermia, muscle rigidity, and altered mental status.
2. It occurs in patients taking neuroleptic medication or, rarely, in association with withdrawal of L-dopa or other dopaminergic agonists.

PATHOPHYSIOLOGY

1. Although a preponderance of reported cases have occurred with the use of potent neuroleptics such as haloperidol, the syndrome has been associated with virtual all dopamine-receptor antagonists and dopamine-depleting agents (e.g., reserpine).
2. It may occur immediately after the first dose of a neuroleptic or in a patient who has been taking neuroleptics for many years. Many cases are associated with a rapid increase in dose.
3. Life-threatening complications of NMS include respiratory failure secondary to muscular rigidity and renal failure secondary to myoglobinuria.

PROGNOSIS

1. NMS is commonly precipitated by dehydration, fever, or environmental exposure to high temperatures in patients taking neuroleptics.
2. These precipitants should be especially avoided in patients taking neuroleptics or dopamine-depleting agents.
3. Withdrawal of dopamine agonists, including carbidopa–L-dopa (Sinemet), should be carried out gradually.
4. If the syndrome is recognized early, the prognosis is excellent. Although mortality rates from NMS as high as 15% to 20% are quoted in the literature, it is clear that with adequate supportive care the mortality is much less.
5. To prevent relapse of NMS, neuroleptic medications must not be reinstituted until the syndrome has resolved completely. Patients may require sedation with benzodiazepines in the meantime. After resolution of all clinical signs of NMS, neuroleptics may be cautiously reinstituted.
6. NMS is not an allergic reaction to neuroleptics, and the occurrence of NMS is not an absolute contraindication to neuroleptic use.

DIAGNOSIS

1. Diagnosis is made in a patient on a neuroleptic drug who developed rigidity and hyperthermia.
2. Laboratory abnormalities may include an elevated serum creatine kinase level, elevated WBC count, and abnormal liver function tests.
3. The CSF is normal, and the EEG shows a generalized slowing.
4. The computed tomography (CT) scan and MRI findings are normal.

TREATMENT

1. Immediate withdrawal of all neuroleptic medications (including those administered as antiemetics) or dopamine-depleting agents (e.g., reserpine, tetrabenazine) is essential at the earliest sign of NMS. In cases associated with withdrawal of dopamine agonists (e.g., L-dopa, bromocriptine, pergolide), reinstitution of dopaminergic therapy and more gradual withdrawal should be undertaken.
2. The mainstay of management is supportive care:
    a. Rehydration and maintenance of adequate urine flow.
    b. Lowering of body temperature with antipyretics, cooling blanket, or tepid water bath as required.
    c. Protection of the airway to endotracheal intubation as required.
    d. In unusual cases, respirator support with muscular paralysis might be required to maintain ventilation in the face of extreme muscular rigidity.
3. The direct-acting muscle relaxant dantrolene is widely used in severe cases of NMS, although there are no systemic studies documenting its benefit.
    a. Muscle relation may facilitate nursing care and aid in lowering body temperature. In addition, to the extent that muscle rigidity contributes to muscle necrosis and myoglobinuria, muscle relaxation can help prevent renal failure.
    b. However, it is clear that muscular rigidity is not the only cause of muscle damage in NMS and that hyperthermia may persist in spite of muscle paralysis.
    c. Doses of dantrolene range from 1 to 10 mg/kg/d IV or by nasogastric tube given in four divided doses. Hepatic toxicity occurs with dosages above 10 mg/kg/d.
4. The dopamine agonist bromocriptine has also been widely used and has theoretical support.
    a. There are no systemic studies documenting its benefit in NMS.
    b. Dosages vary from 2.5 to 10.0 mg IV by nasogastric tube every 4 to 6 hours.
5. Electroconvulsive therapy has shown effectiveness in anecdotal reports. Its role in the treatment of NMS is undefined.

BIBLIOGRAPHY

Ayus JC, Krothapalli RK, Arieff AI. Treatment of symptomatic hyponatremia and its relation to brain damage: a prospective study. *N Engl J Med* 1987;317:1190–1195.

Bouchama A, Knochel JP. Heat stroke. *N Engl J Med* 2002;346:1978–1988.

Brust JC. Acute neurologic complications of drug and alcohol abuse. *Neurol Clin* 1998,16:513–519.

Burn DJ, Bates D. Neurology and the kidney. *J Neurol Neurosurg Psychiatry* 1998;65:810–821.

Canfield RL, Henderson CR, Cory-Slechta DA, et al. Intellectual impairment in children with blood lead concentrations below 10 μg per deciliter. *N Engl J Med* 2003;348:1517–1526.

Perkin GD, Murray-Lyon I. Neurology and the gastrointestinal system. *J Neurol Neurosurg Psychiatry* 1998;65:291–300.

Samuels MA. The neurology of anaemia. *Practical Neurology* 2003;3:132–141.

17. INFECTIONS OF THE CENTRAL NERVOUS SYSTEM

Christina M. Marra

BACTERIAL MENINGITIS

BACKGROUND

Widespread use of *Haemophilus influenzae* type b conjugate vaccines has dramatically decreased the incidence of bacterial meningitis in children but has not affected the incidence in adults.

PATHOPHYSIOLOGY

1. Pathology is characterized by inflammation of meninges and cortical blood vessels.
2. The likely etiology of bacterial meningitis can be predicted on the basis of patient age and clinical characteristics (Table 17-1).

PROGNOSIS

1. Early and late complications of bacterial meningitis can occur.
   a. Early: cerebral edema, communicating hydrocephalus, infectious vasculitis with stroke, dural sinus thrombosis, brain abscess, subdural abscess or effusion, hearing loss.
   b. Late: developmental delay or cognitive deficits, focal neurologic findings other than or in addition to hearing loss, epilepsy.
2. Mortality is highest in *Streptococcus pneumoniae* meningitis and in patients who present with depressed level of consciousness.
3. Dexamethasone decreases neurologic complications in children with *H. influenzae* and *S. pneumoniae* meningitis treated in the developed, but not the developing, world. Dexamethasone improves neurologic outcome and decreases mortality in adults with *S. pneumoniae* meningitis. Dexamethasone should be given before or with first dose of antibiotics (see Treatment, this section).

DIAGNOSIS

1. Clinical findings include fever, neck stiffness, and change in mental status. The very young, very old, and immunocompromised may have minimal symptoms and signs.
2. Cerebrospinal fluid (CSF):
   a. Usually shows neutrophilic pleocytosis, low glucose level, and elevated protein concentrations (Table 17-2).
   b. Gram stain and culture usually positive unless the patient has been treated with antibiotics.
   c. CSF latex agglutination tests can detect antigens of *S. pneumoniae; Neisseria meningitidis* serogroups A, B, C, Y and W135; *H. influenzae* type b; and group B streptococci, but they are often negative when the CSF culture is negative.
   d. CSF polymerase chain reaction (PCR) tests that amplify highly conserved regions of the bacterial *16S RNA* gene provide a potentially rapid diagnostic test but are not yet clinically available.
3. Blood cultures are positive in 30% to 80% of cases and may be positive when CSF culture is negative.
4. Neuroimaging should be performed before lumbar puncture in the following settings:

TABLE 17-1. EMPIRIC THERAPY FOR BACTERIAL MENINGITIS

Patient Characteristic	Likely Organisms	Antibiotics
Neonate[a]	Group B streptococci, Listeria monocytogenes, Escherichia coli	Ampicillin plus cefotaxime
2 mo to < 18 y	Neisseria meningitidis, Streptococcus pneumoniae, Haemophilus influenzae	Ceftriaxone[b] or cefotaxime[c] plus vancomycin[d]
18–50 y	S. pneumoniae, N. meningitidis	Cetriaxone[b] plus vancomycin[d]
> 50 y	S. pneumoniae, L. monocytogenes, gram-negatives	Vancomycin[d] plus ampicillin[e] plus ceftriaxone[b]
Impaired cellular immunity	L. monocytogenes, gram-negatives	Ampicillin[e] plus ceftazidime[f]
Dural disruption or shunt	Coagulase-positive or -negative staphylococci, gram-negatives, S. pneumoniae	Vancomycin[d] plus ceftazidime[f]

[a]Doses depend on age, weight and prematurity. Expert consultation is advised.
[b]Children: 100 mg/kg/day IV or IM divided q12h. Maximum dose 2 gm/day in children 45 kg or less. Adult: 2 mg IV or IM q12h. Maximum dose 4 gm/day in adults.
[c]Children: 200 mg/kg/day IV divided q6h. Adult: 2 gm IV q4–6h. Maximum dose for children and adults is 12 gm/day.
[d]Children: 60 mg/kg/day IV divided q6h. Adult: 1 gm IV q12h. Adjust dose for renal function. Follow levels: trough of 10–15 μg/ml.
[e]Children: 200–400 mg/kg/day IV divided q4h. Adults: 2 gm IV q4h. Maximum dose in children and adults is 12 gm/day.
[f]Children: 150 mg/kg/day IV divided q8h. Adults: 2 gm IV q8h. Maximum dose in children and adults is 6 gm/day.

   a. 60 years of age or older
   b. Depressed level of consciousness
   c. Focal neurologic signs
   d. Papilledema
   e. Patient is immunocompromised
5. Diagnostic approach for bacterial meningitis:
   a. Perform rapid, directed general physical and neurologic examination looking for sources of infection, underlying illness, and contraindications to lumbar puncture.
   b. Draw blood cultures.
   c. Neuroimaging if indicated. Empiric antibiotics should be given prior to

TABLE 17-2. CEREBROSPINAL FLUID FINDINGS IN BACTERIAL AND VIRAL MENINGITIS

CSF Parameter	Type of Meningitis		
	Bacterial	Partially Treated Bacterial	Viral
WBC count	>2,000/uL, >60% PMNs	>2,000/uL, >60% PMNs	<1,000/uL; PMNs in 10%
Glucose	<40 mg/dL	<40 mg/dL	>40 mg/dL
Protein	>200 mg/dL	>200 mg/dL	<100 mg/dL
Gram stain–positive	80%	60%	No
Culture–positive	>90%	65%	No

CSF, cerebrospinal fluid; WBC, white blood cell; PMNs, polymorphonuclear cells (neutrophils).

neuroimaging. If indicated, dexamethasone should be given before or with the first dose of antibiotics.
d. Lumbar puncture: If the patient is clinically worsening or if a delay in lumbar puncture anticipated, give empiric antibiotics. If indicated, dexamethasone should be given before or with first dose of antibiotics. Every effort should be made to obtain CSF within 2 to 3 hours of giving antibiotics.
e. Treat: Base regimen on CSF gram stain findings if patient is neurologically normal, clinically stable, and has not been given oral or parenteral antibiotics. Otherwise, give empiric regimen as soon as lumbar puncture is complete (see Treatment, this section).

TREATMENT

1. Empiric regimens are based on age, clinical setting, and local patterns of antibiotic susceptibility (Table 17-1). In the United States, about 25% of pneumococcal isolates are not susceptible to penicillin.
2. Once culture information is available from CSF or blood, tailor antibiotic regimens to cover specific organisms (Table 17-3).
3. When possible etiologies for meningitis include *H. influenzae* or *S. pneumoniae* in children, or *S. pneumoniae* in adults, give dexamethasone 0.15 mg/kg intravenous (IV) every 6 hours for 2 to 4 days in children and 10 mg IV every 6 hours for 4 days in adults. Dexamethasone should be given before or with the first dose of antibiotics.
4. Patients with *H. influenzae* and *N. meningitidis* meningitis should be placed in respiratory isolation for the first 24 hours of antibiotic therapy.
5. Prophylaxis:
   a. According to the American Academy of Pediatrics. *2000 Red Book: Report of the Committee on Infectious Diseases,* prophylaxis for *H. influenzae* is indicated for:

TABLE 17-3. SPECIFIC THERAPY FOR BACTERIAL MENINGITIS

Organism	Duration of Therapy	Comments
Haemophilus influenzae	7–10 d	Ampicillin resistance is common.
Neisseria meningitidis	5–7 d	If the organism is sensitive, high-dose IV penicillin is appropriate. Penicillin resistance is increasing; clinical significance uncertain.
Streptococcus pneumoniae	14–21 d	Penicillin nonsuceptibility is increasing. If sensitive to penicillin, ceftriaxone, or cefotaxime, discontinue empiric vancomycin. With cephalosporin resistance, use ceftriaxone or cefotaxime plus vancomycin and examine CSF at 36–48 h. If sensitive to rifampin, add rifampin if clinical deterioration, persistent CSF infection or unusually high MIC to ceftriaxone or cefotaxime. Consider adding rifampin to empiric regimen if dexamethasone is used because dexamethasone may decrease CSF penetration of antibiotics.
Listeria monocytogenes	14–21 d	Use ampicillin or penicillin plus gentamicin for severe infections. Use trimethoprim–sulfamethoxazole if penicillin-allergic.

IV, intravenous; CSF, cerebrospinal fluid; MIC, minimum inhibition concentration.

TABLE 17-4. PROPHYLACTIC REGIMENS FOR *N. MENINGITIDIS*

Agent	Dosage According to Age	
Rifampin[a]	≤ 1 mo, 5 mg/kg p.o. q12h for 2 d	> 1 mo, 10 mg/kg (max., 600 mg) p.o. q12h for 2 d
Ceftriaxone	≤ 12 yr, 125 mg IM, 1 dose	> 12 yr, 250 mg IM, 1 dose
Ciprofloxacin[b]	< 18 yr, not recommended	≥ 18 yr, 500 mg p.o., 1 dose

p.o, by mouth; IM, intramuscular.
[a]Do not use during pregnancy; use with caution in women taking birth control pills.
[b]Do not use during pregnancy or for lactating women.

       1) All household members (except pregnant women) if there is a child in the household who is a contact to an index case; and
          a) The contact child is younger than 48 months of age and has not been completely immunized against *H. influenzae;*
          b) If the contact child is immunocompromised, regardless of immunization status;
          c) The contact child is younger than 12 months old. A contact is defined as a person living with an index case or who spent 4 or more hours with an index case for 5 or more of the 7 days before hospitalization of the index case.
       2) The index case if he or she did not receive cefotaxime or ceftriaxone.
       3) Children at nurseries and child care centers who are contacts to an index case, regardless of age, when two or more cases of invasive disease have occurred within 60 days.
    b. Prophylaxis for *H. influenzae* with rifampin should ideally be given within 7 days of contact. In infants younger 1 month, the dose is 10 mg/kg by mouth (p.o.) daily for 4 days. In those older than 1 month, the dose is 20 mg/kg (maximum, 600 mg) p.o. daily for 4 days.
    c. According to the AAP Red Book, prophylaxis against *N. meningitidis* is indicated for:
       1) Household contacts.
       2) People who eat or sleep in the same place as the index patient.
       3) People who have had close contact with the index patient such as through sharing toothbrushes or eating utensils or kissing in the 7 days before onset of illness.
       4) Nursery or childcare center contact in the 7 days before onset of illness.
       5) Health care personnel with direct contact to index patient's oral secretions such as through unprotected mouth-to-mouth resuscitation, tracheal intubation, or suctioning in the 7 days before onset of illness.
       6) The index case if he or she did not receive cefotaxime or ceftriaxone.
    d. Prophylaxis for *N. meningitidis* should be administered within 24 hours of diagnosis of the index case (Table 17-4).

TUBERCULOUS MENINGITIS

BACKGROUND

Tuberculous meningitis is the most common form of nervous system infection by *Mycobacterium tuberculosis.*

TABLE 17-5. OUTCOME OF TUBERCULOUS MENINGITIS BASED ON MRC STAGE AT PRESENTATION

Stage	Clinical Features	Mortality	Neurologic Sequelae
I	Meningeal signs but normal mental status and no focal neurologic findings	< 10%	Minimal
II	Confusion or focal neurologic findings	20%–30%	40%
III	Stupor or coma with hemiplegia or paraplegia	60%–70%	Frequent

MRC, medical research council.

PATHOPHYSIOLOGY

1. May accompany primary infection. This is often the case in children.
2. May also result from reactivation of previous infection. During primary infection, the brain and meninges may be seeded with low numbers of organisms. These foci of infection can develop into larger caseous lesions or "Rich Foci." When a meningeal lesion ruptures into the CSF space, meningitis ensues.
3. Fibrosis of basal meningeal exudate can lead to communicating hydrocephalus. Involvement of the ventricular system can lead to occlusion of the cerebral aqueduct and noncommunicating hydrocephalus. Hydrocephalus is more common in children than adults.
4. Vasculitis may develop in blood vessels traversing the meningeal exudate leading to occlusion and stroke. Stroke is most commonly in the middle cerebral artery distribution.

PROGNOSIS

1. Overall mortality in tuberculous meningitis is about 30%.
   a. Mortality highest in those with low Glasgow Coma Scale score or higher medical research council (MRC) stage at presentation (Table 17-5). Mortality is also greater in those in whom therapy is delayed or interrupted.
2. Neurologic sequelae include hemiparesis or hemiplegia, paraplegia, visual or hearing loss, cognitive changes.
   a. Neurologic sequelae are also highest in those with low Glasgow Coma Scale score or higher MRC stage at presentation and in those who present with focal neurologic findings (Table 17-5).
3. Hydrocephalus may require external ventricular drainage or a permanent shunt.

DIAGNOSIS

1. Symptoms and signs:
   a. Early: low-grade fever, headache, malaise, nausea.
   b. Later: severe headache, neck stiffness, cranial nerve palsies, vomiting, drowsiness, seizures, change in mental status.
   c. Late: coma, brainstem dysfunction.
2. Compared with patients with bacterial meningitis, patients with tuberculous meningitis typically have been sick longer, are more likely to have cranial nerve palsies and are less likely to have elevated peripheral blood white blood cell (WBC) counts.
3. Neuroimaging abnormalities are common: hydrocephalus, meningeal enhancement, mass lesions (tuberculomas, tuberculous abscesses), and infarcts. All patients with suspected tuberculous meningitis should undergo neuroimaging, ideally before lumbar puncture.
4. CSF:
   a. Conventional analysis
      1) WBC count 100 to 500 μL, usually with lymphocytic predominance. If present, polymorphonuclear cells fewer than 50%.

       2) Protein 100 to 500 mg/dL
       3) Glucose less than 45 mg/dL
    b. CSF acid–fast bacillus (AFB) smear positive in about one fourth.
    c. CSF culture positive in about one third. Large-volume CSF and multiple cultures (up to four) increases yield.
    d. CSF PCR specific but not sensitive.
  5. Abnormal chest radiograph findings seen in most children and about one half of adults.
  6. Purified protein derivative (PPD) test is positive in 50% to 80%. If initial PPD is negative, repeat test in 5 to 7 days (two-step test).
  7. Hyponatremia due to the syndrome of inappropriate secretion of antidiuretic hormone (SIADH) or to cerebral salt wasting is common.
  8. Human immunodeficiency virus (HIV)–infected patients are at greater risk of tuberculosis. However, clinical and laboratory findings in tuberculous meningitis generally do not differ between patients with and without concomitant HIV, although PPD less likely to be positive.
  9. Because CSF smear and culture are insensitive, diagnosis is often presumptive and based on compatible clinical findings, CSF profile, risks for tuberculosis, or identification of tuberculous infection at another site.

TREATMENT

  1. Every effort should be made to isolate the organism to allow for determination of drug sensitivities (Table 17-6). This may entail multiple CSF cultures and cultures from non-CNS sites.
  2. Early treatment is important.
  3. Drug-resistant tuberculous meningitis is uncommon. Resistance most likely in individuals noncompliant with previous antituberculous therapy or those from

TABLE 17-6. TREATMENT FOR TUBERCULOUS MENINGITIS

Agent	Dose	Comments
Isoniazid	Adult: 300 mg p.o. qd Child: 10–20 mg/kg/d (max., 300 mg/d) Treat for 9 mo or for 6 mo after cultures are consistently negative, whichever is longer	Add pyridoxine to prevent peripheral neuropathy. Monitor for liver toxicity.
Plus		
Rifampin	Adult: 600 mg p.o. qd Child: 10–20 mg/kg/d (max., 600 mg/d) Treat for 9 mo or for 6 mo after cultures are consistently negative, whichever is longer	Monitor for liver toxicity. Interacts with HIV protease inhibitors and nonnucleoside reverse inhibitors. Replace with rifabutin in consultation with infectious diseases expert.
Plus		
Pyrazinamide	15–30 mg/kg (max. 2 g in children and adults) p.o. qd Treat for first 2 mo of therapy, then discontinue	Monitor for liver toxicity.
Plus		
Ethambutol	15–25 mg/kg (max., 2.5 g) p.o. qd Treat for first 2 mo of therapy, then discontinue	Monitor for optic neuritis.

geographic areas with high prevalence of resistance. In this case, add two additional drugs to which the organism is likely to be sensitive to the regimen in Table 17-6. Consultation with an infectious diseases specialist is recommended.
4. Steroids improve outcome in children and adults. A reasonable dose in children is prednisone 2 to 4 mg/kg/d p.o. for 1 month, followed by a slow taper. A reasonable dose in adults is dexamethasone 4 mg IV or p.o. every 6 hours for 3 to 4 weeks, followed by a slow taper.
5. Paradoxic response: development of CSF polymorphonuclear pleocytosis or development of brain tuberculomas early in course of treatment; does not indicate treatment failure.

FUNGAL MENINGITIS

BACKGROUND

Fungi can cause subacute meningitis that may be clinically indistinguishable from tuberculous meningitis.

PATHOPHYSIOLOGY

1. Fungal meningitis is uncommon in healthy people and most common in those with underlying illness or immune deficiency.
2. Fungal meningitis is more common in adults than children.
3. It is usually, but not always, accompanied by disease in other organ systems, particularly lungs, skin, bones, liver, spleen, and prostate.
4. The most common etiologies are *Cryptococcus neoformans, Coccidioides immitis, Histoplasma capsulatum,* and *Blastomyces dermatitidis.* The latter three are endemic in specific geographic areas. Because meningitis can be a manifestation of reactivation, disease can occur in individuals who reside outside these areas if they previously visited or lived in an endemic area.
   a. *C. immitis*: central California, southern Arizona, southern New Mexico, west Texas, northern Mexico; parts of Central and South America
   b. *H. capsulatum*: Ohio and Mississippi River valleys; parts of Central and South America, Caribbean
   c. *B. dermatitidis*: southeastern and south central states that border the Mississippi and Ohio rivers, the midwestern states and Canadian provinces that border the Great Lakes, and a portion of New York and Canada adjacent to the St. Lawrence River
5. As with tuberculous meningitis, communicating and noncommunicating hydrocephalus can develop.

PROGNOSIS

1. Although most patients with cryptococcal meningitis respond to therapy with an acute mortality of 5%, 25% to 50% of patients with meningitis due to *C. immitis, H. capsulatum* and *B. dermatitidis* die.
2. Worse outcome in immunosuppressed.
3. In cryptococcal meningitis, abnormal mental status on presentation, low CSF WBC count, and high CSF antigen titers are poor prognostic factors in HIV–infected and –uninfected individuals.

DIAGNOSIS

1. Signs and symptoms generally develop over 1 to 2 weeks and include low-grade fever, headache, neck stiffness, malaise, and mental status changes.
   a. Eosinophils may be seen in coccidioidal meningitis
2. Neuroimaging abnormalities include hydrocephalus, meningeal enhancement and, occasionally, infarcts. All patients with suspected fungal meningitis should undergo neuroimaging, ideally before lumbar puncture.
3. CSF:
   a. Conventional analysis:
      1) WBC count 20 to 1,000 cells/μl lymphocytic predominance, but polymorphonuclear cells may be present
      2) Protein 50 to 1,000 mg/dL
      3) Glucose less than 40 mg/dL
   b. Except for cryptococcal meningitis, cultures usually negative.
   c. Antigen and antibody tests:
      1) Except for the cryptococcal antigen test, antibody and antigen tests are specific but less sensitive.
      2) Detection of antibody to *C. immitis, H. capsulatum,* and *B. dermatitidis* in CSF supports diagnosis.
      3) Detection of antigen to *C. neoformans* and *H. capsulatum* in CSF supports diagnosis.
      4) Detection of antibody to *C. immitis, H. capsulatum,* and *B. dermatitidis* in serum supports diagnosis of systemic infection. *C. neoformans* antigen detected in serum in virtually all patients with meningitis.
      5) Detection of *H. capsulatum* antigen in urine supports diagnosis.
4. Diagnosis often presumptive on the basis of compatible clinical findings, CSF profile, detectable serum antibody, and confirmed fungal infection at another site.
5. In some instances, diagnosis may only be established by culture of brain biopsy.

TABLE 17-7. THERAPY FOR FUNGAL MENINGITIDES IN ADULTS

Organism	Induction Therapy	Maintenance Therapy
Cryptococcus neoformans in HIV-uninfected patients	Amphotericin B 0.7 mg/kg/d IV plus flucytosine 150 mg/kg/d p.o. divided into four doses for 4–6 wk	Some experts recommend fluconazole 200 mg/d p.o. for 6–12 mo
C. neoformans in HIV-infected patients	Amphotericin B 0.7 mg/kg/d IV plus flucytosine 100 mg/kg/d p.o. divided into four doses for 2 wk followed by fluconazole 400 mg/d p.o. to complete a 10-wk course	At 10 wk confirm that CSF is sterile. Decrease fluconazole to 200 mg/d p.o. for life or until peripheral blood CD4+ T cells $\geq$ 200 cells/uL for > 6 mo
Coccidioides immitis	Fluconazole 400 mg/d p.o.	Continue for life
Histoplasma capsulatum	Amphotericin B 0.7–1.0 mg/kg/d IV to complete a 35-mg/kg course over 3–4 mo	Fluconazole 800 mg/d p.o. for additional 9–12 mo if patient not HIV-infected, for life if patient HIV-infected
Blastomyces dermatiditis	Amphotericin B 0.7–1.0 mg/kg/d IV for a total dose of $\geq$ 2 g	Fluconazole 800 mg/d p.o. for life if patient HIV-infected

IV, intravenous; p.o., by mouth; CSF, cerebrospinal fluid; HIV, human immunodeficiency virus.

TREATMENT

1. Antifungals (Table 17-7):
   a. Successful treatment of most fungal meningitides involves induction followed by maintenance therapy.
   b. Follow renal function, serum potassium, and hematologic profile carefully in patients treated with amphotericin B.
   c. Follow renal function, hematologic profile, and drug levels in patients treated with flucytosine. Peak serum drug levels should be 30 to 80 μg/mL and always lower than 100 μg/mL.
2. Elevated intracranial pressure (ICP) is an important source of morbidity and mortality in HIV-infected patients with cryptococcal meningitis. Treat with repeated lumbar punctures with removal of enough CSF to yield normal closing pressure. If this strategy does not work, lumbar drain or ventriculoperitoneal shunt is indicated.
3. Hydrocephalus may require ventriculoperitoneal shunt.

VIRAL MENINGITIS

BACKGROUND

Viral meningitis is one of the causes of culture-negative meningitis (Table 17-8). It is more common than all other etiologies of meningitis combined.

TABLE 17-8. CAUSES OF "ASEPTIC" OR CULTURE-NEGATIVE MENINGITIS

Viral	Bacterial
Herpesviruses	Partially treated bacterial meningitis
Herpes simplex virus type 2 and type 1	Rocky Mountain spotted fever
Cytomegalovirus	Spirochetes
Varicella zoster virus	Leptospirosis
Epstein–Barr virus	Syphilis
Human herpes virus type 6	Lyme disease
Human immunodeficiency virus	*Brucella* species
Enteroviruses	*Mycoplasma* species
Echoviruses	*Mycobacterium tuberculosis*
Coxsackieviruses A and B	*Nocardia* species
Numbered enteroviruses	*Chlamydia pneumoniae*
Polio	Endocarditis
Mumps	
Lymphocytic choriomeningitis virus	Noninfectious
Arboviruses	Behçet syndrome
Flavivruses: West Nile, St. Louis	Sarcoid
encephalitis viruses	Vasculitis
California group: La Crosse, Jamestown	Neoplastic meningitis
Canyon, Snowshoe Hare viruses	Drug-induced meningitis
Influenza viruses	
Adenoviruses	

PATHOPHYSIOLOGY

1. In the United States, enteroviruses are responsible for 85% to 95% of cases of viral meningitis. Enteroviral meningitis is most common in the summer and fall, but may be seen year-round in temperate climates.
   a. Eighty percent of cases of enteroviral meningitis occur in young children.
   b. Patients with hypogammaglobulinemia are at risk for chronic enteroviral meningitis and meningoencephalitis.
2. Herpes simplex virus type 2 (HSV-2), and less commonly HSV-1, can cause an acute, self-limiting meningitis.
   a. Most common in young women.
   b. As many as one fourth of patients may have recurrent episodes of meningitis, and these may occur in the absence of cutaneous or mucosal lesions.

PROGNOSIS

1. Most cases of viral meningitis resolve in 2 to 5 days and do not result in sequelae.
2. Increased ICP may be seen in the acute phase.
3. Neonates and patients with hypogammaglobulinemia or agammaglobulinemia may develop severe enteroviral infection that may be fatal.

DIAGNOSIS

1. CSF:
   a. Abnormalities are milder in viral meningitis than in bacterial meningitis (Table 17-2).
   b. Usual pattern is lymphocytic pleocytosis with 10 to 1,000 WBC/μL, although neutrophils can be seen within the first 6 to 24 hours of illness. Glucose level is usually normal and protein level may be normal or mildly elevated, sometimes reaching 100 to 200 mg/dL.
   c. Viral CSF cultures may be positive in 40% to 70% of cases if collected early in illness. Enteroviruses in particular may be cultured from acellular CSF.
   d. PCR is sensitive and specific for diagnosis of meningitis due to enteroviruses, herpes viruses, and some arboviruses.
   e. Identification of IgM to a specific virus in CSF is diagnostic.
2. Identification of serum IgM in a single sample or a fourfold change in IgG concentration in paired serum samples collected 4 weeks apart is diagnostic. This approach is not applicable to enteroviruses unless the specific serotype is known.
3. Culture of throat or stool may identify enterovirus infection, but because enteroviruses may be shed for several weeks after infection, serologic confirmation is required to prove that the isolated virus is the cause of meningitis.

TREATMENT

1. In most cases, only supportive care, including medications for pain, is needed.
2. Pleconaril is a new antiviral drug that is effective against enteroviruses. It is not approved by the Food and Drug Administration (FDA) but is available on a compassionate use basis for life-threatening enteroviral infections.
   a. IV or intrathecal immune serum globulin may be used therapeutically or prophylactically for neonates and patients with antibody deficiencies but efficacy is not proven.
3. The benefit of antivirals such as acyclovir for the treatment or prevention of HSV meningitis is not known.
4. Symptomatic elevated ICP usually responds to lumbar puncture with removal of enough CSF to yield a normal closing pressure.

BACTERIAL BRAIN ABSCESS

PATHOPHYSIOLOGY

1. Brain abscess begins as a localized area of cerebritis that evolves into an encapsulated infection over about 2 weeks. In the setting of concomitant immunosuppression, there may be poorer or slower capsule formation.
2. Brain abscess may be a consequence of contiguous spread of infection, dural disruption, or hematogenous spread (Table 17-9). The source of infection is unknown in 20% to 30%.
3. Most brain abscesses are polymicrobial.

PROGNOSIS

1. Mortality is 15% to 20%.
   a. Prognosis is poorer for patients who present with significantly depressed mental status.
   b. Rupture of abscess into the ventricular system has a mortality of more than 80% and is more common when diagnosis is delayed.
2. About 60% of survivors have no or mild neurologic deficits. Of the remainder, about two thirds will have moderate and one third severe neurologic disability.

TABLE 17-9. LIKELY LOCATION, ETIOLOGY AND EMPIRIC TREATMENT OF BRAIN ABSCESS BASED ON RISK FACTOR OR SOURCE OF INFECTION

Risk Factor or Source	Likely Location	Likely Organisms	Empiric Treatment[a]
Pàranasal sinusitis, teeth	Frontal pole	Aerobic and anaerobic streptococci; other anaerobes; *Staphylococcus aureus,* gram-negatives	Vancomycin, metronidazole[b] and a third-generation cephalosporin[c]
Otitis media, mastoiditis	Temporal lobe, cerebellum	Aerobic and anaerobic streptococci; other anaerobes; gram-negatives	Metronidazole[b] and a third-generation cephalosporin[c]
Penetrating trauma, postoperative	Associated with site of injury or surgery	*S. aureus,* coagulase-negative *Staphylococcus* species, gram-negatives, *Clostridium* species	Vancomycin and a third-generation cephalosporin[c]
Hematogenous; congenital heart disease, pulmonary disease	Middle cerebral artery distribution	*Streptococcus* species, often with additional organisms, depending on site of primary infection	Depends on source, metronidazole[b] and a third-generation cephalosporin[c] are a reasonable start

[a]See Table 17-1 for doses.
[b]Children: 30 mg/kg/d IV divided q 6–8 hr. Adult: 500 mg IV q 6 hr.
[c]Ceftriaxone, cefotaxime, or ceftazidime. See Table 17-1 for doses.

DIAGNOSIS

1. Headache is the most common clinical finding. Focal neurologic abnormalities are seen in one third to one half of cases. Fever is less common and may be absent in more than 50% of patients.
2. Lumbar puncture is rarely helpful and is usually contraindicated.
3. Computed tomography (CT) or magnetic resonance imaging (MRI) show ring-enhancing lesions with central low density and surrounding edema. There may be high signal on diffusion-weighted MRI.
4. Bacteriologic diagnosis rests on culture of abscess material.
5. Blood cultures are rarely positive, but are worth collecting before antibiotics are given.

TREATMENT

1. Control elevated ICP:
   a. Use of steroids is controversial because they may decrease antibiotic penetration into the area of infection. A short course of high-dose corticosteroids is reasonable in the presence of significant cerebral edema.
2. Aspiration or excision reduces ICP and provides a microbiologic diagnosis. Antibiotic therapy can be delayed in clinically stable patients if aspiration can be done quickly.
3. After surgical drainage, parenteral antibiotics generally given for 6 to 8 weeks, followed by 2 to 3 months of oral therapy.
4. Medical therapy alone generally suboptimal, but can be considered for abscesses smaller than 2 cm in diameter, cerebritis without capsule formation, or multiple or surgically inaccessible lesions. Duration of antibiotic regimens are generally longer for patients who do not undergo surgical treatment.
5. Seizures are relatively frequent; consider prophylactic anticonvulsants.

CRANIAL SUBDURAL EMPYEMA

BACKGROUND

Subdural empyema used to be most common in children with bacterial meningitis but is now uncommon because the incidence of childhood meningitis has declined.

PATHOPHYSIOLOGY

1. Subdural empyema now occurs most commonly as a consequence of frontal sinus infection. It is most common in young men.
   a. Veins draining the frontal sinus do not have valves and they drain to the subdural space offering direct access of bacteria or infected clot.
2. Subdural empyema may also occur as a consequence of otitis media, direct trauma, or hematogenous spread. Likely bacterial organisms can be predicted based on the clinical setting (Table 17-10).
3. Because of the anatomy of the subdural space, infection most commonly involves both hemispheres and less commonly the posterior fossa.

PROGNOSIS

1. Mortality is about 10% and is associated with older age and depressed level of consciousness at presentation.

TABLE 17-10. LIKELY ETIOLOGY AND EMPIRIC TREATMENT OF SUBDURAL EMPYEMA BASED ON RISK FACTOR OR SOURCE OF INFECTION

Risk Factor	Likely Organisms	Empiric Treatment[a]
Frontal sinusitis	Aerobic and anaerobic streptococci; other anaerobes; *Staphylococcus aureus,* gram-negatives	Vancomycin, metronidazole and a third-generation cephalosporin
Otitis media	Aerobic and anaerobic streptococci; other anaerobes; gram-negatives	Metronidazole and a third-generation cephalosporin
Penetrating trauma, postoperative	*S. aureus,* coagulase-negative staphylococcus, gram-negatives, *Clostridium* species	Vancomycin and a third-generation cephalosporin
Hematogenous	Depends on site of primary infection	Depends on source, metronidazole and a third-generation cephalosporin are a reasonable start

[a]See Tables 17-1 and 17-9 for doses.

2. Complications include epidural empyema, osteomyelitis, cortical vein or dural sinus thrombophlebitis, cerebritis or brain abscess, brain infarction, brain edema.
3. Epilepsy and focal neurologic sequelae are seen in 10% to 44% of survivors.

DIAGNOSIS

1. Clinical findings include fever, headache, stiff neck, seizures, and focal neurologic signs.
2. May mimic bacterial meningitis.
   a. Lumbar puncture contraindicated because high risk of herniation.
3. Forehead swelling due to subgaleal abscess (Pott puffy tumor) may be seen with concomitant frontal sinusitis, but symptoms and signs of sinusitis may be absent.
4. Contrast-enhanced MRI is the preferred imaging study and shows subdural fluid collection or low density with rim enhancement. Brain edema may not be evident. Findings may be subtle.
5. Bacteriologic diagnosis rests on culture of abscess material.

TREATMENT

1. Surgical drainage required.
   a. If present, infected sinus should be drained and infected bone removed.
2. Parenteral antibiotics generally given for 3 to 6 weeks, followed by at least 3 weeks of oral therapy (Table 17-10).
3. Seizures are frequent and prophylactic anticonvulsants should be given.

CRANIAL EPIDURAL ABSCESS

BACKGROUND

Cranial epidural abscess develops in potential space between dura and inner table of skull. It is less common than subdural empyema and shares similar risk factors.

PATHOPHYSIOLOGY

1. Commonly arises from sinus or otogenic source. Often associated with skull osteomyelitis.
2. Likely bacterial organisms are the same as for cranial subdural empyema and can be predicted based on the clinical setting (Table 17-10).

PROGNOSIS

Better that subdural empyema. Infection more localized; death and neurologic sequelae uncommon.

DIAGNOSIS

1. Clinical findings include fever, headache, periorbital swelling, frontal subgaleal abscesses, neck stiffness, vomiting. Focal neurologic deficits uncommon.
2. Contrast-enhanced MRI preferred imaging study and shows lens-shaped extradural fluid collection with an enhancing rim.

TREATMENT

1. Surgical drainage required.
2. Parenteral antibiotics generally given for 3 to 6 weeks if no osteomyelitis and 6 to 8 weeks if osteomyelitis present, often followed by at least 3 weeks of oral therapy (Table 17-10).

SPINAL EPIDURAL ABSCESS

BACKGROUND

Spinal epidural abscess is uncommon but can cause severe neurologic disability. It is frequently misdiagnosed. Over the last 20 years, the incidence has increased.

PATHOPHYSIOLOGY

1. Most infections caused by *Staphylococcus aureus;* gram-negatives, streptococci less common causes. Rarely caused by anaerobic bacteria and rarely polymicrobial.
2. Infection most commonly by hematogenous route, particularly from skin source. May also result from direct extension or trauma.
3. Thoracic and lumbar epidural space most likely to be infected.

PROGNOSIS

1. Diabetes, injection drug use, spinal procedures, and alcoholism are risk factors.
2. Approximately 15% mortality; 40% to 50% recover completely and the rest have mild or moderate disability.
3. Patients with greater neurologic disability at presentation have poorer outcome. Those with complete paralysis for more than 48 to 72 hours are unlikely to improve, even with aggressive treatment.
4. May be associated osteomyelitis in chronic cases.

DIAGNOSIS

1. Most common clinical findings are fever, back pain, and local tenderness. Meningeal symptoms or signs and focal neurologic findings such as weakness, sensory loss and bowel or bladder incontinence are also seen in some, but not all, patients.
2. Severe neurologic deficits may develop rapidly, even after several weeks of stable illness.
3. Contrast-enhanced spinal MRI is the preferred imaging study. On average, four spinal levels are involved, but infection of the entire spinal epidural space has been described.
4. Peripheral blood leukocytosis and elevated sedimentation rate are seen in most patients.
5. Blood cultures are frequently positive and the results are identical to culture of the epidural space.

TREATMENT

1. Surgical drainage required.
2. Rarely, medical therapy is used alone, but is risky given potential for rapid neurologic deterioration.
   a. Medical therapy alone can be considered for patients without neurologic abnormalities, infection of the entire epidural space, or those completely paralyzed for 3 or more days.
   b. Even if medical therapy alone is used, blood cultures and aspiration of the epidural space should be performed to establish the infecting pathogen.
3. Parenteral antibiotics generally given for 6 to 8 weeks, often followed by at least 4 weeks of oral therapy.
   a. Empiric therapy with vancomycin plus a third-generation cephalosporin (see Table 17-1 for doses).
   b. Tailor subsequent therapy to organism cultured from blood or epidural space.

ENCEPHALITIS

BACKGROUND

Literally hundreds of organisms can cause encephalitis (Table 17-11). The most common causes are viral. Viral encephalitis may occur sporadically or in epidemics. In most instances, the cause of encephalitis is not established.

PATHOPHYSIOLOGY

1. Pathology is characterized by perivascular inflammation in gray matter or at gray–white junction. Neurons may be infected.
2. In the United States, HSV is the most common and most fatal cause of sporadic encephalitis; several hundred to several thousand cases are identified each year.
   a. HSV causes a necrotizing encephalitis that typically involves the orbitofrontal or temporal lobes.
   b. Other than in neonates, most cases are due to HSV-1, but some are due to HSV-2.
   c. HSV encephalitis occurs at any time of year. Bimodal age distribution: 25% to 30% of patients younger than 20 years; 50% to 70% of patients older than 40 years.
   d. About one third of cases are due to primary infection and about two thirds are due to viral reactivation.

TABLE 17-11. SELECTED INFECTIOUS CAUSES OF ENCEPHALITIS

Viral
  Herpesviruses
    Herpes simplex types 1 and 2
    Varicella zoster
    Epstein Barr
    Human cytomegalovirus
    Human herpes virus type 6
    Herpes B
  Arboviruses
    Eastern equine
    Western equine
    Venezuelan equine
    St. Louis
    Japananese
    West Nile
    Powassan
    California
    La Crosse
    Jamestown Canyon
    Colorado tick fever
  Enteroviruses
    Coxsackie
    Echo
  Adenoviruses
  Human immunodeficiency virus
  Influenza viruses
  Nippah
  Hendra
  Mumps
  Measles
  Rabies

Bacterial
  Listeria monocytogenes
  Mycobacterium tuberculosis
  Mycoplasma species
  Bartonella species
  Anaplasma species
  Brucella species
  Whipple disease
  Rickettsia
    Rocky Mountain spotted fever
    Typhus
    Q fever
  Spirochetes
    Syphilis
    Lyme disease
    Relapsing fever
  Infective endocarditis
Fungi
  Cryptococcosis
  Coccidioidomycosis
  Histoplasmosis
Parasites
  Toxoplasmosis
  Cysticercosis
  Malaria

3. Viruses transmitted by the bites of arthropods or "arboviruses" are the most common cause of epidemic encephalitis. Worldwide, Japanese encephalitis virus is the most common cause of arboviral encephalitis. In the United States, West Nile virus is now the most common cause.
   a. Most arboviral infections are subclinical; about one in 140 people infected with West Nile virus develop meningitis or encephalitis.
   b. In the United States, infection is most common in late summer and early fall.

PROGNOSIS

1. Twenty-eight percent of patients with HSV-1 encephalitis die despite treatment and one half have persistent neurologic disabilities.
2. About 6% of patients in the United States with confirmed West Nile infection die. Poliomyelitis and radiculitis are common features of this infection and often lead to persistent disability.

DIAGNOSIS

1. Clinical findings include fever, headache, change in mental status and seizures. Focal findings such as dysphasia and personality changes are common in HSV-1 encephalitis and may also be seen in other etiologies.

2. CSF:
   a. CSF is normal in less than 5%. Usual pattern is lymphocytic pleocytosis with 50 to 1,000 WBC/μL. Neutrophils can be seen early in the course. Glucose level is usually normal and protein usually mildly elevated.
   b. Viral CSF cultures rarely positive.
   c. PCR is sensitive and specific for diagnosis of encephalitis due to enteroviruses, herpesviruses, and some arboviruses.
   d. Identification of IgM to a specific virus in CSF is diagnostic. Identification of serum IgM in a single sample or a fourfold change in IgG concentration in paired serum samples collected 4 weeks apart is diagnostic.
3. Electroencephalogram is often abnormal. Periodic lateralizing epileptiform discharges (PLEDS) common in HSV encephalitis.
4. Hyponatremia common.

TREATMENT

1. Currently, only treatment for encephalitis due to HHV is available.
   a. Treat HSV-1 encephalitis in adults with acyclovir, 10 mg/kg IV when creatinine clearance is normal every 8 hours for a minimum of 14 days.
   b. Treat varicella zoster virus (VZV) encephalitis in adults with acyclovir at 10 to 12.5 mg/kg IV every 8 hours for a minimum of 14 days.
   c. Treatment of other herpesvirus infections of the central nervous system (CNS) is less clearly defined and an infectious disease expert should be consulted.
   d. Continue treatment until CSF PCR is negative.

NEUROLOGIC COMPLICATIONS ASSOCIATED WITH HUMAN IMMUNODEFICIENCY VIRUS

HUMAN IMMUNODEFICIENCY VIRUS–ASSOCIATED DEMENTIA

BACKGROUND

1. HIV-1 causes a subcortical dementia called HIV-1–associated dementia (HAD).

PATHOPHYSIOLOGY

1. In patients not receiving antiretrovirals, HAD typically seen in patients with peripheral blood CD4$^+$ T cell counts below 200/μL. In those taking antiretrovirals, CD4$^+$ T-cell counts may be higher.
2. The cause of HAD is likely related to release of toxic viral gene products or cell products from infected brain macrophages or microglia.

PROGNOSIS

Risks for HAD include the following:
1. Lower peripheral blood CD4$^+$ T cells
2. Higher plasma HIV-1 RNA concentration
3. Not receiving potent antiretroviral therapy
4. Lower hemoglobin concentration
5. Older age
6. Injection drug use

TABLE 17-12. CLINICAL FINDINGS IN PATIENTS WITH HIV–ASSOCIATED DEMENTIA

Cognitive	Motor	Behavioral
Forgetfulness	Balance difficulty	Apathy and social withdrawal
Difficulty concentrating	Leg weakness	Depressed mood
Confusion	—	Irritability
Slow thinking	—	Psychosis, mania

7. Abnormalities on neuropsychologic tests that target executive function
8. Cognitive abnormalities not severe enough to meet criteria for dementia

DIAGNOSIS

1. Clinical findings include cognitive, motor, and behavioral abnormalities (Table 17-12).
2. Patients with HAD perform poorly on neuropsychologic tests that target motor function, attention and concentration, speed of information processing, and visuospatial performance, but these tests have poor sensitivity and specificity for the diagnosis of HAD.
3. Neuroimaging is most useful for excluding other causes of cognitive change:
   a. CT may show atrophy.
   b. MRI may show patchy white matter high intensities on T_2-weighted images.
4. CSF:
   a. Conventional analysis most useful for excluding other causes of cognitive change.
   b. CSF β_2-microglobulin above 3.8 mg/dL in a CSF specimen with normal CSF WBC is specific, but not sensitive, for the diagnosis of HAD.
   c. CSF HIV-1 RNA level greater than simultaneous plasma level supports the diagnosis of HAD.

TREATMENT

1. Patients who are not receiving potent antiretroviral therapy should be started on a regimen that contains agents with good CNS penetration (Table 17-13).
2. Patients who are receiving potent antiretroviral therapy should ideally undergo testing of plasma and CSF for HIV mutations associated with drug resistance and their regimen optimized with regard to both resistance pattern and CNS penetration.
3. Antiretroviral treatment strategies should be developed with the assistance of an expert in HIV treatment.

TABLE 17-13. ANTIRETROVIRAL AGENTS WITH PREDICTED GOOD CENTRAL NERVOUS SYSTEM PENETRATION

Zidovudine (AZT, ZDV, Retrovir)
Stavudine (d4T, Zerit)
Abacavir (ABC, Ziagen)
Lamivudine (3TC, Epivir)
Nevirapine (Viramune)
Efavirenz (Sustiva)
Indinavir (Crixivan)

TOXOPLASMOSIS

PATHOPHYSIOLOGY

1. *Toxoplasma gondii* is an intracellular parasite that exists in three forms:
   a. Replicating organisms, or tachyzoites, that cause active disease.
   b. Nonreplicating organisms, or bradyzoites, that are responsible for latent disease.
   c. Oocysts, infectious form shed in cat feces.
2. Humans acquire infection by ingesting oocysts or by ingesting bradyzoites in undercooked meat.
3. Primary infection is asymptomatic in 90% of immunocompetent individuals and causes a mononucleosis-like illness or regional lymphadenopathy in the rest.
4. HIV–infected individuals with CNS toxoplasmosis develop abscesses, and rarely, meningoencephalitis.

PROGNOSIS

1. The following increase the risk of CNS toxoplasmosis in HIV–infected patients:
   a. CD4$^+$ T cells below 200/μL
   b. Not receiving trimethoprim–sulfamethoxazole prophylaxis
   c. Detectable serum anti-*Toxoplasma* antibody, particularly if titer is high
   d. More than one abscess-like lesion on neuroimaging
2. Most patients respond to therapy, but residual deficits are common and there is an increased risk for subsequent dementia.

DIAGNOSIS

1. Clinical findings include headache, fever, hemiparesis, ataxia, change in level of consciousness, and psychomotor retardation; about 30% have seizures.
2. Ninety percent to 100% of HIV–infected patients with *Toxoplasma* encephalitis will have detectable serum anti-*Toxoplasma* IgG, but IGM rarely detectable.
3. CSF examination is not helpful in establishing the diagnosis.
4. Neuroimaging shows round, isodense or hyperdense lesion(s) in hemispheric gray–white junction, deep white matter, or basal ganglia. More than 90% enhance with contrast in ring, nodular, or homogenous pattern. MRI is more sensitive than CT and often identifies multiple lesions.
5. For patients at high risk for CNS toxoplasmosis (see above), presumptive diagnosis made by response to a treatment trial. Diagnosis is established if clinical improvement occurs within 1 to 2 weeks and radiographic improvement within 2 to 3 weeks.
6. Consider brain biopsy if no response to treatment trial or for patients at low risk for CNS toxoplasmosis (see above).

TREATMENT

1. Synergistic combination of pyrimethamine and sulfadiazine has response rates of 60% to 90% (Table 17-4).
   a. Pyrimethamine causes bone marrow suppression, which is prevented by administration of folinic acid (leucovorin). Patients should not be given folate or multivitamins containing folate because this could make treatment less effective.
2. High-dose, primary therapy is given for at least 6 weeks, and should be continued until there is no evidence of active disease on neuroimaging.
3. After primary therapy, chronic suppressive therapy prevents relapse (secondary prophylaxis). Potent antiretroviral therapy is an important component of maintenance therapy.

TABLE 17-14. PRIMARY AND CHRONIC SUPPRESSIVE THERAPY FOR *TOXOPLASMA* ENCEPHALITIS IN ADULTS

Primary therapy (duration at least 6 wk)

Pyrimethamine		100–200 mg p.o. load, then 75–100 mg p.o. qd
	Plus	
Sulfadiazine		1.5–2 g p.o. q.i.d.
	Or	
Clindamycin		600–900 mg p.o. or IV q.i.d.
	Plus	
Folinic acid (Leukovarin)		10–50 mg p.o. qd

Chronic suppressive therapy or secondary prophylaxis (duration determined by response to potent antiretroviral therapy)

Pyrimethamine		25–50 mg p.o. qd
	Plus	
Sulfadiazine		1 g p.o. t.i.d.–q.i.d.
	Or	
Clindamycin		300–450 mg p.o. t.i.d.–q.i.d.
	Plus	
Folinic acid (Leukovarin)		10–50 mg p.o. qd

p.o., by mouth; q.i.d., four times a day; t.i.d., three times a day.

4. Secondary prophylaxis for *Toxoplasma* encephalitis can be safely discontinued in patients with an increase in CD4$^+$ T cells to more than 200/μL for at least 6 months after beginning potent antiretroviral therapy

BIBLIOGRAPHY

American Academy of Pediatrics. *2000 Red Book: report of the Committee on Infectious Diseases,* 25th ed. Elk Grove Village, IL: American Academy of Pediatrics, 2000.

Aronin SI, Peduzzi P, Quagliarello VJ. Community-acquired bacterial meningitis: risk stratification for adverse clinical outcome and effect of antibiotic timing. *Ann Intern Med* 1998;129:862–869.

Bennett JE, Dismukes WE, Duma RJ, et al. A comparison of amphotericin B alone and combined with flucytosine in the treatment of cryptococcal meningitis. *N Engl J Med* 1979;301:126–131.

Bouza E, Dreyer JS, Hewitt WL, et al. Coccidioidal meningitis: an analysis of thirty-one cases and review of the literature. *Medicine (Baltimore)* 1981;60:139–172.

Carpenter RR, Petersdorf RG. The clinical spectrum of bacterial meningitis. *Am J Med* 1962;33:262–275.

Chapman SW, Bradsher RW Jr, Campbell GD Jr, et al. Practice guidelines for the management of patients with blastomycosis: Infectious Diseases Society of America. *Clin Infect Dis* 2000;30:679–683.

de Gans J, van de Beek D. Dexamethasone in adults with bacterial meningitis. *N Engl J Med* 2002;347:1549–1556.

Dismukes WE, Cloud G, Gallis HA, et al. Treatment of cryptococcal meningitis with combination amphotericin B and flucytosine for four as compared with six weeks. *N Engl J Med* 1987;317:334–341.

Friedman JA, Wijdicks EF, Fulgham JR, et al. Meningoencephalitis due to Blastomyces dermatitidis: case report and literature review. *Mayo Clin Proc* 2000;75:403–408.

Galgiani JN, Ampel NM, Catanzaro A, et al. Practice guideline for the treatment of coccidioidomycosis: Infectious Diseases Society of America. *Clin Infect Dis* 2000;30:658–661.

Hasbun R, Abrahams J, Jekel J, et al. Computed tomography of the head before lumbar puncture in adults with suspected meningitis. *N Engl J Med* 2001;345:1727–1733.

Infections in Neurosurgery Working Party of the British Society for Antimicrobial Chemotherapy. The rational use of antibiotics in the treatment of brain abscess. *Br J Neurosurg* 2000;14:525–530.

Kennedy DH, Fallon RJ. Tuberculous meningitis. *JAMA* 1979;241:264–268.

Luft BJ, Hafner R, Korzun AH, et al. Toxoplasmic encephalitis in patients with the acquired immunodeficiency syndrome: Members of the ACTG 077p/ANRS 009 Study Team. *N Engl J Med* 1993;329:995–1000.

Mathisen GE, Johnson JP. Brain abscess. *Clin Infect Dis* 1997;25:763–779; quiz 780–781.

Morgan H, Wood MW, Murphey F. Experience with 88 consecutive cases of brain abscess. *J Neurosurg* 1973;38:698–704.

Nathoo N, Nadvi SS, Gouws E, et al. Craniotomy improves outcomes for cranial subdural empyemas: computed tomography-era experience with 699 patients. *Neurosurgery* 2001;49:872–877; discussion 877–878.

Nathoo N, Nadvi SS, van Dellen JR. Cranial extradural empyema in the era of computed tomography: a review of 82 cases. *Neurosurgery* 1999;44:748–753; discussion 753–754.

Navia BA, Jordan BD, Price RW. The AIDS dementia complex, I: clinical features. *Ann Neurol* 1986;19:517–524.

Peigue-Lafeuille H, Croquez N, Laurichesse H, et al. Enterovirus meningitis in adults in 1999–2000 and evaluation of clinical management. *J Med Virol* 2002;67:47–53.

Petersen LR, Marfin AA. West Nile virus: a primer for the clinician. *Ann Intern Med* 2002;137:173–179.

Porter SB, Sande MA. Toxoplasmosis of the central nervous system in the acquired immunodeficiency syndrome [see comments]. *N Engl J Med* 1992;327:1643–1648.

Prasad K, Volmink J, Menon GR. Steroids for treating tuberculous meningitis. *Cochrane Database Syst Rev* 2000;3:CD002244.

Raschilas F, Wolff M, Delatour F, et al. Outcome of and prognostic factors for herpes simplex encephalitis in adult patients: results of a multicenter study. *Clin Infect Dis* 2002;35:254–260.

Reihsaus E, Waldbaur H, Seeling W. Spinal epidural abscess: a meta-analysis of 915 patients. *Neurosurg Rev* 2000;23:175–204; discussion 205.

Rotbart HA, Webster AD. Treatment of potentially life-threatening enterovirus infections with pleconaril. *Clin Infect Dis* 2001;32:228–235.

Schuchat A, Robinson K, Wenger JD, et al. Bacterial meningitis in the United States in 1995: Active Surveillance Team. *N Engl J Med* 1997;337:970–976.

Tedder DG, Ashley R, Tyler KL, et al. Herpes simplex virus infection as a cause of benign recurrent lymphocytic meningitis. *Ann Intern Med* 1994;121:334–338.

Thwaites GE, Chau TT, Stepniewska K, et al. Diagnosis of adult tuberculous meningitis by use of clinical and laboratory features. *Lancet* 2002;360:1287–1292.

van der Horst CM, Saag MS, Cloud GA, et al. Treatment of cryptococcal meningitis associated with the acquired immunodeficiency syndrome: National Institute of Allergy and Infectious Diseases Mycoses Study Group and AIDS Clinical Trials Group. *N Engl J Med* 1997;337:15–21.

Wheat J, Sarosi G, McKinsey D, et al. Practice guidelines for the management of patients with histoplasmosis: Infectious Diseases Society of America. *Clin Infect Dis* 2000;30:688–695.

Wheat LJ, Batteiger BE, Sathapatayavongs B. Histoplasma capsulatum infections of the central nervous system: a clinical review. *Medicine (Baltimore)* 1990;69:244–260.

Whitley RJ, Soong SJ, Linneman C Jr., et al. Herpes simplex encephalitis: clinical assessment. *JAMA* 1982;247:317–320.

SUBJECT INDEX

Page numbers followed by f indicate figures; those followed by t indicate tables.